19,50 €

SEARCH FOR NEW DRUGS

MEDICINAL RESEARCH:
A SERIES OF MONOGRAPHS

Consulting Editor: GARY L. GRUNEWALD

VOLUME 1: *Drugs Affecting the Peripheral Nervous System, edited by Alfred Burger*
VOLUME 2: *Drugs Affecting the Central Nervous System, edited by Alfred Burger*
VOLUME 3: *Selected Pharmacological Testing Methods, edited by Alfred Burger*
VOLUME 4: *Analytical Metabolic Chemistry of Drugs, by Jean L. Hirtz*
VOLUME 5: *Biogenic Amines and Physiological Membranes in Drug Therapy, Edited by John H. Biel and Leo G. Abood*
VOLUME 6: *Search for New Drugs, Edited by Alan A. Rubin*

SEARCH FOR NEW DRUGS

Edited by
ALAN A. RUBIN
VICE PRESIDENT-RESEARCH
ENDO LABORATORIES INC.
GARDEN CITY, NEW YORK

1972

MARCEL DEKKER, INC., NEW YORK

COPYRIGHT © 1972 by MARCEL DEKKER, INC.

ALL RIGHTS RESERVED

No part of this work may be reproduced or utilized in any form or by any means, electronic or mechanical, including xerography, photocopying, microfilm, and recording, or by any information storage and retrieval system without the written permission of the publisher.

MARCEL DEKKER, INC.
95 Madison Avenue, New York, New York 10016

LIBRARY OF CONGRESS CATALOG CARD NUMBER: 74-187516

ISBN 0-8247-1593-4

Printed in the United States of America

PREFACE

The search for new drugs is a tantalizing intellectual pursuit which has become more challenging with the passage of time. Success, as measured by the development of clinically useful agents, is elusive partly because of the present availability of effective first generation drugs. In addition, the probability of fortuitous drug discovery has decreased proportionately with the reduced number of attempted clinical trials; the latter situation reflects progressively more stringent governmental regulations and correspondingly higher costs for drug development.

The current need for improved therapy in certain areas of drug research can be satisfied in different ways. If improvement represents solely the diminution of a drug's (or class of drugs) untoward effects, then existing methods may be adequate to realize this goal. On the other hand, it is not likely that efficacy can be enhanced unless new methodology is developed. Are there any alternative testing procedures to those currently in use that offer a reasonable chance for new drug discovery? What are the new conceptual approaches that merit attention?

These are some of the questions that prompted the compilation of this book. The discovery of new drugs is a complex process involving varying proportions of logic, inventiveness, intuition, and chance. But underlying this process is the assumption that a relevant body of information is available to the investigator, information that includes factual as well as speculative and provocative observations.

It is the purpose of this book to provide information regarding the current status of various classes of drugs and to analyze the developmental capabilities of selected areas of drug research. The first three chapters deal with familiar and relatively impenetrable fields; long, arid periods have characterized research on anti-inflammatory, anti-ulcer, and psychotropic drugs. The next four chapters evaluate areas that appear to be on the threshold of new drug development. Drugs affecting beta-adrenergic receptors and atherosclerosis, interferon inducers and fibrinolytic agents all have appeared recently on the therapeutic horizon. Their value at this time is not clearly established except possibly as prototypes or as indicators of research direction. The final two chapters summarize current developments and offer suggestions of future potential in the relatively new fields of aging and memory.

In summary, this book is not organized as a traditional pharmacological review. Its central theme defines areas of methodological and conceptual importance intended to assist investigators in their search for new drugs.

Accordingly, it is anticipated that the contributions presented herein will stimulate discussion, thought, and experimentation in the development of useful therapeutic agents.

Alan A. Rubin

CONTRIBUTORS

Richard H. Adamson, Laboratory of Chemical Pharmacology, National Cancer Institute and Laboratory of Viral Diseases, National Institute of Allergy and Infectious Diseases, National Institutes of Health, Bethesda, Maryland

Samuel Baron, Laboratory of Chemical Pharmacology, National Cancer Institute and Laboratory of Viral Diseases, National Institute of Allergy and Infectious Diseases, National Institutes of Health, Bethesda, Maryland

Walter B. Essman, Queens College, The City University of New York, Flushing, New York

Samuel Irwin, Department of Psychiatry, University of Oregon Medical School, Portland, Oregon

David Kritchevsky, The Wistar Institute of Anatomy and Biology, Philadelphia, Pennsylvania

Frank S. LaBella, Department of Pharmacology and Therapeutics, University of Manitoba, Faculty of Medicine, Winnipeg, Manitoba, Canada

Hilton B. Levy, Laboratory of Chemical Pharmacology, National Cancer Institute and Laboratory of Viral Diseases, National Institute of Allergy and Infectious Diseases, National Institutes of Health, Bethesda, Maryland

Bernard Levy, Department of Pharmacology, University of Texas Medical Branch, Galveston, Texas

Kenneth M. Moser, Department of Medicine, University of California, San Diego, California

Harold E. Paulus, Division of Rheumatology, Department of Medicine, U.C.L.A. Center for the Health Sciences, Los Angeles, California

Jeremy H. Thompson, Department of Pharmacology and Experimental Therapeutics, U.C.L.A. School of Medicine, Los Angeles, California

Michael W. Whitehouse, Division of Rheumatology, Department of Medicine, U.C.L.A. Center for the Health Sciences, Los Angeles, California

CONTENTS

PREFACE iii

CONTRIBUTORS v

I. DRUGS FOR CHRONIC INFLAMMATORY DISEASE
Harold E. Paulus and Michael W. Whitehouse

    Preface 3
    Prologue: By Way of Informing the Reader 4
  I. Introduction 4
  II. Some Relevant Clinical Conditions and the Available Therapy 11
  III. Methodology for Seeking Drugs to Treat Chronic Inflammatory States 40
  IV. Designing New Drugs to Treat Inflammatory States . 54
  V. Immunosuppression with Drugs 77
  VI. Natural Regulators of Inflammation, the Immune Response, and Inflammatory Disease 89
  VII. Some Particular Problems and Pitfalls for Drug Design 96
  VIII. Treating the Individual 101
  IX. Epilogue 102
    References 103

II. GASTROINTESTINAL DISORDERS - PEPTIC ULCER DISEASE
Jeremy H. Thompson

  I. Gastric Physiology 116
  II. Peptic Ulcer Disease 123
  III. Available Drug Therapy 138
  IV. Peptic Ulcer Formation in Animals 155
  V. Future Drugs for the Treatment of Peptic Ulcer Disease 159
  VI. Summary 173
    References 176

III. PSYCHOACTIVE DRUG EVALUATION: PHILOSOPHY AND METHODS

Samuel Irwin

    I. Introduction 201
    II. Approaches to Behavioral Analysis 202
    III. Principles of Exclusion and Inclusion 212
    IV. Observation and Instrumentation 212
    V. Prediction from Normal Subjects 213
    VI. Animal Drug Screening and Evaluation 217
    VII. Drug Assessment in Humans 221
    VIII. Summary 230
    References 231

IV. SELECTIVE BETA RECEPTOR DRUG INTERACTIONS

Bernard Levy

    I. Introduction 233
    II. Selective Beta Receptor Antagonism 237
    III. Selective Beta Receptor Activation 253
    IV. Conclusions 256
    References 257

V. DRUGS AFFECTING ATHEROSCLEROSIS

David Kritchevsky

    I. Introduction 261
    II. Serum Cholesterol Lowering Agents 265
    III. Current Status 274
    IV. Summary 279
    References 279

VI. THE INTERFERON SYSTEM

Richard H. Adamson, Hilton B. Levy, and Samuel Baron

    I. Introduction 292
    II. Biomedical Aspects of the Interferon System 292

	III. Biochemical Aspects of the Interferon System	295
	IV. Pharmacological Aspects of the Interferon System	299
	V. Interferon and Interferon Inducers in Man	305
	VI. Conclusions	310
	References	311

VII. ANTITHROMBOTIC AND THROMBOLYTIC DRUGS
Kenneth M. Moser

I.	Introduction	317
II.	Thrombosis	318
III.	The Natural History of Thromboembolic Disease	322
IV.	The Diagnostic Dilemma	328
V.	The Goals of Thrombolytic Therapy and Approaches to Achieving Them	330
VI.	Lessons of History and the Search for Thrombolytic Drugs	338
VII.	Conclusions	340
	References	340

VIII. PHARMACOLONGEVITY: CONTROL OF AGING BY DRUGS
Frank S. LaBella

I.	Introduction	347
II.	Biological Aging as a Result of Coalescence-Accretion-Stabilization of Body Constituents	349
III.	Hormones	353
IV.	Procaine	357
V.	Procainamide, Diphenylhydantoin, Pemoline, and Inosine-Alkylamino Alcohol Complexes	358
VI.	Antioxidants and Free Radical Scavengers	360
VII.	Lathyrogens	364
VIII.	Centrophenoxine	367
IX.	Immunosuppressants	370

	X. Other Agents	371
	XI. Prospects for Pharmacolongevity	373
	References	377

IX. DRUGS AFFECTING FACILITATION OF LEARNING AND MEMORY

Walter B. Essman

I.	Introduction	385
II.	RNA	389
III.	Uric Acid	392
IV.	Malononitrile Derivatives	392
V.	Magnesium Pemoline	394
VI.	Central Nervous System Stimulants and Analeptics	397
VII.	Cholinergic Agents	399
VIII.	Electrolytes	400
IX.	Status of Behavioral Facilitation and Search for New Drugs	401
	References	402

AUTHOR INDEX	407
SUBJECT INDEX	441

Chapter I

DRUGS FOR CHRONIC INFLAMMATORY DISEASE

Harold E. Paulus and Michael W. Whitehouse

Division of Rheumatology
Department of Medicine
U.C.L.A. Center for the Health Sciences
Los Angeles, California

		PREFACE	3
		PROLOGUE: BY WAY OF INFORMING THE READER	4
I.		INTRODUCTION	4
	A.	Concerning Inflammation, Inflammatory Disease, and Anti-Inflammatory Drugs in General *(Ten Unpalatable Truths)	4
	B.	Goals of a Search for New Drugs to Treat Chronic Inflammatory States * (Table I)	8
II.		SOME RELEVANT CLINICAL CONDITIONS AND THE AVAILABLE THERAPY	11
	A.	Gout	19
	B.	The Rheumatoid Variants	22
	C.	Rheumatoid Arthritis (R.A.)	26
	D.	Systemic Lupus Erythematosus (S.L.E.)	30
	E.	Renal Transplantation	33
	F.	Osteoarthritis (Degenerative Joint Disease)	36
	G.	Psoriasis	37
	H.	Other Skin Diseases	38
	I.	*On Reflection: Strengths and Weaknesses of Current Therapies	39
III.		METHODOLOGY FOR SEEKING DRUGS FOR CHRONIC INFLAMMATORY STATES	40
	A.	Screening Drugs In Vitro	41
	B.	Screening Drugs in Animals	44
	C.	Evaluation of Drugs in that Unique Animal, "Man" ..	50

1

Copyright © 1972 by Marcel Dekker, Inc. **NO PART of this work may be reproduced or utilized in any form or by any means**, electronic or mechanical, including Xeroxing, photocopying, microfilm, and recording, or by any information storage and retrieval system, without permission in writing from the publisher.

IV.		DESIGNING NEW DRUGS TO TREAT INFLAMMATORY STATES	54
	A.	*Some General Considerations	55
	B.	Some Specific Considerations	55
	C.	Some Targets for Drug Action: Mediators of Inflammation and Tissue Injury	64
	D.	More Targets for Drug Action: Mediators of Restitution and Tissue Repair	75
V.		IMMUNOSUPPRESSION WITH DRUGS	77
	A.	*General Strategy and Preamble	78
	B.	The Present Situation	79
	C.	Valuable Properties of Some Current Immunosuppressive Drugs	81
	D.	Adaptation for Further Clinical Use	83
	E.	Some Potential New Leads — Fact and Fancy . .	85
	F.	What Chemical Species Might Be Investigated for Immunosuppressive Activity?	86
VI.		NATURAL REGULATORS OF INFLAMMATION, THE IMMUNE RESPONSE, AND INFLAMMATORY DISEASE	89
	A.	The State of Pregnancy	89
	B.	The State of Jaundice	90
	C.	Endogenous and Exogenous Inhibitors of the Immune Response	90
	D.	Hormones and Tissue Factors	91
	E.	Rindani Agents — Nonsteroid Anti-Inflammatory Factors of Animal Origin	92
	F.	Diet	93
	G.	Anti-Injury Factors	93
	H.	Cartilage Regeneration Factors	94
	I.	*So What?	94
VII.		SOME PARTICULAR PROBLEMS AND PITFALLS FOR DRUG DESIGN	96
	A.	Inadequacy of Present Leads	96
	B.	The Myth of Potency	96
	C.	Vigorous Metabolism of Small Animals	97
	D.	The Induction of Drug Metabolism	97
	E.	Does a Drug Have To Be a Suppressor To Be Effective?	97
	F.	Is the Need for Strict Chemical Similarity a Myth Too?	99
	G.	Chemical Synovectomy	100
	H.	Activation <u>in Situ</u> of Latent Drugs	100
VIII.		TREATING THE INDIVIDUAL	101
IX.		*EPILOGUE	102
		REFERENCES	103

*The asterisk denotes sections providing a rapid overview of this chapter.

I. DRUGS FOR CHRONIC INFLAMMATORY DISEASE

PREFACE

The important difference between the discovery of America by the Indians, by the Norsemen and by Columbus is that only Columbus succeeded in attaching the American continent to the rest of the world.

It is not to see something first, but to establish solid connections between the previously known and hitherto unknown that constitutes the essence of scientific discovery.

To discover does not mean to see, but to uncover sufficiently that many can see and continue to see forever.

— Hans Selye (in The Stress of Life [1]) 1956

These wise words and the title of this book emphasize discovery, the goal, and what must precede its attainment, the act of searching or research. This chapter does not pretend to be a dispassionate, comprehensive survey of the activities of, and publications from, all the laboratories and clinics which have engaged in the search for less inadequate drugs with which to treat some of the many chronic, disabling diseases with an inflammatory component. What we wish especially to share with you is not a mass of data but rather some conclusions derived mainly from our own reading and studies in the clinic and laboratory. It seems to us that new heuristic concepts are urgently needed and they must be clearly formulated today before we can hope to generate tomorrow the requisite experimental data from which to evolve a really new drug, as opposed to an "imitation" of an old one. We have therefore attempted to describe throughout this chapter what we consider to be useful concepts: We offer them as first approximations only, to be questioned and if need be discarded; ideas of no more value than the observations or experiments they engender. What we really wish to encourage is more searching criticism of the ideas underlying the contemporary research effort in this area and a willingness to replace those ideas that are clearly inadequate for the task ahead.

The following words of a great German physicist and an eminent Maltese psychologist indicate that this is not a problem unique to pharmacological research. "Intellect distinguishes between the possible and the impossible: reason distinguishes between the sensible and the senseless. Even the possible can be senseless" (Sir Max Born [1a]). "Ideas have always lived longer than people but today people live longer than ideas. Technology has so speeded things up that ideas may have to be changed within a generation instead of between generations. Yet our culture and education have always been concerned with establishing and communicating ideas, not with changing them" (Edward de Bono [1b]).

Regrettably, too much of the current research endeavor devoted to "anti-inflammatory drugs" imitates rather than originates and is perhaps rather senseless. Few of the scientists and physicians involved seem willing to commit themselves to searching out new and profitable avenues of thought and investigation. These inflammatory remarks are deliberate: They are not meant to be offensive personally but to hurry along the intellectual retooling that is part of the search for the superior "anti-inflammatory" drugs so badly needed in the clinic.

PROLOGUE: BY WAY OF INFORMING THE READER

This chapter is not another detailed review of the property of anti-inflammatory drugs as we know them today. For those who need fully documented, retrospective, surveys, there are many excellent summaries of research relating to the drugs themselves [1-14], inflammation biology [15-21], the rheumatic diseases [22-27], and other clinical disorders which involve a chronic inflammatory condition [28-30]. We have tried to supplement, rather than duplicate, previous reviews and to focus attention especially upon two areas:

i. the present state of the art in treating chronic inflammatory diseases with therapeutic agents, and

ii. those areas where more research might be devoted to searching for the superior drugs of tomorrow — needed to reinforce, if not replace, today's rather inadequate drugs.

Citations of the original literature have been deliberately restricted: They are provided only to give the reader a point of entry into the more recent literature so that by using the I.S.I. Citation Index and other bibliographic aids, he may trace research progress in certain areas. The Arthritis and Rheumatism Abstracts (published monthly by the National Institutes of Health, Bethesda, Maryland), the Bulletin of the Rheumatic Diseases (published bimonthly by the Arthritis Foundation, New York), and the Annual Reports in Medicinal Chemistry (published annually by Academic Press, New York, for the American Chemical Society) provide invaluable coverage of the more significant clinical, biological, and chemical research communications, germane to the subject of this chapter. The "literature of rheumatism" has been recently summarized by Morton and Bywaters [30a].

I. INTRODUCTION

A. Concerning Inflammation, Inflammatory Disease, and Anti-Inflammatory Drugs in General

Inflammation has been defined by Houck [18] as "the vital response of a tissue to injury." It is an essentially protective and normal response to any noxious stimulus which may threaten the well-being of the host, varying from the acute transient and highly localized response to the simplest mechanical injury (such as a pin prick) to the complex, sustained response involving the whole organism which may lead to the immunological rejection of (transplanted) foreign tissues. Normally, the tissue-damaging stimulus initiates a series of biochemical, immunological, and cellular events, which proceed through apparently well-regulated (and logical) steps culminating in physical repair of, and restitution of function to, the injured tissue. When healing is completed, the inflammatory response desists until needed again.

When tissue injury is caused by a single finite event such as mechanical trauma, a thermal or chemical burn, or a single exposure to a nonreplicating antigen, the inflammatory and reparative process progresses smoothly from the injury to healing. In these circumstances, the whole inflammatory process is truly beneficial and provides an example of a complex homeostatic mechanism restoring the affected tissue to its former, normal, "healthy" state. By contrast when the injurious agent is a self-replicating parasite (bacterium, virus, or neoplasm), the ensuing inflammatory response becomes much more complex because some form of tissue injury will continue for as long as the agent itself persists. However, inflammation such as that occurring in a lung infected with the self-replicating noxious agent Diplococcus pneumoniae leads to rapid healing and restoration of normal function as soon as the Diplococci are destroyed (either by the normal immune response or by administered antibiotics).

With certain noxious agents that cannot be destroyed or readily eliminated, the inflammatory response attempts to isolate them from the rest of the organism by forming a granuloma (as seen in pulmonary tuberculosis and silicosis) or gumma (as in syphilis). The ultimate expressions of this type of protective response are the calcified Gohn complexes which contain viable, but "imprisoned," tubercle bacilli, functionally isolated from the host.

Since the startling report by Robert Koch in 1876 that a microbe caused a fatal disease, anthrax, in both cattle and mice, much of the amazing progress in medicine over the past 90 years has been due to the successful identification and isolation of previously unidentified, noxious, etiological agents. Appropriately these then became targets for pharmacological attack. In this way, truly inflammatory conditions ranging from smallpox to leprosy, and from kuru to Whipple's disease have been reclassified according to their etiological agents and the appropriate therapeutics emphasize their eradication: Any anti-inflammatory therapy takes second place to this objective. However there are so many other chronic disabling, inflammatory conditions of as yet unknown etiology, which affect single or multiple organ systems of the body; examples include those affecting the skin (psoriasis, scleroderma), the gastrointestinal tract (ulcerative colitis), the nervous system (multiple sclerosis), and many conditions affecting the connective tissues which are discussed in the next section.

In attempts to modify the persisting inflammatory response, so that it is not injurious to the host, they are treated with a wide variety of agents, chosen empirically to relieve symptoms or suffering with no regard to the underlying causes.

These chronic inflammatory conditions of unknown etiology, with which we are chiefly concerned in this chapter, fluctuate rather unpredictably with spontaneous remissions and exacerbations. The rapidity with which the disease progresses and its prognosis depend on the organ systems involved. Patients with psoriasis may have varying degrees of dermatitis from time to time but their life expectancy is normal and usually they are not seriously disabled. On the other hand, periarteritis nodosum (inflammation of the small or medium-sized arteries) frequently involves the kidneys and other vital organs and soon causes death. "Cures" for these conditions almost certainly will not be found until their causes are unraveled. Many diseases will probably be found to be caused by self-replicating infectious agents which currently escape detection. For example, Whipple's disease has only recently been found to be caused by an intracellular infectious agent and can be eliminated by prolonged tetracycline therapy [31,32]. There have been many tantalizing suggestions that Reiter's syndrome, one of the rheumatoid variants, is also caused by an infectious agent [33]. Other diseases may be due to disorders of the immunological defense system resulting in the production of destructive autoantibodies against "self." There is ample evidence of the presence of autoantibodies in conditions like systemic lupus erythematosus, (autoimmune) hemolytic anemia, and pernicious anemia, but it is not yet clear whether these are secondary to an infectious agent or are actually primary immunological aberrations.

It is possible that some chronic inflammatory diseases may be due to disorders in the regulation of the inflammatory response. Although regulatory mechanisms have not as yet been elucidated, their existence is certainly suggested by the purposeful progression of the various stages of inflammation ending with tissue repair, which must be delicately controlled by some natural mechanism. If this is so, one might expect to find chronic inflammatory diseases due to disorders of these control mechanisms (which are discussed further in Sections IV. B, VI. C, and VI. E), just as hyperthyroidism and Cushing's disease (involving hyperactivity of the thyroid or of the adrenal cortex, respectively) are clinical conditions due to aberrations in control mechanisms involving two endocrine glands.

Although anti-inflammatory drugs may be used to modify the inflammatory response in diseases of unknown etiology, such as rheumatoid arthritis, or to symptomatically relieve inflammation in conditions of known etiology like gout or hay fever, they are unlikely to be curative in the sense of removing the underlying cause of the disease. Ideally, such a drug should not interfere with the normal inflammatory response to invading microorganisms, etc., or the patient will be unable to protect himself against his environment. Almost by definition, however, anti-inflammatory agents are symptomatic therapy and <u>cannot be expected to significantly alter the course of the underlying disease</u>. Agents which truly relieve inflammation by specifically altering or removing a known causative factor are not considered to be anti-inflammatory drugs if one uses this quasidefinition (given above). Extending this admittedly inadequate concept, a "first class" anti-inflammatory drug would completely relieve the signs and symptoms of inflammation even though it

I. DRUGS FOR CHRONIC INFLAMMATORY DISEASE

might not alter its cause; furthermore, it should leave intact the normal, protective, inflammatory responses occasioned by environmental insults, and would have no undesirable side effects or toxicity. Such a drug would be expected to suppress inflammation only while it was administered; unless the underlying disease remitted spontaneously or was "cured" by other therapeutic modalities, it would flare up again when the drug was discontinued. Current anti-inflammatory drugs do satisfy some of these criteria. As one might anticipate, an effective inhibitor of the inflammatory response must inescapably impair part of the body's vital defense mechanisms and so drug potency and toxicity often go hand-in-hand. This is clearly seen in attempts to control another part of the body's vital defense mechanism, the immune response, with synthetic drugs.

Ten Unpalatable Truths about Inflammation and Anti-Inflammatory Drugs

---

1. Inflammation is normally beneficial, being part of a complex protective homeostatic mechanism.

2. When it has achieved its objective, which is the restoration of health and function to an affected tissue, only then is the inflammation naturally terminated. Self-curtailment is usually synonymous with restoration of health.

3. Aberrant, uncurtailed inflammation, however initiated, may cause tissue destruction rather than tissue restoration.

4. Premature termination of the inflammation through drug action does not itself restore the status quo and may fail to halt tissue destruction unless it also eliminates the etiological cause of the inflammatory state.

5. Today's most powerful anti-inflammatory agents — the "supersteroids" — suppress only the manifestations (heat, pain, redness, swelling, etc.) of inflammation and do not treat the underlying cause(s).

6. In addition to this real failure to eradicate the inflammatory stimulus, steroids carry a high price in their alarming side effects, e.g., propensity for precipitating acute infection, ulceration, psychosis, osteoporosis, etc.

7. Other powerful, nonsteroid drugs effective in suppressing only the inflammatory symptoms also carry a high price in their general toxicity.

8. Too readily we accept suppression of symptoms as a (reasonable!) substitute for elimination of the disease process(es).

9. Is this because our views about inflammation (which are generally unfavorable) are misplaced?

10. Or is it because we have failed to define the true targets for drug action?

B. Goals of a Search for New Drugs to Treat Chronic Inflammatory States

There are at least four distinct target areas available for pharmacological attack (Table I). The methods of investigation, realistic goals, and inherent toxicity of therapy will differ for each of these four areas. A clear appreciation of the distinctions between each of these four target areas should prevent unnecessary disillusionment when new drugs fail to accomplish goals which are clearly not included in the area for which they were designed. For example, a drug intended to antagonize one particular mediator of inflammation (e.g., a kinin) should not be expected to eradicate the disease, no matter how efficiently it might moderate the inflammatory symptoms. It seems reasonable to assume that for each individual with a chronic inflammatory disorder, there is some etiological factor which in some way produces tissue injury. This tissue injury triggers the normal protective inflammatory response which attempts to repair the injury and restore normal function to the injured tissue. In the case of chronic inflammation, however, restoration of function is prevented by continuing tissue injury or by some abnormality of the inflammatory response, impairing healing and often leading to progressive loss of function. The four potential targets for pharmacological attack are, therefore:

 i. the etiological factor (Prime Cause);
 ii. mediators of the initial tissue injury released by, or produced in response to, the etiological factor;
 iii. the nonspecific, normal, protective inflammatory response evoked by this tissue injury; and
 iv. the process(es) attempting to restore normal function.

A drug aimed at target (i), if effective, would have much more specificity than drugs aimed at targets (iii) and (iv).

Realistic goals of therapy are therefore as follows:

1. Eradicate the Prime Cause

If the etiological factor can be removed or eliminated from the host, tissue injury should cease and inflammation should progress to healing with either complete restoration of function or some permanent residual disability, e.g., scar formation. This sequence of events is seen most dramatically when chronic infection is eliminated by treatment with appropriate antibiotics, but other examples might include elimination of the foreign antigen in serum sickness or drug allergy, or excretion of the toxic agent in chronic heavy metal poisoning. Obviously there may be as many appropriate drugs as there are etiological agents. Since the manifestations of disease are determined by the host reactions to injury, the same disease may be caused by several etiological agents, each responding to a different specific drug. For example, penicillin may cure pneumonia due to Diplococcus pneumoniae, but have no effect on pneumonia caused by penicillinase-producing Staphylococcus aureus.

I. DRUGS FOR CHRONIC INFLAMMATORY DISEASE

TABLE I
Goals for Therapy of Chronic Inflammatory States

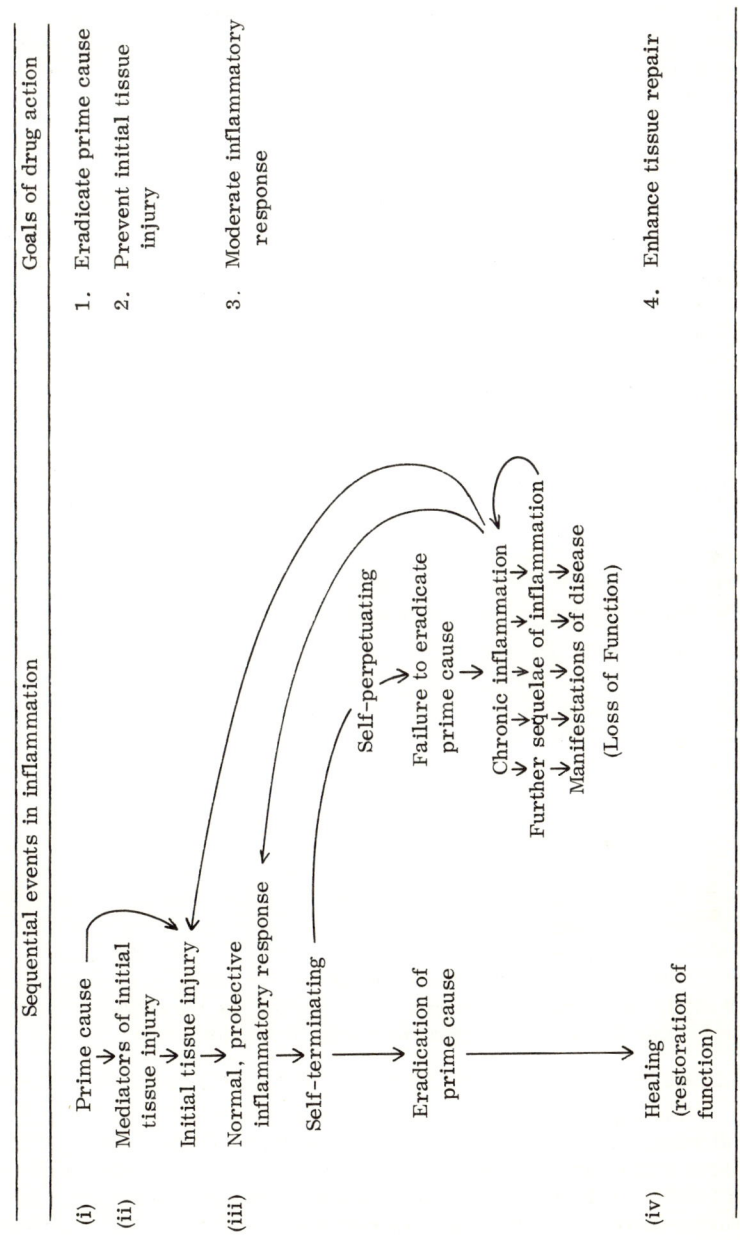

With respect to the chronic inflammatory states, goal (i) is to <u>cure</u> the disease by <u>eliminating</u> the prime cause. It requires a specific attack on a specific etiology. Such specificity has the advantage of not suppressing the beneficial aspects of inflammation, but requires precise knowledge of the prime cause (or exceptional serendipity) and cannot be expected to ameliorate inflammatory diseases caused by other factors.

2. Prevent Initial Tissue Injury

The goal is to intercept, interrupt, or turn off the mediator(s) of the initial tissue injury. Pharmacological attack upon factors incited by the prime cause (and mediating tissue injury) is inherently less specific than eradicating the etiological agent itself. It cannot "cure" disease but does retain the advantage of not interfering with established inflammatory responses. Therefore, all natural defense mechanisms used to protect the host from a hostile environment remain intact, except those dependent upon the particular mediator which is being antagonized pharmacologically. It is necessary to differentiate between (a) mediators elicited by the prime cause and which produce tissue injury, and (b) injurious substances released by damaged tissues which magnify the injury. Examples of the former include the antigen-antibody-complement complexes (which may mediate tissue injury in immunological diseases) and bacterial toxins (tetanus, diptheria). Examples of the latter include histamine, cathepsins, lyosomal constituents, and other amplifying factors within the inflammatory progression participating in the normal, protective inflammatory response.

Successfully intercepting the mediator of initial tissue injury would only prevent the initial tissue injury, could not eliminate the etiological agent, and would not alter the progression of established inflammation to ultimate healing. Currently, this area is being vigorously investigated in the context of immunosuppression. Unless the prime cause is eliminated by the natural host defenses (or in some other way), pharmacological attack on a mediator of initial tissue injury could only prevent injury while the drug was being used; the signs of disease would reappear if the therapy were discontinued. Toxicity, due to interference with needed protective responses, would be expected to be greater than in area 1, but would vary with the nature of the mediator. For example, if it is necessary to "disarm" the entire immunological system to prevent immunologically mediated injury, the inherent and unavoidable toxicity would be rather great. Our concern in attaining goal (ii) should be to increase the specificity of therapy, as for example, in the induction of immunological tolerance to a specific antigen.

3. Suppression of the Final Common Pathway, Established Inflammation

This might be expected to nonspecifically modify the symptoms of any inflammatory state. A drug acting in this fashion would not affect the initial tissue injury and might only moderate, but not prevent the progressive loss of function, unless the prime cause were eliminated in some other way. Furthermore, if the inflammatory responses were completely suppressed, the individual would be defenseless, i.e., unable to protect himself from environmental insults. For these reasons very effective anti-inflammatory therapy, which may be achieved with large doses of corticosteroids, always carries too high a price in terms of undesirable side effects.

Even if we were able to fashion a drug to perfectly counter the effects of any one, or indeed all, of the known (or yet to be discovered) mediators of inflammation, it could hardly be expected to achieve more than relieving the symptoms. Unavoidably it would share the inherent side effects of currently available drugs which are effective in this area.

Therefore Goal (iii) is the development of a drug which will (only) moderate the symptoms of inflammation while avoiding some of the more serious side effects of currently available (steroid and nonsteroid) anti-inflammatory compounds.

4. Enhance Tissue Repair and Aid in the Restoration of Function

If the prime cause cannot be eradicated and the initial tissue injury cannot be prevented, perhaps one could assist the host in its defensive efforts by promoting, or accelerating, repair of the damaged tissue. Some natural factors which may do so are discussed later (Section VI.G). It is difficult to think of any other, readily available, agents which effectively enhance tissue repair without preventing, or at least diminishing, the initial tissue injury; although attempts to treat osteoporosis (osteopenia) with anabolic steroids, fluorides, Vitamin D, and calcium are somewhat feeble efforts in this direction. The lack of effective drugs in this area is not surprising because the task in hand cannot be dealt with adequately if targets (i), (ii), and (iii) are completely ignored.

[Perhaps a more realistic goal might be prevention of abnormal tissue repair which results in excessive formation of nonfunctional scar tissue due to abortive attempts at repair in the presence of ongoing disease. Examples of nonfunctional repair include pulmonary interstitial fibrosis, pyloric obstruction due to chronic duodenal ulceration, and Heberden's nodes of the finger joints due to abnormal proliferation of cartilage and bone in one type of osteoarthritis. Of the available drugs which prevent abnormal tissue repair, the most useful at the present time are the corticosteroids: They seem to act as (Class iii) anti-inflammatory agents, though they do show notable activity in retarding normal growth in animals, presumably by accelerating catabolism at the expense of, and thereby retarding, biopolymer synthesis.]

The inherent shortcomings of drugs developed to attain these four goals are summarized in Table V (p. 56).

II. SOME RELEVANT CLINICAL CONDITIONS AND THE AVAILABLE THERAPY

No attempt will be made in this section to discuss all inflammatory diseases or all of the drugs used to treat them. Such an effort would encompass much of medicine and pharmacology, if a broad definition of inflammation were used. Nor will all rheumatological conditions and their appropriate therapies be discussed. Rather, a few chronic inflammatory conditions have been selected to illustrate (i) the range of factors which may cause the inflammation (ranging from physical irritation in gout to immunological incompatabilities in renal transplanation), and (ii) the interaction of some of these causative agents with those drugs found to be effective clinically. The clinical conditions discussed in this section (subsections A through E) are arranged in the order of an increasing probability that they have an immunopathic etiology. The drugs considered here were chosen merely to exemplify the types of pharmacological activities which have been found useful and beneficial in the clinic. An illustrative classification of disease states and presently available therapy is presented in Table II. Hollander's book [22] and for readers of the German language, a review of "Rheumatherapie" by Werner Moll [34], are recommended as supplemental reading to this section.

Although we wish to stress the fact that chronic inflammatory diseases rarely affect only the joints, it may be helpful to review the anatomy and physiology of a joint prior to discussing specific diseases primarily involving the articular tissues (arthritides).

Most joints are designed to permit controlled movement between two articulating bones. The opposing surfaces of the bones are covered with cartilage, a smooth translucent material which minimizes friction during joint motion. Apposition of the two bones is maintained by the tough fibrous joint capsule as well as by muscles which span the joint. The space between the joint capsule and the articulating cartilages is occupied by the synovial membrane. The synovial membrane has a generous blood supply and secretes synovial fluid, which supplies nutrients to the avascular articular cartilage. Normal synovial fluid also contains hyaluronic acid-protein complexes, macromolecules which are intimately involved in lubrication and decreasing joint friction.

Inflammation of this vascular synovial membrane impairs joint function in a number of ways. The inflamed membrane becomes more permeable to plasma constituents which exude into the joint space, producing a synovial "effusion," which is often described as a "pathological" synovial fluid. Joint friction is increased because hyaluronic acid is not only diluted, but sometimes also chemically degraded by the effusion. Inflammatory cells migrate into the inflamed synovial membrane and into the effusion. When these cells die, they release lytic enzymes which decrease the resilience and slipperiness of cartilage by digesting some of its constituents. With chronic inflammation, the synovial membrane becomes packed with inflammatory cells, hypertrophies, and grows over the already damaged articular cartilage in a form of granulation tissue called "pannus." Wherever pannus grows, it digests and erodes away the cartilage and underlying bone, eventually destroying the joint. Locally, the critical pathological event is the transition from the reversible synovial inflammation (synovitis) to the irreversible pannus overgrowth and subpannus cartilage destruction.

TABLE II

Classification of Disease States and Available Therapy

Disease	Prime cause	Mediator of initial tissue injury	Manifestations of disease	Targets of available drugs [a]		
				Eradicate prime cause	Prevent initial tissue injury	Moderate the inflammatory response

A. Infections

Disease	Prime cause	Mediator of initial tissue injury	Manifestations of disease	Eradicate prime cause	Prevent initial tissue injury	Moderate the inflammatory response
1. Tuberculosis	Mycobacterium tuberculosis	Direct injury Immune response ?	Caseating granuloma	Isoniazid p-Aminosalicylic acid Streptomycin	?	Salicylates
2. Syphilis	Treponema pallidum	Direct bacterial injury Immune response ?	Varied Gumma	Penicillin	?	?
3. Tetanus	Clostridium tetanus	Tetanus toxin	Neuro-muscular spasm	Penicillin	Tetanus antitoxin (active or passive immunization)	Muscle relaxants Curare
4. Infectious mononucleosis	Ebstein-Barr virus	? Immune response ?	Varied	?	?	Corticosteroids
5. Whipple's disease	Bacilli ?	?	Arthritis Enteritis Lymphadenopathy	Tetracycline	?	Corticosteroids

[a] No available agents to enhance tissue repair.

TABLE II

Classification of Disease States and Available Therapy (Continued)

Disease	Prime cause	Mediator of initial tissue injury	Manifestations of disease	Targets of available drugs[a]		
				Eradicate prime cause	Prevent initial tissue injury	Moderate the inflammatory response
B. Physical or Chemical						
1. Silicosis	Silica	Silicic acid	Granuloma	?	?	? Corticosteroids
2. Wilson's disease	Abnormal gene	Copper	Cirrhosis of liver Encephalopathy	?	Penicillamine Dimercaprol	?
3. Gout	Na urate microcrystals	Polymorphonuclear leukocytes	Tophus	Probenecid Allopurinol	Colchicine	Indomethacin Phenylbutazone
C. Immunological						
1. Rheumatic fever	Streptococcal antigen	Antibody cross-reacting with myocardium	Carditis, arthritis, rash, Aschoff body	Penicillin	? (Immunosuppressive)	Salicylates Corticosteroids
2. Glomerulonephritis	Streptococcal or other antigen	Soluble antigen-antibody complex	Nephritis Nephrotic syndrome	Penicillin?	Immunosuppressive	Corticosteroids

	Foreign antigen (drug or serum)	Antigen-antibody-complement	Arthritis, hives, nephritis	Discontinue administration of antigen	Immuno-suppressive ?	Corticosteroids Salicylates
3. Serum sickness						
4. Contact dermatitis	Exogenous antigen	Sensitized lymphocyte	Dermatitis	Avoid the antigen	?	Topical steroids
5. Renal homotransplantation	Homograft antigens	Sensitized lymphocytes Antigen-antibody complex	"Rejection"		Immuno-suppressive (Azathioprine, Antilymphocyte Globulin, etc.)	Corticosteroids
D. Unknown causes						
1. Osteoarthritis	?	?	Arthritis Osteophyte formation Heberden's nodes	?	?	Salicylates Indomethacin Phenylbutazone
2. Rheumatoid arthritis	?	? (globulin-antiglobulin-complement complex)	Synovitis Rheumatoid nodule Vasculitis	?	Immuno-suppressive ?	Salicylates Indomethacin Gold (Corticosteroids)

[a] No available agents to enhance tissue repair.

TABLE II

Classification of Disease States and Available Therapy (Continued)

Disease	Prime cause	Mediator of initial tissue injury	Manifestations of disease	Targets of available drugs [a]		
				Eradicate prime cause	Prevent initial tissue injury	Moderate the inflammatory response
3. Ankylosing spondylitis	?	?	Syndesmophyte Synovitis Iritis, aortitis	?	?	Indomethacin Phenylbutazone
4. Reiter's syndrome	? Mycoplasma ? ? Bedsonia ?	?	Urethritis Arthritis Conjunctivitis Dermatitis	? Antibiotic ?	?	Phenylbutazone Indomethacin Salicylates (Methotrexate ?)
5. Systemic lupus erythematosus	? Virus ?	Probable antigen antibody complex and/ or sensitized lymphocytes	Arthritis, pleuritis Pericarditis Nephritis Dermatitis, carditis Encephalitis, anemia Thrombocytopenia Leukopenia, etc.	?	Immunosuppressive	Corticosteroids Salicylates Anti-malarial drugs Indomethacin

6. Polyarteritis	?	Inflammation of small and medium sized arteries	?	? Corticosteroids
7. Wegener's granulomatosis	?	Arteritis, venulitis Granulomas	?	Corticosteroids Cyclophosphamide
8. Dermatomyositis	Sensitized lymphocyte ?	Dermatitis Myositis	?	Methotrexate Corticosteroids
9. Scleroderma	?	Dermopathy Arthritis Smooth muscle dysfunction (G.I. tract) Pulmonary fibrosis Nephritis, carditis	?	?
10. Psoriasis	?	Dermo-proliferation Arthritis	?	Methotrexate Topical coal tar derivatives, etc.
11. Ulcerative colitis	Antibody ?	Inflammation of bowel	?	Immuno-suppressive ? Azulfidine® Corticosteroids, topical or systemic

---

[a] No available agents to enhance tissue repair.

TABLE II

Classification of Disease States and Available Therapy (Continued)

Disease	Prime cause	Mediator of initial tissue injury	Manifestations of disease	Targets of available drugs[a]		
				Eradicate prime cause	Prevent initial tissue injury	Moderate the inflammatory response
12. Sarcoidosis	?	?	Granuloma	?	Immuno-suppressive	Corticosteroids
13. Chronic active hepatitis	?	? Sensitized lymphocyte	Piecemeal necrosis	?	Immuno-suppressive	Corticosteroids
14. Multiple sclerosis	?	Antibody? Sensitized lymphocyte ?	Demyelination	?	?	Corticosteroids ?

[a] No available agents to enhance tissue repair.

I. DRUGS FOR CHRONIC INFLAMMATORY DISEASE

A. Gout [20, 35]

Gout presents an excellent example of an inflammatory condition which can be well controlled with present day drugs. Its etiology and pathogenesis are fairly well understood, and effective drugs are available to treat both the causative agent and the inflammatory response thereto.

Gout is characterized by acute and chronic inflammatory responses to the deposition of microcrystals of sodium urate (monohydrate) in the joints and tissues. Acute arthritis occurs when the crystals enter the synovial cavity; tophi occur when they are deposited in other tissues. When gout is implicated as a cause of death, it is usually due to renal failure resulting from chronic inflammation secondary to urate crystal deposition in the renal parenchyma. Urate deposits in the tissues when its concentration exceeds its solubility in the extracellular fluid. The extracellular concentration of urate may rise if either the urinary excretion is decreased or if the total metabolic production of urate is increased (Fig. 1). Many causes of underexcretion and overproduction of urate have been established clinically and they include uremia, acidosis, competition of diuretic drugs, excess production in leukemia or psoriasis, and hereditary deficiency of the enzyme phosphoribosyl transferase. Cytostatic drugs, irradiation, and tumor chemotherapy may stimulate nucleic acid catabolism with concomitant rise in urate production from the purine breakdown products.

1. Colchicine [36, 37]

Symptomatic anti-inflammatory therapy of gout was practiced long before hyperuricemia and urate crystal deposition were first described by Garrod in 1848 [38]. Preparations of the autumn crocus were first recommended for

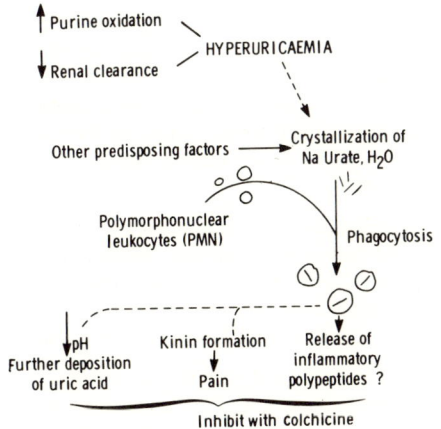

Fig. 1. Pathogenesis in gout.

articular pain by Alexander of Trolles in the Sixth Century A. D., and specifically for acute gout by Baron von Storch in 1763. The active principle, the alkaloid colchicine, was isolated in 1820 by Pelletier and Coventou.

The anti-inflammatory effect of colchicine in acute gouty arthritis is apparently due to its effect on the polymorphonuclear leukocyte. The oxidation of glucose in phagocytizing and nonphagocytizing leukocytes is suppressed by colchicine; this may decrease local lactic acid production. Colchicine also diminishes phagocytosis and interferes with the chemotactic response of leukocytes. It also inhibits the adherence of polymorphs to glass beads and interferes with kinin generation by granulocytes. These effects retard the further emigration of leukocytes into the crystal-containing effusion fluid and diminish the metabolic and phagocytic activity of those polymorphs already present, thus decreasing local lactic acid production and (lysosomal) enzyme liberation, thereby interrupting part of the inflammatory process [39].

Colchicine has a number of other undoubted pharmacological effects such as arresting mitosis, reducing the number of granulocytes in the blood, depressing the respiratory center, neuromuscular function, and the body temperature. However, these effects are not usually seen with normal therapeutic doses of the drug and it is most unlikely that any of these are directly associated with the anti-inflammatory effect. Colchicine is not an analgesic and has no effect on the metabolism, excretion, or solubility of urate, but abolishes the pain of acute gout entirely by its anti-inflammatory action.

It may be given intravenously (1 or 2 mg in 15 ml of 5% glucose in water with a maximum of 5 mg in any 24 h period) or orally (0.6 mg every hour until symptomatic relief is obtained or gastrointestinal toxicity occurs). Significant amounts of colchicine are excreted in the bile and reabsorbed from the intestine, perhaps partly explaining the prominence of intestinal symptoms with overdosage. Colchicine is deacetylated in the liver; both colchicine and its metabolites are excreted in the urine, and some colchicine is also excreted in the stools. Dramatic relief of the pain, swelling, and inflammation of acute gout usually occurs within 6 to 12 h after initiating intensive therapy; complete recovery of joint function occurs within 24 to 48 h. Colchicine, 0.6 mg one to three times daily, is frequently given prophylactically to prevent gouty attacks, even though the underlying hyperuricemia is not altered by this drug.

The primary symptoms of colchicine overdosage are abdominal pain, nausea, vomiting, and diarrhea which may become bloody due to a hemorrhagic gastroenteritis. Burning sensations of the skin and throat may occur and hematuria and oliguria have also been noted. With severe toxicity, paralysis develops and death is usually due to respiratory arrest.

Because diarrhea is frequently caused by therapeutic doses of colchicine, other anti-inflammatory agents are often used to treat acute gout. The most effective substitutes seem to be phenylbutazone (200 mg every 8 h) and indomethacin (50 mg every 6 h) which are both discussed in more detail elsewhere in this section.

I. DRUGS FOR CHRONIC INFLAMMATORY DISEASE

2. Urate Lowering Drugs [20, 35, 36]

The underlying hyperuricemia responsible for gout may be pharmacologically controlled by agents which increase uric acid excretion or by agents which decrease uric acid production.

a. **Uricosurics.** Urate is filtered by the renal glomeruli, reabsorbed in the proximal tubule, and secreted by the distal tubule. Substances which decrease (distal tubular) urate secretion tend to produce hyperuricemia; examples are organic anions like lactate or salicylate (at low doses) and most diuretics. Substances which decrease (proximal tubular) urate reabsorption increase renal urate clearance and lower serum uric acid levels. Salicylates, phenylbutazone, sulfinpyrazone, and probenecid are among the drugs which have been found to inhibit the renal tubular transport of urate. Small doses of these agents <u>decrease</u> urate clearance, presumably by inhibiting its secretion, but larger doses apparently also block reabsorption and thus have a uricosuric effect. Probenecid and sulfinpyrazone are the two most effective uricosuric agents currently used to treat hyperuricemia.

Another type of uricosuric effect is possible which does not require any drug action on the kidney but, rather, the displacement of urate from its binding sites in the body. In plasma, the bulk of the protein-bound urate is associated with the albumin from which it may be displaced rather readily by therapeutic concentrations of salicylate and phenylbutazone [40]. This type of "uricosuric action" may actually precipitate gout by decreasing the solubility of urate in the whole blood plasma, as well as promoting its renal excretion.

b. **Inhibitors of Urate Synthesis [41].** The immediate metabolic precursor of uric acid is xanthine; it is formed from hypoxanthine and is also oxidized to uric acid by the same enzyme, xanthine oxidase, which is present in the liver. A structural isomer of hypoxanthine, allopurinol (4-hydroxypyrazolo (3,4-d) pyrimidine), rather effectively decreases uric acid production by inhibiting xanthine oxidase (Fig. 2). (The 6-hydroxy metabolite of allopurinol, alloxanthine, also inhibits the enzyme.) This raises the levels of xanthine and hypoxanthine in the urine. Perhaps because these two oxypurines are somewhat more soluble than uric acid and are rapidly cleared by the kidneys, there have, as yet, been no reports of xanthine crystal deposition in patients treated with allopurinol. Nature has in fact performed the ultimate experiment of deleting xanthine oxidase in certain patients with xanthinuria with no significant ill-consequences.

Allopurinol is well tolerated in many species. In man, doses up to four times that required to control hyperuricemia (200-600 mg/day) can be safely given orally. There is no evidence for irreversible inactivation of xanthine oxidase and after withdrawing the drug, serum urate levels rise to the predrug levels within a few days. The oxidation of 6-thiouric acid is also inhibited by relatively low doses of allopurinol and the immunosuppressive action (and toxicity) of 6-mercaptopurine may be potentiated three- to six-fold with this drug.

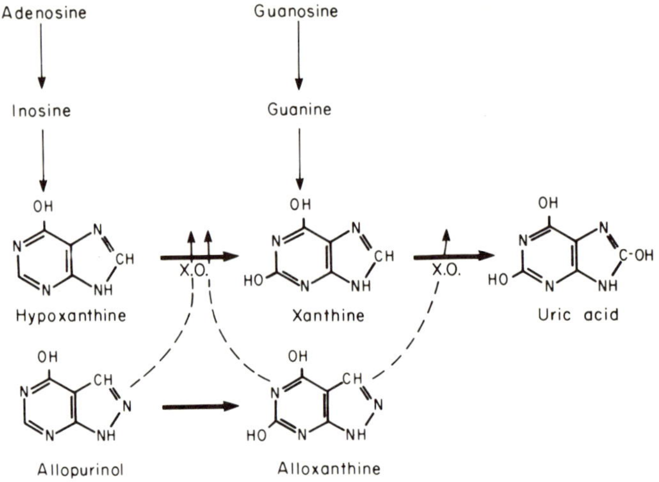

Fig. 2. Purine oxidation by xanthine oxidase (X.O.); inhibition by allopurinol.

Neither the uricosuric agents nor allopurinol have any anti-inflammatory or analgesic effects: So they are not useful for treating the inflammation of gouty arthritis. Thus in gout we see a complete separation of the therapy for inflammation from the therapy for the underlying cause. One can effectively treat the acute inflammatory attack without influencing the underlying hyperuricemia, and conversely, one can effectively lower the blood urate level without altering the course of an acute attack of gouty arthritis.

The causes of the conditions discussed hereafter in this section are not nearly so well understood as that of gout, but the lesson taught by an analysis of gout is equally applicable to them, i.e., successful treatment of the symptoms of inflammation may have no effect on the underlying etiology or the course of the basic disease.

B. The Rheumatoid Variants [20, 42]

The so-called rheumatoid variants are a group of rheumatic disorders characterized by a lack of detectable antiglobulin (rheumatoid factor) and antinuclear antibodies in the serum. Examples include ankylosing spondylitis, Reiter's syndrome, psoriatic arthritis and the arthritis associated with regional enteritis and ulcerative colitis. They do not occur predominantly in females, in contrast to the higher incidence of both rheumatoid arthritis and systemic lupus erythematosus (SLE) in females. Certain clinical characteristics or complications, such as inflammation of the sacroiliac joints and spine, of the iris of the eye (iritis), of the media of the root of the aorta, and dermatological manifestations tend to be shared by some, or all, of this group of variants. Arthritis of the joints in the extremities tends to be

I. DRUGS FOR CHRONIC INFLAMMATORY DISEASE 23

episodic and asymmetrical with an acute onset and relatively less joint destruction than occurs in rheumatoid arthritis.

Arthritis of the sacroiliac joints and spine may progress insidiously to produce complete fusion of the vertebrae of the entire spine. Therapeutically, the inflammation of these variants responds somewhat better to phenylbutazone and indomethacin than it does to salicylates, in contrast to rheumatoid arthritis which responds more satisfactorily to salicylates.

1. Phenylbutazone (Butazolidin^R) [36, 43]

This drug was introduced as an antirheumatic drug in 1949 but, because of the occasional occurrence of agranulocytosis, phenylbutazone's clinical use has declined somewhat since the introduction of indomethacin. It has mild analgesic and antipyretic activity but is rarely used for these activities alone. Its anti-inflammatory activity is readily demonstrated in animal models of experimental inflammation and is not mediated by the adrenal cortex, but more probably by peripheral mechanisms. Its anti-inflammatory potency is greater than that of the salicylates and less than that of indomethacin. Phenylbutazone has a variety of other pharmacological properties. It has a mild uricosuric effect which is mainly mediated by one of its metabolites (Fig. 3). Another principal metabolite, oxyphenbutazone (Tandearil^R) is also a useful anti-inflammatory drug. Both phenylbutazone and oxyphenbutazone may cause significant retention of sodium and chloride ions and sometimes induce peripheral edema or congestive heart failure. They reduce iodine uptake by the thyroid gland, inhibit oxidative decarboxylation of pyruvate, and uncouple oxidative phosphorylation.

Phenylbutazone is rapidly and completely absorbed from the gastrointestinal tract with peak plasma levels being attained in about 2 h [44]. It is slowly and almost completely metabolized by liver microsomes to oxyphenbutazone and a metabolite with marked uricosuric properties [45]. Its biological half-life in man is about 72 h due to marked reabsorption of the unionized molecule in the distal tubules. Both phenylbutazone and its metabolites are strongly bound to plasma proteins. With therapeutic doses of 400 to 600 mg daily, the albumin binding sites become saturated; further increases in dose considerably increase the unbound fraction of the drug in the plasma and the frequency of untoward side effects. These drugs increase the potency of (coumarin) anticoagulants by displacing plasma protein-bound coumarins. Chronic administration of phenylbutazone or of phenobarbital induces hepatic microsomal enzymes and increases the rate of metabolism of phenylbutazone, shortening its effective half-life in vivo and minimizing its side effects.

Epigastric discomfort, nausea, vomiting, and occasionally peptic ulceration may occur in patients taking phenylbutazone. Water and electrolyte retention may result in edema. Skin rashes and serum sickness may occur. The most serious toxic effect is the rare incidence (at least 24 cases between 1954 and 1965 [46]) of agranulocytosis, aplastic anemia, or thrombocytopenia, which have implicated the drug in a number of deaths (and appear to be more frequent with excessive dosage). Overall, some side effect occurs in

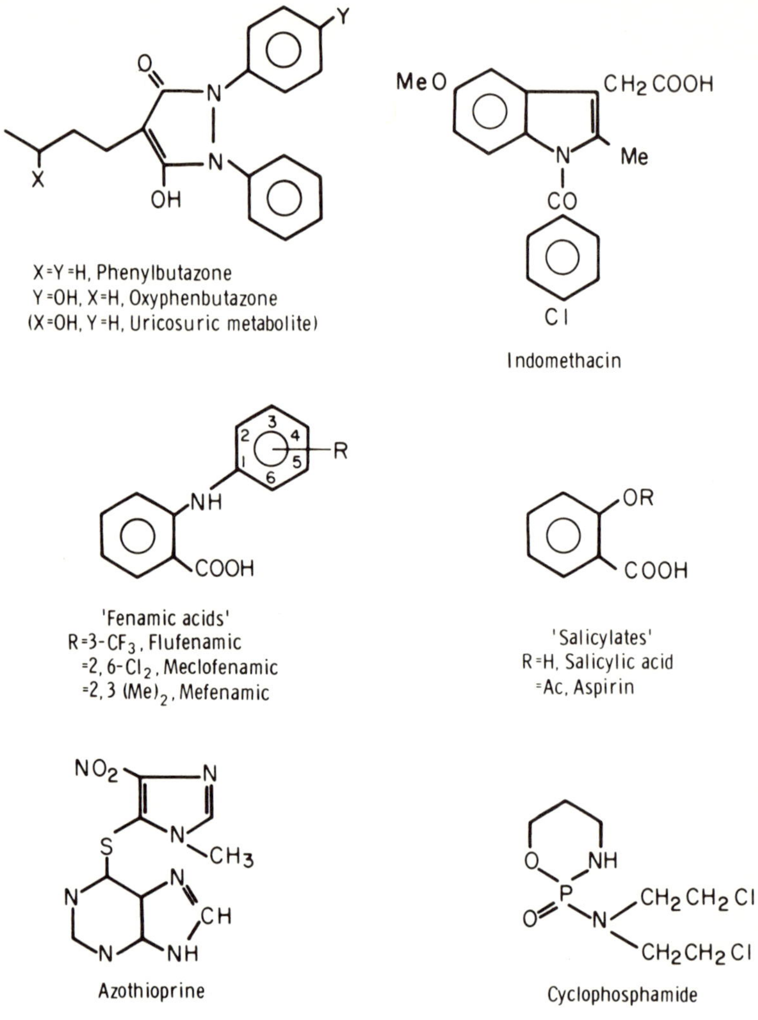

Fig. 3. Nonsteroid drugs currently used to treat rheumatoid diseases.

approximately 40 percent of patients and requires cessation of therapy in about 10 percent.

In the rheumatoid variants, phenylbutazone is used in doses of 200 to 400 mg daily. For acute episodes and for gout, the dose may be increased temporarily to 600 mg daily. Because it may depress the activity of the bone marrow, prolonged therapy with this drug should be avoided unless

I. DRUGS FOR CHRONIC INFLAMMATORY DISEASE

other, less toxic drugs are ineffective. When it is used chronically, the number of blood leukocytes should be monitored regularly.

2. Indomethacin (Indocin^R) [36, 47-52]

Indomethacin is an indole-acetic acid derivative (Fig. 3) first described in 1963. It was originally synthesized by Shen and his associates as a potential antiserotonin drug. Animal studies demonstrated that the drug was a very potent anti-inflammatory agent, particularly against carrageenin-induced edema and exudate formation. It is an effective antipyretic agent and inhibits adjuvant-induced polyarthritis in rats and urate-induced synovitis in dogs. The exact site of action is not known, but in common with other acidic anti-inflammatory drugs, it uncouples oxidative phosphorylation in (isolated) liver mitochondria.

In man, indomethacin is rapidly absorbed and excreted [47]. Peak blood levels occur within 2 h following oral ingestion, and the biological half-life is approximately 24 h. It is 90 to 95 percent bound to plasma proteins. Approximately two thirds of an administered dose is excreted in the urine and the remainder appears in the feces. Plasma indomethacin is thought to be conjugated in the kidney to form the glucuronide which is secreted by the renal tubular cells [48]. Renal clearance of the glucuronide may exceed that of inulin. Probenecid administration decreases the clearance of unconjugated indomethacin and results in somewhat higher plasma levels of the free drug [49]. Recent laboratory studies have suggested that combined dosing with indomethacin and aspirin may actually decrease the anti-inflammatory activity in animals, perhaps due to competition for common binding sites on plasma albumin [50, 51]. The clinical implications of this provocative finding, with respect to combined therapy with anti-inflammatory agents, have not yet been fully evaluated.

Adverse reactions occur primarily in the central nervous system and the gastrointestinal tract and require the withdrawal of this drug in 10 to 15 percent of patients. Headaches, vertigo, light-headedness, and mental confusion occur in 20 to 30 percent of patients, usually at an early stage in this therapy. They are less likely to occur with doses of less than 100 mg daily and may disappear despite continued use of the drug. Nausea, indigestion, epigastric burning, stomatitis or diarrhea have been reported in 25 percent of patients taking indomethacin; both peptic and jejunal ulcers have been reported, and it should not be used in patients with peptic ulcers. Because indomethacin therapy was implicated in several cases of fatal hepatitis in children, its use in children is now contraindicated. It does not seem to show any of the serious hematological toxicity occasionally seen with phenylbutazone, although leukopenia has been reported in a few cases.

In 1968, O'Brien reviewed published reports of clinical trials of indomethacin and concluded that there was no clear reason for preferring it over aspirin for rheumatoid arthritis [52]. It seems to be as effective as phenylbutazone for the treatment of ankylosing spondylitis, the rheumatoid variants, and acute gout. It is also useful for treating patients with osteoarthritis of the hip and selected patients with rheumatoid arthritis. Dosage for chronic use ranges from 50 to 125 mg daily, while acute gout may require 50 to 75 mg every 4 to 6 h during the first day of treatment. Its spectrum of clinical activity is remarkably similar to that of phenylbutazone; a choice between the two agents must be based on individual assessment of the risks of toxicity.

C. Rheumatoid Arthritis (R.A.) [22, 53-55]

It must be admitted that a claim for a role of autoimmunity in the pathogenesis of R.A. receives its strongest support from the absence of any stronger claimant. Nevertheless, despite the circumstantial nature of the evidence, extremely strong support can be adduced for the autoimmune hypothesis. Some of the evidence has been marshalled by Glynn and Holborrow [24].

Interest in the immunological aberrations of the rheumatic diseases was greatly stimulated by the finding of rheumatoid factor (an antiglobulin antibody) in patients with rheumatoid arthritis by Rose and associates in 1948 [56]. Further intensive study has conclusively demonstrated that (depending on the methods used) rheumatoid factor occurs in 70 to 80 percent of adults with rheumatoid arthritis, but has failed to clearly elucidate its role in the pathogenesis of the disease. The demonstration that rheumatoid synovium can produce rheumatoid factor and that leukocytes in the synovial fluid ingest immune complexes (containing rheumatoid factor, globulin, and complement) suggest that these immunological abnormalities may be involved in the mediation of inflammation in rheumatoid arthritis, but the overall picture remains puzzling. This apparent localization of an immunological event in the joint tempts one to conclude that rheumatoid arthritis is a localized disease and accordingly then to restrict therapeutic efforts to the joint. Such reasoning is probably fallacious. It is more likely that the many manifestations of rheumatoid arthritis are expressions of a generalized systemic disease and the joints are merely the most obvious target organ. Monoarticular juvenile rheumatoid arthritis (J.R.A.) is the most benign form of R.A., involving only one joint, and the sedimentation rate (of the erythrocytes in freshly drawn blood) is frequently normal. Certainly it would seem to be an ideal candidate for curative intra-articular or localized therapy. Yet patients with monoarticular J.R.A. have a high incidence of inflammation of the iris of the eye, which may cause blindness if not adequately suppressed. Interestingly, the iritis may occasionally precede the first symptom of arthritis by months or years or it may occur during complete remission of the joint inflammation, in addition to the more usual concurrence of the two clinical findings. This suggests that both the iritis and the arthritis are rather independent dysfunctions of two target organs, resulting from a more generalized pathological process.

Rheumatoid arthritis therefore continues to be an enigmatic clinical condition characterized by symmetrical polyarthritis which occurs more frequently in females and usually has a chronic course with cyclic exacerbations

I. DRUGS FOR CHRONIC INFLAMMATORY DISEASE

and remissions of symptoms. Systemic manifestations vary, but are usually present to some degree. One of the commonest extra-articular symptoms is vasculitis (inflammatory degeneration of the small blood vessels) which may manifest itself in various ways, the most typical example of which is the rheumatoid "nodule." It may progress rapidly to crippling disability, or may "smolder" for years with little apparent deterioration, or it may spontaneously remit at any time. The very variability of the disease and the frequency of these spontaneous remissions make any objective evaluation of drug therapy rather difficult. The symptoms and inflammation of R.A. can be readily suppressed in all patients with corticosteroid therapy and in some patients with intramuscular injection of gold derivatives. Long-term controlled studies have repeatedly shown that joint damage may progress continuously despite an almost complete suppression of symptoms with corticosteroids, and exacerbation tends to occur whenever suppressive therapy is discontinued. These observations clearly indicate that suppression of inflammation <u>does not truly affect</u> the underlying etiology to significantly alter the normal course of the disease [57].

Intensive salicylate therapy, combined with rest and physical therapy, continue to offer the best balance of beneficial anti-inflammatory effect and minimal toxicity for the long-term management of R.A. Indomethacin and phenylbutazone seem to add little to salicylate therapy and the need to use these drugs usually indicates that the patient is not getting sufficient rest. Gold therapy has a delayed effect, but seems to be associated with remissions somewhat more frequently than would be anticipated from the natural history of the disease. The use of corticosteroids is discouraged because of the well-known complications of administering them over a long term. Antimalarial drugs, related to chloroquine, are no longer used extensively because they may cause damage to the retina with prolonged use and they seem to lack any clear advantage over more conservative therapy. In countries where they are available, the fenamates (N-aryl anthranilates, Fig. 3) and certain phenylacetic acid derivatives (e.g., Ibuprofen) are also used to treat R.A. [58-60]. Immunosuppressive (cytostatic) agents such as azathioprine (Imuran ^{R}) and cyclophosphamide (Cytoxan ^{R}, Fig. 3) are currently undergoing clinical trials for R.A. Preliminary reports of their value for this purpose are rather mixed [61-63], although Fosdick reports that complete remissions may be seen in a selected number of patients after 6 to 18 months of therapy [64]. Even if they reliably induce remissions of the disease, the toxicity of the presently available cytostatic agents will probably prove to be too great to allow them to be used very widely and over a long term for treating R.A. However, they clearly point toward another possible pharmacological approach to. treating the disease, working at a more fundamental level than just treating the inflammatory symptoms (see Section V).

1. Aspirin and Other Salicylate Derivatives [36, 65, 66, 66A-C]

Willow and poplar barks which contain salicin, the glucoside of salicyl alcohol, have long been used by the pharmacist-physicians to treat sepsis, pain, gout, and fever. The ancient Greek physicians knew the value of plants containing methyl salicylate (oil of wintergreen). They even made the astute observation that small amounts of poplar bark could exacerbate gout while large amounts would prevent it. Salicylic acid itself was first synthesized in 1860; sodium salicylate became available as a drug in 1875, and acetylsalicylic acid (aspirin, Fig. 3) in 1899. Today, approximately 35 tons of aspirin are consumed daily by citizens of the United States. Even though salicylates have such an ancient heritage, they continue to be the prototype of the nonsteroidal, anti-inflammatory, antirheumatic drug and are still the "yardstick" against which newer agents are assessed.

Aspirin has a very broad spectrum of pharmacological activities. In addition to the anti-inflammatory effects which will be discussed below, aspirin is an analgesic at much lower doses than those needed to demonstrate anti-inflammatory activity. It is an effective antipyretic. It promotes the retention of salt and water. Paradoxically, it elevates the blood glucose levels in normal subjects, but decreases the blood glucose in diabetic patients. It may affect normal activities of the stomach, decreasing gastric motility and increasing pylorospasm. Low doses diminish uric acid excretion while high doses increase renal urate clearance (another paradox!). It may decrease the production of the thyroid-stimulating hormone (thyrotropin) and can displace thyroactive phenols (and perhaps also glucocorticoids) from their respective protein-binding sites. In very high doses, it stimulates the release of corticoids from the adrenal cortex. Many of these activities are undoubtedly mediated by its hydrolysis product, the salicylate anion which is formed rapidly in vivo. (The respective half-lives in man following small doses are aspirin, 20 min; salicylate, 4 h.)

In therapeutic concentrations (0.5-2.0 mM) the salicylate ion uncouples oxidative phosphorylation in the mitochondria. At much higher concentrations, it may inhibit cellular oxidative enzymes. Salicylamide, a useful analgesic, is devoid of useful anti-inflammatory and antirheumatic activity and does not uncouple oxidative phosphorylation.

The anti-inflammatory effects of aspirin seem to be exerted in the early phases of inflammation, especially those associated with vasodilatation and edema formation. Salicylates will prevent the activation of kinin-forming enzymes and antagonize the peripheral effects of the kinins when formed. They inhibit the release of histamine in sensitized animals and modify the effects of intradermal histamine injection. They will also inhibit the response to serotonin injections, both in experimental animals and in man [5].

In the appropriate experimental animals, high doses of the salicylates may suppress antibody production, interfere with antigen-antibody aggregation, and stabilize the capillary permeability in the presence of immunological insults. They may inhibit blood coagulation (increasing the prothrombin time) and decrease platelet (thrombocyte) adhesiveness, a peculiar property of aspirin not shared with the salicylate ion.

It is not clear which, if any, of the many known pharmacological properties of aspirin are responsible for its beneficial effects on rheumatic

I. DRUGS FOR CHRONIC INFLAMMATORY DISEASE

diseases. Despite our present ignorance of this subject, it certainly remains the preferred drug for osteoarthritis, rheumatoid arthritis, and for treating the articular involvement in the other so-called "collagen diseases" like systemic lupus erythematosus and scleroderma.

A list detailing the toxicity of salicylates is certainly as long as one describing their pharmacological effects. It includes allergic reactions, gastrointestinal bleeding, depression of prothrombin, platelet dysfunction, possible increased capillary fragility, hyperventilation with metabolic alkalosis, metabolic acidosis, hyperthermia, tinnitus, deafness, vertigo, and drowsiness. Serious intoxication occurs frequently in children and culminates fatally in 1 to 10 percent of reported cases. Obviously, there is still a need for another inexpensive, broad spectrum, anti-inflammatory agent with efficacy similar to that of aspirin, but with fewer or different adverse effects. Magnesium salicylate (Magon^R) may offer some advantages over aspirin itself, being palatable for oral use but causing less gastric discomfort in many patients.

2. Gold Preparations [22]

The use of organic gold derivatives (frequently misnamed "gold salts") for the treatment of rheumatoid arthritis was first reported in 1927 by Lande [67], and popularized by Forestier [68] in 1929. Because it was known that gold compounds could inhibit tubercle bacilli in vitro, it was reasoned that R.A., another granulomatous disease, might also respond to these compounds. Freyberg has recently thoroughly reviewed the whole subject of gold therapy [22]. He summarized reports of 7700 patients treated with various organic gold preparations and noted that the majority were considered to be significantly improved, although relapses were frequent when the drug therapy was withdrawn. Toxicity occurred in one-third of patients but was severe in only 4.5 percent. He states that several blind studies, especially the Empire Rheumatism Council (E.R.C.) cooperative study in Britain (reported in 1961), have demonstrated significantly greater improvement of treated patients when compared to patients receiving only placebo, acting as controls. The relative frequency of a complete clinical remission during gold therapy is particularly noteworthy. The usual weekly dose contains about 25 mg of gold. The time sequence of the clinical response to gold therapy parallels the metabolism and excretion of gold preparations. When soluble gold compounds are injected intramuscularly, the circulating gold is loosely bound to alpha-1 globulin as a gold-protein complex. Plasma levels rise rapidly and are maintained over at least the next 24 h, but urinary excretion is greatest during the first 2 h and decreases markedly thereafter. With constant weekly dosage, approximately 80 percent of the injected gold is retained in the body after 40 days. It presumably accumulates in the various tissues. It has been found that gold may be continuously excreted in the urine for up to 15 months beyond the last weekly injection. The onset of clinical improvement is very subtle and is usually seen 2 to 3 months after beginning the weekly therapy. If remission occurs, it may persist for 12 to 18 months after injections are discontinued, suggesting that the therapeutic response is related to the quantity of gold retained in the tissues. In the E. R. C. study, the average clinical condition of the gold-treated group of patients was better than that of the placebo-treated group for 13 months following termination of the 3 month course of weekly injections, but by the twenty-fifth month this advantage had all but disappeared. It is still not known if patients who fail to respond to gold derivatives fail to accumulate sufficient gold in the target tissues, or if they are simply resistant to its effects in vivo.

Although gold preparations are chemotherapeutically effective against hemolytic streptococci, tubercle bacilli, and pleuropneumonia-like organisms, the lack of a permanent cure and the probable relationship of therapeutic response to tissue accumulation suggest that gold probably also acts as an anti-inflammatory agent by suppressing the symptoms rather than curing the disease. Persellin and Ziff [69] have shown that gold sodium thiomalate (aurothiomalate) is taken up by tissue macrophages and accumulated in lysosomes. They also showed that the addition of aurothiomalate inhibited the action of acid phosphatase and beta-glucuronidase. Ennis and his associates [70] confirmed these observations and also noted inhibition of cathepsins. The addition of cysteine reversed the inhibition, suggesting that the mechanism of gold inhibition might involve its reversible binding to sulfhydryl groups. However, gold compounds were not found to prevent the release of hydrolases from lysosomes. Ziff has also reported that gold derivatives may inhibit antibody formation by lymphoid cells from rabbits immunized with bovine serum albumin. Although these in vitro observations are interesting, the precise mode of action of these compounds in patients remains uncertain.

Extensive clinical use of gold derivatives is limited by the relatively high incidence of toxicity (hematological, renal, and mucocutaneous), the rather discouraging delay before any therapeutic benefit is apparent, and the fairly large proportion of patients who fail to respond at all. It may well be that the presently available gold preparations are not the most suitable form for clinical use. They were originally developed for treating other diseases (especially tuberculosis) and have really never been "updated," i. e., seriously reformulated, for long-term use in arthritis. Preparations favored today emphasize water solubility for ease of injection, e. g., aurothiomalate (Myochrysin ^{R}) and aurothiosulfate (Sanochrysin ^{R}), but their aqueous solubility might be expected to restrict their distribution in vivo and minimize their entry into cells by mechanisms other than pinocytosis.

D. Systemic Lupus Erythematosus [22, 29, 71]

Systemic lupus erythematosus (S. L. E.) is the immunologist's nirvana because of its many immunological abnormalities. During the course of the disease, a single patient may develop antibodies to many of his own tissue components; thus one or more of the following antibodies: antinuclear, anticytoplasmic, antithyroid, antierythrocyte, and antithrombocyte (platelet), may be demonstrable at various times. The patient may have immunologically mediated disease of the kidneys, skin, joints, heart, formed blood elements, and blood vessels. However, despite its "rich serology" and extensive immunological investigation, the etiology of S. L. E. remains unknown. Recent reports describe the finding of virus-like particles in electronmicrographs of glomerular endothelium from S. L. E. patients [72, 73]. Some further evidence that diseases in Aleutian minks and in NZB mice, which rather closely resemble S. L. E. in man, may be transmitted by a viruslike particle has naturally intensified interest in the possibility that S. L. E. has a viral origin [74].

Clinically, the disease runs an undulating course, involving many tissues simultaneously or independently. The prognosis for the disease varies with the nature of the organs primarily involved. For example, if it is limited to the skin and joints, life expectancy is not decreased, whereas if the kidneys or heart are significantly involved, the prognosis is indeed grave.

The potency of the therapeutic measures required to treat the ongoing disease varies according to the tissue primarily involved. Since no available therapy is curative, the preferred treatment is to use the least toxic agents which will relieve the symptoms without otherwise debilitating the patient. Salicylates or antimalarial drugs, such as chloroquine or hydroxychloroquine, may be the only treatment needed if only arthritis and dermatitis are present. However, if there is any life-threatening involvement of the heart or central nervous system, large doses of corticosteroid drugs may be needed to prevent death. It should be noted that even when steroids have this dramatic effect, they are not really much more effective than salicylates in the sense that they too are incapable of curing the disease and like the salicylates treat only the symptoms. Cytostatic immunosuppressive agents such as azathioprine are being studied in S. L. E. because of their ability to interfere with the immunological mediators of the disease. Preliminary reports suggest that the combination of prednisone and an immunosuppressive drug may delay the progress of early renal lesions, but the ultimate role of such therapy in the general management of S. L. E. still remains to be determined.

1. Adrenal Corticosteroids [22, 36]

The successful molecular manipulation of the cortisol molecule to separate the glucocorticoid effects from the mineralocorticoid effects is a brilliant example of the art of the medicinal chemist. Unfortunately, it has not as yet been possible to separate the therapeutically desirable anti-inflammatory properties of cortisol and its chemical derivatives from the normal effects of endogenously secreted glucocorticoids on the metabolism of carbohydrates and protein. The development of such side effects as hyperglycemia and glucosuria, moon face, "buffalo hump," supraclavicular fat pads, and central obesity is due to exaggeration of the normal (physiological) action of cortisol. These same side effects are also seen when there is excessive production of endogenous corticosteroids, as in Cushing's disease. Excessive gluconeogenesis from protein may cause a negative nitrogen balance, osteoporosis, capillary fragility, cutaneous striae, and possibly also (steroid-induced) myopathy. [There seem to be no particular advantages in using ACTH (adrenocorticotropin) instead of the synthetic (gluco)corticosteroids, even though synthetic human ACTH is now available.] Administration of the drug on alternate days only has been demonstrated to avoid most of the side effects [75, 76] and is advisable if the patient's symptoms can be controlled in this way. The proper dose of corticosteroids is "enough" to suppress the clinical manifestation being treated. If given as prednisone, this may require as little as 2 mg daily for a patient with chronic rheumatoid arthritis, or as much as 500 mg daily for a patient with cerebral vasculitis due to S.L.E. The exact dose is arrived at by clinical titration against the symptoms.

As anti-inflammatory agents, therapeutic doses of glucocorticoids inhibit the entire spectrum of the inflammatory process. In early inflammation, they inhibit capillary dilatation, edema, fibrin deposition, migration of phagocytes into the inflamed area, and phagocytic activity. They also inhibit later manifestations of inflammation such as capillary proliferation, fibroblast proliferation, collagen deposition, and scar formation. Although they cause a marked drop in the number of lymphocytes (lymphocytopenia), especially those in the fixed lymphoid tissues, their therapeutic effects in suppressing immunologically mediated inflammatory diseases are probably due not so much to inhibiting antibody production by the lymphoid tissues as to suppressing the reaction of the other body tissues to (inflammagenic) antigen-antibody complexes, which may be formed and deposited in, or on, these tissues.

It has been difficult to demonstrate suppression of immune processes by glucocorticoids. Even when a delayed hypersensitivity response is modified by a steroid drug, the apparent effect may be due mainly to a nonspecific anti-inflammatory activity, rather than a direct affect upon the underlying immunological phenomena.

With such a broad range of potent anti-inflammatory activity, it is not surprising that glucocorticoids will suppress inflammation due to microbial, chemical, physical, and immunological insults or yet other, unknown causes. If sufficiently large doses are used, all symptoms, signs, and changes in blood composition associated with inflammation are suppressed, even though the causative agent may not be altered (and certainly not eradicated). In fact, if the agent is an infectious microorganism like Mycobacterium tuberculosis, corticosteroid suppression of the inflammatory response may enhance the organism's growth and dissemination. Thus it is easy to appreciate some of the undesirable effects (and real danger) of too efficiently suppressing inflammation, not uncommonly seen with corticosteroid therapy, e.g., increased susceptibility to infection.

If these considerations are appreciated, the appropriate use of corticosteroids (or any other, equally effective, broad-spectrum anti-inflammatory drug) in clinical medicine becomes obvious. Since they have no effect on the underlying causative agent(s) and, indeed, may aid in its dissemination, they really have no place in the therapy of inflammation due to

I. DRUGS FOR CHRONIC INFLAMMATORY DISEASE 33

self-replicating agents. In this respect, it is imperative to note that several controlled studies have demonstrated that joint destruction in rheumatoid arthritis progresses almost as rapidly when inflammation is completely suppressed by corticoids as it does when the inflammation is only incompletely suppressed with salicylates [57, 77, 78]. However, if the actual causative agent of the disease is known to be nonreplicating (as in exogenous asthma) and particularly if the exposure to it has been terminated (as in drug allergy or serum sickness), short-term corticosteroid therapy can suppress the symptoms of inflammation while the inciting agent is eradicated by some other means.

For S.L.E. and other chronic inflammatory diseases of unknown etiology, since the cause of the disease is unlikely to be altered by anti-inflammatory therapy, corticosteroids should be used only to suppress any life-threatening symptoms, e.g., acute damage to the kidneys. When used in this way, they can literally be life saving. The number of deaths due to S.L.E. involvement of the central nervous system has dramatically decreased with aggressive steroid therapy [71] and similar reductions in mortality due to the pericarditis, fever, and hemolytic anemia of S.L.E. have also occurred. Unfortunately, however, many S.L.E. patients die of lupus nephritis, complications of therapy, and uncontrollable progression of disease.

E. Renal Transplantation [79-81]

Although it is not classified as a chronic inflammatory disease, renal homotransplantation is mentioned here because it is a well-studied condition in which the causative factor, immunological incompatibility, is fairly well understood and the time of onset of the inflammatory state can be precisely determined. Rejection of the transplanted organ is clearly initiated by normally protective immunological reactions (meant to be defensive but actually manifest as aggression) but it is mediated by the familiar sequelae of an inflammatory stimulus leading to the cardinal signs of inflammation and, above all, loss of function. Prevention of a "rejection crisis" requires potent immunosuppressive therapy, commonly with azathioprine (and sometimes antilymphocyte globulin also), combined with potent anti-inflammatory therapy, nearly always with corticosteroids. The frequent occurrence of serious infections during such drastic immunosuppression and anti-inflammatory therapy emphasizes the hazards of interfering too efficiently with the natural protective mechanisms of the host. Nevertheless, with appropriate caution, such combination therapy is sufficiently effective for it to be acceptable clinically as an adjunct to renal transplantation.

The mechanisms of action and potential application of immunosuppressives to the rheumatoid diseases and other clinical immunoinflammatory states will be discussed later. It should be noted here that even in the much better understood context or organ transplantation, the production of specific immunological tolerance remains an elusive goal, except for transplants between identical twins. In addition, even with the maximum degree of chronic immunosuppressive and anti-inflammatory therapy which can be tolerated, it probably does not prevent persistent, or episodic, low-grade inflammation in the transplanted organ, so that its physiological function and life expectancy may still be rather limited. Some patients have in fact already required second organ grafts, clearly demonstrating that any inflammation may be too much — just as any flame, no matter how small, is always a fire-risk and the ultimate destruction it may cause cannot be adjudged by its first size. A fire-brigade does not concern itself with reducing the flames to a moderate size; so too, the clinical pharmacologist should seek to extinguish the inflammatory state altogether by deleting either these histo-incompatibility antigens of the donor (the cause of inflammation here) or their recognition by the recipient.

1. Azathioprine (Imuran^R) [36, 82-85]

Azathioprine is the S-(1-methyl-4-nitro)-5' imidazolyl derivative of 6-mercaptopurine (6-MP) which was designed to present this thiopurine in a masked, but metabolically active, form with the hope of thereby influencing its tissue distribution and also perhaps preferentially liberating 6-MP in tumors and lymphoid tissues (which are often rich in the thiols necessary to activate this compound) [82]. It has not found a place in the treatment of leukemia but is firmly established as the customary drug to suppress the immune response during, and after, organ transplantation and, by extension, for the immunosuppressive treatment of the so-called "autoimmune diseases." It has an immunosuppressive effect in mice at lower doses than 6-MP, perhaps due to its further effect of "blocking" those intracellular thiol compounds which react with it to liberate 6-MP itself. It inhibits the synthesis of nucleic acids by interfering with the conversion of adenine to xanthine through the intermediary hypoxanthine (mimicked by 6-MP). 6-MP itself is converted to 6-thiouric acid by xanthine oxidase, and the dose of azathioprine or 6-MP that can be tolerated is diminished considerably when the xanthine oxidase inhibitor, allopurinol, is simultaneously administered [83].

The doses used for chronic immunosuppressive therapy are from 1 to 3 mg/kg/day, the precise dose being determined by balancing its therapeutic effect (no evidence of graft rejection) against its toxicity (usually leukopenia). Clinically troublesome side effects are primarily granulocytopenia, with occasional thrombocytopenia, hepatitis, nausea and vomiting, or idiosyncratic fever or dermatitis requiring cessation of therapy. When given alone, azathioprine is surprisingly well tolerated; combined with prednisone, there is an increased incidence of infections such as herpes zoster, cryptococcosis, or affliction with cytomegalovirus. The tolerated dose is lower in patients with impaired renal function. There appears to be an increased incidence of malignant tumors in patients receiving chronic immunosuppressive therapy, regardless of the drugs used, but this question has not been completely settled as yet.

Clinically, azathioprine is routinely used for organ homotransplantation. It has also been used for the entire spectrum of autoimmune diseases, with varying reports as to its therapeutic efficacy [84, 85].

2. Antilymphocyte Globulin [86-88]

More specific depression of lymphocyte-mediated immunity has been attempted by two methods: (i) administration of heterologous anti-human-lymphocyte globulin and (ii) removal or destruction of circulating thoracic duct lymphocytes by other means.

The administration of heterologous anti-human-lymphocyte globulin (ALG), although not universally practiced, has been used extensively enough to be considered a common, adjunctive, immunosuppressive measure. ALG is prepared by immunizing an animal, usually a horse, with human lymphocytes (usually collected from cadaver spleen tissue). The immune serum is collected, partially fractionated, absorbed with appropriate human red cells, platelets, and plasma to remove unwanted antibodies, and administered intramuscularly to homotransplant recipients. Starzl [86] begins ALG therapy 3 to 5 days before transplantation and continues it, in gradually decreasing doses, for about 4 months. Within 3 days after beginning ALG, previously positive skin tests for delayed hypersensitivity now become negative. Starzl states that mortality and homograft loss were greatly decreased with ALG, renal function was improved, and the quantities of azathioprine and prednisone needed to achieve these results were reduced. (ALG was used in conjunction with these two immunosuppressive drugs.)

ALG is not universally used as an immunosuppressive agent because of a number of problems associated with its use. An injection of foreign proteins may result in serum sickness or anaphylactic reactions, even in a patient receiving immunosuppressive therapy. Failure to absorb all hemagglutinins and antiplatelet antibodies may cause anemia and thrombocytopenia. Pain and swelling at the injection site commonly occur [87]. The risk of ALG enhancing a malignancy (by its immunosuppressive action) is emphasized by a report of the development of a reticulum-cell sarcoma at the site of ALG injection in a patient with a renal transplant [88]. Indeed ALG has been described, not too inaccurately, as an oncogenic agent.

3. Lymphocyte Depletion [89, 90]

Fish and his associates [89] cannulated the thoracic duct of potential renal transplant recipients; the collected lymph was dialyzed against tap water, to destroy the lymphocytes, and then reinfused in the patients to prevent protein depletion. Five patients were treated in this manner for 39 to 108 days, prior to transplanting cadaver kidneys, and from 0 to 68 days after the transplant. Following transplantation, no immunosuppressive drugs or prednisone were given for 19 to 78 days (until the patients recovered from the surgical procedure), when azathioprine and prednisone therapy were begun. Only one of the kidneys was rejected (due to ABO incompatibility) despite the lack of drug therapy. Immunoglobulin levels in blood and lymph remained normal during the period that the circulating lymphocytes were depleted, while skin tests for delayed hypersensitivity diminished in intensity but were not completely abolished. This very provocative study certainly deserves expansion and confirmation.

Depletion of the circulating lymphcytes in rats, by surgical intervention, has been found to ameliorate certain experimental immunopathic diseases, including the lymphocyte-mediated arthritis that can be induced with Freund's adjuvant [90] and the rejection of skin homografts [90a].

F. Osteoarthritis (Degenerative Joint Disease)[22, 91-92a]

"Osteoarthritis is a non-inflammatory disorder of movable joints characterized by deterioration and abrasion of articular cartilage, and also by formation of new bone at the joint surfaces" — Leon Sokoloff in Ref. [22]. Although this definition implies a single disease with a well-defined pathophysiology, clinical experience suggests that the one diagnosis, osteoarthritis, includes several distinct constellations of symptoms. One is seen in weight-bearing joints as the residue of a lifetime of physical labor (or due to injury to a particular joint) and appears to be due to mechanical "wearing out" of the joints. Active inflammation is rarely present, and abortive attempts to repair the damaged joint result in the characteristic pathologic findings of eburnation and osteophyte formation. However, only a small proportion of patients with the characteristic X-ray findings and pathological lesions of degenerative joint disease have notable symptoms, and, with a few exceptions, disability is minimal. When symptoms occur, therapy with analgesic doses of salicylates and physical rest usually suffices.

A contrasting clinical picture is seen in some women at the onset of menopause. Their syndrome was described by Kellgren [91] and more recently emphasized by Peter [92], and consists of rather conspicuous inflammation of the distal joints of the fingers which persists for 1 or 2 years and resolves with the formation of painless Heberden's nodes. Biopsy of the acute lesion shows an infiltration of inflammatory cells into the synovium, sometimes indistinguishable from that seen in rheumatoid arthritis. The other nonweight bearing and weight bearing joints are often extensively involved. A prominent familial predisposition also characterizes the syndrome. Severe impairment of joint function is rare. Therapy of the acute stages usually requires anti-inflammatory doses of salicylates, phenylbutazone, or indomethacin.

Still another picture is seen with osteoarthritis of the hip joint (<u>malum coxae senilis</u>). It may occur as part of generalized osteoarthritis, as a result of a predisposing mechanical derangement (coxae plana, dysplasia of the acetabulum, congenital subluxation, etc.), following avascular necrosis of the femoral head, or spontaneously as an isolated occurrence with no apparent predisposing cause. Regardless of the onset, the end result is degeneration of cartilage, sclerosis of subchondral bone, and marginal osteophyte formation, producing severe pain and marked disability. Treatment is primarily by surgical correction or replacement of the damaged joint, but symptomatic therapy with phenylbutazone, indomethacin and, sometimes, also with mild narcotics, aids in controlling pain.

I. DRUGS FOR CHRONIC INFLAMMATORY DISEASE

These few examples should make it clear that osteoarthritis, which is the most frequently encountered joint disease, really represents a collection of somewhat diverse clinical syndromes which share only a common pathological outcome. Although they are not usually severely disabling or fatal, in aggregate they cause a great deal of discomfort. Patients with osteoarthritis constitute a huge potential market for an effective therapeutic agent.

G. Psoriasis [93]

Psoriasis is a benign skin disease characterized by patches of thick white scales on a base of erythematous skin, which occurs in 1 to 2 percent of white-skinned individuals. It is thought to be genetically determined, being dominantly inherited, with incomplete penetrance. In most patients, for most of the time, the inflammatory component is minimal but episodes of acute severe inflammation (called pustular psoriasis) or of generalized redness (called erythrodermic psoriasis) may occur. Psoriatic epidermis has been demonstrated to renew itself every 48 h, which is excessively rapid compared to the turnover rate of normal epidermis (usually 12 to 14 days). Treatment with the folic acid antagonist, amethopterin (methotrexate), selectively inhibits multiplication of the abnormally replicating basal cells and increases the turnover time toward normal [93]. Psoriasis illustrates the propensity of the chronic inflammatory diseases for involving more than one organ system; in the case of psoriasis, a characteristic type of peripheral joint arthritis which exacerbates or remits when the skin lesions do sometimes occurs.

1. Methotrexate (Amethopterin) [36, 94]

Methotrexate (4-amino-4-deoxy-N^{10}-methyl-folic)acid is a structural analog of folic acid which acts by powerful competitive inhibition of the enzyme, (dihydro)folate reductase, thus decreasing the de novo synthesis of thymidylic acid and inosinic acid, which are essential precursors of DNA and RNA. In this manner it inhibits cellular reproduction. The susceptibility of the various tissues to the cytotoxic effects of methotrexate varies with their rates of cellular turnover. Tissues which are either growing or being rapidly replaced, such as malignancies, bone marrow elements, lymphatic tissue, gastrointestinal mucosa, and skin, are affected more than relatively stable tissues like muscle and bone. Its therapeutic selectivity is based on this fact and on its rapid renal clearance. Depending on the frequency and route of administration, cytotoxicity may be produced continuously (daily oral dosage) or in pulses (weekly intravenous doses).

Methotrexate has established a place for itself in the treatment of acute leukemia, of choriocarcinoma (which it may "cure"), and of psoriasis. More recently, it has been used as an immunosuppressive agent in the treatment of S.L.E. and dermatomyositis. Each of these uses is based on its capacity to selectively inhibit rapidly metabolizing cells. Its considerable toxicity is an extension of the same property and consists of bone marrow depression (with thrombocytopenia and leukopenia), mucosal and gastrointestinal ulceration, hepatic dysfunction, alopecia, and dermatitis. Because of its essentially irreversible inhibition of folate reductase and its rapid clearance by the kidneys, toxicity depends not so much on the size of the dose as it does on the duration of cellular exposure to the drug. Thus, 2.5 mg daily by mouth may not be tolerated for more than 5 to 7 days, while 50 mg intravenously once weekly may cause no toxicity because of the ample "recovery period" allowed by the dosage schedule. Impaired renal function greatly increases the time of cellular exposure and multiplies the hazard of toxicity many fold.

2. Azaribine (Triacetyl-6-azauridine) [95-97]

Azaribine is an acetylated derivative of 6-azauridine; it is readily absorbed from the gastrointestinal tract and then converted by intracellular uridine kinases to 6-azauridine-5'-phosphate. This "false" nucleotide reversibly inhibits the decarboxylation of orotidylic acid to uridine 5'-monophosphate, thus inhibiting the synthesis of pyrimidines. Azaribine has not been particularly promising in the treatment of leukemias and carcinomas but it is rather effective for treating psoriasis and mycosis fungoides [95, 96]. It is of particular interest because of its minimal toxicity with therapeutic doses (150 to 270 mg/kg/day). Leukopenia rarely occurs at this dose and liver toxicity does not seem to be a problem, even in patients with cirrhosis [97]. A moderate anemia may occur, but improves when the drug is temporarily withdrawn.

H. Other Skin Diseases

Most dermatological conditions consist of acute, subacute, or chronic inflammatory reactions to various known and unknown prime causes. They differ from other inflammatory diseases in that the extent and severity of the inflammation (as it involves the skin) is readily assessed visually and also because, by shedding, the skin is sometimes able to rid itself of the actual cause of inflammation. Skin diseases like pemphigus, pemphigoid, and discoid lupus, apparently involve circulating antibodies and do respond to immunosuppressive therapy [98]. Contact dermatitis, on the other hand, is a manifestation of delayed hypersensitivity. There are dermatological manifestations of many bacterial and viral infections, and rashes are often a part of some generalized chronic inflammatory diseases (e.g., rheumatic fever, juvenile rheumatoid arthritis, ulcerative colitis, etc.). Inflammation of the small blood vessels (vasculitis) and inflammatory cell infiltrates are a prominent part of many skin diseases, just as they are in many systemic inflammatory states.

Except for the use of baths, compresses, and mild irritants (such as coal tar ointments) to stimulate shedding and self-renewal of the skin, and ointments to protect it from external irritation, the drug therapy of skin diseases is rather similar to that used for other inflammatory conditions. Thus corticosteroids, antimalarial drugs, or immunosuppressives are used frequently and administered systemically. In addition, if properly formulated

I. DRUGS FOR CHRONIC INFLAMMATORY DISEASE

and administered, topically applied corticosteroids are absorbed sufficiently well to relieve local symptoms while sparing the host much of their systemic toxic effects. Their efficacy is not entirely limited to the skin, however, and the chronic application of steroid-containing creams to large areas of skin may result in adrenal suppression, especially if absorption is enhanced by the use of occlusive dressings. In small animals, topically applied steroids will dramatically reduce the mass of the thymus within a very few days, clearly demonstrating that even a topically applied steroid may carry considerable systemic toxicity [99]. The nonsteroidal acidic anti-inflammatory drugs are not used very often for skin diseases, probably because it is so readily apparent that they are not very effective for this purpose.

I. On Reflection: Strengths and Weaknesses of Current Therapies

1. Present therapy for hyperuricemia is satisfactory. A less toxic, but equally potent, substitute for colchicine would be a valuable addition to therapeutics.

2. Present therapy for the other conditions discussed is a poor compromise between effective relief of symptoms and toxicity.

3. There is still a need for an aspirin substitute. It would have to be cheap, readily available, and free from serious toxicity.

4. Gold drugs must be seriously re-evaluated. They are too effective to remain in limbo. Either they should be relegated to oblivion on account of their sometimes distressing side effects and general toxicity or seriously rehabilitated as useful therapeutic agents. Their remarkable property of effecting more cures or remissions than any other currently available antirheumatic drug should spur interested investigators to invest time, money, and effort in further clinical studies of alternative gold preparations or formulations. Can another metal substitute for gold? The literature contains scattered reference to bismuth, antimony, and copper preparations being effective in inflammatory states. Can they too be "tamed" by reformulation?

5. There is an interesting divergence of the clinical effectiveness of the nonsteroidal anti-inflammatory drugs. Phenylbutazone and indomethacin are more effective than salicylates for the treatment of gout and the so-called rheumatoid variants, while salicylates are more effective for rheumatoid arthritis. (Incidentally, patients with R.A. almost invariably prefer aspirin to the narcotic analgesics.)

6. Use of today's cytostatic immunosuppressive drugs for temporary relief of symptoms cannot be justified (because of excessive toxicity), unless the symptoms threaten to shorten the life of the patient. The same statement may be applied equally well to the corticosteroids.

7. We badly need a drug which relieves the symptoms of inflammation, but does not irritate the gastrointestinal tract.

8. For all of the rheumatological conditions, our therapeutic depth and versatility is much too shallow. For example, if a patient becomes allergic to allopurinol, there is no alternative xanthine oxidase inhibitor; or if a patient with rheumatoid arthritis develops a duodenal ulcer, there are no effective anti-inflammatory agents available for his treatment (except gold preparations and antimalarial drugs, both of which have a delayed onset of action).

9. A "low-potency" antimetabolite such as azauridine may be much more manageable than a very toxic antimetabolite like methotrexate. Further clinical studies of other, not too toxic and perhaps somewhat less effective antimetabolites should certainly be encouraged.

III. METHODOLOGY FOR SEEKING DRUGS FOR CHRONIC INFLAMMATORY STATES

It should now be apparent from the preceding discussion that the chronic inflammatory conditions include a large variety of diseases and syndromes, each caused by one or more factors (which are known for only a few diseases but unknown for many more). Their common attribute is the participation of the inflammatory response in the production of symptoms and tissue malfunction. Therefore any drug which effectively suppresses inflammation in all of these diverse conditions must almost certainly act at such a late stage in the inflammatory process that it must also suppress the normal, protective, inflammatory response to other noxious stimuli in the environment. It is also clear that existing, broad-spectrum, anti-inflammatory drugs (from the corticosteroids to the salicylates) cover the full range of clinical potency, but are rather limited in their usefulness because the very properties which contribute to their therapeutic effect, undoubtedly contribute to their toxicity also.

Past experience certainly suggests that it is unlikely that a truly nontoxic, yet potent, broad-spectrum anti-inflammatory agent can be developed. However, some improvements may be possible within the present range of potency, perhaps by deliberate manipulation of selected drugs to <u>eliminate</u> some of their untoward side effects, and also by greater precision in their clinical use (e.g., by carefully establishing individual serum drug levels and more precisely monitoring toxicity).

Dramatic improvements in the therapy of chronic inflammatory diseases are more likely to arise by specifically focusing attention on <u>individual</u> diseases rather than by screening for <u>general</u> anti-inflammatory activity. The ideal agent would eradicate the prime cause (stage 1, Table I). Failing this, the second-best drug would act before inflammation is initiated by the original tissue insult or injury (stage 2, Table I) and so would not interfere with established inflammation. Such an agent could be completely overlooked by the screening methods currently emphasized, which detect the effect of a compound on induced inflammation (more appropriate to stage 3, Table I).

I. DRUGS FOR CHRONIC INFLAMMATORY DISEASE 41

The theoretically ideal drugs might be found either from knowing more of the etiology (stage 1) or pathophysiology (stage 2) of individual diseases, or by empirical screening of many compounds in animal or in vitro models which, fortuitously, correctly simulate the specific disease. Undoubtedly quite different models will be needed for each disease, or group of diseases, depending on their causes. What models might be appropriate and how can they be developed? These two questions should be asked continually until very much more satisfactory answers can be given to them than we can give them today.

A. Screening Drugs in Vitro

Just how may in vitro studies, especially those conducted at the biochemical level, contribute to the discovery of new drugs for treating inflammatory diseases (Table III)? This is a very different question from, though it is often confused with, the assumption (hope or belief, might be a better description) that in vitro studies may afford some insight into the mode of action of anti-inflammatory drugs. It ought to be self-evident that any in vitro studies conducted for either of these purposes (i.e., drug-prospecting or analysis of action) should be carried out with isolated tissue, cellular or subcellular preparations which are both (i) drug-sensitive and (ii) sufficiently viable to retain some of the characteristic "pacemaker" events which sustain the ongoing disease process(es). Accepting these criteria, we might conclude that many of the in vitro drug studies described in the literature (and even some of those listed in Table III) are largely, or even wholly, irrelevant.

To measure drug binding to platelets may be of little significance as such, but to then show that drug-impregnated platelets now resist complement- or neutrophil-mediated lysis (liberating inflammagenic amines and enzymes) may be of tremendous significance. Likewise, showing that drugs bind to albumin or xanthine oxidase in vitro may mean very little until it can be shown, for example, that urate is displaced from the albumin both in vitro and in vivo by the drug, or that urate synthesis is inhibited in vivo. Again, demonstrating that a compound is cytostatic in vitro is not very meaningful until it can be shown that it is a useful inhibitor of the in vivo lymphoproliferative response to an antigen, and therefore a potential immunosuppressive agent.

These examples should indicate that in vitro studies can rarely do more than suggest what a compound might do in vivo. They never substitute for, though they may usefully complement, whole animal studies. Even when an in vitro system is used to search for molecules resembling (in their drug action) a reference drug, it must be realized that an enormous number of "false positives" may be found, i.e., drugs active in vitro but inactive in vivo.

A series of closely related chemical compounds may differ widely with regard to their absorption, biodistribution, biotransformation, and excretion (ignoring for the moment, differences in metabolism of any one compound in different animal species). Until current methods of predicting drug activity (within a given series of compounds), based wholly on physicochemical

TABLE III

Summary of Some In Vitro Systems which Detect Anti-Inflammatory (AID) or Immunosuppressive (IS) Drugs

Property	Method of recognition	Possible significance
Binding to plasma albumin	Inhibit thermal denaturation of albumin	
	dye binding (e.g., HBABA, DNSA)	Drug may block other ϵ-NH$_2$ groups (e.g., in histidine decarboxylase)
	chemical reactivity of ϵ-amino groups at neutral pH (e.g. with 2,4,6-trinitrobenzaldehyde)	May displace urate from albumin ($\rightarrow$ "uricosuric" action)
	Changes in optical properties (O.R.D., etc.)	May displace thyroxine, corticoids?
Binding to organelle surfaces:		
erythrocytes	Protection against hypotonic or thermal injury	Uncertain
platelets	Prevent combination with antiplatelet antiserum	Possible application of drug in thrombotic disease
	Minimize collagen- or ADP-induced aggregation	Prevent release histamine, serotonin from platelet stores
lysosomes (usually from liver)	Enzyme release in mild injury/shock is minimized	Stabilize lysosomes in vivo?
Uptake by cells (yeast, lymphocytes, Ehrlich's ascites, HeLa, etc.)	Partitioning measured with radioactive drug	Indicates biological partition coefficient
	Spectrophotometric determination of residual drug in medium, etc.	Serves to exclude those potential drugs which are too hydrophilic, ionic, etc.

Inhibit Cellular Metabolism: oxidative phosphorylation	With isolated mitochondria → low ADP/O ratios	Far reaching, if drug "shuts down" energy production
synthesis of biopolymers in intact cells (fibroblasts, lymphocytes) or tissue slices (cartilage, etc.)	Incorporation uridine-5-^{3}H into RNA, thymidine-^{14}C or -^{3}H into DNA. choline-^{14}C or ^{32}Pi into phospholipids. aminoacids-^{14}C or -^{3}H into protein. glucose-^{14}C and/or ^{35}S into mucopolysaccharides	Equivalent to a rapid antigranuloma or immunosuppressor assay Locate area of drug action, e.g., cytarabine and hydroxyurea inhibit DNA synthesis selectively
Inhibition of growth	Effect on replication of cultured mammalian cells, bacteria, etc.	
Inhibition of leukocyte activation	lymphocyte response to mitogens/antigens polymorph response to urate crystals, latex particles, chemotactic agents	Detect cytostatic agents (IS), uncoupling agents (nonsteroid, acidic AID) [Fail to detect drugs requiring <u>in vivo</u> activation, e.g., cyclophosphamide]

properties [100], are sufficiently refined to take into account these in vivo variables there will be no adequate alternative to the "sweat-and-toil" approach to screening drugs in vivo.

No doubt it is unrealistic to expect in vitro screening methods to precisely select drugs which will be useful in the infinitely more complex situation of human disease. However, such studies should certainly not be discounted altogether. Their relative simplicity makes them well suited for extending our basic knowledge of the various individual biochemical and cellular events which, coordinated with many other (presently unknown) events, produce inflammatory disease in the intact organism. Indeed, most of the exciting advances of the past decades (for example, description of the kinin system, the role of lysosomes and lysosomal enzymes, the lymphokines, the complement system, etc.) only occurred when it became possible to isolate a particular part of the inflammatory response in vitro. Here it could be studied in detail without the distraction, and overriding complications, of other aspects of the dynamic situation in vivo. Undoubtedly, many further discoveries in the field of inflammation physiology will be made by similar in vitro studies, and any knowledge of how a drug might affect the appropriate in vitro system should aid further drug design. We must be careful, however, that we do not naively assume that each newly discovered chemical, or cellular, mediator of inflammation is the crucial one, and that if we could only block it, we should then "cure" chronic inflammatory disease!

B. Screening Drugs in Animals

1. Search for Antietiological Agents

Our lack of knowledge of the prime cause of most chronic inflammatory diseases certainly makes it most difficult to find suitable animal models with which to screen potential drugs. For conditions like gout or organ homotransplantation, in which the cause of inflammation is known, it has not been particularly difficult to devise some appropriate animal models to study the effects of potential therapeutic substances. For any of the other conditions (of as yet unknown etiology), more effort will have to be expended in first developing, and then adapting for (drug) screening purposes, realistic models which somehow reflect the presumed causes of the disease in question.

The human diseases which we hope to treat occur sporadically in certain, more susceptible, members of an outbred population, the remainder of whom are presumably less susceptible to the etiological agents in question. One of the problems presented to the host's defenses may be that the inducing agents have such a "low profile" that they are not recognized as "foreign"; consequently the ensuing inflammatory process may be directed not against the etiological agent itself but, rather, against the host constituents which have been altered by the agent and are now recognized as "foreign" (e.g., autoantigens). If we wish to find a drug to treat such an elusive parasite, the animal disease model used to screen various compounds should also have a "low profile" etiological agent. This situation is more likely to be found in

I. DRUGS FOR CHRONIC INFLAMMATORY DISEASE

a spontaneously occurring disease than in one which can be artificially induced. (In contrast, the cause of an artificially induced, well-recognized, disease state in a laboratory animal is likely to be quite "foreign" to the host, and therefore much more easily attacked pharmacologically.) Some models of inflammatory diseases involving low profile etiological agents are available in large and small animals, and others could probably be found if sought. They include:

i. A lupus-like disease which occurs in certain highly inbred strains of mice (e.g., NZB/Bl). These animals demonstrate many of the characteristics of the human disease, i.e., L.E. cells, chronic renal inflammation, hemolytic anemia, and dysproteinemia [101].

ii. The polyarteritis which occurs in certain strains of Aleutian minks with accompanying glomerulonephritis, hypergammaglobulinemia, and plasma cell proliferation [102].

iii. Scrapie [103], which is a naturally occurring central nervous system disease of sheep and may be a model for at least one human brain disease, kuru, and perhaps also for multiple sclerosis.

Scrapie, as well as the diseases of NZB/Bl mice [104] and of Aleutian minks [105], is caused by a chronic virus-like infection. The scrapie agent has been transferred to goats, mice, and rats. Other animal models of slow-virus infections are being found, and they are likely to be useful models for the screening of drugs directed against "low-profile" viral agents [105a].

iv. Canine systemic lupus erythematosus has been described by Lewis [106] as a spontaneously developing disease characterized by hemolytic anemia, thrombocytopenia, membranous glomerulonephritis, symmetrical polyarthritis, and the consistent occurrence of antinuclear antibodies and L.E. cells. It responds to high doses of corticosteroids in a manner similar to human S.L.E. and relapses when they are withdrawn.

Mycoplasmal infections of animals may be associated with chronic inflammation [19, 107] of joints, pericardium, respiratory, or genital organs (M. arthritides in rats, M. hyorhinis in swine, M. gallisepticum in turkeys). A psitticosis-lymphogranuloma venereum agent causes a chronic polyarthritis of sheep [108].

Such an animal model of chronic inflammatory disease could be used to screen compounds for efficacy in attaining any of the "goals of therapy" outlined earlier in this chapter. If we are screening for an agent to eradicate the prime cause, however, the following conditions should be satisfied:

i. Relapse should not occur when therapy is withdrawn (after a reasonable course of treatment).

ii. The inflammatory response to other insults should remain intact.

Attempting to eradicate the cause of a disease for which the etiology is unknown is admittedly a difficult task. Empirically screening large numbers of compounds for possible pharmacological activity is a time-honored method of pharmaceutical research, however, and has probably disclosed more useful drugs than the more sophisticated approach of rationally designing a compound for a particular need. While screening for antietiological activity would certainly add additional tests to the many already in use, it might be much more productive than all the "traditional" anti-inflammatory screens which, at best, are likely to disclose only a "more-effective aspirin" or a less toxic corticosteroid.

2. Search for Drugs to Prevent the Initial Tissue Injury

If we are unable to eradicate the prime cause of chronic inflammatory disease, perhaps we can find a drug which will prevent the initial tissue injury, before the inflammatory response has been triggered. Such a drug, which we might call a "desensitizer," could not eliminate the etiological agent, so that there would probably be a relapse when the drug was discontinued. Since this hypothetical desensitizer, if specific, would only act prior to the inflammatory response, normal protective inflammation elicited by other causes would not be prevented.

The models described in the previous section could probably also be used to detect such desensitizing activity, which would be distinguished from antietiological activity (discussed in Section III.C.1) by recurrence of the disease when the drug was withdrawn. In addition, a number of models have been developed in which a mediator of initial tissue injury is given in a controlled manner to cause a reproducible inflammation. Examples include the injection of sodium urate microcrystals in experimental gout and the induction of immunological injury by controlled administration of antigen (adjuvant arthritis, immune arthritis, experimental allergic encephalitis (E.A.E., experimental allergic thyroiditis, experimental allergic myositis, homograft survival studies, etc.), of antigen-antibody complexes (passive Arthus reaction), or of sensitized lymphocytes (e.g., passive transfer of E.A.E. and adjuvant arthritis) into carefully selected host animals (Table IV).

The value of these models in drug prospecting could be enhanced by also screening any effective compounds in vivo for possible impairment of the host's natural defenses against infection. The ideal drug should not increase susceptibility to infection, whereas all effective immunosuppressives might be expected to do so. A model which could be readily adapted for this purpose has been described by Triopathy and Mackaness [109]. A known quantity of bacteria (Listeria monocytogenes) is injected into test animals who are then sacrificed at intervals. Samples of the spleen or liver are cultured and the number of surviving Listeria determined. If a drug interferes with natural defenses against infection, larger numbers of viable bacteria are found in these organs of the test animals than in those of matched animals used as controls.

TABLE IV

Summary of Some Animal Models Used to Screen Drugs for Anti-Inflammatory Activity

Description	Elicited by	In	Measure	When	Mediated by	Responds to	Comments
Acute response to injury	Ultraviolet light	Guinea pig (shaved skin)	Erythema	1–4 h	Histamine + ? Platelets ?	Acidic AID Inhibitors of glycolysis	Steroid-insensitive
	Warm water (45–60 °C)	Rat foot Rabbit	Foot swelling	10 min–3 h	Histamine SH-protease Kinins ?	Antihistamine MAO inhibitors	
	Edemagenic agents:						
	Carrageenin (50–100 μg)	Rat foot	Foot swelling	2–4 h	Kinins Complement ? Prostaglandins	Vasostimulants Steroids, certain bases (thiazines, amidines) Acidic AID	Inhibition rarely > 80% Flat dose-response curve for many compounds
	Dextran	Rat foot or peritoneum	Foot swelling		Serotonin Histamine ?	Serotonin antagonists, steroids	Resistant to PB
	Turpentine	Rat pleural cavity		½–3 h	Histamine	Antihistamines Antimalarials	
('Experimental gout')	Sodium urate crystals	Dog knee joint or rat foot	Swelling	4–8 h	Polymorphs (PMN)	Indomethacin Colchicine Anti-PMN serum	Transient since these animals oxidize urate

Granulomatous response	Foreign implants: cotton pellets (may be impregnated)	Rat abdomen or dorsal areolar tissue	Granuloma weight	3–12 days		Steroids	Poor response to salicylate, PB
	plastic sponges air sac (containing an irritant, e.g., croton oil)		Granuloma weight Exudate volume	7–10 days		Limited data Steroids, PB Estradiol-17β Adrenaline	Salicylate ineffective
Cathepetic arthritis	(a) Lysosomal enzymes (from leukocytes, liver) (b) Polyene antibiotics, e.g., filipin	Rabbit knee joints	Synovial proliferation Leukocyte infiltration Cartilage degradation	12 days	Cathepsins	6-aminohexoic acid	Injury apparent after 24 h
Immune arthritis	Second dose antigen injected into joint	Pre-immunized rabbits	Synovial proliferation Leukocyte infiltration Cartilage degradation Complement depletion in joint fluid		Antibody-antigen complex complement	Steroids	Not practicable for wide screening of drugs

I. DRUGS FOR CHRONIC INFLAMMATORY DISEASE

TABLE IV

Summary of Some Animal Models Used to Screen Drugs for Anti-Inflammatory Activity (Continued)

Description	Elicited by	In	Measure	When	Mediated by	Responds to	Comments
Adjuvant-induced (poly)	Dead Mycobacteria (0.5 mg) in mineral oil (complete Freund's adjuvant)	Rats (only) tail, 1 paw, or lymph node	Swelling all paws, weight loss, "inflammation units"[a] drop in serum albumin	14 days	"Pathophoric" lymphocytes	Immunosuppressors[b] Estrogens Acidic AID Steroids Gold?	Ameliorate established disease Chloroquine inactive
Allergic thyroiditis (E.A.T.)	Thyroglobulin + adjuvant	Rats, rabbits, guinea pigs lymph nodes or foot pad	Thyroid mass	14 days	Antibody lymphocytes?	Immunosuppressors[b]	
Allergic encephalomyelitis (E.A.E.)	Spinal cord (guinea pig, bovine) + adjuvant	As for E.A.T.	Weight loss, paralysis of tail and hind limbs (death)	9 days onward	Pathophoric lymphocytes Antibody?	Immunosuppressors[b] Gold	Rat does not respond to bovine cord; rabbit and guinea pigs do.

[a] Material in the (diluted) plasma, mainly α_2 – glycoprotein and fibrinogen, which gives a turbidity on heating at 56°C for 30 min.

[b] Including anti-lymphocyte globulin: AID is anti-inflammatory drug, PB is phenylbutazone, and PMN is polymorphonuclear leukocyte.

3. Search for Drugs Acting after the Initial Tissue Injury ("Traditional" Anti-Inflammatory Drugs)

Drugs which moderate the inflammatory response to tissue injury (acting at stage 3, Table I) would be expected to modify the symptoms of inflammation present in the models described in both of the preceding sections. In addition, tissue injury may be induced by a multitude of chemical or physical irritants; inhibition of the resulting inflammation may be used as a measure of the anti-inflammatory potency of the test drug. A number of animal models of this type are listed in Table IV and are discussed elsewhere [4,6,110-114]. They have traditionally provided the primary screen for an anti-inflammatory effect; if a compound cannot inhibit rat paw edema, it is unlikely to be considered as a potential drug for chronic inflammatory disease. It should be obvious that the ideal and second-best drugs which prevent the initial tissue injury (acting at stages 1 or 2) are more desirable in proportion to their lack of effect in the traditional edema/erythema/granuloma-dependent assays. It is not surprising, therefore, that few such drugs are being developed at the present time (while the latter assays still constitute the primary screen).

These methods seem quite satisfactory for finding more drugs with the same anti-inflammatory properties as those currently available. To achieve any "advances" with this approach, much more emphasis will have to be placed on rigorously eliminating the undesirable side effects displayed by today's anti-inflammatory drugs. Some of the intrinsic natural inhibitors of inflammation such as the "Rindani factors" or even chalones (discussed in Section VII) should be readily perceived in these "standard" models of induced inflammation. They offer the potential advantage of (i) avoiding some of the nonspecific toxicity of the presently available drugs, (ii) possible normal occurrence (and function?) in humans, and (iii) their (presumably) specific site of action. However like the drugs they might replace, they still carry the inherent danger of too effectively blocking the normal, protective, inflammatory response.

C. Evaluation of Drugs in that Unique Animal, "Man"

The ultimate test of every new drug, of course, is its effectiveness and toxicity when it is used to treat a disease in patients. Just as the methods used for screening drugs in animals must be varied to meet the specific therapeutic goal, the design of human clinical studies also must be consistent with the designated therapeutic goal.

1. Evaluation of Antietiological Agents (Eradicating the Prime Cause)

The distinguishing characteristic of an effective antietiological agent should be its ability to produce a "cure" which persists even when all treatment is discontinued. It is quite possible that the prime causes of the various chronic inflammatory states may be exposed to the effect of a drug only intermittently, and a rather long course of administration may then be needed to

I. DRUGS FOR CHRONIC INFLAMMATORY DISEASE 51

ensure the complete elimination of the prime cause(s). It is also possible that a single diagnostic entity, like rheumatoid arthritis, may be caused by any one of a number of different etiological factors; if only one of these factors were susceptible to the drug being tested, only a minority of patients with this diagnosis (rheumatoid arthritis) would benefit from it. Since successful eradication of the prime cause would have no effect on the existing inflammation, there would be a definite time lag before the symptoms and clinical signs abated, during which the existing injury was being repaired.

For these reasons, clinical evaluation of an antietiological drug requires a fairly long study — probably at least one year. Since the criterion for success is cure of the disease, sustained despite withdrawal of therapy, the parameters to be evaluated may be fairly gross and should include complete cessation of active inflammation. Because of the propensity of the pertinent diseases to remit spontaneously, a control group of patients receiving only "placebo" is essential to establish the significance of the apparent drug action. A careful search should be made for a drug-responsive clinical subgroup of patients who are cured by the drug, even though statistically the overall drug-treated group may be only slightly better than the control (untreated) group because the agents causing the disease in other clinical subgroups are resistant to the drug being evaluated. Since none of the standard therapeutic measures is curative, there is no need to discontinue them during the trial. A considerably greater degree of toxicity would be acceptable in a truly curative drug than in one which merely relieved symptoms, and side effects should be evaluated with this in mind.

2. Evaluation of Drugs Which Might Prevent Initial Tissue Injury

The same sort of clinical study described in the previous section could be applied equally well to recognize and evaluate this second type of drug ("desensitizer"), except that one could now expect recurrence of clinical disease when the therapy was withdrawn. Specific studies of the effect of the drug on primary and secondary humoral antibody production and upon cellular immunity could be carried out to demonstrate immunosuppressive potency, but they are really of minor importance when compared with more direct demonstrations of the clinical suppression of the disease state in question. The price, in terms of undesirable side effects, of this less specific therapy is likely to be greater than that of an eradicator of the prime cause, and must be carefully evaluated in terms of the potential disability and life expectancy associated with less effective therapy. Subgroup responses, if present, are likely to be larger and more easily discerned when one treats a general mediator rather than a specific etiological agent.

3. Evaluation of Classical Anti-Inflammatory Agents

Since drugs of this type do not pretend to cure the underlying disease, or even to completely prevent tissue injury (or progressive loss of function), and because a number of effective nonsteroidal and steroidal agents are available, the emphasis here must be largely on (lack of) toxicity, as well as efficacy. Long term studies should not be needed to demonstrate any beneficial effects (2 to 4 weeks should be sufficient), and these agents should be effective in a wide variety of conditions. The parameters by which the drug is evaluated will show qualitative changes only, so that precise measurement is necessary. Fairly large numbers of patients may be needed to demonstrate any statistical significance when the drug-treated group is compared to a control group in which considerable spontaneous improvement may have occurred. Since our requirement is for less toxic therapy, even though it may be no more effective than the "standard" therapy, it is unfair to discard a new drug merely because it does not demonstrate statistical superiority to a standard treatment. This is especially true of trials of drugs for rheumatoid arthritis, in which the control group is almost always permitted ad lib aspirin and frequently also continues with corticosteroids and other drugs. Lack of superiority to such a control group should not eliminate a drug from consideration. It is preferable that the control group should be truly placebo-treated, although this may be difficult when one of the standard drugs is as readily available as aspirin. Careful evaluation for undesirable side effects is essential and requires large numbers of patients and frequent clinical and laboratory follow-up studies.

In our own clinical studies of patients with rheumatoid arthritis we have included some, or all, of the following qualitative and quantitative responses to the drug under investigation. (This list is not meant to be exhaustive but merely to indicate what measurements are feasible, practicable, and occasionally meaningful.)

Evaluation of	Parameters	Comments

A. Disease activity	1. Subjective
	  a. Duration of morning stiffness
	  b. Intensity of pain
	  c. Quantity of supplementary analgesic tabs (codeine) required
		Rather gross parameters

	2. Objective
	  a. Ring size of selected PIP joints[a]
	  b. Range of motion of selected joint
	  c. Grip strength
	  d. Number of tender joints
		Moderately sensitive indicators of degree of inflammation present

I. DRUGS FOR CHRONIC INFLAMMATORY DISEASE

Evaluation of	Parameters	Comments

	3. Laboratory
	  a. Hematocrit
	  b. Erythrocyte sedimentation rate
	  c. Rheumatoid factor
		Useful only in medium to long term study

B. Toxicity of drug	1. Subjective Symptoms of nausea, headache, gastrointestinal distress, etc.	
	2. Objective Examine for rash, etc.	

	3. Laboratory
	  a. Complete blood count
	  b. Urinalysis, creatinine
	  c. Alkaline phosphatase, SGOT, SGPT, bilirubin in serum
	  d. Quantitation of blood lost in stools.
		Markers of
		
		kidney function
		
		liver function

C. Induced inflammation (nonimmune)	1. Trafuril [b] erythema assay	Evaluate early acute inflammation
	2. Subcutaneous injection of microcrystalline sodium urate	Evaluate subacute inflammation
	3. Rebuck skin window preparation	Evaluate cellular response to inflammation
D. Induced inflammation (immune)	1. Intradermal test for delayed hypersensitivity (PPD [c] mumps, etc.)	

Evaluation of	Parameters	Comments
	2. Rebuck skin window preparation (with diphtheria toxoid applied)	
E. Humoral antibody response (during drug administration) to subcutaneous antigens	1. Primary response to keyhole limpet hemocyanin	
	2. Secondary response to tetanus toxoid (IgG antibody) and typhoid vaccine (IgM antibody)	
F. Delayed hypersensitivity	1. Primary sensitization with intradermal keyhole limpet hemocyanin or topical 2,4-dinitrochlorobenzene	
	2. Secondary response to PPD^c, mumps, etc.	

^{a} PIP stands for proximal interphalangeal.

^{b} Trafuril^R is tetrahydrofurfuryl nicotinate (a topical rubefacient).

^{c} PPD is purified protein derivative for tuberculin sensitivity.

IV. DESIGNING NEW DRUGS TO TREAT INFLAMMATORY STATES

No drug can be designed without some knowledge of what it should do and how this might be achieved. Our present anti-inflammatory agents seem to have all been discovered by accident and it is very unlikely that we can expect many further change observations in the clinic to supply the chemical leads for novel antiarthritic drugs, now that so few new compounds are being examined in man. Can we rationally anticipate what a novel antiarthritic drug might do? If so, can we then (and only then) instruct the organic chemist what type of compound he should make (regardless of the patent literature at this stage)? This section considers some features of present anti-inflammatory drugs and the inflammatory response with a view to reassessing the strategy for pharmacologically controlling both the response and its pathogenic consequences.

I. DRUGS FOR CHRONIC INFLAMMATORY DISEASE

A. Some General Considerations

Even in this era of the logical, rational scientist, the search for, and design of, new anti-inflammatory agents seems to be afflicted with, and impeded by, more than its fair share of fuzzy thought and ill-conceived rationales to sustain the considerable research effort now being expended in this area. Much of this effort seems to reflect the hope that, if only the crucial mediator of inflammation can be found, then it will be a relatively simple matter to design its antagonist; thus, with one clean stroke, "curing" all inflammatory diseases forever. Unfortunately, the real world is not that simple. Both the normal (protective) inflammatory response and the normal immune response are just as essential to life as the proper function of the heart, liver, or any other vital organ. When any of these vital functions is significantly impaired by drugs, poisons, or illness, retribution is swift and certain.

Therefore, before embarking on a discussion of drug design, we would like once again to direct attention to the goals of therapy which were discussed earlier (Section I.B). We especially wish to emphasize that certain limitations or constraints are implicit in pursuing these goals, and it is unrealistic to expect to avoid these constraints while successfully achieving the therapeutic goal (see Table V). A careful consideration of these limitations, which are inherent and shared by all drugs aimed at a particular target or goal, should save the drug designer from the unnecessary but almost inevitable disillusionment which follows from unrealized expectations; these having been rather unrealistic in the first place.

For example, the isolation and synthesis of a natural regulator of inflammation (discussed in Section VII) would be a valuable advance in its own right but might be of real therapeutic benefit if this regulator avoided many of the (nontherapeutic) side effects of today's anti-inflammatory drugs. Nevertheless the inherent benefits and limitations of successfully attaining its goal (in this case, moderating the inflammatory response), as outlined in the accompanying Table V, make it obvious that even the therapeutic application of an almost "perfect" natural regulator of inflammation can not cure chronic inflammatory disease.

These constraints should be kept clearly in mind throughout the subsequent discussion (Sections IV-VI) and the ideas presented therein must all be viewed in the perspective provided by Table V.

B. Some Specific Considerations

The causes of chronic inflammation are still not well defined. By contrast there is a considerable body of knowledge about the various physiological consequences of an inflammatory stimulus, the signs of which were first summarized so elegantly by Celsus (30 B.C.-A.D. 38), a Greek, in Latin,

TABLE V

Constraints in the Development of Drugs for Chronic Inflammatory Diseases[a]

Goal	Benefits of effective drug	Inherent disadvantage of effective drug	Currently available drugs (e.g.)	Drugs that are still needed (awaiting discovery)
1. Eradicate prime cause	1. Cure disease due to the specific prime cause 2. Protective, immune, and inflammatory responses remain intact	No effect on similar conditions due to other prime causes (even though they might be closely related — if the drug is sufficiently specific)	Antibiotics Probenecid (II.A.2a) Allopurinol (II.A.2b)	Antiviral agents (IV.D)? ?
2. Prevent initial tissue injury	1. Prevent progression of tissue injury 2. Normal inflammatory response (to burns, physical injury, etc.) remains intact	1. Benefit restricted to period of therapy — relapse if discontinued 2. Less specific — may disrupt entire immune response (predisposing to infections, etc.)	Immunosuppressives (II.E.1,2; II.G1,2) Antitoxins Colchicine (II.A.1)	Anticomplement agents (IV.C.2) Very specific immunosuppressors (V)

I. DRUGS FOR CHRONIC INFLAMMATORY DISEASE

3. Moderate inflammatory response	1. Relieve symptoms of the inflammation 2. Prevent the destructive (amplifying) inflammatory sequelae to initial tissue injury 3. Immune response may remain intact 4. Control many inflammatory states, regardless of their causes	1. Benefit restricted to period of therapy — relapse if discontinued 2. Initial tissue injury (due to prime cause) continues — also consequent loss of function; e.g., R.A. treated with corticosteroids 3. Normal, protective, inflammatory response inhibited — may cause delayed healing, etc.	Corticosteroids (II.D.1) Acidic nonsteroidal anti-inflammatory drugs salicylates (II.C.1) phenylbutazone (II.B.1) indomethacin (II.B.2) ibuprofen gold preparations (II.C.2) antimalarials	Antineutrophil ⎫ Antimacrophage ⎬ (IV.C) Antilymphocyte ⎭ Antikinins Antienzymes (lysosomal, cathepsins, etc.) Natural regulators of inflammation: (Chalones?, Rindani agents?) (VI.D, E)
4. Enhance tissue repair	1. Repair damage of incompletely controlled inflammation 2. Retard degenerative effects of aging	Hyperplasia, if not "turned off"	None really effective? (IV.D) Cartilage regeneration factors (VI.H)?	

a̲ Figures in parentheses refer to sections of this chapter where these topics are discussed in more detail.

("calor, tumor, rubor et dolor") as heat, swelling, redness, and pain. To this list of descriptions, Galen (A. D. 130-200), another Greek physician, subsequently added yet another sign, functio laesa, loss of function. This most important "after-thought" deserves especial emphasis when we consider the pharmacological approach to inflammation. Most of the present day drugs seem to have been designed for Celsus: They primarily treat the original symptoms. But after Celsus came Galen's revision: In a revised pharmacology of the inflammatory diseases, can we give first place to maintenance and restoration of function?

One of Celsus's contemporaries was Virgil (70-19 B. C.), the great poet of the Roman republic, who wrote in his discourse on husbandry: "felix, qui potuit rerum cognoscere causas" (Georgics, ii, 490) which can be translated as "it is a fortunate man who has been able to learn the causes of things." Perhaps we are not so fortunate today, knowing so little of the etiology of many inflammatory states. Eventually we may learn many, if not all, of the causes of arthritis. Meanwhile as we have seen in Section II, it is only for gouty arthritis that we have adequate remedies (because we know its cause). As emphasized throughout this chapter, the only certain cure for all other arthritides and inflammatory disorders is extirpation of the causative agent. Until we have the means to do so (i.e., curative agents), can we find any improvements upon our present palliative anti-inflammatory agents? Operationally, such an improved drug would have to afford either more long-range benefit to the patient than our most powerful palliative drugs (the corticosteroids) or less adverse side effects than present steroids.

The past 20 year's experience with corticosteroids has repeatedly disclosed that tissue destruction within a rheumatoid joint may proceed largely unchecked, as determined radiologically, even as the patient temporarily recovers joint mobility and the clinical signs abate. No matter how powerful the drug may be in disposing of the symptoms, if the patient (or test animal) ends up permanently crippled, this drug has failed. The steroids fail their ultimate test in the clinic when both the patient and the physician become disillusioned by the progressive loss of function accompanying steroid therapy. The current nonsteroid anti-inflammatory agents can be seen to be insufficient both in the clinic and in the rat adjuvant arthritis assay, for they only ameliorate the symptoms without altering the course of both the natural human and the experimental rat arthritides. Removing the drugs leads to a rapid exacerbation of symptoms, clearly indicating that the diseased state here was never "turned off," but only suppressed.

The nearest approximation to a chemical cure for the adjuvant arthritis and related, chronic, tissue-destroying inflammatory states (allergic thyroiditis, encephalomyelitis, etc.) is provided by the corticosteroids and immunosuppressive agents [115-119]. These drugs inhibit the onset, severity, and progression of these experimental diseases by primarily depressing the interaction of the etiological agent with the lymphoid tissues and with the exception of the steroids (and possibly, cyclophosphamide [117]) fail to control established disease. Though "failures" in this respect, the immunosuppressive drugs nonetheless command attention at the present time

I. DRUGS FOR CHRONIC INFLAMMATORY DISEASE

because some of them, if judicially used, may benefit certain patients with rheumatoid disease. There is hope that future research may improve their suitability as therapeutic agents in arthritis and auto-intolerant states in general. These drugs are therefore considered in further detail in Section V.

It is no accident that some of the greatest advances in therapeutics could only have been made by students of physiology. No mammoth sifting of plant and microbial products, the traditional el dorado of the drug hunter, could have led to the facile elimination of diabetes as a medical problem or given us some of the currently preferred drugs for treating the adrenogenital syndrome (prednisolone), thrombosis (Arvin, an enzyme from the venom of the Malayan pit viper), certain forms of cancer (L-asparaginase), and homograft rejection (antilymphocyte globulin). These therapeutic agents were developed only because physiologists had first unraveled some of the essential, normal feature of the homeostatic regulation of the blood glucose, cortisol production, blood clotting, tumor nutrition, and immune surveillance, respectively. With this lesson in mind, any dedicated soul interested in the development of new drugs for inflammatory diseases might make it his urgent business to learn all that he can of the subject of normal (vis a vis, abnormal) inflammation. This should no longer be regarded as the exclusive preserve of the experimental pathologist, who may in fact be studying the relatively unimportant aspects of inflammation; namely, how the signs are manifested and thereby disclosing only more loci of action of antisymptomatic drugs (for which there is no real need in the clinics). The mass of information in the accompanying Table VI should not be allowed to distract attention from the salient fact that the most important feature of normal inflammation is that it is regenerative, not destructive; self-regulating, not continual, or (to relapse into medical jargon) acute, not chronic. Some of the natural factors which might act as autoregulators are discussed elsewhere in this chapter (Section VI). For the present, let us ask some questions about these putative intangible factors which somehow "switch off," or otherwise limit, the ongoing inflammatory response: Can they be exploited as such in therapeutics? Even if the answer is "no," can they be imitated or their action reinforced with other types of chemical compounds which might then serve as "inflammalytic agents" and transform a chronic (intractable) inflammatory condition into a tractable one? Such agents need not necessarily be inflammalytic of themselves: They could be either small or large molecules able to bring about at least one of the following "events" in vivo:

i. induce, or boost, the biosynthesis of a natural inflammalytic agent; and/or

ii. potentiate its activity by displacing it from tissue stores (where it is inactive); and/or

iii. potentiate its activity by blocking its catabolism or excretion (so extending its useful half-life in vivo).

To aid further thought on this subject, it may be helpful to reflect how both synthetic chemicals and natural products can reinforce the natural defense mechanism combating viral infections, by boosting interferon production

TABLE VI

Outline Summary of the Pathophysiology of Inflammation

Sequelae to the inflammatory insult [a]	Source	Cause	Prevented by	Antagonized by
Liberation of:				
Amines (histamine, 5-HT)	Mast cells, platelets, basophilic LK	First injury Anaphylotoxins Platelet adhesion	Decarboxylase inhibitors [b] Inhibitors of mast cell metabolism	Antihistamines Antiserotonins
Kinins	Plasma kininogens	Activation of kininogen-ases	Aryl amidines antiproteases (anti-esterases) [c]	Natural kinin-ases Chymotrypsin Nonsteroid AID [d]
Other permeability-increasing factors	Cell lysosomes Vasculature Lymph nodes		Steroids?	
Complement activation: Anaphylotoxins Chemotaxins for LK Cell destruction	Plasma (intestine) (liver)	injury Ag/Ab complexes	Fumaropimaric acid Aryl amidines Prior depletion with acidic polysaccharides	

I. DRUGS FOR CHRONIC INFLAMMATORY DISEASE

Event	Location/Source	Mediator	Drug/Treatment
Infiltration of leukocytes:			
Polymorphs ... early	Marrow	Chemotaxins	
Monocytes (phagocytic cells) ... later		MIF	
Lymphocytes ... later	Lymph nodes	Normal Lc circulation	
	Marrow		
Increase in blood glycoproteins, fibrinogen, etc. ("acute phase reactants")	Liver Intestine?	Circulating enzymes	AID?
Release cathepic enzymes	Lysosomes of granular LK	Drop in pH	Steroids
			Other AID?
			6-aminohexoic acid gold?
			Chloroquine?
Stimulation lymphoid tissues:			
("activated") LK (Lc + macrophages)		Auto-Ag, ("non-self")	Immunosuppressive drugs
		Exogenous Ag	Anti-Lc-Ab steroids
antibody synthesis			Ag excess
			Ab excess
Complement fixation		Ag-Ab complex	
Proliferative response:			
Fibroblasts	Adjacent tissues	Loss of chalones	Chalones
Epithelial cells			Steroids
Lymphoid cells (see above)			Cytostatic drugs

[a] The abbreviations used are as follows: LK, leucocytes; AID, anti-inflammatory drugs; Ag, antigen; Ab, antibody; Lc, lymphocyte. MIF, (macrophage) migration inhibiting factor(s). The event are not necessarily in this chronological order of involvement.

[b] Acidic AID, steroids?, hydrazines, and oxyamines

[c] Certain bases (e.g., quinine), DFP

[d] In guinea pig lung preparations.

(see Chapter VI). Since the sequelae to an inflammatory stimulus are so numerous (see Table VI), there may well be several endogenous regulators of inflammation acting more or less independently. If so, this gives considerable scope for developing a possible range of exogenous inflammalytic agents or adjuncts for any, or all, of these endogenous regulators. A few synthetic drugs are known which behave as anti-inflammatory agents in intact animals but fail to do so in adrenalectomized or thymectomized animals. Do the adrenals and thymus then produce endogenous inflammalytic agents, only in suboptimal quantities, until further stimulated by one of the drugs in question?

Passing on, we must ask yet a few more questions. For what other reasons than lack of endogenous inflammalytic agents, might an inflammation fail to regress? If there are positive causes of chronicity, what might they be? The simplest is probably persistence of the initial inflammatory stimulus which somehow never becomes muted but instead might even become more inflammagenic. If this involved a persistent antigen, the immune response to it might continually amplify the consequent immunoinflammation. Another phenomenon amplifying the inflammatory response would be the substitution for the original inflammatory stimulus of others that it might engender. Even if the original initiating stimulus were eliminated, the inflammatory response to it would still be self-perpetuating if its products either accumulated continuously or were cycled (see Fig. 4) to effectively "scale up"/ "escalate" the degree of inflammation. Examples of such cycles (exhibiting positive feedback control), which might aggravate or reinforce an inflammatory state, are given below:

i. liberation of lysosomal or extracellular inflammagenic enzymes which then release inflammatory amines or kinins;

ii. liberation of other, histolytic enzymes which degraded the adjacent tissues releasing (i) immunological adjuvants, such as oligonucleotides, (ii) other molecules, sufficiently large to activate the Hageman factor (thereby initiating further kinin production), and (iii) other molecules now recognized as "non-self," to trigger off an immune response;

iii. stimulation, by the original inflammatory insult, of fibrinogen and kininogen synthesis (in the liver) or antibody production by lymphoid tissues so that fibrin-, kinin-, or antibody-mediated injury might be added to the original inflammation;

iv. complement activation to generate permeability factors, anaphylotoxins (releasing histamine), chemotaxins (concentrating inflammatory leukocytes), and cell lysins (releasing catabolic enzymes, new antigens, etc.), or perhaps alternatively, promoting the immune response by facilitating the entry of antigen into antibody-forming cells [120].

Any drug which could interrupt one of these positive feedback loops (see Fig. 4) would deserve intensive study as a potential anti-(chronic)-inflammatory agent. To distinguish this type of drug action from that of many

I. DRUGS FOR CHRONIC INFLAMMATORY DISEASE

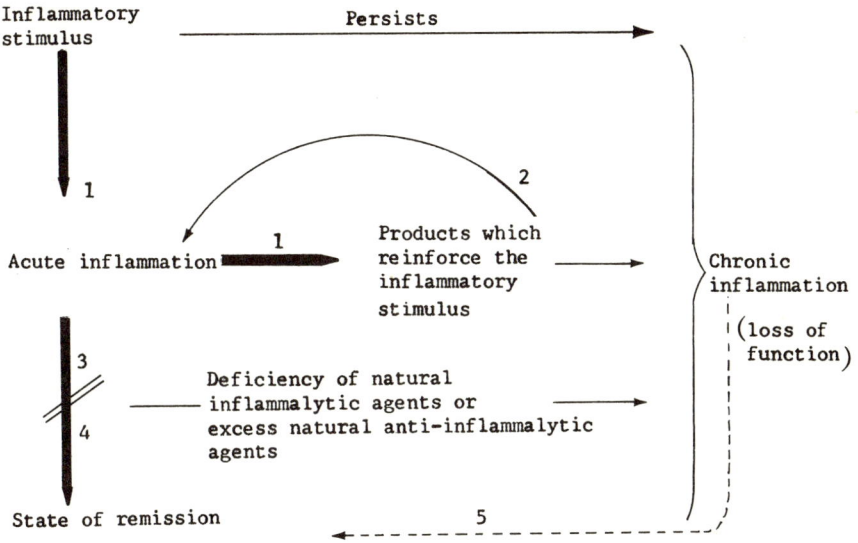

Fig. 4. Mechanisms sustaining chronic inflammation: (postulated) sites of action of drugs to moderate it. (1) "Conventional anti-inflammatory agents (those disclosed in acute assays, e.g., carrageenin-induced edema). (2) "Antireinforcement" drugs. (3) Exogenous inflammalytic agents. (4) Potentiators of endogenous inflammalytic agents. (5) A wonder drug!

conventional suppressive anti-(acute)-inflammatory agents (AAI) we should find a new description: Provisionally we suggest anti-(reinforcement) inflammatory (ARI). The original literature now contains many references to the possibility that some of the currently used antiarthritic drugs stabilize lysosomes (e.g., corticosteroids, chloroquine) or inhibit some of their contained enzymes (e.g., phenylbutazone, gold preparations), based upon their activities demonstrable in vitro. If further data could be accumulated to adequately demonstrate such activities in vivo, we might then understand why certain drugs which seem to act in the clinic, such as gold derivatives, immunosuppressors, and chloroquine, and here designated as ARI's, have not been hitherto classified as "genuine" anti-inflammatory agents since they fail to qualify in fact as AAI's (in pharmacological assays emphasizing the acute inflammatory response). Drugs behaving as both AAI's and ARI's such as the steroids and to a lesser degree, phenylbutazone, demonstrate rapid and powerful action in the clinic and in certain chronic inflammatory states in animals. (In assessing the potency of phenylbutazone in small animals and comparing it with that of the steroids, it must be remembered that the half-life of phenylbutazone in man is approximately 12 times that in the rat [121] while the half-life of prednisolone in man is not quite so different from that in the rat.)

To summarize this section: In therapy, a drug suppressing any of the molecular or cellular events leading to chronic inflammation (falling within goals 2 and 3) could be placed in at least one of the five categories, indicated under Fig. 4, if it does not eradicate the original inflammatory stimulus (goal 1). The fact that we have neither suitable reference (lead) compounds nor adequate in vivo pharmacological assays for compounds listed as acting at loci 2, 3, and 4 (perhaps we should include 5, also) should not be allowed to deter the requisite further thought and experimental endeavor being devoted to this all-important question: How to find new, clinically effective, antirheumatic/anti-inflammatory drugs that are really an advance upon those now available? Finally, knowing that considerable remodeling of the tissue architecture must take place at the seat of inflammation which (if ill-controlled) may impede or destroy the normal tissue function (e.g., granuloma formation, invasion of joint cartilage by overgrowing pannus, tissue erosion by histolytic enzymes), it may be necessary to treat not just the inflammatory state and its immediate sequelae as perceived by Celsus' four signs but also its ultimate consequences (goal 4) as described by Galen, loss of function. The drugs of choice for this purpose, perhaps inhibitors of growth or catabolism, may differ markedly from the ideal inhibitors of acute or chronic inflammation.

C. Some Targets for Drug Action: Mediators of Inflammation and Tissue Injury

This section will almost certainly be obsolete at the time of publication. Its purpose is merely to indicate some of the cellular and molecular events in a sustained inflammatory state that are poorly controlled by today's available drugs.

1. Microvascular Histamine Synthesis

In a series of papers published throughout the past decade, Schayer has presented considerable evidence that histamine may be an endogenous dilator of microvascular smooth muscle, being continuously generated in situ by an inducible histidine decarboxylase and subject to natural antagonism by glucocorticoids that reduce the dilator action of this "nascent" histamine [122]. This histidine decarboxylase is activated following a local or systemic stimulus, attains near maximal activity within 4 h; the rate of activation closely paralleling the rate of development of the second (or delayed) phase of an acute inflammatory response. Schayer has shown that the duration of this enzyme activation depends on the persistence of the stimulus: Thus in turpentine-injected rats paws, increased histidine decarboxylase activity was apparent even after 10 days, though it could not be determined whether or not this represented augmentation by enzyme(s) carried in by infiltrating leukocytes, etc. The only drugs known as yet to block the activation of this histidine decarboxylase are inhibitors of protein synthesis such as puromycin, cycloheximide, and tenuazonic acid [123]. When these particular drugs were tested against the turpentine-induced inflammation, they showed powerful anti-inflammatory activity — all the more remarkable as neither indomethacin nor cortisol have much effect on this particular type of inflammation. Though Reilly and Schayer [124] have indeed shown that other histidine decarboxylases (e.g., in the stomach, mast cell, liver, etc.) are readily inhibited in vivo by certain amines or hydrazines which effectively block these enzymes in vitro at micromolar concentrations, the basal (i.e., preinduction) level of the microvascular histidine decarboxylase seems to be resistant to these enzyme inhibitors. This may reflect the failure of these drugs to normally penetrate the vascular smooth muscle or endothelial cells, but it is not clear what changes may occur in the permeability of these cells to drugs as they become permeable to blood constituents in response to various dilators including histamine. The real questions here are: (i) whether or not histamine generation after an inflammatory response can be regulated by another class of drugs, other than the very toxic inhibitors of de novo protein synthesis; and (ii) are there other drugs beside glucocorticoids which may antagonize these dilator effects of histamine at lower, and more realistic, concentrations than those which must be used in order to antagonize this effect with conventional antihistamines?

These questions assume further significance with Schayer's identification of histamine as a probable growth factor for mouse lymphoid tissues and the activation of histidine decarboxylase in lymph nodes (but not thymus) following a variety of stresses [125]. Thus any effective antagonism of either the lymphoid (microvasculature?) decarboxylase or the suspected growth-promoting action of histamine would probably influence immunoinflammation, sustained by lymphoid activation, as well as the more acute inflammatory events primarily involving enhanced permeability of the microvascular bed. Histamine has also been implicated as a growth promoter of connective tissues [126] and it is rather interesting that serotonin has also been found to stimulate the growth of mouse and human fibroblasts in culture [127].

Theoretically both cortisol [128] and certain nonsteroid acidic anti-inflammatory drugs [129] might be capable of blocking certain histamine and serotonin receptors. Some ramifications of this hypothesis are examined in Section VII. F as possible leads for designing new drugs.

2. The Complement System

The 11 identified protein components of complement together constitute approximately 10% w/w of the human serum globulins. They are therefore continually available to all the body tissues and undoubtedly play an important role in the defense mechanisms of the body when directed against exogenous and injurious agents. When activated, some or all of these complement components may also cause extensive tissue injury in the host. Thus complement is a rather powerful but impartial instrument; an inflammatory mediator normally benefitting the host but on occasions also injuring him as well.

The recent tremendous advances in defining the biochemical and pathogenic activities [130] of the various individual complement components have already given some indications of (a) those steps in complement activation that may be regulated naturally, (b) other "pacemaker" events which can be inhibited by synthetic chemicals (possible prototypes of novel anticomplement drugs), and (c) where, along the sequence of events in complement activation, the agents are generated which initiate "immunological injury." The problem now is to find (i) those drugs which can selectively inhibit complement activation in vivo without systemic toxicity and (ii) other drugs which might antagonize the complement-derived pathogenic or inflammatory factors, once formed.

Mediators of complement-sustained injury include:

i. A C3-derived anaphylotoxin (C3a), a basic polypeptide with a molecular weight of approximately 7000, causing smooth muscle contraction and increased capillary permeability (both antagonized by antihistamines) and directed migration (chemotaxis) of polymorphonuclear leukocytes. The anaphylotoxic (histamine-liberating) and chemotactic activities evidently reside in different regions of the C3a molecule since trypsin rapidly destroys the anaphylotoxic, but not the chemotactic, activity.

ii. A C5-derived anaphylotoxin (C5a) with a molecular weight of about 10,000 (human origin) or 15,000 (guinea pig origin) and like C3a exhibiting both anaphylotoxic and chemotactic activities. Smooth muscle desensitized to C3a (by repeated application of C3a) will still respond to C5a and vice versa, suggesting that C3a and C5a react with different tissue receptors, are chemically distinct, and would probably require different drugs to antagonize their respective binding to histamine-releasing tissues. However both C3a and C5a are inactivated by the same thermolabile inhibitor, presumed to be an enzyme, in human serum [131].

iii. A (C4-derived?) "kinin," distinguished from other known kinins by its high molecular weight of the order of 15,000.

iv. Cytolysin composed of C5-9 activated by cell-bound antibodies which have successively bound C1, C4, C2, and C3.

v. Cytolysin(s) that are not dependent on cell-bound antibody for their formation. They too are activated by C1, C4, C2, and C3, combined in free solution or upon a cell surface.

vi. Target cell damage mediated by human monocytes that have bound and reacted with complement as far as C3 only. [The normal sequence of complement activation is surface bound (+ activated) C1a + C4 + C2a + C3 + (C5,6,7) + C8 + C9 where a (or $\overline{C}$) are activated components derived from corresponding inactive precursors (and subcomponents).]

vii. Target cell damage mediated by human lymphocytes that have bound complement components up to C7.

I. DRUGS FOR CHRONIC INFLAMMATORY DISEASE

viii. Platelet binding to a soluble (circulating) antigen-antibody complex that has fixed complement, then followed by lysis of the platelets releasing histamine, serotonin, and other vasoactive materials such as lysosomal enzymes, etc.

ix. Lysis of platelets, caused to adhere (but not lyse) by antigen-antibody complexes interacting with only the first four complement components, then subject to "injury" by neutrophilic leukocytes.

x. Platelet attachment to the complex formed by antibody bound to particle or membrane antigens and the first four complement components, releasing only histamine and serotonin without rupture of the platelets.

Complement activation is subject to rigid constraints in time and space. With the exception of C1, the individual components rapidly lose their capacity to bind to each other following appropriate (enzymic) activation, so restricting the membrane-damaging effect of complement to the immediate vicinity of the vascular site where C1 activation was triggered off. Natural regulators in serum include an inhibitor of the protease (esterase) activity of activated C1 and inactivators of natural C4 and active (cell-bound) C3 and C6.

The very first step in complement activation is usually through the association of a C1 subcomponent (C1q) with the heavy chain (Fc) portion of an IgG or IgM molecule contained in antigen-antibody complexes or γ-globulin aggregates. Minor chemical modifications of an IgG molecule, e.g., reaction of only one tryptophane residue with 2-hydroxy-5-nitrobenzyl bromide [132], may abolish its ability to bind C1q (and activate the whole complement sequence). Can this be emulated with more specific drugs than tryptophane-alkylating agents, such as perhaps a synthetic polypeptide reproducing part of the immunoglobulin-recognition sequence in C1q, or even with C1q fragments obtained by chemical or enzymatic degradation (but unable to combine with C1r and C1s to reconstitute $\overline{C1}$)? C1q has a rather unusual composition for a plasma protein, containing 19 glycine residues and 2 or 3 hydroxylysine residues per 100 aminoacid units, more reminiscent of a structural protein like collagen or enamel protein. It also contains a lot of carbohydrate (15 percent). Perhaps these relatively unique features might be exploited pharmacologically. Soluble collagen precursors will bind certain drugs like colchicine or vinca alkaloids [133]. Can such collagen-associating drugs be used to hinder the interaction between C1q and an immunoglobulin? Are there any carbohydrate-complexing reagents, like concanavalin A (a protein from jackbeans), which might bind selectively to C1q in vivo?

Other points of pharmacological attack are suggested by the presence of a key thiol group in C2 and a reactive disulfide group in C1; ready dissociation of the $\overline{C5,6,7}$ complex by 10 mM α-glutamyl-L-tyrosine; noncompetitive inhibition of $\overline{C1}$ with diisopropylfluorophosphate; and the inhibition of C1 binding (and therefore activation → $\overline{C1}$) by 6-aminohexoic (ϵ-aminocaproic) acid.

The disparity in quantities of the individual complement components present in serum might also perhaps be exploited. C8 and C9, both essential for cytolytic activity, are normally the least abundant (less than 10 μg/ml) and might be particularly amenable to neutralization in vivo by exogenous antibodies. [These particular antibodies might be expected to be least likely to trigger off complement-derived cytolysin production after combining with their appropriate antigens.] The individual components are also stated to be of disparate origin: Thus C1 is believed to be synthesized in the intestinal epithelium and both C3 and C4 are reported to come from macrophages. If this is wholly substantiated, then the individual components might be selectively regulated by somehow controlling their biosynthesis in the different organs.

Of the few effective complement inhibitors in vitro, the one most intensively studied, fumaropimaric acid, is too toxic to be of any value in vivo. Baker and his colleagues at Santa Barbara have explored using modified trypsin inhibitors as irreversible complement inhibitors [134-136] and some of these seem to be moderately effective in vivo at subtoxic doses [137]. Cobra venom has long been used as a complement inhibitor and, more recently, as a suppressor of the immune response in organ transplantation. If some means can be found to detoxify this venom, either by rigid purification of the anticomplement principle from all other toxic components or by simple chemical modification (attenuation) to eliminate its neurotoxicity, etc., such a "biological" preparation might offer some advantage over a purely synthetic drug — not only in potency but also by having a shorter half-life in vivo. It is instructive to consider how the cobra venom principle actually inhibits complement: Apparently it activates a natural (but latent) inactivator of C3 in serum, a β-globulin. Perhaps similar activators (enzymes?) are available from "nicer/cleaner" sources than a venom. If the C3-inactivator truly plays the role of an inflammalytic agent, then we have here a "blueprint," as it were, of how to boost a natural regulator of inflammation.

3. Proteolysis

Local proteolytic events may contribute to either the perpetuation or the resolution of inflammation. For this reason it is difficult to guess the outcome of any program to develop new antiproteolytic drugs as regards their potential therapeutic utility in inflammatory states. If such a drug were to prevent the destruction of adjacent tissue (histolysis), kinin generation or perhaps, fibrin deposition, it might be of real benefit. If however, it inhibited tissue débridement (essential for normal tissue repair), kinin destruction, and normal platelet aggregation, the injury might be exacerbated. We must remember the paradox that while exogenous proteases (e.g., from pancreas, streptococcus spp., plant juices, etc.) may act as anti-inflammatory agents, one of the body's (defensive?) responses to inflammation is increased hepatic synthesis of glycoproteins, some of which have antiprotease activity (see Section VI. G).

In a swollen knee joint, one can find extracellular proteases [138] which have originated from the plasma transudate, from infiltrating leukocytes

I. DRUGS FOR CHRONIC INFLAMMATORY DISEASE

(e.g., eosinophils bearing profibrinolysin, neutrophils containing cathepsins D and E) and from such other cell types as chondrocytes, synovial cells, etc. Immunoglobulins are rather resistant to digestion by these synovial fluid enzymes. By contrast, albumin is readily degraded and this may facilitate de novo protein synthesis and wound repair by delivering a pool of aminoacids and peptides. At the same time, any albumin-bound anti-inflammatory drugs (almost inactive while bound) would be "unloaded" in situ, thereby enhancing their potency, so that albuminolysis could locally liberate these active drugs. However albumin-bound urate might also be unloaded too as the albumin is degraded: This would certainly favor further urate deposition and probably augment the inflammation in a gouty joint.

This discussion will indicate that there can be no single, "blanket" approach to regulating local proteolytic activity. Where it may be advantageous to inhibit it in one disease state (osteoarthritis perhaps), it may be just the thing not to do in another (gout?). The same may be true of other histolytic enzymes, e.g., nucleases.

4. Contributions of Leukocytes

The leukocytes collectively constitute a most important motile "organ system," intimately involved with nearly all the phases of the inflammatory and immune response to both exogenous and endogenous irritants and antigens. It is rather arresting therefore to find that for this one system (and in contrast to the situation regarding most of the other vital systems of the body), the pharmacologist has no rational armamentarium of effective drugs to offer the clinician. It is true there is an ad hoc leukocyte pharmacology, partly sketched out in Table VII, but it is certainly an impoverished thing when compared to the corpus of knowledge constituting each of the "pharmacologies" we associate with the endocrine, gastrointestinal, cardiovascular, and central nervous systems, for example. Presently available drugs which qualify for consideration in any putative "leukocyte pharmacology" are more notable for their toxicity than their pharmacodynamic action and for their distinctly empirical (vis a vis, rational) use in treating diseases other than leukemia. Drugs primarily acting on platelets may provide the exception to this generalization as there is already an adequate experimental basis upon which to construct a rational platelet pharmacology [139].

In recent years there has been much interest in the biological role of lymphocytes in so-called "cellular immunity," involving delayed hypersensitivity, certain autointolerant states, and the rejection of homografts. Lymphocytes contributing to these phenomenon have been variously described as "sensitized," "activated," "primed," "pathogenic," "committed," etc. A population of sensitized lymphocytes may have special capabilities beyond just synthesizing antibodies, including production of various factors mediating cellular immunity, designated "lymphokines" [140]. The production of these is triggered when a sensitized cell comes into contact with the appropriate antigen or sensitizing agent (Fig. 5). These lymphokines include macrophage-inhibiting factors (MIF), cytotoxins, permeability enhancing

TABLE VII

Towards a "Leukocyte Pharmacology": Examples of Drug Action on Various Leukocytes[a]

Cell type	Relationship to inflammation	Some effective drugs	Drug action
Platelets (thrombocytes)	Source inflammagenic amines vascular injury	Acidic, nonsteroid AID 2-chloro-AMP	Inhibit aggregation
Granulocytes:			
Polymorphnuclear (neutrophils)	Source of histolytic and kinin-generating enzymes, cationic permeability factors, etc.	Colchicine	Depress metabolic activation by urate crystals
		Vinca alkaloids 6-Mercaptopurine Methotrexate	Delete from blood (poison marrow synthesis)
Eosinophils Basophils	Activate fibrinolysis Carry histamine	Corticosteroids	Delete from blood
Lymphocytes[b]			
in bone marrow	Recruited for reinforcing immune response and injury	Cyclophosphamide	(Relatively resistant to steroids); renders unadaptive
in lymphoid tissues (nodes, spleen, Peyer's patches)	Conscripted for cellular immunity and antibody synthesis	Corticosteroids	Nucleolysis (especially in thymus)
		Antilymphocyte globulin	Delete node and circulating cells
short-lived circulating long-lived circulating	Aggressor cells if stimulated? Carry immunological memory?	Corticosteroids ?	Lymphopenic response Relatively resistant to steroids

I. DRUGS FOR CHRONIC INFLAMMATORY DISEASE

Monocytes (large mononuclear, phagocytic cells)	Abundant at site of inflammation	6-Mercaptopurine — Delay infiltration Inhibit proliferation of precursor cells?
Macrophages	Accumulate in granulomatous response "Processing" particulate antigens	Corticosteroids — Depress cell migration? Estrogens — Increase number of macrophages in spleen

[a] Excluding drugs causing idiosyncrasies, e.g., severe marrow depression (agranulocytosis, etc.) in only a small percentage of the total population. AID stands for anti-inflammatory drugs.

[b] Nonphagocytic, mononuclear cells with small cytoplasm.

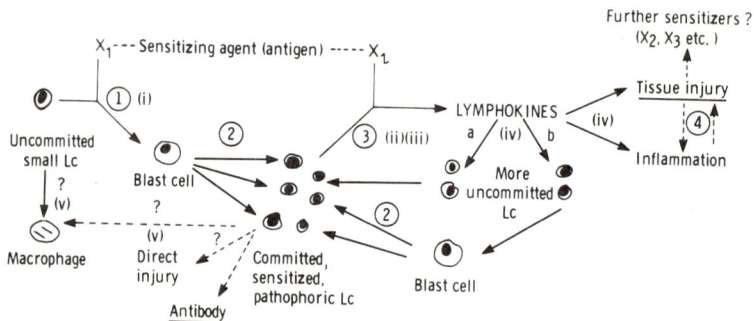

Fig. 5. Involvement of lymphocytes (Lc) in tissue injury: Some sites of action of present (1-4) and needed (i-iv) drugs. Key: a - transfer factor, b - mitogenic factor.
1. Immunosuppressor - harsh sensitization-inhibitor,
2. Immunosuppressor - cytostatic agent,
3. Anti-lymphocyte globulin (also at 1?),
4. Anti-inflammatory agent,
i. 'Soft' sensitization-inhibitor,
ii. Inhibitor of Lc + X interaction - "desensitizer,"
iii. Lymphokine-antagonist — inhibitor of their synthesis,
iv. Lymphokine-antagonist — inhibitor of their action,
v. Inhibitors of intercellular transformation.

(inflammagenic) factor(s), mitogens for other lymphocytes, "interferons," "transfer factor(s)," etc. [141].

There is good evidence that the rat adjuvant-induced arthritis, allergic encephalomyelitis, and thyroiditis are mediated by a population of "pathophoric" lymphocytes [90] which can passively transfer these diseases to other inbred animals at the appropriate time (8-11 days after initiating disease in the donor animals). Antilymphocyte globulins and many immunosuppressive drugs, which effectively inhibit lymphocyte "activation," will arrest the development of these three experimental autoallergic inflammatory diseases (see Section V); providing pharmacological evidence for a key role of the lymphocytes in initiating and/or sustaining these disease states. What is badly needed now is an answer to the question: Is it possible to use less drastic drugs than the conventional immunosuppressors to control these autoallergic diseases in rats and related sustained inflammatory states in man? Present therapy in this regard is rather like using a sledgehammer or piledriver to crack open a walnut. Can we hope to find less "crushing" drugs (more akin to a conventional nutcracker) for regulating pathophoric lymphocytes? Much more consideration should be given to trying to find (i) "softer" and safer sensitization inhibitors, to prevent lymphocyte activation in the first place, and (ii) lymphokine antagonists to block the effects of these (re)active principles on their respective target cells.

I. DRUGS FOR CHRONIC INFLAMMATORY DISEASE

Drugs of the first category (inhibiting sensitization) are considered in the subsequent section (V), devoted to immunosuppressive agents. A drug within the second category ("lymphokine antagonist") would theoretically be much more suitable, probably less toxic, and certainly much more specific for dealing with an ongoing disease in which a certain proportion of the lymphycyte population has already been sensitized, "programmed" (as it were) for tissue injury, and become pathogenic. Is it feasible to "desensitize" a committed cell before it begins to make lymphokines? This would necessitate either "gagging" or "anesthetizing" the cell so that it could not combine with, or otherwise recognize, its trigger antigen or whatever-it-may-be that it is especially sensitive to. This may be just what an antilymphocyte globulin does anyway, but are there any foreseeable alternatives to using an antibody for this purpose?

These questions are not just rhetorical: There is so much current research activity devoted to elucidating the chemical nature of (a) the lymphokines and (b) antigen recognition, that it will surely not be very long before pharmacologists could attempt to design potential inhibitors based on the (then) known chemistry of the active, or recognition, sites, respectively. It should prove to be a very exciting phase of drug development and may help to establish leukocyte pharmacology once and for all on a genuinely rational basis.

Macrophages may also be sensitized to manufacture or release pyrogens, interferon, cytotoxins, and other injurious agents. There may indeed be a considerable overlap between drugs, designed to curb sensitized lymphocytes and other drugs to curb those activities of macrophages which promote and sustain injury to the host. Since macrophages may perhaps develop from cells very closely resembling "lymphocytes," any drugs that might arrest this intercellular transformation would certainly be of the greatest interest, as tools of research, if not perhaps in the clinic. Again, perhaps this is another activity of antilymphocyte globulin _in vivo._

We have tried to outline the rational development of a new lymphocyte and macrophage pharmacology by pointing to where we have no adequate drugs to regulate some, or all, of the potentially injurious activities of these cells. The same intense scrutiny should be applied to the activities of other leukocytes, whose role in inflammation and immunity is more fully discussed elsewhere [17, 20, 142].

Before we leave this topic of leukocyte pharmacology, we should briefly consider how these various projected (and conjectured) new drugs might be discovered. Discounting serendipity for the moment, it will almost certainly require intensive screening of various chemicals (at first rather chosen at random) for ability to regulate these various activities of leukocytes insofar as they can be studied _in vitro_. This will probably necessitate intensively culturing cells _in vitro_ after they have been withdrawn from the animal, preferably at various intervals after suitably activating them _in vivo_, thereby avoiding one possible pitfall of studying spurious responses (e.g., false activation) that may be obtained only _in vitro_. Drugs of interest _in vitro_ would then have to be studied carefully in vivo and most would be found wanting. This tedious approach, which we sincerely hope might be circumvented, does at least indicate just where a new drug might be acting ab initio, which is about the chief merit of any in vitro screening program.

5. Contributions of Synovial Cells

The synovium which lines the joint cavity and acts as the bridge between the blood and the joint (synovial) fluid is nevertheless a specialized organ. It actively secretes the hyaluronate-protein complex responsible for the characteristic lubricant property of the synovial fluid. In a similar manner, the ciliary body of the eye is a bridge between the blood and both the aqueous and vitreous humors. Both the synovium and the ciliary body are frequently inflamed in some chronic inflammatory conditions such as Reiter's disease, ulcerative colitis, and ankylosing spondylitis.

The normal synovium is composed of at least two types of cells (A, B) lining the synovial cavity: The A cell corresponds to a resident macrophage and the B cell is a secretory fibroblast. Behind this lining there are supporting structures (other fibroblasts, extracellular fibers) and vascular endothelium. In inflammation, various leukocytes accumulate within the synovial tissue and may synthesize antibodies and lymphokines, found in the synovial fluids of inflamed joints.

Certain activities of this multicellular organ have been studied in in vitro cultures of "synovial cells," the viable cellular residue rather resembling fibroblasts in their morphology obtained from minced synovium.

Synovial cells taken from inflamed synovial tissue of patients with rheumatoid arthritis show persistent differences from synovial cells taken from normal subjects [143], notably in their response to hydrocortisone [144] and in resisting viral infection [145] — suggesting the presence of resident viruses in the rheumatoid-derived cells. Cultured rheumatoid cells have been found to secrete a collagenase which is not inhibited by the normal enzyme inhibitors present in serum and synovial fluid [146]. Collectively, such observations suggest that a synovial cell may be transformed, may now generate harmful products (enzymes), or may escape normal regulation. Can these aberrant activities be suppressed or normalized with exogenous agents which do not directly affect the other elements of inflammation?

This brief discussion should make it clear that the study of drug action on both normal and rheumatoid synovial cell cultures may be very rewarding.

6. Contributions of Endothelial Cells

The endothelial cells, which form the inner surface of all blood vessels and are the sole component of the capillaries, are seldom considered in discussions of inflammation. Yet, three of the cardinal signs of inflammation (rubor, calor, and tumor) are direct manifestations of changes in the small blood vessel. Vasculitis is recognized frequently in chronic inflammatory conditions. Furthermore, all of the noncellular elements (antibodies, complement, fibrinogen, etc.) and most of the cellular components (leukocytes,

I. DRUGS FOR CHRONIC INFLAMMATORY DISEASE 75

platelets, etc.) of inflammation are actively mobilized at the inflammatory site only after they have passed through, or between, endothelial cells. When we speak of "increased capillary permeability" we are really referring to increased endothelial cell permeability. Platelet adherence to, and polymorph margination upon, the walls of small vessels in an area of inflammation may well be precipitated by changes in the endothelial cells. There appears to be some specialization of endothelial cells by function. For example, the (kidney) glomerulus is merely a collection of specialized endothelial cells which are exceptionally permeable to a plasma transudate (the glomerular filtrate), and the postcapillary venules of lymphoid tissues are lined by a particular type of endothelial cell through which blood-borne lymphocytes readily migrate. Inflammation due to antigen-antibody complexes is frequently localized in the subendothelial basement membrane and may be observed as "lumpy-bumpy" or "linear" deposits with fluorescent immunohistological studies [147]. In the early phases of experimentally induced serum sickness, marked endothelial proliferation and thickening has been noted in the aorta of rabbits. Finally, the formation of new capillaries by endothelial budding from existing vessels is a vital part of healing and restoration of function.

Therapeutic thought has been directed primarily at the mediators (histamine, kinin, serotonin) of the vascular changes in acute inflammation rather than at the targets of these mediators, the endothelial cells themselves. A comprehensive cellular pharmacology should not neglect these particularly vital cells, even though we know so little of the mechanisms by which they regulate the interchange of solutes and hematogenous cells between the extracellular fluid and the bloodstream. Are there special drugs which can selectively desensitize their response to preformed inflammatory agents? Is this a key function of present day anti-inflammatory drugs?

D. More Targets for Drug Action: Mediators of Restitution and Tissue Repair

While the organism is alive and vital, the restitutive response is almost immediately set in motion by the inflammatory response: Indeed this is probably the prime purpose of inflammation. Just as cities are rebuilt by new buildings rising from the wastelands created by the demolition crews and just as a retreat may necessarily precede an advance, so the site-clearing tissue destruction, accompanying inflammation, may be essential for laying down healthy new tissue to replace the old, injured area. It might be just as wise to consider boosting some of these restitutive and reparative mechanisms as it is to halt the various factors constituting the biological "demolition crew." A side issue here is the possible need to curb an overenthusiastic reparative response leading to the synthesis of malstructured, poorly functional, repair tissue such as a grossly acellular, collagen-filled scar replacing highly cellular areolar and epithelial tissue.

Paradoxically, it may be necessary to boost the tissue injury in order to raise the reparative response to a new, exalted, level. Weissman and Hirschorn [148] have indicated how the release of catheptic enzymes from lysosomes might degrade nuclear histones, thereby derepressing the synthesis of new DNA and initiating cell division. Other mitogenic stimuli may include histamine [126], bradykinin [149], and nucleotides; the latter serving as (immunological) adjuvants to boost lymphoproliferative responses. These of course are all products of tissue inflammation, breakdown, or injury. Exogenous proteases may facilitate the resolution of inflammation: Do they achieve this by yet other means than a general ground-clearing operation (débridement) or boosting the adaptive synthesis of antiprotease globulins (to neutralize overactive tissue or leukocytic proteases)?

We would like to see more attention being given to the search for what we can only call restorative agents; agents to selectively "pep-up" the anabolic or defensive activities of a tissue under onslaught, however caused. Nature has probably provided further regulators for this purpose which the drug designer might well imitate (see Section VI) and supply exogenously when the natural supply shows signs of being insufficient. (This would certainly seem to be a kinder approach than inflicting further injury to boost the deficient supply.)

Restoration of the status quo would of course be tremendously facilitated by eradication of the injurious, etiological agent. Again, paradoxically, catabolism may have to precede anabolism. Are there means to boost the manufacture of opsonins, the phagocytic activities of macrophages, and other mechanisms for disposing of the biological "garbage" like inflammagenic antigen-antibody complexes? Instead of trying to poison the lysosomal enzymes with various drugs (e.g., gold preparations), perhaps they should be activated a little more to assist with the "garbage disposal." If there are no other means to dispose of the etiological agent than by a heightened immune response to it, are there safe means to boost antibody production (perhaps with a toxoid) and lymphocyte emperipolesis (to encounter and recognize intracellular crypto-antigens)?

We just do not seem to have at the present time much in the way of eradicative agents other than endocrine replacements, nutrients (where deficient, e.g., L-dopa for Parkinson's disease), antibiotics, and antiparasitic drugs; surely a rather serious shortcoming of contemporary pharmacology. One approach to cancer therapy is to boost the natural defense mechanisms, particularly the immunological component. As discussed elsewhere in this book, one approach to antiviral therapy is to boost another defense mechanism, interferon production. These are both eradicative measures, the agents promoting them being forerunners perhaps of a new family of eradicative drugs. In essence, these would instruct the body's defenses (actually the offensive arm) to perform rather more actively: The leverage they might exert could be tremendous.

There is some presumptive evidence for an intracellular microorganism being present in rheumatoid synovial cells, (see Section IV.C.5). Several investigators [72, 73, 150] have recently recently reported the presence of

I. DRUGS FOR CHRONIC INFLAMMATORY DISEASE

virus-like endothelial cytoplasmic inclusions in patients with S. L. E., dermatomyositis, and idiopathic thrombocytopenic purpura, suggesting that additional investigation of a possible viral etiology for collagen diseases is warranted.

Thus if some of the chronic inflammatory diseases are really caused by self-replicating agents, their chronicity may be due to the host's inability to recognize these agents as foreign [151-153]. As a (non)consequence, the host fails to activate his normal immunological and inflammatory defense mechanisms against this causative agent. Perhaps these "infections" are acquired in utero or even transmitted with the genetic material and therefore tolerated because they antedate the fetal development of the system for immune recognition, or perhaps they are merely very successful parasites which have evolved in such a way that they generally elude detection and rejection by the host. In any event, in certain individuals (who develop chronic inflammatory disease), the unrecognized parasite may alter normal proteins, etc., produce tissue injury, kill cells, or in some other way initiate an immunological reaction against the altered normal inflammatory response to tissue injury. Because the host is unable to recognize and eliminate the parasite, the defensive immunological and inflammatory processes are sustained and become destructive in themselves. Therapy directed against these processes may produce symptomatic improvement while it is administered, but does not and cannot be expected to eliminate the disease. However, the frequent occurrence of remissions and occasional spontaneous "cures" of chronic inflammatory diseases, coupled with the apparent lack of susceptibility of large segments of the population, suggest that there is some effective natural means of dealing with such parasites. A useful pharmacological approach to this problem might be to enhance the host's ability to recognize the parasite as being truly "foreign" so that it could be eliminated in the usual way. This might be done by chemically altering some component of the parasite or, perhaps more realistically, by immunization with a similar (but recognizably foreign) antigen, causing the production of cross-reacting antibodies.

Again we come up against the fundamental problem: What types of assays would be most suitable for detecting restorative and eradicative agents with which to treat chronic tissue injury? We honestly do not know, but unless sought for, they certainly won't be found.

V. IMMUNOSUPPRESSION WITH DRUGS

There are a number of excellent general surveys of the immune response and its suppression [154-157]. In this section we will focus attention not so much on the present day drugs themselves but primarily upon some of the principles which must be considered in the development of any new immunosuppressors.

A. General Strategy and Preamble

Although immunoglobulins have a rather distinctive molecular architecture which sets them apart from most other globular proteins, their synthesis follows the same general pattern as that of other proteins. Consequently attempts to suppress protein synthesis as such in antibody-forming cells by antibiotics (e.g., puromycin, cycloheximide) or amino acid antagonists (e.g., 4-fluorophenylalanine) can hardly be expected to specifically affect only immunoglobulin synthesis in vivo. However on exposure to antigen, antigen-sensitive cells in the lymphoid tissues are stimulated to proliferate after a suitable induction period and then to differentiate, yielding eventually either a population of antibody-producing cells (plasma cells or circulating lymphocytes) or "sensitized" lymphocytes, either of which may contribute factors initiating and sustaining the removal of, or attack on, the original antigen. At this time of induction and subsequent early proliferation, these antigen-sensitive cells are very sensitive targets for drugs which block DNA synthesis if these are administered at the time of, or within 48 h after, exposure to antigen. These agents would be expected to preferentially block only that small fraction of the total lymphoid cell population stimulated to divide by a given antigen and to spare all other antigen-sensitive cells not undergoing concurrent stimulation. Since certain powerful antigens may induce some production of antibody without cell division, this strategy of controlling cellular proliferation, does not block the immune response entirely. The ideal immunosuppressant would be one that could delete the response to a single antigen, or complex of antigens, without affecting any other immunological responses. At the time of writing, we are aware of only one such ideal, specific immunosuppressant: This is anti-Rh antiserum, used to prevent erythroblastosis fetalis (fatalis too!).

It is really beyond the scope of this chapter to discuss in any detail other modes of suppressing the immune response that do not employ conventional drugs as such. These include irradiation, early thymic ablation, passive transfer of antibodies which either react with potentially all the circulating lymphocytes (antilymphocyte globulin) [158, 159] or only with a unique antigen (and presumably compete with the corresponding antigen-sensitive cell for the antigen in question), administration of chemical carcinogens [160] or oncogenic viruses [161], and induction of immunological paralysis by massive infusion of antigen. The use of antibodies to suppress the immune response will be referred to in another section (VI. C). In general, drugs are superior to irradiation in that they primarily affect the reproducing cell population whereas radiation destroys lymphocytes and causes reproductive lesions regardless of whether the cells are proliferating or not. Even cells that are not multiplying at the time of irradiation tend to "store" the lesions and exhibit the radiation injury when they attempt to divide. As a consequence, radiation-induced immunosuppression is rather persistent and certainly unselective.

I. DRUGS FOR CHRONIC INFLAMMATORY DISEASE

B. The Present Situation

Most of the drugs currently available that we can describe as immunosuppressors were originally developed for use in cancer chemotherapy. A partial listing of them is given in Table VIII. The European description of these drugs as "cytostatica," rather than cytotoxic agents, serves to emphasize that their prime action is to minimize cellular proliferation rather than to poison the established cell population. However the immune response involves many more events than just the proliferation of certain lymphoid cells. A purely antiproliferative drug would not be a very suitable agent to regulate, for example, the recognition and "processing" of an antigen which must precede the stimulus to proliferate. Likewise the same antiproliferative drug would be of restricted value in regulating those events in the immune response which only take place after lymphoid cells have proliferated and/or

TABLE VIII

Some Antitumor and Immunosuppressive Drugs [165]

Type of drug	Cellular adaptation leading to resistance [a]
Alkylating agents	Reduced drug uptake Increased drug destruction Change in intracellular thiols (one drug target) Increased repair potential
Folate analogs	Increased activity of dihydrofolate reductase Reduced drug uptake or access
Purine analogs	Loss of anabolic enzymes (which activate the drug) Reduced drug access
Pyrimidine analogs	Loss of anabolic enzymes Changes in structure of the drug-sensitive enzyme
Actinomycin D	Drug loses its ability to penetrate the nuclear membrane
Mitomycin C	Increased drug breakdown
L-Asparaginase	Increased levels of asparagine synthetase

[a] Though the mechanism of resistance to all these drugs was established using tumor cells that were originally drug-sensitive, all these drugs are also immunosuppressive and in long-term use would probably elicit similar resistance in drug-sensitive lymphoid cells.

differentiated, e.g., antibody synthesis, complement fixation, production of cytotoxins by activated lymphocytes, etc.

Certain antimetabolites such as the 6-thiopurines apparently seem to act as immunosuppressors by interfering with the process of "antigen-priming" or induction of the immune response, rather than by acting as antimitotic agents to prevent cellular proliferation. Accordingly the effect of these drugs is exceptionally time-dependent when a single antigenic insult is administered. The immunodepressive effect of certain chemical carcinogens (e.g., 3-methylcholanthrene) is likewise very time-dependent, usually being manifested only when the carcinogens are administered before the antigen.

The fact that certain cytostatic agents do sometimes also affect nonproliferative events in the immune response serves to remind us again of the truth of the fact that there are indeed very, very few, purely monovalent drugs, i.e., with a single, unique site of action. Even a supposedly monovalent cytostatic drug like amethopterin (Methotrexate R), designed to block the enzymic resynthesis of tetrahydrofolate from dihydrofolate (and hence thymine and DNA synthesis), may apparently affect other cellular events in an immunologically stimulated lymph node, such as protein and RNA synthesis and the activity of other enzymes besides dihydrofolate reductase [162]. The converse is certainly true, namely that drugs with polyvalent action affecting many enzyme systems will also, at high enough concentrations, inhibit cellular proliferation. Thus many acidic anti-inflammatory drugs with no significant potential as antitumor agents nonetheless inhibit growth of microorganisms or ascites tumor cells [163] and the synthesis of nucleic acids in cultured mammalian cells [164] at levels not far removed from those attainable in plasma after chronic dosage in man or laboratory animals.

There are at least four contraindications to using the immunosuppressors, as we know them today, in clinical situations where there is no threat to normal life processes, because of:

i. their toxicity to other cells which are being continually replaced, especially those with proliferation rates comparable to that of a stimulated lymphoid cell population. The gastrointestinal mucosa and bone marrow are therefore particularly susceptible to cytostatic agents.

ii. their very effectiveness in "disarming" the immune response may permit the resurgence of a latent infection (e.g., tuberculosis, often reactivated by corticosteroid therapy) and lower resistance to further infection.

iii. their potential oncogenic effect. Unless the incipient tumor is also sensitive to the cytostatic drug used to obtain immunosuppression, it may no longer be held in check. This is a particularly serious problem in using antilymphocyte globulins which only affect the proliferation or activation of lymphocytes and cannot control the growth of nonlymphoid tumors.

I. DRUGS FOR CHRONIC INFLAMMATORY DISEASE

iv. the development of drug resistance by animal cells to many of the most powerful cytostatic agents (see Table VIII), necessitating the use of two or more of these drugs in combination or in succession.

In addition, almost all cytostatic drugs have further, equally undesirable, side effects — some of which carry further risks to the patient's well-being. For example, cyclophosphamide which has been intensively studied in many patients with otherwise intractable rheumatoid disease, frequently causes cystitis with its attendant risk of chronic hemorrhage from the bladder mucosa. At present the high price which must be paid, in terms of these unfortunate and often severe side effects, really only justifies the systemic use of the currently available cytostatic agents when there is no other way to help the patient in a life-threatening situation, e.g., glomerulonephritis of systemic lupus disease.

However before we relegate this class of drugs to the category of "impossible/untameable," let us consider some of their real merits, when compared to the other drugs now available to treat arthritis and auto-allergic states, and see whether or not some of these excellent qualities might be put to good use in designing new drugs, or new formulations of old drugs, for future use.

C. Valuable Properties of Some Current Immunosuppressive Drugs

For convenience we will discuss these under a number of separate categories which do not all necessarily apply to one given drug.

1. Fundamental Action

In general, these drugs act at a rather more fundamental stage than the conventional anti-inflammatory drugs and can often literally suppress inflammation prior to activation of its cascade-like mechanisms. This is certainly more positive than merely suppressing the symptoms of inflammation, without affecting either its course or development. (Unfortunately, both steroids and nonsteroidal anti-inflammatory agents primarily relieve the symptoms only.) When administered over a suitable, restricted time interval, most of the immunosuppressive drugs including antilymphocyte globulins, will prevent the induction of adjuvant-induced (poly) arthritis in rats and experimental auto-allergic states (like thyroiditis and encephalomyelitis) in a number of small animal species. By contrast, conventional anti-inflammatory drugs must be given continuously to suppress the adjuvant arthritis and do not prevent the development of these (experimental) auto-allergic diseases. However, although these diseases in experimental animal models (produced by a single, discrete, and known insult) are undoubtedly prevented by properly timed cytostatic therapy, we should be very careful about concluding that a similar type of therapy can be applied to human diseases in which the etiological insult is yet unknown, may be acting continuously, and certainly precedes any opportunity to treat it.

2. Reversibility of Action (Toxicity)

Where the immunosuppressor is an antimetabolite, being an analog of a purine, pyrimidine, amono acid, or enzyme, it is perfectly feasible to counteract much of the drug's activity by subsequently administering the "normal" metabolite, i.e., the compound whose metabolism is being antagonized by the drug in question. In this fashion, the duration of drug action can be limited, as first the drug and then its antagonist are given to the patient at suitable time intervals. This approach has been particularly successful in treating childhood leukemia and applied to inhibition of the immune response [166, 167] using relatively high and rather toxic doses of methotrexate followed by a salvage dose of the natural metabolite, folinic acid (5N-formyltetrahydrofolic acid). In principle this approach of "overdosage" and then "rescue" should be applicable to other antimetabolites and has been explored in at least one other instance with "cycloleucine" (1-aminocyclopentane-1-carboxylic acid) as the drug and L-valine as its antagonist [168]. Cycloleucine itself will inhibit both the adjuvant arthritis in rats and the allergic encephalomyelitis, though it is rather toxic, causing considerable weight loss.

3. Potency

Since these drugs can often be given at intervals for a short period only and still be effective, many of the more chronic side effects associated with the anti-inflammatory drugs can be avoided, e.g., gastric ulceration, development of an allergy to the drug. To suppress the adjuvant arthritis in rats, immunosuppressors need be given in doses of the order 0.1-5 mg/kg/day and then for only a few days. By contrast, with the exception of indomethacin and certain derivatives of hydrocortisone, the anti-inflammatory drugs must usually be given to rats in doses of the order 20-100 mg/kg/day for at least 15 days to bring about the same degree of inhibition of the arthritic symptoms. Particularly noteworthy is the fact that on withdrawing the anti-inflammatory drugs, the disease progresses with flare-up of symptoms. This occurs also when the steroids or indomethacin are withdrawn. (However, for human applications, potency is a minor consideration; the degree of efficacy at subtoxic doses is the crucial factor.)

4. Capacity to Induce Immunological Tolerance

One method of eliciting a state of tolerance to a given antigen in an adult animal is simply to administer it in such massive amounts that it overwheims the responsive mechanisms. Unfortunately it does not seem practicable for clinical use to induce tolerance through this principle of immunological exhaustion. The problem probably is not the induction of tolerance; this is routinely done by allergists when they "desensitize" an individual who is allergic to a known antigen, e.g., ragweed pollen, horse serum, penicillin, etc. The limiting factor in inflammatory disease is identification and isolation of the antigen(s) involved. A subtler, and clinically more feasible way to induce tolerance is to use only moderate amounts of antigen in combination with an immunosuppressive drug. A toxic dose of an irreversible immunosuppressor, such as an alkylating agent, given at this time will then selectively delete primarily those cells (within the whole lymphoid population constituting the immunological memory or capabilities of an animal) which respond to this one antigen. The hope is that cells sensitive to other antigens will not be affected to anything like the same extent as they should be receiving a much smaller stimulus from their appropriate antigens (from invading microorganisms, tumors, etc.) at the time of tolerance induction. There is no doubt this combination of faith and theory sometimes works, that tolerance is induced for a limited period at least, and that the immunosuppressive drug is a key feature of the whole operation.

5. Potential Antiviral Activity

Inhibition of nucleic acid synthesis by cytostatic drugs may suppress the replication of DNA or RNA viruses to a greater degree than it suppresses host nucleic acid synthesis. Viral replication may be more susceptible to suppression at certain stages of its life cycle. If this were true and if some of the inflammatory diseases in fact are mediated by viral agents, then it is possible that we might stumble upon a truly curative agent among the antimetabolites. The report of prolonged complete remissions of rheumatoid arthritis occurring after 6 to 18 months of cyclophosphamide therapy [169] encourages further cautious speculation in this direction.

6. "Steroid-Sparing" Action

With their rather more specific site of action, immunosuppressive drugs have a somewhat narrower spectrum of toxicity than the broadly acting corticosteroids. Many clinical studies have now demonstrated that giving an immunosuppressor, e.g., chlorambucil, aminopterin, cyclophosphamide in very judicious doses to steroid-dependent patients will often permit quite a considerable reduction in the daily dose of steroids (sometimes by as much as 70 percent) required to maintain the patient in a given state of freedom from arthritic disability, further renal damage in lupoid disease, etc. Thus it is possible by replacing part of the steroid requirement with an immunosuppressor to avoid some of the side effects of chronic steroid therapy (osteoporosis, diabetes, psychosis, Cushing's syndrome, etc.). However, it must be noted that the combination of immunosuppressors with corticosteroid therapy may introduce other problems of drug toxicity due to both the potency and broad spectrum of activity, and the fact that the one drug may greatly enhance the toxicity of the other.

D. Adaptation for Further Clinical Use

The use of more powerful doses of these drugs over very limited periods of time (reinforced with use of an appropriate drug antagonist such as the normal metabolite, when available) is an active area of drug development at the present time. This is partly stimulated by the realization that it will be particularly difficult to introduce into the clinic many new cytostatic agents while the very many stringent demands of governmental regulatory agencies such as the U.S. Food and Drug Administration continue to prevail. The virtual impossibility of finding a powerful cytostatic agent without significant side effects (e.g., hair loss) and without long-term toxicity make the chances of a new cytostatic agent coming into the American clinics, for other than very restricted use (e.g., in leukemia), very slight indeed. It therefore becomes very expedient to find better ways to use those drugs already permitted in the clinic.

If it were possible to extract from a patient's own tissue some local antigen to which he was especially sensitive, then this state of autosensitivity might be treated by attempting to make the patient tolerant to this one antigen. The key to this approach is of course to find the antigen in question, whether it be a locally restricted microorganism or a true autoantigen that is no longer recognized as "self" by the patient's own lymphocytes as they conduct their immunological surveillance for an incipient tumor or invading microorganisms. There are techniques for screening a tissue extract for a potential crypto-antigen by incubating the tissue preparations in vitro with a population of lymphocytes which may be already sensitized to this one antigen. Following antigen recognition by these cells, they would transform and either form blast cells or produce any one of several identifiable factors not produced by unstimulated cells, such as the macrophage inhibition factor, cytotoxins, etc. A response by the patient's own blood lymphocytes, not given by a normal (nonrheumatoid) subject's lymphocytes, to an extract of the rheumatoid patient's synovial tissue would be strong presumptive evidence that the patient's lymphocytes were hypersensitive to a particular synovial antigen. With some purification, this putative antigen might then be used, in conjunction with a brief but intense period of immunosuppressive therapy, to induce tolerance.

If the cells which uniquely responded to this putative antigen were also chiefly present in the inflamed arthritic joint, constituting as it were an "extra-nodal lymph node," then there is much to be said for administering just the immunosuppressor alone into the joint because the antigen would already be there in abundance "doing its thing" and "turning on" the appropriately sensitized cells. Indeed, intrasynovial cytolytic therapy might liberate a relatively large quantity of the presently unidentified antigen responsible for the disease, and, if combined with a properly timed "pulse" of systemic immunosuppressor, might induce tolerance similar to that produced in experimental animals by properly timed administration of an antigen (to activate a particular clone of lymphocytes) and a cytostatic drug (to delete that clone of specifically activated cells). One added benefit from directly administering the immunosuppressor intra-articularly would be that the proliferation of the synovial tissue which is one of the responses to the local injury, regardless of whether or not it were sustained immunologically, would also be suppressed.

The real problem here is to find drugs which are not too painful when injected into the joint, which are not too rapidly resorbed therefrom with risk of systemic toxicity, and which do not, of themselves, trigger off any further joint injury (as the steroids may when injected as microcrystals,

I. DRUGS FOR CHRONIC INFLAMMATORY DISEASE

intra-articularly). Some notable preliminary reports have originated from Europe describing the intra-articular use of chloroquine (which binds to DNA), metal derivatives, and a podophyllotoxin derivative, Proresid^R (presumably with antimitotic activity) [170]. If rather more emphasis were given in the appropriate research laboratories to administering some of the compounds under investigation by intra-articular injections into larger animals like the rabbit, with less emphasis on oral dosing of smaller animals like the rat, we might hope for more progress in the near future toward the development of locally active, powerful, cytostatic agents for use in rheumatoid arthritis. Development of the jet-injector for intra-articular therapy [171] may minimize one difficulty. Another difficulty though is the long-held objection to injectable drugs in general, but this must be recognized as the shibboleth that it is. Of what real merit are second-best, palliative drugs that can be taken orally like aspirin but must be taken in larger doses, when so much more benefit might be obtained from a short course of injections of another, superior drug? The continued use of, and demand for, gold preparations (which must be given parenterally) to treat advanced rheumatoid disease should occasion further thought on this subject.

E. Some Potential New Leads — Fact and Fancy

The current great interest in finding ways to prevent rejection of a tissue graft periodically throws up a new idea for using some of the established immunosuppressive agents, including antilymphocyte globulins, in yet another mode. The whole field of transplantation biology with its especial goal of readily inducing tolerance to the tissue graft deserves careful attention from the would-be immunopharmacologist. Another fruitful source of leads, especially in defining new chemicals with the requisite intrinsic activity for potential immunosuppressor activity, is the whole massive research effort devoted to cancer chemotherapy and antiviral agents.

The problem of selectively restricting drug action to a lymphoid population and sparing the marrow and epithelial mucosa requires much more research upon the biodistribution of a potential immunosuppressor and comparative studies of the biochemistry of all rapidly growing tissues within the same animal. The idea of locally activating potential immunosuppressant drugs in one tissue was brilliantly presented by the Merck chemists with their preparation of steroid glucosaminides for selective hydrolysis by those (connective) tissues rich in glucosaminidases [172]. Can this idea be adapted to favor drug action on lymphoid cells only?

The use of an antigen to selectively stimulate a lymphocyte has been brilliantly exploited for tolerance induction. Can this same antigen be immobilized, injected where it might do no harm, and then used to act as a "lure" to attract specifically sensitized cells to that site and localize tissue injury where it might be less harmful? If the "lure" were also compounded with a truly cytotoxic agent (also immobilized), then we might have the situation corresponding to the control of certain insect populations based on the appropriate sex-attractant bringing the males to a trap where they are killed with an insecticide or other means. In each case the same toxic agent is used on a selected population which would otherwise be used, in the absence of a "lure," on the whole population at large (insects or lymphocytes). Just as the widely detrimental effects of an old, hard-line insecticide like DDT can now be severely restricted by this strategy, so too the virtues of an immunosuppressive agent could be exploited without poisoning the whole animal. This idea of using an antigen "sump" of exogenous origin to which sensitized lymphocytes might "home" and perhaps do less harm there than when they combine with the alternative, endogenous antigen depots may have been proved in practice already. In a fascinating experiment, Currey has demonstrated that deposition of killed tubercle bacilli in the peritoneal cavity greatly ameliorates the severity of the rat adjuvant arthritis induced by sensitizing the animal to the same tubercle bacilli [173].

If the immunogenic amino acid sequences of some of the most common autoantigens could be unraveled, we might hope that they would be eventually synthesized chemically to obtain truly "false antigens" for induction of tolerance, trapping sensitized cells, and other therapeutic manipulations of the autosensitive state. A forerunner of what might come was the announcement of the 16-amino acid sequence of part of the bovine encephalitogenic protein which is sufficient for inducing the allergic encephalomyelitis in guinea pigs [174].

To return to considering micromolecules for a moment. How is it that a thiazolidinone drug (I.C.I.-43,823) can uniquely suppress the adjuvant arthritis in rats, but show no anti-inflammatory activity or any other immunosuppressor activity [175]? Does it chemically resemble some feature of the arthritogenic fractions of the adjuvant? Does it have some specific desensitizing effect not based on any molecular similarities to the arthritogen? Above all, does its selective activity encourage us to search for yet other, unique, "odd-ball" immunosuppressants?

F. What Chemical Species Might Be Investigated for Immunosuppressive Activity?

1. Natural Products

Obviously any compounds, uncovered by programs studying natural products for potential carcinostatic activity, deserve to be studied in an immunosuppressor test system and if active therein, to be used as leads for synthesizing new compounds to delineate a structure-action relationship.

A good assay, from the point of view of ruthlessly eliminating all but the most effective compounds, is to test a candidate compound for its ability to prevent allergic encephalomyelitis in a highly susceptible (usually inbred) rat strain [176]: This requires dosing groups of at least four animals with the compound for perhaps 5 days and affords an all-or-none type of end point within the next 10 days (see Table IV). Further confirmation may then be sought by testing the compound for activity in suppressing allergic thyroiditis and/or adjuvant arthritis in rats, and promoting survival of

I. DRUGS FOR CHRONIC INFLAMMATORY DISEASE

transplanted tissues (homografts) such as colored goldfish scales [177]. Assays of this type, though time consuming, also usually afford some evidence of adverse toxicity, weight loss, etc.

A more economical, but less stringent, assay for potential cytostatic activity in vivo is to study the effects of the compound on cultured mammalian cells and/or upon the synthesis of biopolymers in isolated, surviving animal cell populations. Little material is needed for this type of first assay and indications of drug activity are rapidly disclosed — certainly within a 3-day time period. Unfortunately many quite selective inhibitors of DNA or protein synthesis in vitro subsequently fail to exhibit any useful activity in vivo, being either too toxic or, as is so frequently the case, quite inactive in the whole animal. This is a fundamental shortcoming of all in vitro screening techniques: It is not possible as yet to forecast with any certainty how effective a drug will be when it is subject to the dynamic interplay of such factors as absorption, competition from endogenous regulators, distribution in vivo, biotransformation, and excretion.

2. Nucleosides

Cytosine arabinoside (cytarabine, Cytosar ^{R}) is quite a useful immunosuppressor and antileukemic drug which inhibits the rat adjuvant arthritis [178] and may ameliorate (but not prevent) allergic encephalomyelitis [179]. Its 5'-adamantoyl conjugate (U-26516) shows enhanced, long-lasting, activity perhaps because it is degraded less rapidly in vivo than cytarabine itself [180]. Many seemingly rather unnatural nucleosides actually occur naturally and exhibit antibiotic activity, e.g., cordycepin, formycin, angustomycin, sangivamycin, showdomycin, and nucleocidin. There is still considerable scope for the synthetic organic chemist to compose variations upon nature's themes in this area and also to devise suitable potentiating agents which can block nucleoside catabolism in vivo. An example of this latter manipulation is the raising of the effective level of cytarabine in vivo by coadministering tetrahydro-uridine to inhibit deoxycytidylate aminohydrolase, the enzyme which rapidly inactivates cytarabine by deamination [181].

3. Other Analogs of Nucleic Acid Precursors

These encompass the range from such antibiotics as 6-diazo-5-L-oxonorleucine (DON) and azaserine (both glutamine antagonists) to compounds synthesized as potential antiviral agents, new antifolate drugs, etc. In light of recent reports that L-asparaginase (the enzyme which destroys L-asparagine) inhibits the immune response, it would be interesting to study the effects of L-asparagine analogs such as 5-diazo-4-oxo-L-norvaline which might block asparagine utilization. Since glycine may neutralize the activity of L-asparaginase [182] and is an essential building block in the biosynthesis of purines, it may be worth investigating glycine antagonists again for possible immunosuppressive activity.

4. Small Molecules not Designed To Be Antimetabolites

Though in fact they may effectively regulate nucleic acid biosynthesis by interrupting transcription or duplication of the genome, these are not specifically antimetabolites. In this category we would have to include biological alkylating agents, other radiomimetic drugs, selective cell poisons such as a drug primarily influencing nuclear enzymes (e.g., pyruvaldehyde combining with key nuclear thiols) involved in glycolysis, respiration, phosphorylation, protein or polynucleotide synthesis while (relatively) sparing similar enzymes in the extranuclear compartment of the cell. Some apparent cell selectivity may be gained when the extranuclear compartment is relatively small as in resting lymphocytes. Such thiol poisons as 4-nitrobenzofurazan [183] and the cucurbitacins [184] undoubtedly seem to be more effective in suppressing DNA synthesis in lymphocytes, than in many other cell types, because there is less "cytoplasmic buffer" (thiols) to neutralize the drug in a lymphocyte than in most other animal cells.

3-Acetyl-5-(p-fluorbenzylidene)-4-hydroxy-2-oxo-2,5-dihydrothiophene (ICI-47,776) is an experimental immunosuppressive agent which suppresses lymphocyte respiration [185] but only inhibits the immune response in rats, not in mice or guinea pigs [186]. It does however affect human, mice, and guinea pig lymphocytes in vitro. Perhaps we should remember this rather remarkable, species-specific drug before deciding that any other drug found to be active in vitro but inactive in small animals in vivo, is of no further interest as a potential drug in man. A further lesson we might learn is that ICI-47,776 could not have been anticipated to be such an active drug (effective at $10 \mu M$ in vitro), since it bears little formal resemblance to any known constituent of a metabolic pathway. The discovery of such a novel drug cannot be intelligently predicted at present. Any new knowledge which might eliminate the random screening of miscellaneous chemicals needed to disclose drugs with activity like I.C.I.-47,776 should immediately justify the research investment required.

For blocking nuclear transcription, very little may be required in the way of chemically reactive groups. If the drug can form a "molecular clamp" across the double-stranded DNA helix, preventing its unraveling for self-duplication or the informational transfer (transcription) to concurrently synthesized RNA molecule, then bulk and physical binding will be more important than the presence of individual atomic clusters (the chemist's functional groups). A molecule like 2,3-dianisylindole (indoxole) or its analog, diphenylindole, with only a rather nonreactive imine group in the pyrrole moiety, can nevertheless display remarkable potency in arresting lymphocyte metabolism [164] — perhaps not by interaction with DNA, but certainly by combination with some regulatory molecular species within the cell or on its surface.

To a chemist, few compounds could be less interesting than some of the polynuclear benzenoid hydrocarbons with their lack of key functional groups: To a biologist, few molecules match them for their frightening activity in inducing cancer and probably in achieving this, overwhelming the normal immune surveillance. We might well remember the recent renaissance of a whole area of inorganic chemistry engendered by Bartlett's discovery in 1961 that the rare, so-called "inert," gases could form chemical compounds.

A study of the interaction of chemically nondescript and functionally unreactive micromolecules with sorptive biopolymers (in contexts other than induction of anaesthesia by the rare gases) may yet revivify our whole approach to the regulation of biological phenomena by exogenous chemicals. Put simply, can the medicinal chemist afford to ignore even nonfunctional chemical compounds as potential new drugs for regulating membrane phenomena, the genome, and cell differentiation in lymphoid cells?

5. Large Molecules

Large molecules might be introduced into (or onto) lymphoid cells to reprogram their biosynthetic activities. Perhaps this is one effect of antilymphocyte globulins *in vivo*. Stimulating interferon production with synthetic polyribonucleotides seems to divert certain impressionable lymphocytes from engaging in other responses and may perhaps partly explain why poly I:poly C copolymers can suppress both an acute inflammation and the rat adjuvant arthritis.

Can "artificial histones" be developed for insertion into responsive cells to repress gene activation? Is it feasible to mimic the other, nonhistone, regulatory proteins in the nucleus or if these promote biopolymer synthesis (which certain nuclear phosphoproteins appear to do [187]), to antagonize them? The possibilities are really only limited by our imagination, after due allowance has been given to predictable side effects (such as immunogenicity and the fact that many basic peptides will liberate histamine from mast cells).

VI. NATURAL REGULATORS OF INFLAMMATION, THE IMMUNE RESPONSE, AND INFLAMMATORY DISEASE

A. The State of Pregnancy

The amount of hydrocortisone circulating in the plasma rises appreciably in pregnancy. One of the reasons that corticosteroids were first studied as possible antirheumatic drugs by Hench and his colleagues at the Mayo Clinic in the late 1940's was because these investigators were so struck by the natural, but temporary, remission of the arthritic symptoms during pregnancy.

However there are other factors which also change in pregnancy and which might act as natural antiarthritic agents. Estrogens have been shown to ameliorate the adjuvant-arthritis in rats [188-190], and the levels of estrogen in both plasma and urine rise almost continually in pregnancy. By contrast, progesterone is reported to have no effect on the rat adjuvant arthritis [190].

The remission of the inflammatory symptoms of rheumatoid disease is usually most marked during the third trimester of pregnancy which is also the time when the γ- and β-globulins are increased. Evidence has been presented that pregnancy serum contains protein factor(s) which can stabilize both liver and leukocyte lysosomes [191] and, it is inferred, lessen tissue injury caused by release of lysosomal enzymes.

The specific maternal (immunological) tolerance of the fetus during pregnancy [192] suggests that further studies of the immunological role of the placenta may be quite productive. The prevalence of rheumatoid arthritis and systemic lupus erythematosus in women during the reproductive age, the tendency to remit during pregnancy, and the frequent exacerbation of these diseases following delivery, may be due to temporary imbalance of mechanisms promoting and inhibiting immunological intolerance.

B. The State of Jaundice

In addition to his interest in pregnancy as a cause of remissions of rheumatoid arthritis, Hench [193] was also fascinated by the remission which occurred in patients with jaundice, regardless of its cause. Before the advent of cortisone, there was sufficient interest in the possible protection afforded by jaundice that at least one investigator actually transmitted infectious hepatitis to a group of patients as a therapeutic measure [194, 195]. Delayed enzymatic transformation of cortisol to (biologically inactive) reduced 17-hydroxycorticosteroids occurs during jaundice and may account for some of the antirheumatic effects of jaundice [196]. Thus far, none of the normal bile constituents has been found to be an effective anti-inflammatory agent. Unfortunately, little has been added to our knowledge of this subject in the past 25 years but there is some recent evidence that ligation of the bile duct may diminish subsequent inflammation of a rat's paw with carrageenin [197].

C. Endogenous and Exogenous Inhibitors of the Immune Response

An "autoimmune" component of an inflammatory disease state may, like many other biological phenomena, be under some form of self-regulatory control. This might help to explain the spontaneous remission of symptoms which is so frequently seen in rheumatoid disease, between the intervals of "flare-up" or exacerbated disease.

If antibody production is involved, then this may in some instances be controlled by the end-product, the antibody itself. Some insight into this type of autoimmunoregulation, or feedback control, has been obtained in recent years, not only by studying the effect of an antibody (i.e., γ-globulin) upon its own synthesis [198, 199] but also from wider studies of the action of cell-secreted products, such as hormones and enzyme-precursors (e.g., chymotrypsinogen), upon the very cells which synthesize them.

Other immunoregulatory macromolecules (not γ-globulins) have been detected in serum, including α-globulins with ribonuclease activity. One of the latter has been identified as an α_2-glycoprotein. This has prompted the synthesis of "artificial" complexes of pancreatic RNA-ase, some of which display immunosuppressive activity in vitro and/or in vivo, whereas "native" pancreatic RNA-ases are not immunosuppressive [200, 201].

I. DRUGS FOR CHRONIC INFLAMMATORY DISEASE

Flare-up of the disease symptoms presumably reflects exacerbation of the disease process and, in the context of an immunologically sustained disease this might be due to reimmunization or resensitization. The immunogen here may be either a new endogenous (auto)antigen, perhaps arising as a result of previous injury, or an exogenous antigen such as an infectious particle. If a competing antigen is available at this time, then the immunological response to the original auto-, or other, antigen may be diminished or even perhaps "turned off" altogether. In this fashion, not only may antibody production be controlled but also the raising of a further population of pathophoric, sensitized, and aggressive lymphocytes may likewise be hindered. Under certain conditions, essentially those of coimmunization, an exogenous antigen like hen egg albumin can prevent the sensitization of a rat to the arthritogenic component of the Freund's adjuvant [202] and so inhibit the development of adjuvant-induced arthritis. There is evidence that nonprotein polymers (e.g., synthetic polynucleotides) can also inhibit this rat arthritis [203], perhaps by a similar process of desensitization. Nucleic acid complexes are known to have immunosuppressive properties [204] and the phenomenon of immunodepression by mammalian viruses and plasmodia has been clearly documented [205]. Indeed the question has been asked, "can parasitic infections suppress autoimmune disease?" in the light of epidemiological findings of a rarer-than-expected incidence of rheumatoid and autoimmune disorders in West African people [206].

D. Hormones and Tissue Factors

To be successful, an immunological response requires a biological "scale-up"; that is, a limited number of committed lymphoid cells must reproduce their kind and differentiate to form antibody-producing cells or a new population of sensitized, perhaps pathophoric, lymphocytes. Without some form of control and given a sufficient supply of nutrients, such a proliferative response might proceed almost indefinitely, much to the detriment of the host. One form of control is that of physical restraint: There are anatomical and other factors which impose some limit as to how far the spleen or a lymph node may expand in volume in conjunction with mounting an immunological response. Another, tighter, form of control is through a negative feedback mechanism involving inhibition by the end-product, as indicated in the previous paragraphs — at a critical concentration of circulating antibody and perhaps also with a critical number of committed lymphocytes, there is some recognition that the immunological response should be moderated or even severely curtailed. Yet another type of control may involve hormone-like suppressors of natural origin.

Only recently has it been generally realized, largely due to the writings of Professor Bullough (a zoologist at the University of London) that a new class of tissue hormones exists, the "chalones," which act as natural antimitotic agents [207, 208]. They are secreted within a tissue and are specific for that same tissue, so that in one sense they do not qualify as hormones under the strict classical definition, not being blood-borne. Quite remarkably, although they are tissue-specific, they are not species-specific: Thus an epithelial chalone prepared from pig skin will inhibit the proliferation of epithelial cells derived from other animals. The epithelial chalone is a glycoprotein, a type of biopolymer which is not usually highly antigenic. If other tissue chalones are also glycoproteins, there is some hope that chalones of animal origin may be of some eventual use in man. Other macromolecular animal products, which are normally feeble antigens, have been invaluable in medicine as endocrine supplements (e.g., insulins, corticotrophins, calcitonins, etc.) and we might anticipate a bright future for chalone therapy as well.

A number of, as yet, poorly characterized factors have been isolated from certain lymphoid tissues, with properties which suggest they might suppress the (immuno)inflammatory response [209-211]. When sufficient evidence has been obtained to establish that these factors are not behaving as competitive antigens or as systemic toxins, in the sense of depressing the proliferation or turnover of nonlymphoid cells, then they might be considered potential chalones for the lymphoid tissues.

Further research might be expected to establish (or disprove) the existence of connective tissue chalones, specific for fibroblasts and related cells, e.g., chondrocytes.

The recent elucidation of previously unsuspected hormonal regulators like the prostaglandins [212] and (thyro)calcitonins [213] encourages the belief that other hormonal regulators of the inflammatory response might yet be found. These might either prove to be therapeutically useful as such, or if they were promoters of inflammation, some knowledge of their chemical constitution would at least suggest what sort of molecule should be constructed to serve as a potential antagonist. We might also note that "new" properties may still be found for the "old" hormones. For example, there is considerable indirect evidence that thyrotrophin and somatotrophin may each promote the immune response.

E. Rindani Agents — Nonsteroid Anti-Inflammatory Factors of Animal Origin

Countless contributors to the medical literature over the past 2500 years have commented upon the fact that many irritant substances will inhibit inflammation. Indeed one school of thought has held the view that the anti-inflammatory effects of many drugs, including tars and turpentine, is to be ascribed simply to their counterirritant actions. Lader et al. [214] seem to have been the first workers to indicate that an irritant injected at one site could release a substance which acted as an anti-inflammatory agent at another site in the body.

Although the existence of natural anti-inflammatory agents in animal tissues (other than ACTH or the corticosteroids) had long been suspected, it was not until Rindani's work was published in 1956 [215] that they were considered sufficiently "real" to warrant serious investigation. Since then, a number of studies have amply confirmed the anti-inflammatory properties of inflammatory exudates obtained from both animals [216, 217] and humans [218]. The purification of at least one of these factors from rat tissues by Billingham et al. [219] indicates that it is a protein which may be an α-globulin. Since anti-inflammatory activity is also present in the serum of animals suffering an inflammatory reaction, the factor may be synthesized in the liver as one of the "acute phase reactants" and travel to the inflammatory site via the blood stream. Further investigation of such endogenous anti-inflammatory factors should certainly aid our understanding of the natural regulation of inflammation.

It should be noted that a Rindani agent need not necessarily be extracellular. For example, eosinophilic leukocytes seem to carry antihistamine activity sufficiently powerful to protect guinea pigs from the usually fatal bronchospasm induced by a histamine aerosol [220].

F. Diet

Putrefaction products derived from tryptophane have been shown to be arthritogenic when injected into joints [221]. The possible role of the aromatic amino acids in exacerbating the symptoms of certain connective tissue diseases, e.g., scleroderma, has been discussed elsewhere [222]. By contrast, there are many indications that other dietary components may cause some remission of symptoms. It is not feasible in the present context to explore this subject further, beyond noting that many folk-remedies for arthritis do lay emphasis on fruit products (cider vinegar, citrus pectin, etc.) or seafoods (shellfish especially). Can the folk memory be mistaken all the time? There very probably must be some factual foundation for many of these "half-truths" to persist as they do around the world. Are there in fact "Rindani agents" widely spread throughout the plant and animal kingdom, some of which may defy digestion following ingestion and therefore be available from the diet if absorbed from the gut? Perhaps other dietary components can control the enteric production, and intestinal absorption, of putrefactive metabolites.

G. Anti-Injury Factors

The rapid termination of the action of known inflammagens such as histamine, serotonin, and the kinins by the appropriate oxidative or hydrolytic enzymes clearly indicates that higher animals have a very well-developed capacity to overcome, and survive, the effects of (initially) excessive production or release of these inflammagens. It appears that the body is normally well prepared to deal with other injurious agents as well, particularly most of the tissue-destroying enzymes. In many forms of experimental injury, such as following thermal burns or the application of corrosive chemicals, there is a marked rise in the globulin components of the blood, the so-called "acute reactants," and an accompanying decline in the albumin levels.

Among the post-injury blood factors there is a notable rise in the titre of α-globulins with antienzyme activity, especially toward hydrolytic enzymes such as proteases [223] and to a lesser extent, nucleases. High levels of an α_2-macroglobulin are found in the serum of rats suffering adjuvant arthritis, in pregnant females, and in newborn rats [224]. The latter are very resistant to induction of arthritis with Freund's adjuvant [225] and we have already noted the amelioration of arthritic symptoms in pregnant women (see Section VI.A).

Tissue antiproteases of both animal and vegetable origin will suppress certain aspects of inflammation [226]. It will be very interesting to know what relationship these may have to the Rindani-type of natural anti-inflammatory agents. It would also be interesting to know if other tissue-injuring agents, such as the various macromolecular permeability factors, were likewise neutralized by an appropriate globulin (or other blood proteins), or if catabolic enzymes (analogous to chymotrypsin and the kininases) were present in the tissues or circulation to ensure their rapid destruction.

H. Cartilage Regeneration Factors

One of the tissues first affected in arthritis is articular cartilage. In osteoarthritis (also known as degenerative arthritis), there is slow thinning of the cartilage matrix, usually termed erosion though the erosive agent(s) are still unknown. One theory holds that they are present within the tissue; being the autolytic enzymes activated by a reduction in the ambient pH, such as cathepsins B and D [227] or another family of enzymes active at neutral pH and perhaps sensitive to salicylate [228]. In rheumatoid disease, normal cartilage is eroded by an overgrowth and ingrowing of chronic inflammatory tissue called pannus. In both types of arthritis, cartilage regenerates at an insufficient rate to replace that lost.

There are at least two factors which can stimulate the biosynthesis of a cartilage matrix by chondrocytes. One of these is the so-called "sulfation factor" [229], present in the serum and muscle [230] and apparently regulated by the pituitary growth hormone, somatotrophin. Another factor is present in young cartilage and is commercially available, in combination with a marrow extract, under the name of Rumalon ® (RobaPharm, Basel, Switzerland). Biochemical studies have shown that mucopolysaccharide synthesis in articular cartilage tissue, healing wounds, and cultured fibroblasts is indeed stimulated by addition of Rumalon itself or of certain macromolecular subfractions prepared therefrom [231-233]. The recent studies of the Bonn School of Pharmacology indicate that one of the active principles may be a mucopolysaccharide-peptide complex. Preparations of sulfation factor and Rumalon, respectively, stimulate thymidine and uridine incorporation into the nucleic acids of cartilage cells, suggesting that they affect chondrocyte metabolism at a rather fundamental level.

I. So What?

Armed with this information about natural regulators of rheumatoid symptoms and the immune process, we should ask ourselves if any of these regulators could be used either as novel therapeutic agents or at least as

I. DRUGS FOR CHRONIC INFLAMMATORY DISEASE

"blueprints," providing some intellectual guidelines for the development of new drugs. Of course we must have considerable faith in natural products to do so. This should in no way diminish our present faith in the art of the synthetic organic chemist, who may now be required to modulate or simplify the activity of such a natural regulator through molecular manipulation. The real question is, are we in any position to ignore these, and other possible, signposts in nature? If not, then we suggest that attention be given to some of the following possibilities:

i. Establishing whether or not estrogens ameliorate rheumatoid arthritis.

ii. If they do, finding ways to "de-estrogenize" these steroids yet retain the potential (antirheumatic?) activity, so that they might be used in a wider context. We might hope to repeat a previous "success story" — the separation of the anabolic and androgenic activities of steroids related to testosterone.

iii. Desensitization of that fraction of the lymphoid cell mass which is sensitive to a rheumatogenic antigen (if indeed such an entity exists). This might involve deliberate parasitization with a benign, feebly antigenic, microorganism or if a rheumatogenic antigen is ever found, finding some means to confer adaptive immunity, or tolerance, to it.

iv. Development of new blood products such as antiproteases, the lysosomal-stabilizing protein(s), etc., again for use in replacement therapy.

v. Development of lymphoid and fibroblast chalones as potential agents for replacement therapy, to be used whenever it is clear that the patient's own adaptive mechanisms are insufficient to moderate an untoward immune response or connective tissue hyperplasia.

vi. Finding ways to consistently boost the endogenous production of such blood borne anti-injury factors: Just as certain drugs may induce in the liver an increase in those enzymes which metabolize them, so perhaps small quantities of a potentially injurious agent, like an exogenous protease, might be used to elicit (amplified) production of an antiprotease globulin by the liver.

vii. That those who study the epidemiology of disease be asked to give more weight (in the design of their data-collecting protocols) to investigating possible dietary factors, which may benefit the population at large but be in short supply to those with advanced disease. More nutritional studies of the relationship between the severity of say, the rat adjuvant arthritis, and the dietary composition would be of real value; if only to find out whether or not we are right in generally assuming that nutrition is a "dead science," of little relevance to modern medicine and no help to pharmacology.

viii. Further development of growth or repair factors for partly destroyed connective tissues, such as the sulfation factor and the active principle(s) in the commercial cartilage extract (Rumalon).

ix. Further development of the natural anti-inflammatory agent(s) present at an inflamed site.

[By development, we mean making available sufficient quantities of these several factors in a reasonably pure form for adequate therapeutic trials in animals and eventually in man.]

VII. SOME PARTICULAR PROBLEMS AND PITFALLS FOR DRUG DESIGN

The following observations are certainly not unique to, but are certainly relevant for, finding new drugs to treat inflammatory states and the concomitant tissue injury. If we can learn anything from a retrospective survey of past and present drugs to guide our drug-prospecting today, it should certainly include noting the following facts.

A. Inadequacy of Present Leads

Following in the time-honored tradition that "nature may know best" and accepting that a natural product may provide an adequate lead; a great deal of effort has gone into producing anti-inflammatory drugs resembling salicylates on the one hand, and cortisol (hydrocortisone) on the other — doubtless because these were originally (in the 1950's) the best anti-inflammatory drugs available from the plant and animal kingdom, respectively. Pharmacological assays came to be devised and assessed, based solely on their ability to detect these natural leads. For this reason, and probably this reason only, we have today a plethora of "salicylate-like" nonsteroid drugs and, of course, a whole range of "supersteroids." Nor can we hope to break out of this mold until we break away from the types of assays that are eminently satisfactory for recognizing a new "salicylate," or a new "steroid-like" drug, but little else. With conceptually poor chemical leads and inadequate assays, can we really expect to achieve "the exciting breakthrough" that everyone is hoping for?

B. The Myth of Potency

This has to be combated at two levels, the qualitative and the quantitative. Salicylates and steroids are indeed remarkable drugs for the number of individual pharmacological activities they can manifest: They are in fact pluripotent/multivalent. How many, if any, of their known activities should be reproduced in a "new" anti-inflammatory drug?

Do we in fact need such a broad spectrum of activities to moderate the symptoms of chronic inflammation? Would drugs with a narrower spectrum actually benefit the patient more, being less toxic and perhaps also less blunt in their action? Within reasonable limits, the quantity of a drug

I. DRUGS FOR CHRONIC INFLAMMATORY DISEASE

required to produce a desired effect is of little consequence to the patient. The crucial factor limiting dosage is rarely the number of tablets to be swallowed; almost always, it is the occurrence of undesirable side effects or toxicity. Of what comfort is it to the patient to know that dexamethasone is eight times as potent as prednisone, if three tablets a day of either steroid cause him to become Cushingoid?

Medicine did not advance greatly with the discovery that certain cortisol derivatives exhibited anti-inflammatory potencies of the order 10^3 times that of cortisol itself; unfortunately, the side effects were also greatly potentiated as well. The net result was some academic excitement but little to further assist the clinician in his patient care.

Since many patients are now daily swallowing up to 5 g of aspirin, they will not be upset unduly by being given large quantities of a reasonably priced aspirin-substitute with a higher therapeutic index (i.e., more freedom from side effects). A less potent drug would be more useful to them if it had a wider margin of safety between the therapeutic dose and the toxic dose. Therapeutics is not like electronics: The trend does not have to be consistently towards miniaturization (of the dose at least) to constitute progress.

C. Vigorous Metabolism of Small Animals

It is humbling to realize how improbable it is that one of today's standby and standard drugs, phenylbutazone, would have been discovered by just relying on its performance in small animals. The reason: Its short half-life in these animals compared with that in man. How many other "feeble performers" have been discarded in drug-screening programs conducted only in rats, mice, or other animals, whose metabolism of foreign compounds may be so much faster than man's? The marginally active compounds in these small animals may possibly be the most suitable for further trials in larger animals: Many of the most active compounds in the minianimal may prove to be too potent in a larger one, if their metabolism is indeed much slower in the larger species. This brings us to another, related problem.

D. The Induction of Drug Metabolism

This has been well exemplified by phenylbutazone which, upon repeated administration, induces or enhances its own metabolism in small animals. The implication is clearly that such a drug may become less toxic, the longer it is administered. For this reason, if no other, we should be slow to discard a drug on the basis of its initial toxicity alone (in high, acute-doses).

E. Does a Drug Have To Be a Suppressor To Be Effective?

It is rather arresting to find that some of today's useful anti-inflammatory drugs are able to induce the synthesis of other, potentially valuable, agents. Three examples should suffice to establish this point:

i.   A highly water soluble gold preparation, aurothioglucose, stimulates the biosynthesis in vivo of mucopolysaccharide sulfates in the mesenchymal tissues [234]. This is one of the normal reparative events which may actually govern the overall synthesis of new connective tissue. (By contrast, conventional anti-inflammatory drugs all inhibit mucopolysaccharide synthesis.)

ii.   Three, chemically unrelated, anti-inflammatory drugs (namely cortisol, oxyphenbutazone, and indomethacin) are reported [235] to each induce the synthesis of a collagenase (active at pH 5) and some neutral proteases by rat skin fibroblasts in vivo and mouse 'L' cells (a fibroblast) in tissue culture. One of the proteases resembles chymotrypsin and could therefore destroy kinins, so functioning as an anti-inflammatory agent.

iii.   It is well known that anti-inflammatory steroids (related to cortisol) initiate liver gluconeogenesis from noncarbohydrate precursors. At low concentrations (less than $1 \mu M$), cortisol may also stimulate other metabolic events such as albumin synthesis by cultured liver cells [236] and antibody production by lymph node cells in tissue cultures [237]. These effects of cortisol in promoting tissue anabolism are in marked contrast to some of its other effects in stimulating catabolism and acting as a suppressor rather than a promoter. Many of the suppressive or deleterious effects are only observed at much higher steroid concentrations though there are some notable exceptions, such as inducing cytolysis of thymocytes in vitro by $0.27 \mu M$ cortisol [238, 239]. Even in this latter situation, there is evidence that the cortisol actually initiates some metabolic event(s), linked to respiration and dependent on phosphate ions, which destroys the nuclear structure of these thymic lymphocytes.

One point is clear however. The great potency of the steroids (compared to the suppressive nonsteroid drugs) may be simply related to the fact that one steroid molecule, binding at the right regulatory site in the nucleus (or even perhaps on the outer cell membrane), will trigger the synthesis of many molecules of RNA; each of which, in turn, directs the synthesis of many molecules of protein. The net effect is a biological cascade with amplification at each step. From the point of view of drug design, could there be a more economical way to carry out biological regulation than this type of activation or its converse, namely drug-induced repression of RNA synthesis?

The real problem again is: How does one try to intelligently anticipate the discovery of such drug-induced capabilities? How may chemicals be screened in large numbers for such, apparently bizarre, activities? This takes us into the area of "chromosomal pharmacology," the interactions of a drug with a genome. The possibilities are both frightening and very exciting, even if it is rather frustrating at the moment not to know how to do the right experiments.

F. Is the Need for Strict Chemical Similarity a Myth Too?

By tradition, and rarely questioned, an antimetabolite is supposed to "look" rather like the molecule it antagonizes, the normal enzyme substrate or cofactor. Consider the following: the binding to, and blockading of the active site of, trypsin by thionine [240]; the very similar inhibition of chymotrypsin by Biebrich scarlet [240] (which fails to bind chymotrypsinogen) or by anti-inflammatory acidic drugs such as phenylbutazone and the fenamic acids [241]. The conventional (admittedly abnormal) substrates for each of these proteolytic enzymes are amide or ester derivatives of the appropriate basic and aromatic amino acids respectively. None of these inhibitors bear much recognizable structural resemblance to the substrate but they certainly recognize, and consequently occlude, a considerable portion of substrate-binding sites of these two enzymes. Enzymes resembling trypsin in their substrate-specificity have been widely implicated in inflammagenesis: The list includes thrombin, Hageman factor, at least one cathepsin, plasmin, and the kininogenases. This raises the question of whether or not some of these chemically unrelated compounds, such as thionine, should be used as starting points for further molecular modification to develop new antitryptic drugs (rather along the lines that Baker et al. [242] have modified some of the conventional substrates of serine-type proteases to obtain very effective irreversible inhibitors in vitro). The fundamental point here though is the apparent nonresemblance of the "lead" compound to its intended drug receptor (itself designed to recognize and complement another type of molecule), in this instance the active site of the tryptic enzyme. It may seem rather irrational to the medicinal chemist to take as his lead compound a chemically foreign, but nevertheless effective, antimetabolite but can we afford to neglect any lead of this sort. It may indeed be short-sighted to work with only chemically similar (i.e., strict) antimetabolites, unerringly recognized by inspecting their chemical structures.

Earlier we noted that oxyphenbutazone, indomethacin, and cortisol could all independently induce the synthesis of the same enzymes by fibroblasts, strongly suggesting that all three drugs activated the same part of the (latent) genome. It has been calculated that a hypothetical receptor for histamine, in one of its two favored conformations (corresponding to the N-N interatomic distance 4.55 Å), should also be able to bind cortisol, a phenylbutazone metabolite, the fenamic and salicylic acids; while a hypothetical serotonin receptor (N-N distance 5.84 Å) should also be able to accommodate cortisol and the phenylbutazone metabolite (but differently disposed to their manner of combining with the postulated histamine receptor) and an indomethacin metabolite, 5-methoxy-2-methylindol-3-yl acetic acid [129]. These speculations are partly supported by some observations indicating that salicylate (5 mM), phenylbutazone (0.2 mM), and indomethacin (0.05 mM) may each antagonize the constrictor effects of serotonin and histamine on the mesenteric vein of rats and guinea pigs, respectively [243]. The question now is: Is it mere coincidence that these various lines of evidence should all suggest that these chemically diverse species, represented here by phenylbutazone, indomethacin, cortisol (and perhaps salicylate as well), could fulfill the geometric and stereochemical requirements of histamine or serotonin antagonists or both? Certainly only one of these molecules, indomethacin, bears much formal resemblance to either of these amines (in this case, serotonin).

If this line of speculation is at all valid, it might indicate that whole new classes of antihistamines and antiserotonins may be devised or awaiting discovery. The need for some molecular rigidity implied in these discussions (to match the postulated receptors) may then explain why there are, as yet, no clinically useful aliphatic nonsteroid anti-inflammatory drugs, apart from the various gold preparations.

G. Chemical Synovectomy

A variety of substances have been injected into inflamed joints in attempts to destroy the diseased synovium. High concentrations of toxic drugs can be achieved locally with doses that are small enough so that little, if any, generalized toxicity occurs. This is the case for example when nitrogen mustard [244] and one of its pharmaceutical derivatives, thiotepa [245], are injected intra-articularly. Although both of these drugs are easily absorbed into the circulation, they can be used in small enough doses to avoid systemic toxicity. If the drug can be completely localized within the synovium, the doses used can be increased without fear of extra-articular toxicity. Both radioactive colloidal gold [246], which is restricted to the joint by its size, and osmic acid [247, 248], a tissue fixative for electron microscopy, are reported to localize in synovial and subsynovial macrophages and remain in these cells for rather long periods of time.

All these drugs appear to act by destroying the chronically inflamed synovium, which is then replaced by normal synovial lining cells, in a manner similar to the regeneration occurring following surgical synovectomy. One disadvantage of using these drugs is the temporary, but marked, exacerbation of inflammation which occurs during the first few days following the injection although these, admittedly, rather noxious drugs apparently cause no injury to the articular cartilage. If these synovial poisons could be administered in a masked form, perhaps attached to a slowly metabolized macromolecule which was too large to leak through the synovium, the same long-term therapeutic benefit might be obtained without the discomfort associated with acute and massive tissue destruction. This problem of chemical latentiation of an effective drug deserves further consideration.

H. Activation in Situ of Latent Drugs

Previously in this chapter we have referred to the *in vivo* activation of cyclophosphamide, azathioprine, and steroid glucosaminides (generating respectively an activated nitrogen mustard, 6-mercaptopurine and a 21-hydroxy cortisol analog). The activation of these three "masked" drugs

I. DRUGS FOR CHRONIC INFLAMMATORY DISEASE

is not confined by any means just to the site of inflammation. Is it possible to refine this approach whereby one or more of the enzymes concentrated at the inflammatory site(s) is harnessed to simultaneously activate a "pharmacogen," thereby preferentially liberating an active drug at, or near, the site(s) of inflammation? This pharmacogen could be a small molecule, specifically a drug conjugate with one or more biolabile linkages, or it could be a drug-macromolecule complex. Elsewhere (Section IV. C. 3), we have wondered if albuminolysis would liberate (albumin-bound) anti-inflammatory anions. Are there other macromolecules which could serve as drug carriers, "unloading" the active drug only when they interact with products of inflammation? Can leukocyte populations be paralyzed locally at the site of inflammation and not systemically, by the in situ unloading (or administration from outside) of a drug attached to a molecule that the leukocyte would phagocytose or pinocytose?

VIII. TREATING THE INDIVIDUAL

Because of the heterogeneity of the human population, the absorption, metabolism, toxicity, or therapeutic activity of any one drug may vary greatly in individual patients. Individuals also differ markedly in their reactions to the same prime cause, so that the same etiological agent may produce seemingly different diseases in different patients. Conversely, a variety of prime causes may initiate similar clinical symptoms and findings and appear to constitute a single disease entity.

Therefore, the drug designer should not be dismayed when the fairly reproducible results of preclinical testing in highly controlled strains of laboratory animals are not easily confirmed in clinical trials. The clinical pharmacologist, and the Food and Drug Administration, are both being rather unrealistic (and unreasonable) if they require that all new drugs demonstrate activity in all patients with a particular inflammatory disease (of unknown etiology). Those conducting a clinical trial should rather search for a group of drug-responsive patients, perhaps obscured by a larger number who are drug-resistant. More emphasis should certainly be placed on the correlation of patient responses with serum drug concentrations, rather than merely with the administered dose. Serum drug levels, or some other measurable parameter of drug action, should be used much more frequently by the clinician as a reasonable, perhaps objective, guide to dosage.

It would be especially helpful to the clinical pharmacologist if this fact were borne in mind when, of necessity, only one drug can be chosen for clinical investigation from several potential candidates of equal suitability in small animal studies. All other factors being equal, the drug most easily determined in the serum should be the drug of choice at this stage, since it will lend itself to the most detailed studies in the clinic of absorption, half-life in vivo, and recognition of the therapeutic blood levels. If the chemist can anticipate this need, by designing drugs with strong chromogenic, or fluorophoric, groups to facilitate their analysis, so much the better.

Finally, as every good clinician knows, each patient has his own disease; so this therapy must be individualized, and his responses to various, alternate, therapeutic agents may reveal as much about his particular disease, as the traditional diagnostic laboratory studies. For this reason the aim of every research program should be <u>to find, not one drug, but a family of drugs</u> which could be offered as alternatives (perhaps attaining different goals) from which the physician can choose the <u>one</u> most appropriate for <u>each</u> individual at <u>each</u> stage of the disease.

IX. EPILOGUE

It is not feasible here to summarize the data and concepts enumerated in the previous eight sections but the following points certainly deserve re-emphasis:

1. For most of the inflammatory diseases, drugs are needed to treat more than just the manifestations of inflammation. Even if these seem to primarily involve single organs, e.g., joint(s), skin, lymph nodes, etc., therapy may be required to control other, systemic factors.

2. Pharmacological assays which recognize a drug solely by its effects on acute local inflammation, however induced, are almost certainly insufficient for disclosing:

    a. eradicators of the prime cause (goal i);

    b. interceptors of the chemical and cellular mediators which initiate the earliest tissue injury (goal ii);

    c. interceptors of the "vicious" cycles which help to transform an acute, protective state of inflammation into an unregulated, destructive chronic inflammatory disease;

    d. restorative agents (goal iv).

3. Even the adjuvant-induced rat arthritis, as commonly studied for 2 or 3 weeks only and scored by the acute symptoms of the delayed, secondary phase, is still inadequate for unambiguously disclosing drugs categorized above as (a) through (d). Observations of the effect of a drug on rat arthritis over this time period (2 to 3 weeks) cannot really be extrapolated to predict drug efficacy in controlling ongoing <u>chronic</u> human disease.

4. It is not too much of an exaggeration to state that the drugs most needed in the clinic (e.g., like gold preparations) are those likely to be now eliminated in the preliminary screens (e.g., carrageenin-induced acute edema) which employ an acute inflammatory model and focus only on attaining Goal 3. For example, the drugs of choice to treat gout (allopurinol and probenecid) fail to survive even the "first line" screen employed in very many laboratories at the present time.

5. We must expunge the naive hope (in reality, a hindrance) that there will ever be a single universal panacea for all chronic inflammatory diseases.

I. DRUGS FOR CHRONIC INFLAMMATORY DISEASE

6. Before a rational pharmacology can be constructed for each of these diseases, they must be understood to be in fact a family of variants, each of which in turn may have a variety of causes, may progress (and alter) with time, and may manifest itself differently in different individuals. Accordingly, we must realize that a population of patients all presenting with similar inflammatory signs, or loss of function, will actually offer a range of opportunities for therapeutic intervention, only a few of which will be appropriate for any one individual. Translating this therapeutic ideal into practice requires the drug designer to provide a range of effective and target-specific drugs, from which the one most appropriate to the individual patient's needs would be selected by the physician.

7. Even for therapeutic attack on a single target, a plurality of drugs must be available so that the physician will be able to suit the therapy to the patient's idiosyncrasies, particularly his tolerance of any given drug at the particular stage of his disease.

8. Ehrlich originally proposed that the ideal drug would be a "magic bullet," selecting its target and effectively eliminating its pathogenic activity. This analogy is still appropriate today even when enormously destructive alternatives to a bullet are available. A pharmacological "overkill" is no substitute for pharmacological "sharpshooting." It is time that we seriously questioned whether or not powerful drugs with the breadth of action and potency of the supersteroids (or carcinostatic immunosuppressors) should be emulated, or regarded as trend-setters for future developments, particularly in the therapeutic care of patients without life-threatening inflammatory disease.

REFERENCES

1. Hans Seyle, The Stress of Life, McGraw-Hill, New York, 1956.
1a. Max Born, My Life and Views.
1b. Edward de Bono, The (Sunday) Observer Magazine, London, 1969.
1c. W. G. Spector and D. A. Willoughby, The Pharmacology of Inflammation, The English Universities Press, London, 1968 (Also Grune and Stratton Inc., New York, 1968).
2. M. Weiner and S. J. Piliero, Ann. Rev. Pharmacol., 10, 171 (1970).
3. W. Kuzell, Ann. Rev. Pharmacol., 8, 357 (1968).
4. C. A. Winter, Ann. Rev. Pharmacol., 6, 157 (1966); Progr. Drug Res., 10, 139 (1966).
5. R. Domenjoz, Advan. Pharmacol., 4, 143 (1966); also in Ankylosierende Spondylitis, D. Steinkopff Verlag, Darmstadt, 1969, p. 343.
6. S. S. Adams and R. Cobb, Progr. Med. Chem., 5, 59 (1967).
7. M. W. Whitehouse, Progr. Drug Res., 8, 321 (1965).

8. I. F. Skidmore and K. Trnavsky, Acta Rheumatol. Balneol. Pistiniana, 3, 1967.
9. T. Y. Shen, in Topics in Medicinal Chemistry (J. L. Rabinowitz and R. M. Myerson, eds.), Vol I, Interscience, New York, 1967, p. 29.
10. K. J. Doebel, Pure Appl. Chem., 19, 49 (1969).
11. K. J. Doebel, M. L. Graeme, N. Gruenfeld, L. J. Ignarro, S. J. Piliero, and J. W. F. Wasley, Ann. Rept. Med. Chem., 1968, Academic Press, New York, p. 207.
12. T. Y. Shen, Ann. Rept. Med. Chem. 1966, Academic Press, New York, 1967, p. 217; Ann. Rept. Med. Chem. 1967, Academic Press, New York, p. 215.
13. R. A. Scherrer, Ann. Rept. Med. Chem. 1965, Academic Press, New York, p. 224.
14. H. J. Sanders, "Arthritis" in Chem. Eng. News, July 22, July 29, August 12, 1968.
15. B. W. Zweifach. L. Grant, and R. T. McCluskey (eds.), The Inflammatory Process, Academic Press, New York, 1965.
16. J. C. Houck and B. K. Forscher (eds.), Chemical Biology of Inflammation, Suppl. to Biochem. Pharmacol., Pergamon, Oxford, 1968.
17. W. G. Spector, Intern. Rev. Exptl. Pathol., 8, 1 (1969).
18. J. C. Houck, Ann. N. Y. Acad. Sci., 105, 767 (1963).
19. K. W. Walton, Intern. Rev. Exptl. Pathol., 6, 285 (1968).
20. E. M. Hersh and G. P. Bodey, Ann. Rev. Med., 21, 105 (1970).
21. D. J. McCarty, Ann. Rev. Med., 21, 357 (1970).
22. J. L. Hollander (ed.), Arthritis and Allied Conditions: A Textbook of Rheumatology, 7th ed., Lea and Febiger, Philadelphia, 1966.
23. J. J. R. Duthie and W. R. M. Alexander, Rheumatic Diseases (University of Edinburgh Pfizer Medical Monographs #3), Williams and Wilkins, Baltimore, 1968.
24. W. S. C. Copeman (ed.), Textbook of the Rheumatic Diseases, 4th ed., Livingston, Edinburgh, 1969.
25. J. L. Decker (ed.), Primer on the Rheumatic Diseases, The Arthritis Foundation, New York; also serialized in J. Am. Med. Assoc., 190, 127, 425, 509, 741 (1964).
26. A. G. S. Hill (ed.), Modern Trends in Rheumatology, Vol. 1, Butterworth, London, 1966.
27. J. Rotstein (ed.), Rheumatology, an Annual Review, Vol. 1 et seq., S. Karger, Basel, 1967.

I. DRUGS FOR CHRONIC INFLAMMATORY DISEASE

28. L. E. Glynn, Intern. Rev. Connective Tissue Res., 2, 213 (1964).
29. M. Samter and H. L. Alexander (eds.), Immunological Diseases, Little, Brown, and Co., Boston, 1965.
30. P. A. Miescher and H. J. Müller-Eberhard (eds.), Textbook of Immunopathology, 2 vols., Grune and Stratton, New York, 1968.
30a. L. T. Morton and E. G. L. Bywaters, Ann. Rheumatic Diseases, 28, 669 (1969).
31. J. Caroli, C. Julien, J. Etévé, A. R. Prévot, and M. Sébald, Semaine Hop. Paris, 39, 1457 (1963).
32. C. T. Ashworth, F. C. Douglas, R. C. Reynolds, and P. J. Thomas, Am. J. Med., 37, 481 (1964).
33. D. K. Ford, Can. Med. Assoc. J., 99, 900 (1968).
34. W. Moll, Progr. Drug Res., 12, 165 (1968); Klinische Rheumatologic, 2nd ed., S. Karger, Basel, 1967.
35. J. H. Talbott, Gout, 3rd ed., Grune and Stratton, New York, 1967.
36. L. S. Goodman and A. Gilman (eds.), The Pharmacological Basis of Therapeutics, 3rd ed., Macmillan, New York, 1965.
37. S. L. Wallace and N. H. Ertel, Bull. Rheumatic Diseases, 20, 582 (1969).
38. A. B. Garrod, Trans. Med. Chir. Soc., 31, 83 (1848).
39. S. E. Malawista and V. T. Andriole, J. Lab. Clin. Med., 72, 933 (1968).
40. R. Bluestone, I. Kippen, and J. R. Klinenberg, Brit. Med. J., 4, 590 (1969).
41. R. W. Rundles, J. B. Wyngaarden, G. H. Hitchings, and G. B. Elion, Ann. Rev. Pharmacol., 9, 345 (1969).
42. R. H. Ferguson and H. F. Polley, Med. Clin. N. Am., 52 (3), 503 (1968).
43. H. K. von Rechenberg, Phenylbutazone, Edward Arnold Ltd., London, 1962.
44. J. J. Burns, R. K. Rose, T. Chenkin, A. Goldman, A. Schulert, and B. B. Brodie, J. Pharmacol. Exptl. Therap., 109, 346 (1953).
45. J. J. Burns, R. K. Rose, S. Goodwin, J. Reichenthal, E. C. Horning, and B. B. Brodie, J. Pharmacol. Exptl. Therap., 113, 481 (1955).
46. J. F. Fraumeni, Jr., J. Am. Med. Assoc., 201, 828 (1967).
47. H. B. Hucker, A. G. Zacchei, S. V. Cox, D. A. Brodie, and N. H. R. Cantwell, J. Pharmacol. Exptl. Therap., 153, 237 (1966).

48. R. E. Harman, M. A. P. Meisinger, G. E. Davis, and F. A. Kuehl, Jr., J. Pharmacol. Exptl. Therap., 143, 215 (1964).
49. M. D. Skeith, P. A. Simkin, and L. A. Healey, Clin. Pharmacol. Therap., 9, 89 (1968).
50. D. W. Yesair, L. Rogers, and C. J. Kensler, Federation Proc., 27, 531 (1968).
51. D. W. Yesair, L. Remington, M. Callahan, and C. J. Kensler, Biochem. Pharmacol., 19, 1591 (1970).
52. W. M. O'Brien, Clin. Pharmacol. Therap., 9, 94 (1968).
53. C. L. Short, W. Bauer, and W. E. Reynolds, Rheumatoid Arthritis, Harvard University Press, Cambridge, 1957.
54. J. H. Bland, ed., Rheumatoid Arthritis. Med. Clin. N. Am., 52(3) (1968).
55. R. W. Moskowitz, Med. Clin. N. Amer., 52(3), 623 (1968).
56. H. M. Rose, C. Ragan, E. Pearce, and M. O. Lipman, Proc. Soc. Exptl. Biol. Med., 68, 1 (1948).
57. C. A. Berntsen and R. H. Freyberg, Ann. Internal Med., 54, 938 (1961).
58. A. J. Glazko, Ann. Phys. Med. (Suppl.), 8, 24 (1966).
59. S. S. Adams, R. G. Bough, E. E. Cliffe, B. Lessel, and R. F. N. Mills, Toxicol. Appl. Pharmacol., 15, 310 (1969).
60. M. K. Jasani, W. W. Downie, B. M. Samuels, and W. W. Buchanan, Ann. Rheumatic Diseases, 27, 457 (1968).
61. W. H. Dodson and J. C. Bennett, J. Clin. Pharmacol., 9, 251 (1969).
62. J. Baum and J. Vaughan, Ann. Internal Med., 71, 202 (1969).
63. M. Mason, H. L. Currey, C. G. Barnes, J. F. Dunne, B. L. Hazleman, and I. D. Strickland, Brit. Med. J., 1, 420 (1969).
64. W. M. Fosdick, J. L. Parsons, and D. F. Hill, Arthritis Rheumat., 11, 151 (1968).
65. Medical Staff Conference, Calif. Med., 110, 410 (1969).
66. Proc. Conf. on Effects of Chronic Salicylate Administration, New York, June 13-14, 1966, R. W. Lamont-Havers and B. M. Wagner, eds., U. S. Govt. Printing Office, Washington, D. C., 1969.
66a. M. J. H. Smith and P. K. Smith, The Salicylates, A Critical Bibliographic Review, Interscience, New York, 1966.
66b. M. L. Tainter and A. J. Ferris, Aspirin in Modern Therapy, A Review, Bayer Co., New York, 1969.
66c. H. O. J. Collier, Advan. Pharmacol. Chemotherop., 7, 333 (1969).

67. K. Lande, München Med. Wochschr., **74**, 1132 (1927).
68. J. Forestier, Bull. Mem. Soc. Med. Hop. de Paris, **45**, ser. 4, 323 (1929).
69. R. H. Persellin and M. Ziff, Arthritis Rheumat., **9**, 57 (1966).
70. R. S. Ennis, J. L. Granda, and A. S. Posner, Arthritis Rheumat., **11**, 756 (1968).
71. E. L. Dubois (ed.), Lupus Erythematosus, McGraw Hill, New York, 1966.
72. W. L. Norton, Arthritis Rheumat., **12**, 320 (1969).
73. F. Györkey, K-W. Min, and P. Györkey, Arthritis Rheumat., **12**, 300 (1969).
74. R. C. Williams, Arthritis Rheumat., **11**, 593 (1968).
75. G. L. Ackerman and C. M. Nolan, New Eng. J. Med., **278**, 405 (1968).
76. R. R. MacGregor, J. M. Scheagren, M. B. Lipsett, and S. M. Wolff, New Eng. J. Med., **280**, 1427 (1969).
77. Empire Rheumatism Council, Ann. Rheumatic Diseases, **16**, 277 (1957).
78. Medical Research Council and Nuffield Foundation, Brit. Med. J., **2**, 695 (1955).
79. D. A. Ogden, K. A. Porter, P. I. Terasaki, T. L. Marchiero, J. H. Holmes and T. E. Starzl, Am. J. Med., **43**, 837 (1967).
80. R. J. Glassock, D. Feldman, E. S. Reynolds, G. J. Damin, and J. P. Merrill, Medicine, **47**, 411 (1968).
81. T. C. Moore and D. M. Hume, Ann. Surg., **170**, 1 (1969).
82. G. B. Elion, S. Callahan, S. Bieber, G. H. Hitchings, and R. W. Rundles, Cancer Chemotherapy Rept., **14**, 93 (1961).
83. G. B. Elion and G. H. Hitchings, Advan. Chemotherap., **2**, 91 (1965).
84. C. C. Corley, H. E. Lessner, and W. E. Larsen, Am. J. Med., **41**, 404 (1966).
85. I. Lorenzen, C. Brun, and A. Videbaek, Acta Med. Scand., **185**, 501 (1969).
86. T. E. Starzl, New Eng. J. Med., **279**, 700 (1968).
87. P. S. Russell, Ann. Internal Med., **68**, 483 (1968).
88. S. D. Deodhar, A. G. Kuklinca, D. G. Vidt, A. L. Robertson, and J. B. Hazard, New Eng. J. Med., **280**, 1104 (1969).

89. J. C. Fish, H. E. Sarles, A. R. Remmers, K. R. T. Tyson, C. C. Canales; G. A. Beathard, M. Fukushima, S. E. Ritzmann, and W. C. Levin, Surg. Gynecol. Obstet., 128, 777 (1969).

90. D. J. Whitehouse, M. W. Whitehouse, and C. M. Pearson, Nature, 224, 1322 (1969).

90a. D. D. McGregor and J. L. Gowans, Lancet, i, 629 (1964).

91. J. H. Kellgren, Bull. Rheumatic Diseases, 4, 46 (1954).

92. J. B. Peter, C. M. Pearson, and L. Marmor, Arthritis Rheumat., 9, 365 (1966).

92a. L. Sokoloff, The Biology of Degenerative Joint Disease, University of Chicago Press, Chicago, 1969.

93. G. D. Weinstein and P. Frost, Natl. Cancer Inst. Monograph, 30, 225 (1969).

94. H. H. Roenigk, Jr., W. Fowler-Bergfeld, and G. H. Curtis, Arch. Dermatol., 99, 86 (1969).

95. P. Calabresi, R. Turner, and E. Lefkowitz, Proc. Am. Assoc. Cancer Res., 5, 10 (1964).

96. M. Slavick, J. Elis, H. Raskova, M. Gutova, M. Duchkova, M. Kubikova, and V. Sercek, Pharmacol. Clin., 2, 120 (1970).

97. P. Calabresi and R. Turner, Ann. Internal Med., 64, 352 (1966).

98. A. Ebringer and I. R. Mackay, Ann. Internal Med., 71, 125 (1969).

99. G. DiPasquale, C. L. Rassaert, and E. McDougall, J. Pharm. Sci., 59, 267 (1970).

100. C. Hansch, Ann. Rept. Med. Chem. for 1966 (C. K. Cain, ed.), Academic Press, New York, 1967, p. 347

101. J. East, Vox Sanguinis, 16, 318 (1969).

102. J. B. Henson, J. R. Gorham, Y. Tanaka, and G. A. Padgett, Lab. Invest., 19, 153 (1968).

103. E. J. Field, Intern. Rev. Exptl. Pathol., 8, 129 (1969).

104. R. C. Mellors and C. Y. Huang, J. Exptl. Med., 124, 1031 (1966).

105. L. Karstad, Current Topics Microbiol. Immunol., 40, 9 (1967).

105a. J. Hotchin, Current Topics Microbiol. Immunol., 40, 33 (1967).

106. R. M. Lewis, in Animal Models for Biomedical Research, Proceedings of a Symposium (C. W. McPherson, ed.), National Academy of Sciences, Washington, D. C., 1968, pp. 21-34.

107. G. Jasmin, in Ref. 27, Vol. 1, p. 107 (1967).

108. J. L. Shupe and J. Storz, Am. J. Vet. Res., 25, 943 (1964).

I. DRUGS FOR CHRONIC INFLAMMATORY DISEASE

109. S. P. Triopathy and G. B. Mackaness, J. Exptl. Med., 130, 1 (1969).
110. R. A. Good, J. Finstad, W. A. Cain, A. Fish, D. Y. Perey, and R. A. Gatti, Federation Proc., 28, 191 (1969).
111. P. Stastny and M. Ziff, in Ref. 27, Vol. 1, p. 189 (1967).
112. L. Levy, Surv. Ophthalmol., 11, 444 (1966).
113. C. H. Lack, Med. Clin. N. Am., 52 (3), 667 (1968).
114. W. G. Spector and D. A. Willoughby, Evaluation of Drug Activities: Pharmacometrics (D. R. Lawrence and A. L. Bacharach, eds.), Academic Press, New York, 1964, Chap. 39.
115. E. M. Glenn, Proc. Soc. Exptl. Biol. Med., 129, 860 (1968).
116. M. E. Rosenthale, L. J. Datko, J. Kassarich, and F. Schneider, Arch. Intern. Pharmacodyn., 179, 251 (1969).
117. P. Y. Paterson and M. A. Hanson, J. Immunol., 103, 1311 (1969).
118. J. H. Brown, N. L. Schwartz, H. K. Mackey, and H. L. Murray, Arch. Intern. Pharmacodyn., 183, 1 (1970).
119. G. J. Possanza and P. B. Stewart, Clin. Exptl. Immunol., 6, 291 (1970).
120. R. S. Schwartz, Ann. N. Y. Acad. Sci., 123, 64 (1965).
121. J. J. Burns, T. F. Yü, P. G. Dayton, A. B. Gutman, and B. B. Brodie, Ann. N. Y. Acad. Sci., 86, 253 (1960).
122. R. W. Schayer, Perspectives Biol. Med., 10, 409 (1967); Medical College Virginia Quart., 4, 107 (1968).
123. R. W. Schayer and M. A. Reilly, Am. J. Physiol., 215, 472 (1968).
124. M. A. Reilly and R. W. Schayer, Brit. J. Pharmacol., 34, 551 (1968).
125. R. W. Schayer, Endocrinology, 81, 1357 (1967).
126. G. Kahlson and E. Rosengren, Physiol. Rev., 48, 155 (1968).
127. R. J. Boucek and T. R. Alvarez, Science, 167, 898 (1970).
128. L. B. Kier, J. Med. Chem., 11, 915 (1968).
129. L. B. Kier and M. W. Whitehouse, J. Pharm. Pharmacol., 20, 793 (1968).
130. H. J. Müller-Eberhard, Advan. Immunol., 8, 1 (1968); Ann. Rev. Biochem., 38, 389 (1969).
131. V. A. Bokisch, H. J. Müller-Eberhard, and C. E. Cochrane, J. Exptl. Med., 129, 1109 (1969).
132. D. Griffin, D. K. Tachibana, B. Nelson, and L. T. Rosenberg, Immunochemistry, 4, 23 (1967).

133. M. Nimni, Arthritis Rheumat., 12, 684 (1969).
134. B. R. Baker and M. Cory, J. Med. Chem., 12, 1049, 1053 (1969).
135. B. R. Baker and J. A. Hurlbut, J. Med. Chem., 12, 415 (1969).
136. B. R. Baker and E. H. Erickson, J. Med. Chem., 12, 408 (1969).
137. M. Cory, M. Glovsky, and M. W. Whitehouse, to be published.
138. M. I. Barnhart, C. Quintana, H. L. Lenon, G. B. Bluhm, and J. M. Riddle, Ann. N. Y. Acad. Sci., 146, 527 (1968).
139. F. Michal and B. G. Firkin, Ann. Rev. Pharmacol., 9, 95 (1969).
140. D. C. Dumonde, R. A. Wolstencroft, G. S. Panayi, M. Matthew, J. Morley, and W. T. Howson, Nature, 224, 38 (1969).
141. H. S. Lawrence and M. Landy (eds.), Mediators of Cellular Immunity, Academic Press, New York, 1969.
142. D. S. Nelson, Macrophages and Immunity, North-Holland Co., Amsterdam, 1969.
143. C. Smith and D. Hamerman, Arthritis Rheumat., 12, 639 (1969).
144. C. W. Castor and E. L. Dorstewitz, J. Lab. Clin. Med., 68, 300 (1966).
145. A. I. Grayzel and C. Beck, J. Exptl. Med., 131, 367 (1970).
146. E. D. Harris, Jr., J. M. Evanson, D. R. DiBona, and S. M. Krane, Arthritis Rheumat., 13, 83 (1970).
147. C. G. Cochrane and F. J. Dixon, in Ref. [30], p. 94.
148. G. Weissman and D. T. P. Davies, Arthritis Rheumat., 12, 703 (1969).
149. A. D. Perris and J. F. Whitfield, Proc. Soc. Exptl. Biol. Med., 130, 1198 (1969).
150. W. L. Norton, E. E. Velayos, and L. B. Robison, Arthritis Rheumat., 12, 320 (1969).
151. M. F. Barile, Hosp. Practice, 3 (10), 41 (1968).
152. J. J. van Loghem, Vox Sanguinis, 10, 1 (1965).
153. R. M. Herriott, Progr. Med. Virol., 11, 1 (1969).
154. A. E. Gabrielson and R. A. Good, Advan. Immunol., 6, 91 (1967).
155. R. S. Schwartz, Progr. Allergy, IX, 246 (1965); Hosp. Practice, 4 (2), 42 (1969); also Ref. [30], p. 227 (with Y. Borel).
156. E. Sorkin (ed.), The Immune Response and Its Suppression: Vol. 15 of Antibiotica et Chemotherapia, Karger, Basel, 1969.
157. G. B. Elion and G. H. Hitchings, Accounts Chem. Res., 2, 202 (1969).

158. Ciba Foundation Study Group #29, Anti-Lymphocytic Serum, Churchill, London, 1967.
159. P. B. Medawar, Hosp. Practice, 4 (5), 26 (1969).
160. J. Stjernswärd, Ref. [156], p. 213.
161. M. N. Salaman, Ref. [156], p. 393.
162. J. L. Turk, Brit. Med. Bull., 23 (1), 4 (1967).
163. T. Wagner-Jauregg and J. Fischer, Experientia, 24, 1029 (1968).
164. M. W. Whitehouse, J. Pharm. Pharmacol., 19, 590 (1967).
165. J. A. Stock, Chem. Brit., 6, 11 (1970).
166. M. C. Berenbaum and I. N. Brown, Immunology, 8, 251 (1965).
167. M. S. Mitchell, M. E. Wade, R. C. DeConti, J. R. Bertino, and P. Calabresi, Ann. Internal Med., 70, 535 (1969).
168. F. J. Gregory, S. F. Flint, H. W. Ruelius, and G. H. Warren, Cancer Res., 29, 728 (1969).
169. W. M. Fosdick, J. L. Parsons, and D. F. Hill, Arthritis Rheumat., 12, 663 (1969).
170. See, for example, the Abstracts of the 12th Intern. Congr. Rheumatology, Prague, 1969.
171. D. Banaski, Z. Rheumaforsch., I, 425 (1969).
172. R. Hirschmann, R. G. Strachan, P. Buchschacher, L. H. Sarett, S. L. Steelman, and R. Silber, J. Am. Chem. Soc., 86, 3903 (1964).
173. H. L. F. Currey, Ann. Rheumatic Diseases, 29, 314 (1970).
174. E. H. Eylar and G. A. Hashim, Proc. Natl. Acad. Sci., 61, 644 (1968).
175. B. B. Newbould, Brit. J. Pharmacol. Chemotherap., 24, 632 (1965).
176. M E. Rosenthale, L. J. Datko, J. Kassarich, and F. Schneider, Arch. Intern. Pharmacodyn., 179, 251 (1969).
177. L. Levy, Proc. Soc. Exptl. Biol. Med., 114, 47 (1963).
178. E. M. Glenn, Proc. Soc. Exptl. Biol. Med., 129, 860 (1968).
179. M. E. Greig and A. J. Gibbons, Arch. Intern. Pharmacodyn., 182, 364 (1969).
180. G. D. Gray, M. M. Mickelson, and J. A. Crim, Biochem. Pharmacol., 18, 2163 (1969).
181. G. W. Camiener, Biochem. Pharmacol., 17, 1981 (1968).
182. W. L. Ryan and H. C. Sornsen, Science, 167, 1512 (1970).

183. M. W. Whitehouse and P. B. Ghosh, Biochem. Pharmacol., 17, 158 (1968).

184. M. W. Whitehouse and R. W. Doskotch, Biochem. Pharmacol., 18, 1790 (1969).

185. T. J. Franklin and B. Higginson, Biochem. J., 102, 705 (1967).

186. G. E. Davies, Immunology, 14, 393 (1968).

187. E. L. Gershey and L. J. Kleinsmith, Biochem. Biophys. Acta, 194, 519 (1969).

188. E. M. Glenn, Am. J. Vet. Res., 27, 339 (1966).

189. M. N. Mueller and A. Kappas, Proc. Soc. Exptl. Biol. Med., 117, 845 (1964).

190. P. Toivanen, K. Määttä, R. Suolanen, and R. Tykkyläinen, Med. Pharmacol. Exptl., 17, 33 (1967).

191. K. H. Hempel, L. A. Fernandez, and R. H. Persellin, Nature, 225, 955 (1970).

192. L. Green and G. I. Urbach, Can. Med. Assoc. J., 99, 469 (1968).

193. P. S. Hench, Proc. Staff Meeting Mayo Clinic, 13, 161 (1938).

194. F. Gardner, A. Stewart, and F. O. MacCallum, Brit. Med. J., 2, 677 (1945).

195. F. O. MacCallum and W. H. Bradley, Lancet, ii, 228 (1944).

196. E. Englert, Jr., H. Brown, S. Wallach, and E. L. Simons, J. Clin. Endocrinol., 17, 1395 (1957).

197. B. Silvestrini, S. Burberi, and B. Catanese, Japan. J. Pharmacol., 18, 421 (1968).

198. R. J. W. Ryder and R. S. Schwartz, J. Immunol., 103, 970 (1969).

199. H. Wigzell, in Ref. [156], p. 82.

200. J. F. Mowbray, A. W. Boylston, J. D. Milton, and M. Weksler, in Ref. [156], p. 384.

201. R. C. Davis, S. R. Cooperband, and J. A. Mannick, J. Reticuloendothelial Soc., 7, 43 (1970).

202. C. M. Pearson and F. D. Wood, Immunology, 16, 157 (1969).

203. M. A. Kapusta and J. Mendelson, Arthritis Rheumat., 12, 463 (1969).

204. R. C. Davis, S. R. Cooperband, and J. A. Mannick, J. Immunol., 103, 1029 (1969).

205. M. H. Salaman, Proc. Roy. Soc. Med., 63, 11 (1970).

I. DRUGS FOR CHRONIC INFLAMMATORY DISEASE

206. B. M. Greenwood, E. M. Herrick, and A. Voller, Proc. Roy. Soc. Med., 63, 19 (1970).
207. W. S. Bullough, in The Biological Basis of Medicine (E. E. Bittar and N. Bittar, eds.), Vol. 1, Academic Press, New York, 1968, p. 311.
208. O. H. Iversen, in Homeostatic Regulators (G. W. Wolstenholme and J. Knight, eds.), J. and A. Churchill, London, 1969.
209. N. Radiou, F. A. Zydeck, and P. L. Wolf, Experientia, 25, 643 (1969).
210. J. F. Moorhead, E. Paraskova-Tschernozenska, A. J. Pirrie, and C. Hayes, Nature, 224, 1207 (1969).
211. W. S. Bullough and E. B. Lawrence, Europ. J. Cancer, 6, 525 (1970).
212. S. Bergström, Science, 157, 382 (1967).
213. D. H. Copp, Ann. Rev. Physiol., 32, 61 (1970).
214. C. Laden, R. Q. Blackwell, and L. S. Fosdick, Am. J. Physiol., 195, 712 (1958).
215. T. H. Rindani, Indian J. Med. Res., 44, 673 (1956).
216. G. DiPasquale and R. J. Girerd, Am. J. Physiol., 201, 1155 (1961).
217. P. Lallouette, R. Richou, A. Schwartz, and H. Richou, Compt. Rend., 270 D, 876 (1970).
218. M. E. J. Billingham, B. V. Robinson, and J. M. Robson, Brit. Med. J., 2, 93 (1969).
219. M. E. J. Billingham, B. V. Robinson, and J. M. Robson, Brit. J. Pharmacol., 35, 543 (1969).
220. D. Lee, J. Pathol., 99, 96 (1969).
221. I. Nakoneczna, J. C. Forbes, and K. S. Rogers, Am. J. Pathol., 57, 523 (1969).
222. M. W. Whitehouse, in Ref. [7], p. 400.
223. M. Steinbuch and C. Blatrix, Rev. Franc. Etudes Clin. Biol., 13, 142, 179 (1968).
224. D. Branceni and J. Gonin, Rev. Franc. Etudes Clin. Biol., 14, 754 (1969).
225. E. M. Glenn and J. Gray, Am. J. Vet. Res., 26, 1180 (1965).
226. R. Vogel, I. Trautschold, and E. Werle, Natural Proteinase Inhibitors, Academic Press, New York, 1968.
227. S. Y. Ali, L. Evans, E. Stainthorpe, and C. H. Lack, Biochem. J., 105, 549 (1967).

228. O. D. Chrisman, Clin. Orthop., 64, 77 (1969).
229. W. H. Daughaday, J. N. Heins, L. Srivastava, and C. Hammer, J. Lab. Clin. Med., 72, 803 (1968).
230. K. Hall, A. Holmgren, and U. Lindahl, Biochim. Biophys. Acta, 201, 398 (1970).
231. W. Weigel and B. Jasinski, Pathol. Microbiol. (Basel), 25, 400 (1962).
232. A. J. Bollet, Arthritis Rheumat., 11, 663 (1968).
233. D. A. Kalbhen, K. Karzel, and R. Domenjoz, Pharmacology, 1, 33 (1968).
234. H. Wagner, G. Junge-Hülsing, W. Wirth, and W. H. Hauss, Z. Rheumaforsch., 28, 287 (1969).
235. J. C. Houck, V. K. Sharma, Y. M. Patel, and J. A. Gladner, Biochem. Pharmacol., 17, 2081 (1968).
236. F. C. Bancroft, L. Levine, and A. H. Tashjian, Jr., Biochem. Biophys. Res. Comm., 37, 1028 (1969).
237. C. T. Ambrose, J. Exptl. Med., 119, 1027 (1964).
238. A. F. Burton, J. M. Storr, and W. L. Dunn, Can. J. Biochem., 45, 289 (1967).
239. J. F. Whitfield, A. D. Perris, and T. Youdale, Exptl. Cell Res., 52, 349 (1968).
240. A. N. Glazer, J. Biol. Chem., 242, 3326, 4528 (1967).
241. I. F. Skidmore and M. W. Whitehouse, Biochem. Pharmacol., 16, 737 (1967).
242. B. R. Baker, Ann. Rev. Pharmacol., 10, 35 (1970).
243. B. J. Northover, J. Pathol. Bacteriol, 94, 204, 206 (1967); Brit. J. Pharmacol. Chemotherap., 31, 483 (1967).
244. E. D. Henderson and F. F. Nathan, Southern Med. J., 62, 1455 (1969).
245. N. Pace, A. Gristina, and T. G. Kantor, Arthritis Rheumat., 12, 321 (1969).
246. M. Makin and G. Robin, Proc. Roy. Soc. Med., 61, 908 (1968).
247. L. Dazziano, J. Gagnon, and C. A. Laurin, Can. Med. Assoc. J., 101, 24 (1969).
248. A. Kajander and A. Ruotsi, Ann. Med. Internal Fenniae., 57, 87 (1967).

Chapter II

GASTROINTESTINAL DISORDERS — PEPTIC ULCER DISEASE

Jeremy H. Thompson

Department of Pharmacology and Experimental Therapeutics
U.C.L.A. School of Medicine
Los Angeles, California

I.	GASTRIC PHYSIOLOGY	116
	A. Anatomy	116
	B. Gastric Secretion	116
II.	PEPTIC ULCER DISEASE	123
	A. Definition	124
	B. Pathology	125
	C. Symptoms	127
	D. Etiology	128
III.	AVAILABLE DRUG THERAPY	138
	A. Introduction	138
	B. Antacids	139
	C. Antimuscarinics	142
	D. Musculotropic Antispasmodics	145
	E. Gastric Mucin	145
	F. Licorice Derivatives	148
	G. Antipepsins	152
	H. Synthetic Estrogens	153
	I. Miscellaneous	153
IV.	PEPTIC ULCER FORMATION IN ANIMALS	155
	A. Pylorus-Ligated (Shay) Rat	155
	B. Stress-Induced Ulcers	156
	C. Drug-Induced Ulceration	157
	D. Mann-Williamson Ulcers	158
	E. Miscellaneous	158
V.	FUTURE DRUGS FOR THE TREATMENT OF PEPTIC ULCER DISEASE	159
	A. Drugs Acting on the Central Nervous System	160
	B. Drugs Acting on the Gastrointestinal Tract	160
VI.	SUMMARY	173
	A. Inhibition of Hydrochloric Acid Secretion	174
	B. Neutralization of Hydrochloric Acid	175

Copyright © 1972 by Marcel Dekker, Inc. **NO PART of this work may be reproduced or utilized in any form or by any means,** electronic or mechanical, including Xeroxing, photocopying, microfilm, and recording, or by any information storage and retrieval system, without permission in writing from the publisher.

C. Pepsin and Mucous Production 175
D. Cell Kinetics 175
REFERENCES 176

I. GASTRIC PHYSIOLOGY

Food is swallowed down the esophagus (gullet). In the stomach it is mixed with hydrochloric acid, the proteolytic enzyme pepsin, and mucus, and then passed at a slow, controlled rate into the duodenum. In the duodenum and small bowel the food (chyme) is digested and absorbed.

A brief review of the functional anatomy of the stomach and of gastric secretion will facilitate an understanding of the etiology and treatment of peptic ulcer disease, and moreover, it will serve as a framework for a discussion of future possibilities in drug development.

A. Anatomy

The gross anatomy of the stomach and duodenum is indicated in Fig. 1. The mucosa in the fundus and body of the stomach has deep glands which contain hydrochloric acid-secreting (parietal, oxyntic) cells, pepsin-secreting (chief) cells, and mucosubstance-secreting (mucous) cells (Fig. 2). In the gastric antrum and cardiac regions, the glands secrete mucus. Gastrin (Table I), the polypeptide hormone which stimulates acid secretion, is produced by cells in the gastric antrum [1]; only about one cell in a 100 synthesizes the polypeptide. The stomach has a rich blood supply; parasympathetic and sympathetic innervation comes from the vagus nerve and the celiac plexus, respectively.

B. Gastric Secretion

Gastric juice is a highly complex fluid, but for the purposes of this chapter only hydrochloric acid, pepsin, and mucosubstances will be discussed.

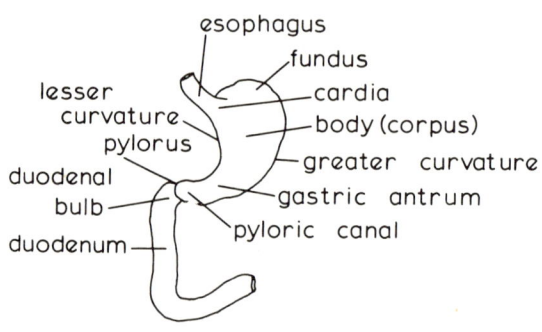

Fig. 1. Gross anatomy of the human stomach and duodenum.

II. GASTROINTESTINAL DISORDERS – PEPTIC ULCER DISEASE

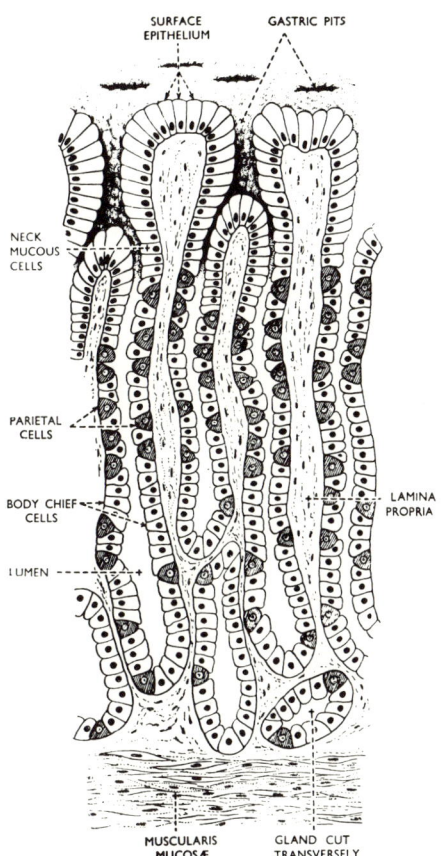

Fig. 2. Diagram of glands in the mucosa of the body of the human stomach. (Reproduced, with permission, from G. H. Bell, J. N. Davidson, and H. Scarborough, Textbook of Physiology and Biochemistry, E. and S. Livingstone Ltd., London, England, 1961, p. 236, Fig. 16.9.)

Since the overall mechanisms and control of gastric secretion are complex, only the points of direct importance will be presented.

1. Hydrochloric Acid

The quantity of gastric acid secreted at any moment is dependent on the interplay of many stimulatory and inhibitory factors [2]. Classically, gastric acid secretion has been divided into two periods, Interprandial (interdigestive, basal, unstimulated, spontaneous) and postprandial (digestive, stimulated) secretion, with postprandial secretion further separated into cephalic, gastric,

TABLE I

Structures of Gastrointestinal Polypeptide Hormones[a]

Gastrin

		1	2	3	4	5	6	7	8	9	10	11	12	13	14	15	16	17
Man [515]	[b]	Glu-	Gly-	Pro-	Trp-	Leu-	Glu-	Glu-	Glu-	Glu-	Glu-	Ala-	Tyr[c]	-Gly-	Trp-	Met-	Asp-	Phe-NH$_2$
Hog [516]							-Met-											
Dog [1, 517]							-Met-		-Ala-									
Cow and Sheep [517, 518]							-Val-			-Ala-								
Cat [518]							-(Glu$_4$-			-Ala)-								

Synthetic gastrin-like
pentapeptide [519]   N-t-butyloxycarbonyl-β-Ala-Trp-Met-Asp-Phe-NH$_2$

Caerulein [435]

$$\overset{SO_3H}{|}$$
[b] Glu -Glu-Asp-Tyr-Thr   -Gly-Trp-Met-Asp-Phe-NH$_2$

Pancreozymin-
Cholecystokinin
[451, 520]

Lys-(Ala-Gly-Pro-Ser)-Arg-Val-
(Ileu-Met-Ser)-Lys-Asp-(Asp-Glu-His
Leu$_2$-Pro-Ser$_2$)-Arg-Ileu-(Asp-Ser)-Arg-Asp-Tyr-Met

$$\overset{SO_3H}{|}$$
-Gly-Trp-Met-Asp-Phe-NH$_2$

Secretin [452]

		1	2	3	4	5	6	7	8	9	10	11	12	13	14	15	16	17	18
	[d]	His-	Ser-	Asp-	Gly-	Thr-	Phe-	Thr-	Ser-	Glu-	Leu-	Ser-	Arg-	Leu-	Arg-	Asp-	Ser-	Ala-	Arg-

19 20 21 22 23 24 25 26 27
-Leu-Gln-Arg-Leu-Leu-Gln-Gly-Leu-Val-NH$_2$

Glucagon [452] $\underline{d}$ His-Ser-Gln-Gly-Thr-Phe-Thr-Ser-Asp-Tyr-Ser-Lys-Tyr-Leu-Asp-Ser-Arg-Arg

1 2 3 4 5 6 7 8 9 10 11 12 13 14 15 16 17 18

19 20 21 22 23 24 25 26 27 28 29

-Ala-Gln-Asp-Phe-Val-Gln-Try-Leu-Met-Asn-Thr

$\underline{a}$ Except where amino acids are indicated, the sequence for gastrins of different species are similar. Amino acid sequences within brackets have not yet been elucidated.

$\underline{b}$ The N-terminal residue of the gastrins and caerulein is in the pyroglutamyl form.

$\underline{c}$ Gastrins from all species exist in two forms, I and II. In form II, SO_3 is attached to Tyr- in position 12.

$\underline{d}$ The amino acid residues common to both secretin and glucagon are underscored.

and intestinal phases; this is an artificial division indicating only the region in which a stimulus acts.

Interprandial secretion occurs in the absence of all intentional stimulation; in man it contains acid but in varying amounts [3]. The cephalic phase of postprandial secretion is mediated via the vagus nerve. Stimuli are the taste, sight, smell, or swallowing of food. Vagal impulses produce acid release by direct cholinergic stimulation of parietal cells [4], and indirectly, by the cholinergic release of gastrin [5]. Gastric secretion in the gastric phase of postprandial secretion has the same two components as seen in the cephalic phase. Both components can be activated by either long vago-vagal reflexes [6] or by short nerve reflexes within the mucosa [7, 8]. Intestinal gastrin is the mediator of acid secretion during the intestinal phase [9], but it has limited importance.

The precise mechanism of acid secretion is unknown [10, 11] but when the parietal cells are secreting at maximal rate gastric juice is nearly an isotonic solution of hydrochloric acid with a concentration of about 150 mN [10]. Schemes of acid secretion and associated metabolism are presented in Figs. 3 and 4. Recent evidence suggests cyclic AMP as being the final link in gastrin- and histamine-induced secretion [12-14].

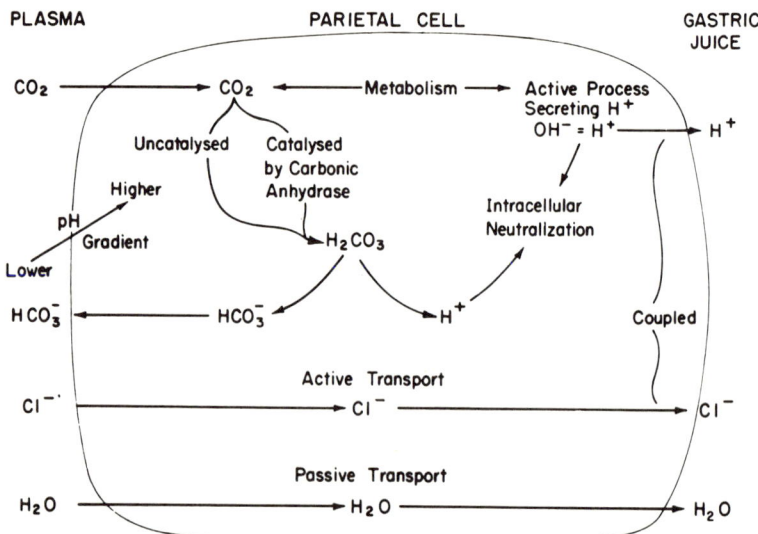

Fig. 3. A scheme of the metabolic basis for hydrochloric acid secretion. (Reproduced, with permission, from H. W. Davenport, "Metabolic Aspects of Gastric Acid Secretion," in Q. R. Murphy (Ed.), Metabolic Aspects of Transport across Cell Membranes, p. 296, Fig. 103, University of Wisconsin Press, Madison, Wisconsin, 1957.)

II. GASTROINTESTINAL DISORDERS — PEPTIC ULCER DISEASE

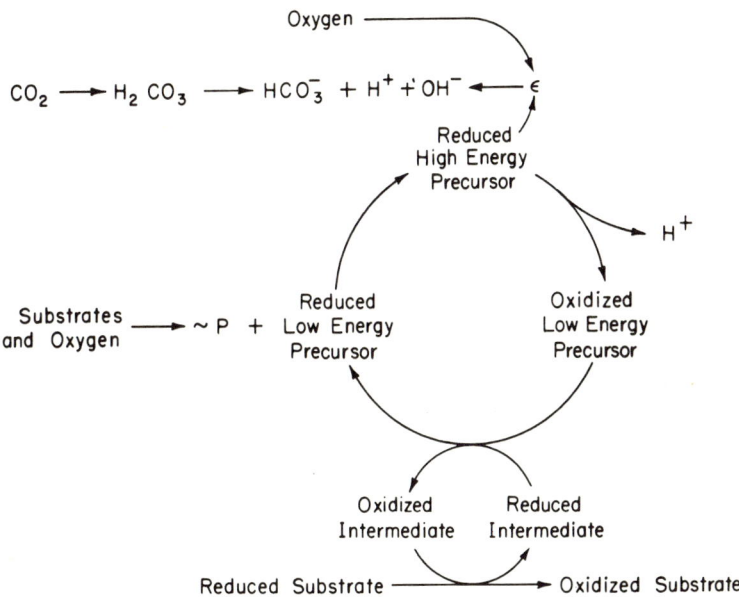

Fig. 4. Role of CO_2 in intracellular neutralization during secretion of hydrochloric acid by the gastric mucosa. (Reproduced, with permission, from H. W. Davenport, Physiology of the Digestive Tract, 2nd ed., Year Book Medical Publishers, Chicago, Illinois, 1966.)

The early discovery that hydrochloric acid could inhibit its own secretion [15] suggested the presence of important local auto-regulatory mechanisms in gastric physiology. Subsequently, liberation of gastroduodenal humoral agents have been shown to produce inhibition of gastric acid secretion; however, the concept of nerve reflex participation is still unresolved [16].

High gastric antrum acidity will effectively block local gastrin release regardless of the stimulus used [17, 18]; a nerve reflex is probably involved, but it is not known whether the mechanism is an all or none phenomenon [16]. Two suggested mechanisms dependent on decreasing pH might be either an alteration of the gastrin releasing mechanism itself or an alteration of gastrin releasing substances.

Apart from controlling gastrin release, acid in the gastric antrum may also release an antral "chalone" into the blood stream which in turn inhibits acid secretion [19]. No conclusive evidence for the existence of such a substance has been produced [16]. pH sensitive receptors are present in the gastric antrum [20] but their precise function is unknown.

An acid sensitive receptor mechanism is located within the duodenal bulb [21] which inhibits the gastric acid response to exogenous and endogenous gastrin [16, 22]. This suggests that the humoral agent involved acts at or near the parietal cell; no evidence is available suggesting that gastrin release is inhibited. A good correlation has been shown between the magnitude of secretory depression produced on the one hand, and the level of duodenal acidity achieved [23] or the rate of acid absorption on the other hand [24]. A humoral agent is probably responsible, and in animals an intact vagus nerve may have a "permissive" effect on the inhibition produced, but is not essential [22]. A local nerve reflex may be involved in the release of the humoral agent [25] which is possibly secretin and/or cholecystokinin-pancreozymin (Table I) [22, 26, 27].

In normal and duodenal ulcer patients, submaximal histamine-stimulated gastric secretion was inhibited by duodenal acidification [28, 29], but the inhibition was greater in normal individuals; maximal histamine-stimulated secretion however was not inhibited in the ulcer patients whereas inhibition occurred in normal individuals [28, 29]. This suggests that failure of acid-induced inhibitory mechanisms may be a contributory factor in peptic ulcer genesis [28, 30, 30a].

Fats and fatty acids when in an absorbable form may liberate a "chalone," enterogastrone, from intestinal mucosa, which depresses exogenous and endogenous gastrin-induced gastric acid secretion and gastric motility [9, 24, 25]. In general, the pattern of fat-induced secretory inhibition is similar to that occurring following duodenal acidification with one exception; fat is an effective inhibitor when applied throughout the intestine [24], whereas the acid-sensitive mechanism is confined to the duodenal bulb [21].

Introduction of hypertonic solutions into the duodenum results in reduction in gastric acid secretion, but the effect is not as strong as that produced by acid or fat [24]. As yet, there is no evidence that osmoreceptor mechanisms are important clinically in the control of acid secretion [16], or in ulcer etiology.

2. Pepsin(ogen)

Pepsinogen, the inactive precursor of pepsin, is synthesized and stored in the gastric chief cells [31]. Pepsinogen is composed of pepsin and peptide moieties; the terminal moiety is an inhibitor. Below pH 5.4 the pepsin-inhibitor complex dissociates, and below pH 4.0 the inhibitor is rapidly digested [32]. Using different isolation and substrate techniques "pepsin" can be fractionated into a number of proteolytic "enzymes" [10, 31, 33], but their separation and distinction for a study of this kind is unimportant.

Pepsinogen is synthesized on the endoplastic reticulum and then transported to the Golgi complex where it is encapsulated. Encapsulation is not obligatory in the path of secretion, and the stomach can secrete pepsin continuously for many hours despite histological evidence of enzyme depletion [35].

During the basal state, pepsin stores remain intact and the small continuous secretion is probably an "overflow" from continued synthesis. The most powerful stimulus to pepsin secretion is vagal stimulation, no matter how produced; complete inhibition is produced by atropine.

The immediate response to an adequate stimulus is a rapid discharge of stored pepsin; loss of enzyme granules stimulates pepsin synthesis by a positive feedback mechanism ensuring continued secretion. When secretion is inhibited, pepsinogen accumulates in the cell. Histamine and gastrin stimulate pepsin secretion in man but probably by different mechanisms since the effect of gastrin can be reduced 75 percent by atropine [31].

3. Mucosubstances

Gastric mucin is the viscous secretion of the stomach [36]. It is derived from the surface epithelium columnar cells, and the mucous neck cells of the cardiac, fundic, and pyloric gland areas [37]. It is far from homogenous, containing glycoproteins, mucopolysaccharides, and mucopolysaccharide-protein complexes [38-40].

As yet, primarily due to problems of collection and analysis, the principal mucosubstances have not been isolated or chemically characterized. Furthermore, it is not known how all the substances interrelate in normal secretion, or from what cells each component arises. The two major fractions are the acidic mucoprotein-pepsin complex and the neutral glycoprotein-mucoprotein complex [40].

The acidic mucoprotein-pepsin complex characterizes a group of acidic mucosubstances and proteins of relatively high negative charge arising primarily from the fundic area and rich in sialic acid and sulfated amino polysaccharides; carbohydrate composition is small. Pepsin and intrinsic factor are associated with this fraction [40]. The neutral glycoprotein-mucoprotein complex characterizes a group of neutral mucosubstances and proteins with low negativity and γ-globulin-like mobility. This fraction is high in carbohydrate and also contains some sialic acid. The neutral glycoprotein is of a fucomucin and sialomucin type and is related to blood group substances [40]; gastrone activity is associated with this fraction.

Secretion of alkaline mucus is spontaneous. It is increased by mechanical irritation of the mucosa and by sympathetic and parasympathetic stimulation [10, 37, 39]. However, atropine has equivocal blocking activity [39]. Mucus secretion is strongly stimulated by serotonin [41, 42].

II. PEPTIC ULCER DISEASE

Peptic ulcer disease is a familiar entity in American society since about $3\frac{1}{2}$ million people develop the condition each year [43, 44]. Ulcers have increasingly become the butt of humorists, and having an ulcer is often considered a status symbol, conferring on the victim the stamp of success, and conjuring up a picture of the busy junior executive who is always <u>with it,</u>

rushing around and <u>doing it now</u>, and like a Pinkerton agent, never sleeping. Peptic ulcers, however, are no laughing matter; in 1965, they were ranked twelfth as a cause for work absenteeism and fifteenth in the causes of death in this country [45]. Furthermore, it has been estimated that ulcer disease results in an annual economic loss of about $1 billion [44, 46], and the money spent on antacids in the United States alone has risen from about $79 million in 1964 to about $100 million in 1968 [47].

The history of man's understanding of peptic ulcer disease has been long and colorful [48]. Symptoms due to gastric ulcer were recognized by Hippocrates (460 BC), and engravings on the pillars at the temple of Aesculpius at Epidaurus, which date back to the Fourth Century, BC, describe complications of gastric ulcer [48].

Peptic ulcers are of worldwide distribution but the precise incidence is unknown. Estimates are probably conservative since symptomatology is periodic in nature and often confused with other disease states. One interesting phenomenon, however, is the changing pattern of incidence [49]; environmental factors must be responsible.

A. Definition

Peptic ulcer can be defined as a sharply circumscribed, benign, nonspecific ulcer, involving the mucosal, submucosal, and muscular layers, occurring in areas of the digestive tract exposed to acidic gastric juice containing pepsin. Peptic ulcers can develop in the esophagus, stomach, duodenum, the small bowel adjacent to the gastroenterostomy opening, or in a Meckels diverticulum, or at any other mucosal site where there is functional, heterotopic gastric mucosa. This chapter is concerned only with gastric and duodenal ulcers.

<u>Are gastric and duodenal ulcers the same disease?</u> This question is controversial. The age, sex, and social class distributions [50], the relationships to blood groups and secretor status [51], and the patterns of gastric secretion, motor activity, and number of parietal cells [52] are different between the two ulcer groups, suggesting that they may be separate entities. Furthermore, during this century there has apparently been a decrease in the incidence of duodenal ulcer, whereas the incidence of gastric ulcer has remained unchanged [49, 53]. However, gastric and duodenal ulcers occur in the same individual with greater frequency than can be considered by chance alone [54-56]. In this situation it is usually considered that the gastric ulcer follows the duodenal ulcer, possibly mediated via retarded gastric emptying and gastritis [57]; in support of this is the fact that gastric secretion has been shown to increase after gastric ulcers have healed [58].

Thus, at present, the evidence points to the two ulcer states being, if not similar, at least related.

B. Pathology

In man, most peptic ulcers occur on the posterior wall of the lesser curvature of the stomach within 6 cm of the pylorus, or on the anterior or posterior walls of the first 4 cm of the duodenum, the duodenal bulb (Fig. 5). Post bulbar ulcers are rare (Fig. 6). Ulcers are conveniently separated into acute erosions, and acute and chronic peptic ulcers.

Acute erosions do not penetrate the submucosa (muscularis mucosae). They are often multiple and may arise from small hemorrhages. Healing is usually rapid and complete, but occasionally an acute erosion may develop into a chronic ulcer. Erosions often occur in the presence of gastritis; they are commonly associated with brain injury, sepsis, stress, and burns [59].

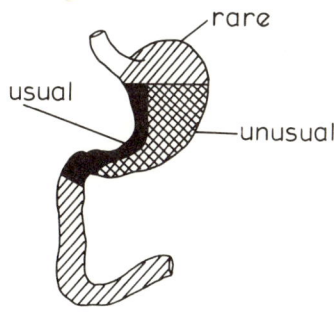

Fig. 5. Location of gastric and duodenal ulcers in man.

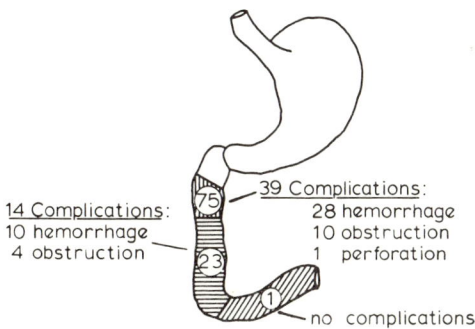

Fig. 6. Location and complications of postbulbar duodenal ulcers in man. (Reproduced, with permission, from J. A. Ramsdell et al., Ann. Intern. Med., 47, 700 (1957), Fig. 1, p. 701.)

Hemorrhage may be severe. Acute gastric erosions are probably common. In fact they may be a normal occurrence or arise from a virus infection analagous to aphthous stomatitis.

Acute and chronic peptic ulcers differ from acute erosions in that they penetrate the muscularis mucosae. They usually occur as a single, round-to-oval, punched out crater. The distinction between them is primarily a histological one based on evidence of chronicity in the form of <u>fibroplasia</u> and <u>cellular infiltration</u>. Acute ulcers are chiefly important in that they may perforate into the peritoneal cavity or give rise to hemorrhage.

Microscopically, the ulcer bed is composed of three blending layers: a fibrinous exudate infiltrated with leucocytes and erythrocytes; a layer of granulation tissue with a varying infiltrate of lymphocytes, plasma cells, and occasionally eosinophilic leucocytes; and a layer of fibroplasia. Acute ulcers are characterized by local edema, vascular engorgement, and thrombosis. The ulcer edge may be undermined and there is little fibroplastic reaction. An acute ulcer heals from the base upwards by the growth of granulation tissue and fibroblasts which are then covered by a layer of epithelium growing in from the margins. Depending on the severity of the ulceration, some glandular formation may redevelop, and the mucous containing cell is the first to reappear in a regenerating gastric gland [60]. Because the muscularis mucosae is penetrated, scarring results; however, this is usually minimal, and several weeks after healing, the site of the acute ulcer may not be apparent.

Chronic ulcers are characterized by a marked fibroplastic reaction in the ulcer bed. Vascular thrombi may be <u>organized</u>, and there is usually evidence of arteritis, periarteritis, and subintimal fibroplasia. Nerve fibers and ganglia may be completely destroyed. Adjacent mucosa may be normal, atrophic, inflammed, or cicatrized. Edema is usually less than that seen in acute ulcers and mucosal folds can be seen running up to the crater edge. Acute inflammatory changes and healing are seen side-by-side. Healing follows the same general pattern as that of an acute ulcer, but the process is slower and greater scarring results. The fibroplastic core which forms the base of the ulcer is relatively avascular and therefore cannot support adequately the regenerating epithelium. Thus, cellular differentiation is slow or nonexistent, and down-growing pouches of epithelium are likely to become cut off by the fibroplastic tissue, becoming sequestered with subsequent cystic degeneration. Pathological changes in experimentally induced ulcers in animals show some differences [61].

<u>Hemorrhage</u> may result from any ulcer. Normally hemostasis is produced by vascular constriction and thrombus formation. Fatal hemorrhages, however, may occur, particularly from multiple superficial erosions, and from chronic peptic ulcers when a major vessel in the ulcer bed becomes eroded. Since the blood vessels in the bed of a chronic peptic ulcer are encased in a dense mass of fibrous tissue, they have limited ability to contract. Disorders of gastric fibrinolysin production may be important as a cause of

gastric ulcer hemorrhage [62] and subclinical scurvy (avitaminosis C) may render patients more susceptible to aspirin-induced hemorrhage [63].

Ulcer perforation into the peritoneal cavity is more frequently seen with acute peptic ulcers. Initially a chemical peritonitis results, but bacterial contamination quickly follows. A perforation, particularly into the lesser peritoneal sac may become sealed off with the formation of an abscess. Ulcer penetration or local perforation into the pancreas or other adjacent tissue is not unusual, particularly in chronic ulcer disease. Stomal or anastomotic ulcers may develop following gastroenterostomy [64].

Gastrointestinal obstruction may result from one of two ways; acute active duodenal ulcers or juxtapyloric gastric ulcers may produce reflex pyloric sphincter closure (pylorospasm), and the marked fibroplastic reaction found with chronic ulcer healing may produce obstruction of the gastric lumen (hourglass constricture), or of the pyloric canal (pyloric stenosis).

Duodenal ulcers probably never become cancerous. In the case of gastric ulcers the problem is less clear and is confused by two facts; first, stomachs prone to develop gastric ulcer are also prone to develop cancer, and second, a cancer may initially present symptomatically as a gastric ulcer.

C. Symptoms

The majority of patients with chronic peptic ulcer disease present with a characteristic symptomatology.

Pain, the commonest symptom, is of a "burning," "gnawing," "hunger-type" quality, and is felt in the epigastrium. It occurs after meals [for example, $\frac{1}{2}$-2 h (gastric ulcer) and 1-3 h (duodenal ulcer later)], and is relieved by food, alkalis, or vomiting. Nocturnal pain is almost pathonomonic of duodenal ulcer. When penetration occurs, for example, to the pancreas, the pain becomes continuous, nonrelievable (by food and alkalis), and radiates through to the back. In uncomplicated peptic ulcers, the episodes of pain are classically periodic [65].

"Heartburn" is a burning retrosternal pain and results from acid regurgitation into the esophagus; occasionally, acid regurgitation reaches the mouth. Heartburn may be accompanied by a sudden discharge of saliva (water brash).

The mechanism of pain production is controversial [66]. Ever since the classical experiments of Lennander et al. [67], who showed that the bowel was only sensitive to stretching, and that burning, cutting, and pinching were innocuous, investigators have clung to the theory that local muscle spasm was responsible for ulcer pain [68]. However, the direct local effect of acid on nerves in the ulcer crater is probably more important [69, 70]; alternatively, acid may act indirectly by local release of histamine, bradykinin, or serotonin [71]. These hormones are present abundantly in bowel mucosa and may well have a modulating influence on afferent impulses in the splanchnic nerves.

Nausea and vomiting may occur when the pain is severe. They are more common in uncomplicated gastric as compared to duodenal ulcers. Copious vomiting usually indicates pylorospasm or cicatrical obstruction.

Appetite usually remains excellent since food relieves ulcer pain. In the elderly gastric ulcer patient, anorexia may be prominent.

D. Etiology

Since the detailed description of peptic ulcer in 1828 [72], theories concerning etiology have abounded, but a generally acceptable unifying hypothesis has not yet been advanced. Quincke [73] was probably the first to use the term "peptic ulcer," and certainly the importance of acid and pepsin in etiology has been stressed in the very name of the disease. However, although a peptic ulcer does not form in the absence of acid, as originally stated in 1910 by Schwarz [74], many other variable factors determine whether or not an ulcer will form when both acid and pepsin are present; it is fallacious to consider that there is a single "cause."

According to Shay [75], the development of chronic peptic ulcer is determined by the algebraic sum of defensive and aggressive factors acting on gastric secretion and the gastroduodenal mucosa (Fig. 7); an extension of this thesis (Figs. 8 and 9) has recently been proposed by Bralow [45]. To explain the propensity of some anatomical sites to peptic ulceration, Oi et al. [76] have recently proposed a "dual control mechanism" based on the relationship of nonacid- to acid-secreting mucosa, and the position and arrangement of gastric muscle bundles.

In the following paragraphs an attempt has been made to summarize some of the pertinent etiological factors in peptic ulcer disease since an understanding of ulcer etiology is an essential prerequisite to a rational approach to drug treatment and ulcer prevention. Only classical or key references are cited since the literature on peptic ulcer disease is enormous. Methodology is not discussed, since this is more appropriately obtained from the original sources. Chronological reviews should be consulted for more detailed information [45, 75, 77-79].

1. Environmental Factors

a. Geographical differences. Peptic ulcers are found world-wide but few thorough studies are available to indicate actual incidence [80]. Comparisons between gastric ulcer : duodenal ulcer ratios have shown, generally speaking, that duodenal ulcers are more common; two exceptions have been identified [81, 82]. Regional differences in ulcer ratio have been found in the United Kingdom [53], India [83], and Nigeria [84]. Duodenal ulcer may be more common in the U. S. than in the United Kingdom [80].

b. Diet. Heavy sugar consumption [85, 86] and a diet high in refined cereals [86-88] may contribute to peptic ulcer disease. Other dietary factors may be partly responsible for the changing incidence of peptic ulcer

II. GASTROINTESTINAL DISORDERS — PEPTIC ULCER DISEASE

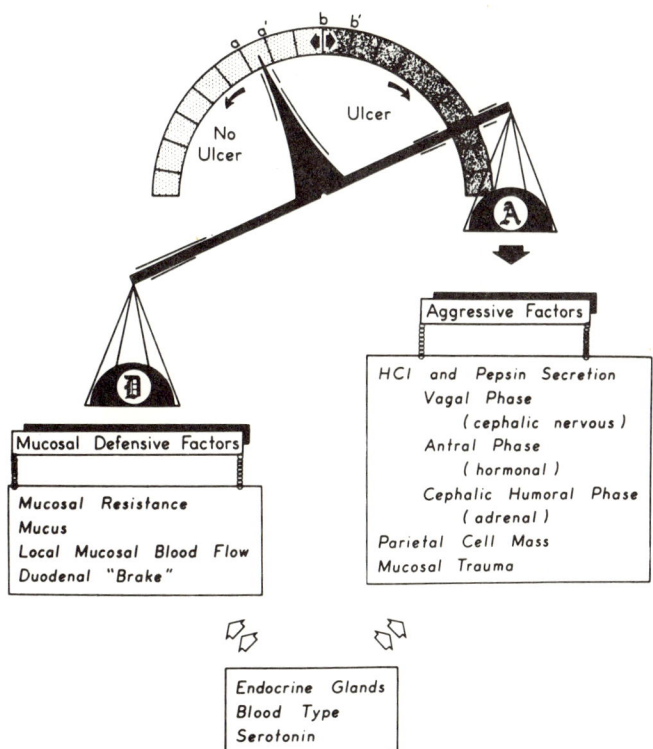

Fig. 7. Etiology of peptic ulcer. (Reproduced, with permission, from H. Shay, "Etiology of Peptic Ulcer," in G. McHardy (Ed.), <u>Current Gastroenterology</u>, Paul B. Hoeber, Medical Department, Harper and Row, New York, 1962, p. 277, Fig. 1.)

seen in this century. Intensive epidemiological studies of so-called primitive peoples while adjusting to the ways of the western civilization may be of value in evaluating the importance of dietary factors in ulcer etiology.

c. Occupation. In the United Kingdom [50], duodenal ulcer is more common among physicians and business executives than other professions. Similarly, in the United States duodenal ulcer is more frequently found in female physicians than in the general female population [49]. In the United Kingdom, duodenal ulcer has a low incidence in agricultural laborers [50].

d. Tobacco, Alcohol, and Drugs. Doll et al. [89] have shown that the proportion of life-long smokers is higher among patients with peptic ulcer disease than controls, and that the overall mortality from duodenal ulcer is greater for smokers than for nonsmokers. Gastric ulcers heal more rapidly

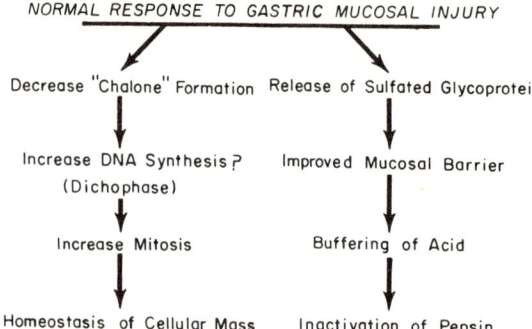

Fig. 8. Normal response to gastric mucosal injury. Acute injury to normal gastric mucosa may set in motion concomitant response which increases cellular mitosis and neutralizes secondary aggressive factors of acid and pepsin. (Reproduced, with permission, from S. P. Bralow, "Current Concepts of Peptic Ulceration," Am. J. Digestive Disease, 14, 655 (1969), p. 669, Fig. 2.)

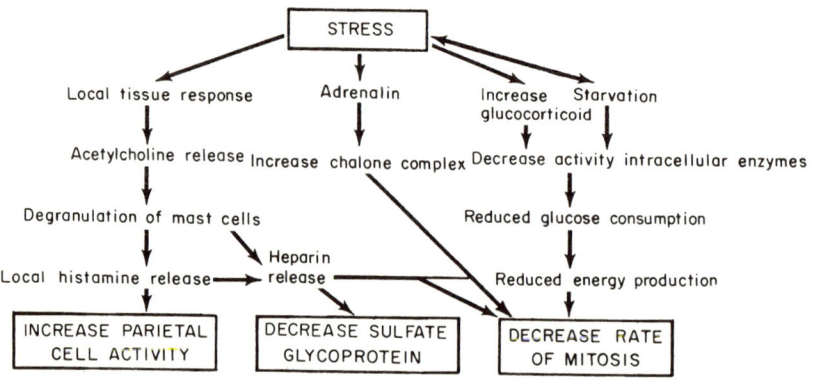

Fig. 9. Ulcerogenic response to gastric mucosal injury. When injury is more severe or chronic the initiation of decrease in rate of mitosis, decrease in secretion of sulfated glycoproteins, and increase in parietal cell activity may result in ulcer formation. These three functions are intimately related at the neck of the gastric gland. Both mitosis and glycoprotein secretion occur at the base of the duodenal crypt. (Reproduced, with permission, from S. P. Bralow, "Current Concepts of Peptic Ulceration," Am. J. Digestive Disease, 14, 655 (1969), p. 670, Fig. 3.)

in those who stop smoking than those who do not [90] and nicotine and aqueous extracts of tobacco smoke condensate have been shown to stimulate gastric acid and pepsin secretion [91, 92].

II. GASTROINTESTINAL DISORDERS – PEPTIC ULCER DISEASE

Alcohol is both a gastric secretory stimulant [2] and a mucosal irritant [93].

Aspirin ingestion is frequently followed by multiple small, superficial gastric erosions which bleed [94]. Recently, Davenport has suggested [95] that as it is absorbed, aspirin increases mucosal permeability by damaging the gastric lipid-protein layers. The resulting increased permeability allows hydrogen ions to back diffuse into the mucosa producing further damage to capillaries sensitized by histamine release.

Aspirin may also increase epithelial cell exfoliation [96], reduce the secretion of mucus [42], and alter its composition [97] and physiochemical properties [98, 99]. Aspirin has been shown to inhibit oxidative phosphorylation [100] and the synthesis of connective tissue polysaccharides in fibroblasts in vitro [101].

Antacids and antimuscarinic agents reduce aspirin-induced gastric mucosal damage [102].

Several other commonly used drugs have been shown to induce or activate peptic ulcers in both animals and man, and a variety of mechanisms has been postulated [14, 42, 95, 103-106]: (a) production of local tissue damage (phenylbutazone, cinchophen); (b) stimulation of hydrochloric acid secretion (caffeine, theophyline, alcohol, reserpine); (c) interference with epithelial cell renewal (corticosteroids, 5-fluorouracil); (d) reduction of mucus secretion (phenylbutazone, ACTH and glucocorticoids, cinchophen, and serotonin antagonists); and (e) activation of histidine decarboxylase (indomethacin, phenylbutazone, acetylsalicylic acid, and fluphenamic acid).

2. Constitutional Factors

a. Race. One good example of racial differences is the rarity of peptic ulcer in the South African Bantu whereas the white South African has an incidence similar to that in the United Kingdom [57]. Racial factors are intimately associated with geographical, dietary, and hereditary factors.

b. Age. Peptic ulcers occur at all ages. The annual expectation of developing an ulcer is almost constant at a rate of 3.2 ulcers/1000 men [50]. In women peptic ulcer incidence rises to a maximum of about 6 percent at 55 years [107].

c. Sex. About 80 percent of peptic ulcers occur in men [53]. Ulcers are rare in women during the reproductive years and particularly during pregnancy, but after the menopause the incidence increases sharply [107, 108]. In the case of acute gastric erosions causing massive hemorrhage, and in peptic ulcers in children before puberty, the sex distribution is equal.

d. Heredity. There is more than twice the incidence of peptic ulcer in close relatives of peptic ulcer patients than in the population as a whole [109]. Furthermore, gastric and duodenal ulcers are apparently inherited independently [110]; the inheritance for gastric ulcer is linked to a recessive gene

[111]. Heredity may partly explain the increased incidence of peptic ulcer in some patients since stomach size, parietal cell mass, and blood group, for example, are among the important but variable factors influencing the frequency and severity of the disease.

3. Hydrochloric Acid Secretion

Peptic ulcer does not develop in the absence of acid secretion (achlorhydria) [112, 113]. Acid hypersecretion due to stimulation of the vagus nerve [114] with or without an increased number of parietal cells [52, 115, 116] is present in some patients with the disease. However, the concentration of acid is not the critical factor in ulcerogenesis since many individuals have hypersecretion and no ulcer, and many patients with ulcers have normal or subnormal secretion [117]; there does seem however to be a threshold of acid secretion below which duodenal ulcers will not occur [117].

Acid must be present to maintain an ulcer, but hypersecretion by the parietal cells although increasing ulcer liability is not by itself sufficient. One possible exception to this may be the Zollinger-Ellison syndrome [118]; however, even here, other humoral or constitutional factors may be operating.

4. Number of Parietal Cells

In spite of the fact that gastric parietal cells secrete hydrochloric acid at a concentration of about 150 mN [10], interest in the total number of parietal cells is of relatively recent origin [116, 119]. Early reports showed that there was a relationship between acid response to a test meal and the number of parietal cells [120], and that on the average, the number of parietal cells was higher in duodenal ulcer patients than in controls or those with gastric ulcer [116, 119]. It is well known that the maximal histamine response as defined by Kay [115] yields a satisfactory estimate of the number of parietal cells [52, 121], and that both the number of parietal cells and the maximal acid output are about twofold greater in the majority of patients with duodenal ulcer than in healthy controls [52, 115, 116, 121]. According to Cox [116] the number of parietal cells in healthy men and women is about 1.09 and 0.82 x 10^9, respectively. In patients with duodenal ulcer this is increased to the level 1.52 - 1.90 x 10^9 [52, 116]. The number of parietal cells in patients with gastric ulcer is usually low, 0.63 - 0.80 x 10^9 [52, 116], probably reflecting evidence of gastritis. In spite of the varying number of parietal cells, the maximal histamine response/billion parietal cells is essentially constant [75].

Due in part to pyloric obstruction and gastric dilation, patients with duodenal ulcer tend to have larger stomachs than either normal or gastric ulcer patients [122], and acid hypersecretion may be due to an increased number of parietal cells [123]. This is supported by experiments in rats with induced pyloric obstruction [124]. However, the greater stomach size and number of parietal cells could be the result of chronic hyperstimulation [116, 125]. In rats both histamine and synthetic gastrin (ICI-50123) have

II. GASTROINTESTINAL DISORDERS — PEPTIC ULCER DISEASE

been shown to increase the number of parietal cells [124, 126, 127], whereas chronic treatment with antimuscarinic agents has given controversial results [128-130]. Vagotomy is not followed by a reduced number of parietal cells [131].

5. Mucosal Resistance

Resistance to digestion by acid and pepsin is an inherent property of normal mucosa. It was recognized in 1772 by John Hunter [132] who suggested that mucosal resistance was due to an "unknown living principle." When resistance is lowered, ulceration may develop even in the presence of subnormal acid and pepsin secretion. Factors associated with producing diminished resistance are: nutritional deficiencies [133], fungal infection [134], alcohol and drugs [95], mucosal injury [121], decreased mucosal blood flow [135], and gastritis [136-138]. Gastritis may result from regurgitation of duodenal contents [137-140] or from an autoimmune attack [141]; however, in the case of autoimmunity, the antigastric antibodies probably arise as the result of mucosal damage and are not the prime cause [138].

The commonly accepted idea that gastritis in gastric ulcer patients produces acid hyposecretion [142] with return to normal production on ulcer healing [58] may be artifactual since hydrogen ions can back diffuse into damaged mucosa and exchange with sodium ions [95]. Back diffusion may increase tissue damage and cause hemorrhage [95, 143, 144].

6. Mucosubstances

Following Claude Bernard's suggestion that gastric mucous protected the underlying mucosa from damage [145], the integrity of the gastric mucous-producing cells and their secretion have been generally accepted as an important defense mechanism [42, 146, 147]. Mucosubstances are a heterogenous mixture of mucoproteins of which only several components have been separated [38, 42, 148]; as well as mucous itself, soluble blood group substances [149], gastrone [150], and sulfated glycoproteins [148, 151, 152] are of direct interest. The mucous lining is normally in a state of dynamic equilibrium, since mucous lost from the surface mucosa is rapidly replaced.

Mucous adheres tenaciously to the epithelium, thereby protecting it not only because of its buffering and absorbant properties [153], but also because it is relatively impermeable to injurious substances such as pepsin, drugs, and toxins. Ulcers result if the mucous layer is breached [146, 154]. A number of potent anti-inflammatory agents, ACTH, cortisone, aspirin, indomethacin, and phenylbutazone, which frequently cause ulcers, all reduce mucin secretion [42]; in addition, the mucous secreted is qualitatively altered by a selective decrease in its sialic acid content. This reduction in sialic acid content may be directly important, since mucosubstances without a terminal sialic acid moiety are less resistant to acid and pepsin digestion than normal mucous [155]. Growth hormone increases mucous production, a fact which may explain why this hormone can inhibit ulcer formation in rodents in spite of increased acid and pepsin output [156].

"Gastrones" are substances present in saliva and gastric juice which inhibit gastric acid secretion [150]. Gastrone activity of human anacid gastric juice has been shown to reside in two separate fractions [157]. One of these fractions has a molecular weight of between 10,000 and 40,000; it is a nondialyzable glycoprotein, with γ-globulin-like properties and is susceptible to peptic digestion. The second component has a molecular weight of over 100,000 and resembles the mucosubstances in carbohydrate content, electrophoretic mobility, and resistance to peptic digestion; in the pylorus-ligated rat the glycoprotein fraction was more potent in inhibiting gastric acid secretion than the high molecular weight fraction.

Sulfated glycoproteins are released by drugs such as urecholine [148, 152], and by forming a complex with cellular proteins they reduce peptic activity [151]. Direct intracellular combination with pepsin(ogen) may also be important [158].

So far there is little evidence that peptic ulcer patients have either a quantitative or qualitative abnormality in mucous production [134, 157, 159, 160]; however, reduced gastrone activity [161] and increased gastric mucus viscosity [162] have been found in some patients with duodenal ulcer.

7. Blood Group and Secretor Status

Peptic ulcers are more likely to develop in individuals with Blood Group (BG) O phenotype [163-165] and the relative risk for developing a duodenal or gastric ulcer among BG O as compared to BG A, B, or AB, is 1.28:1, and 1.16:1, respectively; the risk is higher still for anastomotic (stomal) peptic ulcers [165]. BG associations for gastric ulcer differ depending on the anatomical location: Patients with gastric ulcers in the body of the stomach and no duodenal ulcer are more likely to be of BG A phenotype, whereas patients with prepyloric gastric ulcers, or gastric ulcers and duodenal ulcers are more likely to be of BG O phenotype [166, 167].

About 75 percent of all individuals are "secretors," that is, they secrete BG ABH antigens in body secretions such as saliva and gastric juice [51]. The ability to secrete is an inherited dominant trait which is independent of the inheritance of the BG phenotype; there may not however be a perfect correlation between gastric cell BG composition and host BG [168]. ABH nonsecretors have up to a 40 percent greater risk of developing peptic ulcer than have secretors [169, 170]. In the case of BG O and nonsecretor status, the genes are additive [171, 172] and the risk of duodenal ulcer is greater than twofold when compared to BG A, B, or AB secretors [51, 169]; in addition, the risk of ulcer complications is greater [173-175]. Why secretors are relatively protected is not known, but it may be related to gastric mucous quality and mucosal resistance, since the mucopolysaccharide BG substances are present in mucosal cells of secretors and relatively absent in nonsecretors [176, 177]. However, failure to secrete the specific ABH antigens is compensated for by an increase in secretion of the nonspecific Le (Lewis) antigen. Since there are only minor differences in the composition of ABH and Le BG antigens [178], the total quality of salivary BG substances as

II. GASTROINTESTINAL DISORDERS — PEPTIC ULCER DISEASE

measured by fucose content is constant independent of secretor status [51]. This suggests that the relative immunity enjoyed by the secretor is not due to the protective action of the BG substance itself but to some other mechanism, possibly immunological [51]. Similarly, there is no evidence that the H substance of BG O affords less protection against ulceration [179]; however, gastric mucosal cell loss following aspirin ingestion is greater in patients with BG O and in ABH nonsecretors than in controls [180].

The output of acid and pepsin in relationship to BG and secretor status is controversial [171, 179, 181, 182], but according to Ventzke and Grossman, acid hypersecretion in patients with duodenal ulcer is unlikely to be determined by BG or secretor status [183].

8. Mucosal Blood Flow

An intact mucosal blood flow is essential for normal mucosal secretion and cellular integrity and renewal. Virchow [184] was one of the first to suggest that ulcers resulted from reduced mucosal blood flow ("aseptic vascular occlusion") but, although the vasoactive substances epinephrine [135], 5-hydroxytryptophan, and serotonin [185, 186] produce ulceration, the lesions are superficial and tend to heal rapidly. In rats, release of mast cell histamine, heparin, and serotonin by stress has been suggested as a prime cause of ulcer production [187].

Peptic ulcer formation has been blamed on mucosal anoxia resulting from embolization of end arteries [188] or from shunting of blood through arterio-venous anastomoses [189]; neither of these mechanisms, however, has been satisfactorily proved. A vascular diathesis predisposing to ulceration has also been suggested [190].

An increase in gastric vein free plasmin levels associated with an increased mucosal plasminogen activator has recently been found in peptic ulcer patients; these changes associated with abnormal fibrinolysis have been suggested as contributory factors in ulcer genesis and ulcer bleeding [62].

9. Epithelial Cell Kinetics

In normal individuals, gastric mucosal cell loss as calculated from the DNA content of gastric juices occurs at the rate of about one-half million cells/min [191] and renewal occurs from the rapidly growing germ cells at the base of the gastric pits [191, 192]. In states of tissue damage such as gastritis, the mitotic rate increases [191]. As yet, reduction in mitotic rate has not been found in peptic ulcer patients; however, stressed animals demonstrate a diminished cell renewal [193-196] which occurs in both histologically normal and ulcerated mucosa [193, 194]. The cause for this reduced activity is not known, but many factors such as ACTH, glucocorticoids, and heparin [196, 197], starvation [194], and hormones [61, 198] depress mitosis and can be theoretically applied to peptic ulcer in man. Mitosis under normal conditions is controlled by specific tissue inhibitors (chalones) or stimulators [195] but little is known about these agents in the gut.

10. Endocrine Glands

The major endocrine glands constitute a closely integrated system making it difficult to determine the effect of individual hormones upon gastric secretion and peptic ulcer production. Only a few general comments will be made; reviews should be consulted for more information [79, 199]. Cyclic 3',5'-AMP (adenosine-3',5'-phosphate) may be one of the final links in hormonal action [200, 201]. It is synthesized by adenyl cyclase and degraded by cyclic nucleotide phosphodiesterase to inactive 5'-AMP (adenosine-5'-phosphate). Tissue levels of cyclic 3',5'-AMP are increased by ACTH [202], glucagon [203], pitressin [204], and parathormone [205] which augment the activity of adenyl cyclase, and by methyl xanthines (theophylline and caffeine) which inhibit cyclic nucleotide phosphodiesterase [106, 206].

a. Pituitary.
Posterior pituitary hormone probably plays no role in normal gastric secretion; however, it may produce acute gastric erosions in animals, probably from reduced mucosal blood flow. Hypophysectomy removes control of several endocrine glands and is usually followed by involutional changes in many tissues; reduction in gastric secretion has been reported in the rat [126] and man [207].

b. Adrenal medulla.
Catecholamine release from the medulla has a far greater influence on other body systems than on gastric secretion. Local catecholamine release in the gastric mucosa reduces blood flow and produces ulceration [135] and epinephrine has been shown to reduce gastric juice volume and acid output in man [208].

c. Adrenal cortex.
Corticosteroids are "permissive" for gastric secretion under normal circumstances [209-211]. There is achlorhydria in Addisons disease [212] and replacement therapy restores secretion [213]. Conversely, gastric secretion is increased in Cushings disease and returns to normal following adrenalectomy [214]. In animals, the fall in acid output after adrenalectomy is not associated with a change in the number of parietal cells, but just reflects a general metabolic disorder [215, 216]. Corticosteroids have been shown to alter gastric mucous [42] and increase the number of parietal cells.

As far as peptic ulcer is concerned, it is important to separate the possible role of adrenal hormones under normal physiological conditions, including "stress," and the clinical situation occurring when massive doses of steroids are used, often with other drugs such as aspirin and phenylbutazone, etc. Gray et al. [217] considered that emotional and physical stress stimulated increased acid and pepsin secretion via the hypothalamic-pituitary-adrenal-gastric axis, but this is a normal physiological reflex, and in the absence of other contributory factors would be unlikely to produce peptic ulcer. Certainly excretion of 17-ketosteroids and 17-hydroxycorticosteroids are normal in peptic ulcer patients [218].

Massive doses of glucocorticosteroids increase the risk of peptic ulcer formation and increase the risk of perforation and hemorrhage from one already present. It is unlikely that these effects are mediated through an alteration of acid/pepsin secretion. Alteration of the gastric mucous barrier and a general "anti-inflammatory" action are probably more important [219]. It is not clear whether the ulceration seen with massive steroid therapy bears any relationship etiologically to the usual ulcer developing in otherwise healthy people.

d. Thyroid. Thyroxine is probably essential for normal gastric secretion, but its mode of action is unknown [199].

e. Parathyroid. Peptic ulcer is common in hyperparathyroidism [220]. The mechanism is not clear but is probably due to the elevated serum calcium level and not a direct effect of the parathormone [221]; calcium infusions in man have been found to increase acid and pepsin output by vagal stimulation [222]. Parathyroid hyperplasia may be associated with hyperplasia of other endocrine glands, the multiple adenoma syndrome, or the polyglandular syndrome [223, 224].

f. Pancreas. The Zollinger-Ellison syndrome due to uncontrolled gastrin production by pancreatic tumors [118] has achieved widespread recognition; gastrin-induced acid hypersecretion is presumably the cause of ulceration seen in this condition [225]. Patients with the Zollinger-Ellison syndrome have a 6- to 8-fold increase in the number of parietal cells [226].

Excessive insulin production has been found in some patients with duodenal ulcers and vagal overactivity has been blamed for ulcer formation [227].

Glucagon (Table I) is a 29-amino-acid peptide secreted by the α- (A-) cells of the pancreatic islets [228]. In man, it inhibits spontaneous gastric acid and pepsin secretion [229] and in dogs the hormone inhibits both vagus-stimulated and gastrin-stimulated secretion [199, 230, 231]; histamine-stimulated secretion is not inhibited [230]. Glucagon-induced gastric secretory inhibition is not dependent on hyperglycemia [230] and the hormone resists passage through the liver [230].

g. Ovary. Female sex hormones (estrogens) are protective against peptic ulcer formation since women are less likely to develop peptic ulcer during the reproductive years, but after the menopause ulcer incidence abruptly increases [108]. In addition, perforated peptic ulcer is rare in pregnancy [108], and cinchophen-induced ulcers in dogs are inhibited by estrogens [232]. In rats, prednisolone-induced gastric ulcers heal more rapidly during pregnancy [233], possibly due to increased epithelial cell renewal [234]. Stilbesterol is therapeutically effective in treating peptic ulcer in men [235].

11. Emotional Stress and Anxiety

The concept that peptic ulcers develop more frequently in the oversensitive, overconscientious, overanxious individual is by no means proven [236, 237]; however, anxiety, resentment, frustrations, and emotional or physical stresses are etiologically important in that they lead to ulcer intractability [75, 236, 238].

The pathway through which "stress" operates is not clear; parasympathetic overactivity or the endocrine glands may be responsible. Recently chronic stimulation of the anterior hypothalamus in cats was found to produce an increase in the total number of gastric parietal and chief cells [239], and in monkeys chronic hypothalamic stimulation increased the sensitivity of the parietal cells to submaximal histamine stimulation; pepsin production and adrenal glucocorticoid output were not affected [240].

12. Association of Peptic Ulcer with Other Diseases

Clues to the etiology of peptic ulcer have been sought in association of the disease with other conditions. However, since peptic ulcers are common, they have been associated with almost every disease other than those characterized by anacidity [112, 113]. Peptic ulcer is commoner in patients with alcoholic cirrhosis [241] and biliary cirrhosis [242]; this may be due to a reduced capacity to neutralize the duodenal contents. Peptic ulceration has been reported to follow portocaval shunting [243], and an increased number of parietal cells with augmented acid secretion has been demonstrated [244]. Patients with tissue anoxia from chronic pulmonary disease, particularly emphysema and cor pulmonale are likely to develop peptic ulceration; similarly aortic stenosis and arteriosclerotic heart disease seem to be predisposing factors [245]. Peptic ulcer develops in about 20 percent of patients with rheumatoid arthritis; however, this may partly be due to concomitant drug therapy [246].

III. AVAILABLE DRUG THERAPY

A. Introduction

The overall medical treatment of peptic ulcer disease is controversial since spontaneous remission has made it difficult to evaluate the benefit of any single regimen. The prime objectives of treatment, however, are the relief of symptoms, particularly pain, acceleration of ulcer healing, and prevention of relapse. In general, pain relief is secured by protecting the mucosa from acid and pepsin digestion using antacids and antimuscarinic drugs and by the relief of emotional stress with sedatives. Acceleration of ulcer healing and prevention of relapse are more difficult to evaluate, and apart from the deleterious effects of tobacco smoking [90] little is known about these phenomena. Dietary control is probably relatively unimportant [247], but variations in gastric pH are less when diets are given two-hourly than when given four-hourly [248]; thus, frequent feeding is probably more important than the actual diet. Surgical removal of the gastric antrum and vagotomy are efficient methods of reducing acid secretion but will not be considered here.

1. Hydrochloric Acid

Attempts to reduce parietal cell secretion have not been entirely successful. The popular concept that "stress" and emotional factors stimulate acid secretion prompted the use of <u>sedatives</u> and <u>tranquilizers</u> in the treatment of peptic ulcer. These drugs certainly reduce tension and worry by depression of the limbic system [249], but they have little action in reducing gastric acid secretion. Antimuscarinic drugs have achieved some popularity in reducing interprandial and postprandial secretion since they are partly under cholinergic control. However, to effectively reduce acid secretion they need to be given in doses which produce symptoms of systemic parasympathetic blockade. Carbonic anhydrase inhibitors are of no practical value since parietal cell carbonic anhydrase is present in excess [10]. Furthermore, there is a theoretical disadvantage to their use in that they may increase pepsin release [35]. Because histamine induces copious gastric acid secretion, innumerable antihistamine preparations have been tested for possible antisecretory effects. To date, none has shown any therapeutic value [250]. Parenthetically, there is no conclusive evidence as yet that histamine plays a role in normal gastric acid secretion [2]. Thus, there is no drug which effectively prevents hydrochloric acid secretion at the parietal cell, and the majority of drugs used are antacids which neutralize and buffer preformed hydrochloric acid.

2. Pepsin and Mucosubstances

Anti-muscarinic drugs have been used to reduce pepsin secretion. However, the same limitations apply as described in the previous paragraph. Several antipepsins have been used and are discussed below. Carbenoxolone sodium probably acts by increasing mucus production.

B. Antacids

1. Mechanism of Action

The most important mechanism of antacid action is direct chemical neutralization of preformed hydrochloric acid.

$$AB + CD \rightarrow AD + CB \tag{1}$$

Most antacids contain a weakly basic moiety which is sufficient to elevate the gastric pH above 4.5 (see below) but not strong enough to produce mucosal damage. Other less important mechanisms of action with aluminum antacids are absorption of HCl, and absorption and inactivation of pepsin. Some antacids, by forming a colloidal suspension, protectively coat the mucosa and ulcer crater.

2. Principles of Use

Antacids are used to raise the gastric pH to about 4.5, at which point the proteolytic enzyme pepsin becomes inactive [251], and to relieve pain. Complete acid neutralization is not desirable since this results in rebound acid secretion due to excessive release of pyloric gland area gastrin and an increased gastric emptying. The efficiency of an antacid depends upon the quantity of acid secreted, the neutralizing capacity of the drug (drug solubility and rate of buffering), and the rate of gastric emptying. Of these variable factors, the rate of gastric emptying is the most important [252, 253] and no antacid can be relied upon to give effective neutralization for longer than an hour; in many instances, a shorter period is operative.

3. Classification

Classically, antacids have been grouped into "systemic" or "nonsystemic" agents depending on whether the cationic fraction is absorbed or retained in the bowel lumen, respectively; cationic absorption produces alkalosis and an expanded extracellular fluid volume, a situation which is exaggerated by chloride loss (gastric suction or vomiting). Confusion exists, however, in this separation, since certain nonsystemic antacids, notably calcium carbonate, occasionally produce systemic alkalosis [254]. The usual explanation proposed to account for lack of a systemic effect with a nonsystemic antacid, for example magnesium hydroxide, is that after the magnesium ions neutralize hydrogen ions in the gastric lumen, they subsequently combine with bicarbonate ions in the small bowel, forming relatively insoluble magnesium carbonate. Recently Schroeder [255] has confirmed this theory, and has further shown that concomitant administration of an ion exchange resin with a high affinity for magnesium ions readily produces systemic alkalosis from absorption of excessive bicarbonate ions. Schroeder has proposed a similar etiological mechanism involving calcium phosphate formation [255] to account for the systemic alkalosis occurring with calcium carbonate therapy [254].

There is a bewildering plethora of antacids available [253, 256, 257]. Sodium bicarbonate is the only important systemic antacid; the nonsystemic antacids most frequently used are basic compounds of calcium, magnesium, and aluminum. Milk, anion exchange resins, and gastric mucin are of less importance.

4. Clinical Use

Antacids are considered the mainstay of treatment for two reasons: Theoretically, by neutralizing HCl antacids should increase the rate of ulcer healing since acid is a prerequisite for ulcer formation; in addition, antacids are the most effective agents available for relief of ulcer pain.

To date, there are no well-controlled clinical trials which convincingly show antacids increase the rate of ulcer healing [258] or reduce recurrence rate. However, experimental evidence suggests that healed duodenal ulcer mucosa is less likely to break down than normal mucosa [259].

Practically, antacid solutions or fine suspensions are preferred over solids or coarse powders; liquid preparations permeate gastric contents more easily, whereas solids may sediment out [260]. Nonsystemic antacids are preferred over systemic agents; however, excessive sodium absorption may be a problem [261].

Although there are many observable differences between the various antacids in vitro, the major factors in selecting one for clinical use are unrelated to neutralizing ability since gastric emptying controls the duration of action; thus, important considerations for antacid selection are, patient

II. GASTROINTESTINAL DISORDERS — PEPTIC ULCER DISEASE

acceptance (palatability), cost, ease of administration, and adverse effects.

Antacids are effective only if taken over long periods of time, and the rapid relief of ulcer pain (usually occurring within days of commencing therapy) is not an indication for a reduction in dosage. Antacids are more likely to achieve good results in acute ulceration. Furthermore, attention to diet, rest, sedation, antimuscarinic drugs, and the removal of irritant drugs are often just as important.

a. Sodium Bicarbonate. Sodium bicarbonate is a cheap, easily obtained antacid. It neutralizes acid rapidly due to its high solubility:

$$NaHCO_3 + HCl \rightarrow NaCl + H_2O + CO_2 \qquad (2)$$

About 12 mEq acid are neutralized by 1.0 g, but large doses are required therapeutically since the drug rapidly leaves the stomach.

Sodium bicarbonate may produce systemic alkalosis, and CO_2 liberated in the stomach by acid neutralization may accentuate ulcer pain and may lead to perforation in gastric ulcer.

b. Precipitated Calcium Carbonate. Calcium carbonate is an effective and inexpensive antacid. It buffers acid rapidly, 1.0 g neutralizing about 20 mEq acid. Calcium carbonate has a more prolonged action than sodium bicarbonate and reacts thus:

$$CaCO_3 + 2HCl \rightarrow CaCl_2 + H_2O + CO_2 \qquad (3)$$

The $CaCl_2$ forms insoluble calcium soaps in the bowel lumen, and the chloride is absorbed. Calcium carbonate has a chalky taste which may be intolerable to some patients. Calcium soaps may produce constipation or even fecal concretion. Nausea can be troublesome, but CO_2 production is rarely important. The milk-alkali syndrome [262] may occur with soluble alkalis, for example, sodium bicarbonate, or with excessive calcium and milk ingestion. In the latter case, calcium absorption is facilitated by the lactose and galactose of milk.

c. Magnesium Antacids. Magnesium hydroxide. Magnesium hydroxide is a 7.0-8.5 percent aqueous suspension. It is almost insoluble, but in the stomach the magnesium chloride formed on acid neutralization is soluble. About 2.7 mEq acid are neutralized by 1.0 ml.

Magnesium oxide. Magnesium oxide is less popular than other magnesium preparations in spite of its efficiency; about 50 mEq acid are neutralized by 1.0 g. Magnesium oxide acts slowly since it must first be converted into magnesium hydroxide in the stomach. Two chemically identical preparations are available, a light form and a heavy form. Light magnesium oxide is more bulky, but since it has a greater rate of dispersion than heavy magnesium oxide it is therapeutically preferable.

Magnesium trisilicate. Magnesium trisilicate is a compound of magnesium oxide, silicon dioxide, and water and acts slowly, owing to poor dispersion and solubility. It is a relatively poor acid neutralizer, 1.0 g neutralizes about 10 mEq acid:

$$2MgO \cdot 3SiO_2 \cdot n(H_2O) + 4HCl \rightarrow 2MgCl_2 + 3SiO_2 + n + 2H_2O \qquad (4)$$

In the small bowel, the magnesium chloride converts to magnesium carbonate and the chloride is adsorbed. The gelatinous consistency of the silicon dioxide, liberated as an end-product of the acid neutralization, may protectively coat the ulcer crater. In addition, silicon dioxide adsorbs acid and pepsin.

Adverse effects of magnesium antacids are minimal. Laxation is common, necessitating use of these agents with calcium or aluminum preparations which produce constipation. Rarely, excessive magnesium absorption occurs; this may produce symptoms of hypermagnesemia in the presence of impaired renal function.

d. Aluminum Hydroxide. Aluminum hydroxide gel is a varying mixture of the oxide, the hydrated oxide, and the carbonate. Different proprietary preparations may therefore produce different responses in vivo. On average, 1.0 ml neutralizes about 2 mEq acid, and because they are poorly soluble, both the oxide and the hydrated oxide react slowly with acid:

$$Al(OH)_3 + 3HCl \rightarrow AlCl_3 + 3H_2O \qquad (5)$$

Aluminum chloride is an acid salt, but it never depresses the gastric pH below about 3.5. In addition to its neutralizing properties, the aluminum ion may exhibit a mild astringent action and may precipitate and inactivate pepsin; mucous production is stimulated and a demulcent mucosal coating effect has been noted. Aluminum hydroxide forms insoluble complexes with dietary phosphates which produce constipation and excessive fecal loss of phosphate. Usually this phosphate loss is insignificant since the peptic ulcer patient has an excess of phosphate in the diet. However, if phosphate intake is low, or if absorption is poor, aluminum phosphate gel may be used, though it is a less effective antacid.

Adverse effects of aluminum hydroxide are constipation and phosphate loss. Nausea and gastric irritation from the astringent action of the aluminum ion may be intolerable to some patients. Chronic therapy may produce osteomalacia and an iron deficiency anemia.

e. Polymeric Antacids and Exchange Resins. Several polymeric antacids such as sodium carboxymethylcellulose and various ion exchange resins have been briefly used in therapy [255]. These drugs react with hydrogen ions in the stomach and become reconstituted in the small intestine. Because of their poor antacid properties, and their cost, bulk, and unpalatable gritty taste, they are rarely used.

C. Antimuscarinics

Anticholinergic drugs are either antinicotinic or antimuscarinic, depending on whether they primarily block the action of acetylcholine at ganglionic synapses and the neuromuscular junction, or at the neuro-effector

II. GASTROINTESTINAL DISORDERS — PEPTIC ULCER DISEASE

junction of all postganglionic cholinergic fibers, respectively. For the purposes of this discussion, only the antimuscarinic agents will be considered. Since the main actions of all members of this group are similar to those of the parent drug atropine, they are often called atropine-like or atropinic. All parasympathetic neuro-effector junctions are not equally sensitive to the antimuscarinic drugs. The order of sensitivity varies little between different drugs, but there are some variations in their potency on different organ systems. In general, doses of antimuscarinic agents that depress gastric secretion do so in the face of systemic parasympathetic blockade. Thus, clinically there tends to be overactivity of the sympathetic nervous system as a compensatory mechanism. Some antimuscarinic agents have a central effect which probably results from actions on cholinergic receptors pharmacologically similar to those at the parasympathetic postganglionic junction.

1. Mechanism of Action

Antimuscarinic drugs competitively antagonize the effects of acetylcholine by attachment to the postganglionic receptor mechanism and by preventing access of the transmitter. The attachment of the antimuscarinic compounds is primarily by the amino alcohol portion and there may be transient receptor stimulation on attachment.

2. Principles of Use

Antimuscarinic agents are theoretically desirable as adjuncts in the treatment of duodenal ulcer disease for two reasons. On the one hand, they have the potential of reducing vagal and antral mechanisms of gastric acid secretion, and on the other hand, they reduce gastric motility, thereby potentiating the effect of antacids by retarding gastric emptying [263] and reducing ulcer pain. Practically, oral therapy with antimuscarinic compounds fails to effectively block gastric secretion in doses that do not produce marked systemic side effects [37]. In addition, these drugs do not alter the incidence of ulcer complications or ulcer recurrence [263-266]; however, two possible exceptions have been described [267, 268]. Antimuscarinics should not be used by themselves but can be combined with antacids if the latter have failed to control symptoms and if no contraindications to their use are present.

3. Classification

The lack of selectivity by atropinic drugs for those parasympathetic functions which might profitably be blocked in treatment of disease has led to the development of numerous separate agents [269]. The antimuscarinic drugs in general can be separated into natural alkaloids (atropine and scopolamine) and numerous derivatives (Tables II and III). As far as reduction in gastric secretion is concerned, no one drug has been proved superior, and apart from a few possible exceptions, none is more effective than atropine [79, 260, 270, 330].

The quaternary ammonium derivatives are in general poorly absorbed after oral administration. Thus, their action is unpredictable and therefore

TABLE II

Natural Belladonna Alkaloids and Synthetic Congeners[a]

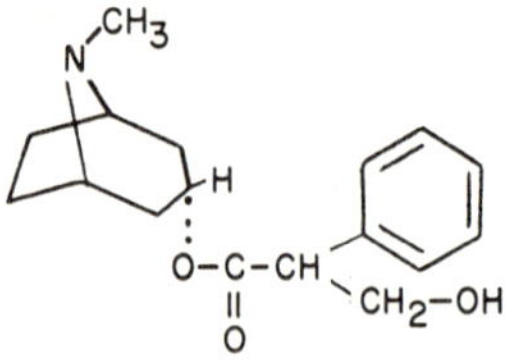

Atropine

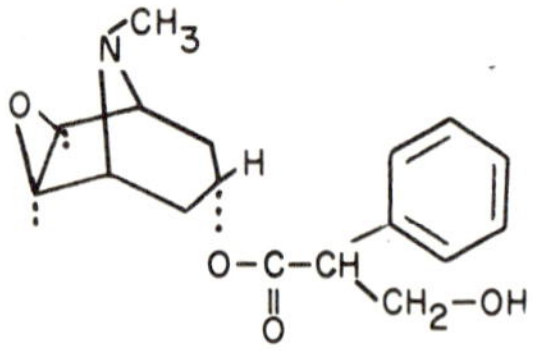

Scopolamine

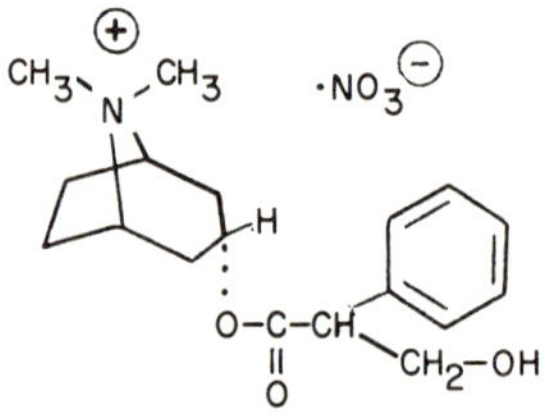

Atropine methylnitrate

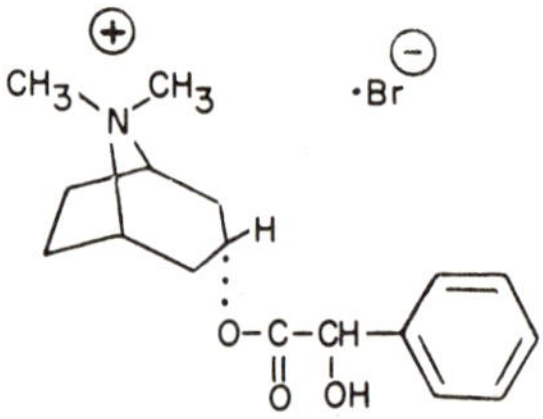

Homatropine methylbromide

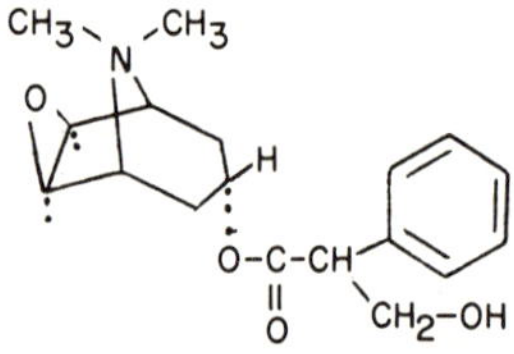

Scopolamine methylbromide

[a] Reprinted in part with permission of The Macmillan Company from *The Pharmacological Basis of Therapeutics*, 4th ed. (Louis S. Goodman and Alfred Gilman, eds.), Copyright 1970 by The Macmillan Company.

unreliable, but they tend to have a longer duration of action then the natural alkaloids. It is generally believed that the quaternary ammonium compounds exhibit a greater effect on the gastrointestinal tract than other atropinic

II. GASTROINTESTINAL DISORDERS — PEPTIC ULCER DISEASE

drugs. This belief may have arisen from the additional antinicotinic effects possessed by these compounds, but to date there is very little convincing evidence to prove specificity [271]. Quaternary ammonium compounds have almost no effect on the central nervous system since they have little or no tendency to pass across the blood-brain barrier.

4. Adverse Effects

Adverse effects of the antimuscarinic agents are either attributable to their pharmacological action or to hypersensitivity reactions. <u>Antimuscarinic effects</u> include dryness of the mouth and nose, dryness of the skin and flushing, and mydriasis and cycloplegia are fairly common. Tachycardia may be important insofar as cardiovascular compensatory mechanisms may be compromised, particularly in the patient who is bleeding. Reduction in smooth muscle tone may produce urinary retention and constipation, and if pyloric stenosis or esophagitis are present, exaggerated gastric retention or esophageal reflux, respectively. Conjunctivitis and increased intraocular tension are important complications, particularly in the elderly patient. Relief of ulcer pain in the absence of healing has also been described [272], and reduction of bronchial secretions may lead to inspissation of residual secretions which may be dangerous in patients with chronic respiratory disease; with overdosage, a toxic psychosis may appear.

The quaternary ammonium derivatives may have some additional ganglion blocking (antinicotinic) side effects, such as impotence and postural hypotension, and in large doses, a curareform paralysis.

<u>Hypersensitivity reactions</u> are rare. Usual manifestations are generalized erythematous skin rashes which occasionally exfoliate.

D. Musculotropic Antispasmodics

These drugs, although smooth muscle relaxants, should not be classified as antimuscarinic agents (Table IV). They reduce smooth muscle spasm by a nonspecific relaxant action on the muscle itself; competitive antagonism of acetylcholine is not involved but minimal antimuscarinic effects are occasionally seen on glandular elements and the cardiovascular system with massive doses. Structural resemblance to atropine is minimal, but <u>adiphenine</u> and <u>amprotropine</u> are chemically related to local anesthetics, and, in fact, possess some local anesthetic activity. The two other members of this class are <u>carbofluorene</u> and <u>dicyclomine</u>. These drugs have no demonstrable effect on gastric secretion. Clinical trials on their antispasmodic activity have been disappointing [271].

E. Gastric Mucin

Gastric mucin has been used in the treatment of peptic ulcer disease since it is frequently assumed that the gastric mucous barrier is deficient in this condition. Gastric mucin is available as an alcoholic (defatted)

TABLE III

Synthetic Antimuscarinic Compounds Commonly Used in
Peptic Ulcer Disease [a]

Generic Names	Chemical Structures
Diphemanil	
Glycopyrrolate	
Methantheline	
Oxyphencyclimine	
Oxyphenonium	

II. GASTROINTESTINAL DISORDERS — PEPTIC ULCER DISEASE

Pipenzolate

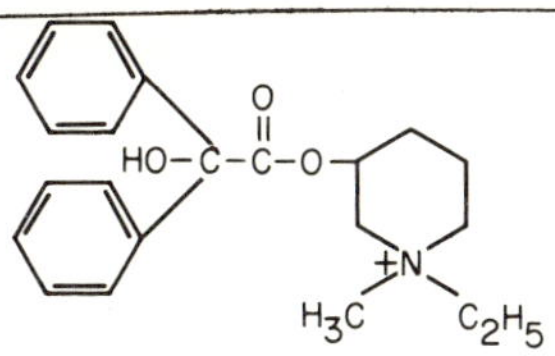

Poldine

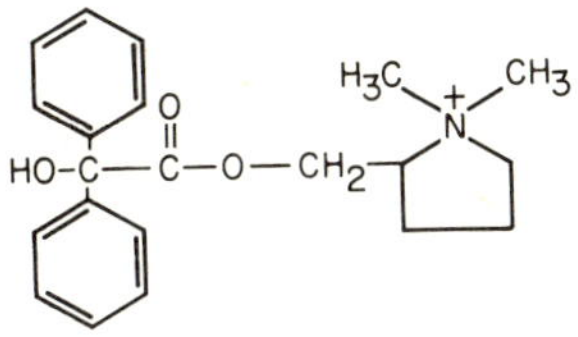

Propantheline

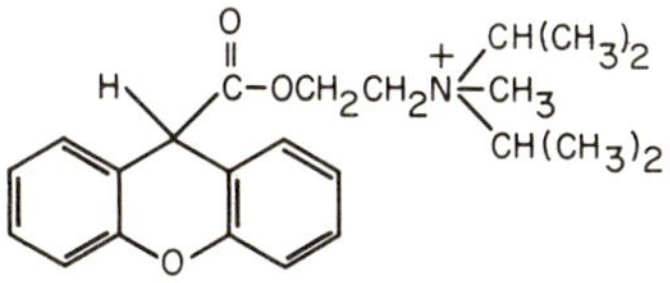

Tricyclamol

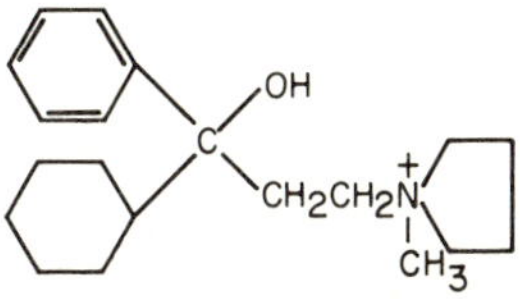

Valethamate

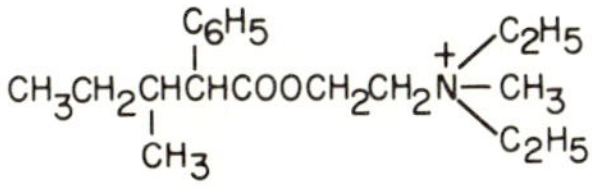

[a] All drugs except oxyphencyclimine are quaternary compounds.

Reprinted in part with permission of The Macmillan Company from *The Pharmacological Basis of Therapeutics,* 4th ed. (Louis S. Goodman and Alfred Gilman, eds.). Copyright 1970 by The Macmillan Company.

TABLE IV

Musculotropic Antispasmodics[a]

Generic names	Chemical structures
Adiphenine	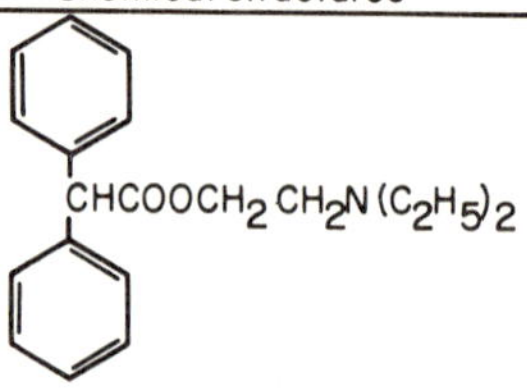 (C$_6$H$_5$)$_2$CHCOOCH$_2$CH$_2$N(C$_2$H$_5$)$_2$
Amprotropine	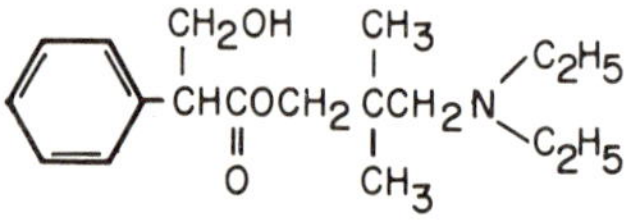 C$_6$H$_5$-CH(CH$_2$OH)COOCH$_2$-C(CH$_3$)$_2$-CH$_2$N(C$_2$H$_5$)$_2$
Carbofluorene	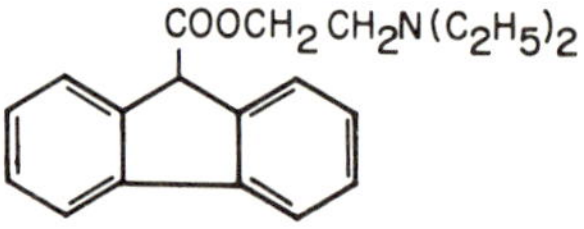 (fluoren-9-yl)COOCH$_2$CH$_2$N(C$_2$H$_5$)$_2$
Dicyclomine	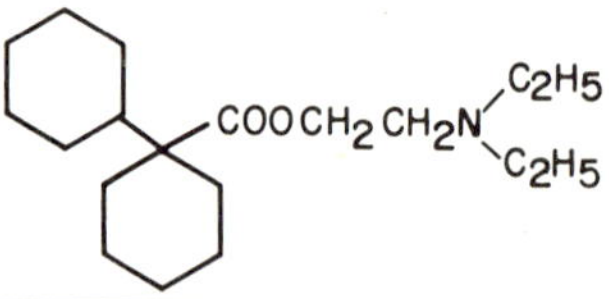 (C$_6$H$_{11}$)$_2$C(COOCH$_2$CH$_2$N(C$_2$H$_5$)$_2$)

[a] Reprinted in part with permission of The Macmillan Company from *The Pharmacological Basis of Therapeutics,* 4th ed. (Louis S. Goodman and Alfred Gilman, eds.). Copyright 1970 by The Macmillan Company.

precipitate prepared from hog stomach. It is not homogenous but contains primarily degraded mucins and mucoproteins. By itself, and combined with antacids and anion exchange resins, gastric mucin was shown to have only limited benefit in peptic ulcer disease since it is a poor acid neutralizer; the reported antipeptic activity is probably due to its content of sulfated glycoprotein [273, 274]. There seems little objective evidence for the use of exogenous gastric mucin, based on its inefficiency and poor antacid properties. It is also bulky, costly, and has a disagreeable salty taste and peptone odor. Vegetable mucilages are equally ineffective [274].

F. Licorice Derivatives

Two separate drugs have been prepared from licorice, carbenoxolone sodium and deglycyrrhizinated licorice.

II. GASTROINTESTINAL DISORDERS — PEPTIC ULCER DISEASE

1. Carbenoxolone Sodium

Carbenoxolone sodium is the water soluble, disodium salt of the hemisuccinate of β-glycyrrhetinic acid (Table V). It is synthesized from glycyrrhetinic acid, in turn obtained from glycyrrhizic acid, a glycoside extracted from liquorice. The agent acts locally on the mucosa and thus since absorption occurs primarily in the stomach, poor results were initially obtained in the treatment of duodenal ulcer. Three preparations of the drug are now available for peptic ulcer disease. Biogastrone® for gastric ulcers, Biogastrone® electuary for esophagitis, and Duogastrone®, a position release form, for duodenal ulcers. All preparations contain carbenoxolone sodium, but Duogastrone is formulated in a special gelatin capsule designed to release the active ingredient in the gastric antrum for discharge into the duodenum [275].

Carbenoxolone sodium has been hailed as the most significant contribution to the treatment of gastric ulcers in this century [276]. However, its beneficial effects in duodenal ulcer await proof.

a. Pharmacology. On parenteral administration only, carbenoxolone sodium has anti-inflammatory activity about one-third as strong as hydrocortisone in intact, but not adrenalectomized animals [277]; this may be due in part to reduced catabolism or displacement from plasma protein binding sites of endogenous glucocorticoids [278-279]; carbenoxolone sodium has no effect on urinary 17-oxycorticoid excretion [280]. Carbenoxolone sodium inhibits mitochondrial oxidative phosphorylation and histidine decarboxylase activity *in vitro* [281].

In general, the metabolic effects of carbenoxolone sodium are retention of sodium chloride and water and hypokalemia; it is not clear if the hypokalemia is due to potassium loss, or to redistribution between the extracellular and intracellular compartments [282-285]. These mineralocorticoid effects are due to an intrinsic aldosterone-like activity of the drug and not to release of aldosterone from the adrenal [277, 285]; it is possible that in addition, carbenoxolone sodium displaces aldosterone from plasma protein binding sites [279]. Both of the effects of carbenoxolone sodium on salt and water retention and on gastric ulcer healing can be reversed by spironolactone [286, 287], but hydrochlorothiazide just blocks carbenoxolone sodium-induced salt and water retention [286, 287]. The mechanism of spironolactone-induced reversal of ulcer healing is not known, but is unlikely to depend on an action of aldosterone on gastric acid and pepsin secretion [288]. Carbenoxolone sodium has no glucocorticoid activity in normal patients, but in the prediabetic, the drug may impair glucose tolerance with development of insulin resistance [284].

In man, carbenoxolone sodium is absorbed mainly from the stomach [289]. Plasma protein binding is almost 100 percent, a phenomenon which may displace other bound agents [279]. Metabolism to inactive compounds is primarily by sulfuric and glucuronic acid conjugation. Conjugates are excreted in the bile and are partly reabsorbed or hydrolyzed; urinary excretion is minimal [279].

TABLE V

Synthesis of Carbenoxolone

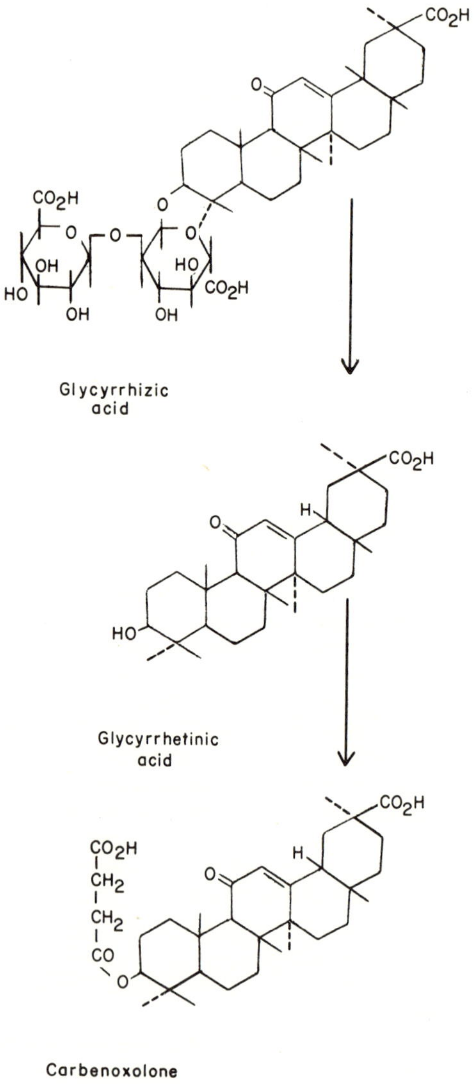

Glycyrrhizic acid

Glycyrrhetinic acid

Carbenoxolone

II. GASTROINTESTINAL DISORDERS — PEPTIC ULCER DISEASE

b. <u>Mechanism of Action.</u> Carbenoxolone sodium has no effect on gastric secretion [290] or gastric motility [291], but it has been shown to increase the healing of some types of experimentally induced gastric ulcers in rats and guinea pigs [277, 291a, 292]. The mechanism of action is not known for certain, but probably involves increased mucus production. Experiments in animals [291a, 292] and man [293, 294] have suggested that carbenoxolone stimulates increased mucus turnover and discharge. It is unlikely that carbenoxolone directly influences epithelial cell renewal since pathological examination of resected stomachs from patients taking the drug has indicated normal patterns of ulcer healing [295]. It has been suggested that ulcers treated and healed with carbenoxolone are less likely to break down compared to ulcers healed with conventional outpatient measures [295a].

c. <u>Adverse Reactions.</u> Following oral administration, carbenoxolone sodium is of low toxicity, but local necrosis is produced on parenteral administration of concentrations greater than 1 percent [277]. Decreasing the dose from 300 to 150 mg/day reduces the risk of adverse reactions [287]. Edema following salt and water retention can generally be controlled by chlorothiazide diuretics, but aldosterone antagonists should not be used since they also block the ulcer-healing properties of the drug [286]. In the elderly patient, or after prolonged exposure, carbenoxolone sodium may produce reversible elevation of serum transaminases and alkaline phosphatase [282]. Myopathies and muscular weakness due to potassium loss and a decrease in plasma C-reactive protein have also been recorded [282, 283]. These side effects have also been reported following excessive ingestion of licorice [296].

d. <u>Clinical Use.</u> A carefully controlled clinical trial in a group of selected gastric ulcer patients has shown that carbenoxolone sodium increased ulcer healing in 39 percent of patients against 17 percent in the control group; in addition, the average healing was 75 percent following the drug as compared with 37 percent in the control group [286]. However, 50 percent of ulcers failed to heal, even with prolonged treatment, and carbenoxolone sodium did not reduce relapse rate [286]. Other clinical trials have shown the benefits of carbenoxolone in the treatment of gastric ulcer [280, 290, 297-299] and reflux esophagitis [300]; however, although Duogastrone has been found effective in duodenal ulcer disease [301-303], failures have been reported [304, 305]. Thus, problems of dose and mode of administration in the case of duodenal ulcer need attention.

Widespread acceptance of this drug will be hastened by proof of effectiveness in larger clinical trials. However, as yet we have no information on relapse rate, on possible long-term side effects, or why some patients with gastric ulcer disease fail to respond.

2. <u>Deglycyrrhizinated Licorice</u>

Glycyrrhizinic acid is the basic substance used in the production of carbenoxolone sodium. It has been suggested, however, that deglycyrrhizinated licorice is not only free of the adverse effects of carbenoxolone sodium but is still effective in peptic ulcer disease. Two clinical trials using deglycyrrhizinated (about 3 percent glycyrrhizinic acid) licorice (Caved-(S)®) in patients with gastric and duodenal ulcer disease support this idea [306, 307]. Deglycyrrhizinated licorice exhibits spasmolytic activity [306] and has been shown to depress gastric acid secretion [308]. It may therefore have a different mode of action to that of carbenoxolone sodium.

G. Antipepsins

Antipepsins are drugs which inhibit peptic activity independent of changes in gastric pH. Several agents have been investigated but to date no evidence is available to indicate that antipepsins significantly alter the course of peptic ulcer disease [286, 309-311].

1. Antacids

Some aluminum, magnesium, and bismuth antacids may inactivate or adsorb pepsin [312], but this is probably unimportant.

2. Alkyl Sulfates

These are surface active detergents which denature protein (pepsin). Therapeutic results have been unsatisfactory [313].

3. Sulfated Polysaccharides

Several natural sulfated polysaccharides (heparin, "poly-hydromanuronic acid," chondroitin sulfate, and carrageenin) possess antipeptic and antiulcerogenic properties [314-316]. Synthetic derivatives (heparinoids) have been developed which variably retain certain biological properties of the natural compounds [317]. In general, of all the physical and chemical parameters evaluated, high molecular weight and high degree of sulfation were the most significant predeterminants of antipepsin, antiulcer, and anticoagulant properties. Amylopectin sulfate was one exception, possessing minimal anticoagulant activity. Some of the sulfated polysaccharides depress acid secretion in animals, possibly by complexing with histamine [318, 319].

a. Amylopectin Sulfate (Depepsen)®. Amylopectin sulfate is the sodium salt of sulfated potato amylopectin. It has 1.6 sulfate groups/glucose unit, a molecular weight of 2 to 8 x 10^7, and contains 15-16.5 percent sulfur. Depepsen inhibits pepsin by direct combination but has no action on gastric acid secretion or motility or on intestinal enzymes [320]. It has been shown to reduce cortisone- and histamine-induced ulceration in animals. It has no anticoagulant or anticholinergic properties [314]. Depepsen has given variable results in the treatment of gastric ulcer in man; in general, it is not as effective as conventional antacid and antimuscarinic agents [286, 310, 311, 320]. Addition of antimuscarinic drugs with Depepsen increases efficacy and has been reported to prevent the recurrence of duodenal ulcers; Depepsen may have most value in treating patients in whom antimuscarinic drugs are contraindicated [310]. Since sulfated polysaccharides are present in gastric secretion, the possible interaction of Depepsen with other components of gastric mucus should be investigated.

II. GASTROINTESTINAL DISORDERS — PEPTIC ULCER DISEASE

H. Synthetic Estrogens

In men with duodenal ulcer symptoms of less than 10 years duration, stilbestrol (0.5 mg twice daily for 6 months) produced a five-fold increase in healing rate [235]; in addition, stilbestrol reduced relapse rate when patients were evaluated within five years of stopping the drug. Similar effects of stilbestrol have been noted in a subsequent study [321]. Stilbestrol has no effect on basal or maximal histamine-stimulated secretion of acid or pepsin [321], but stimulates mucus production [321] and cell renewal [234]. Unfortunately synthetic estrogen therapy is not generally suitable, since unpleasant feminizing effects occur. Future research may yield more specific analogs with less feminizing activity (see below).

Healing of gastric ulcers is unaffected by stilbestrol therapy (0.5 mg/day) [90, 286, 322].

I. Miscellaneous

1. Sedatives and Tranquilizers

Sedation with barbiturates should probably be reserved for those patients with concomitant anxiety, restlessness, or insomnia. Ataractics should be given only if indicated by specific symptomatology. Since these drugs do not directly influence gastric secretion, they do not have direct therapeutic value. Controlled trials have shown no benefit of phenobarbital in the medical treatment of gastric [90] or duodenal ulcer [285].

2. Gastric Irradiation

Deep X-irradiation may rarely be used as an adjunct to intensive medical therapy. The objects are to reduce hydrochloric acid and pepsin secretion by destruction of parietal and chief cells. Effects are manifest within 1 to 6 weeks after therapy, but rarely persist for longer than about 6 months [323]. It is a treatment worth considering in the rare patient with intractable symptoms for whom surgery is contraindicated [324]. No drugs are yet available which can selectively potentiate the effect of X-irradiation or lessen the hazards of overdosage.

3. Gastric Freezing

This involves the circulation of 95 percent alcohol at $-12°C$ through a balloon in the stomach. Gastric freezing should not be confused with gastric cooling, a technique used in the treatment of gastric bleeding; cooling temperatures of 5 to $10°C$ only are used. The objects of gastric freezing are to reduce hydrochloric acid and pepsin secretion by destruction of parietal and chief cells and relief of pain by destruction of mucosal nerve elements.

This form of treatment originally hailed as a major advance in therapy is now unpopular since relief of symptoms in only temporary and serious side effects of the freezing are common [325, 326].

4. Local Anesthetics

The use of local anesthetics is theoretically justifiable on two counts: (1) to block gastrin release from the gastric antrum [327, 328], and (2) to reduce ulcer pain [69, 70].

Oxethazine (Table VI) is one member of a class of potent anesthetic agents [329]; it is said to be 4000 times as potent as procaine. Oxethazine HCl is a weak base (pKa 6.25), and therefore relatively un-ionized at pH 1. Combined with aluminum hydroxide gel (Oxaine®) it is effective in relieving pain in peptic esophagitis [330, 331] and heartburn of pregnancy [332]. Clinical response in peptic ulcer disease other than esophagitis has not been too satisfactory [332-335].

5. Diuretics and Carbonic Anhydrase Inhibitors

Carbonic anhydrase is a metaloprotein containing zinc. It has a wide distribution within the body, significant levels occurring in the kidney, pancreas, gastric mucosa, eye, and red blood cells. In the gastric mucosa, it is present in and around the parietal cells and catalyses one step in the formation of hydrochloric acid (Fig. 4). It would be logical to try and control this enzyme using carbonic anhydrase inhibitors but results in animals and man have not been promising [336-339]. This results from several facts: Carbonic anhydrase is not essential for acid secretion; the enzyme is present in gastric mucosa in very high concentration, making complete inhibition almost impossible [10]; and carbonic anhydrase inhibitors are not available with a selective action on the gastric enzyme, and thus, side effects are considerable.

Recently, a significant reduction in histamine-stimulated gastric acid output in man was observed with a low salt diet alone or in combination with the diuretic furosemide [340]; depletion of sodium chloride was suggested as the probable cause of reduced acid output.

TABLE VI

Oxethazine, a Local Anesthetic

IV. PEPTIC ULCER FORMATION IN ANIMALS

Peptic ulcer is primarily a disease of man, since spontaneous ulceration with hemorrhage and perforation has only been identified in swine [341], marmosa [342], and an inbred strain of NZB mice [343]. Thus, as yet there is no ideal animal experimental model for human peptic ulcer disease since colonies of swine and marmosa are both impractical and uneconomical, whereas the duodenal lesions in NZB mice are probably primarily due to an autoimmune phenomenon rather than acid and pepsin digestion. The occurrence of spontaneous peptic ulcer disease in these three animal species, however, offers hope that in the future a species of small laboratory animals with a high incidence of spontaneous ulceration might be selectively inbred.

Because of the absence of a suitable model, many techniques of producing gastrointestinal ulceration in animals have been devised. However, we are primarily concerned in this discussion with those techniques with direct applicability to the rapid and effective screening of potential therapeutic agents.

Practical test systems in general involve either prevention of ulcer formation or healing of induced standardized ulcers. In light of our imperfect knowledge of ulcer etiology, about the most that can be asked for is that the method used consistently produce recognizable ulceration in the gastroduodenal area, and that either the development or healing of this lesion be modified by regimens effective in man.

The pathology of peptic ulcer disease in man was outlined in Section II. In general, the two important differences between ulceration in animals and man are the location of the ulcer and its natural history [61, 344, 345]. In animals, most experimentally induced ulcers occur in the stomach, whereas in man, although stress ulcers occur in the stomach [59], the duodenum is preferentially affected. The natural history is also importantly different in that experimentally induced ulcers in animals are simple erosions which do not penetrate the muscularis mucosae and therefore heal rapidly without scar formation; peptic ulcers in man often perforate, often become chronic, and when healing occurs, heal with scarring.

The usefulness of experimentally induced ulcer techniques is limited since it is usually only possible to determine the end result of altered ulcer incidence, and not how this has been achieved. Thus, for practical purposes, these tests should be combined with tests on gastric acid, pepsin, and mucous secretion.

The present discussion of experimentally induced ulceration briefly reviews the major simple and practical techniques available. Chronological reviews should be consulted for more detailed information [61, 344-347].

A. Pylorus-Ligated (Shay) Rat

Pylorus ligation in the rat was found by Shay et al. in 1945 [348] to result in gastric ulceration. Originally, however, the preparation had been introduced as a technique of gastric juice collection. The technique involves ligation of the pylorus under anesthesia, allowing accumulation of hydrochloric acid in the stomach over a period of at least 18 hours. Per unit time, the pylorus-ligated rat secretes more acid than a fistula animal due to stimulation of vago-vagal reflexes [349], and the lesions produced are hemorrhagic glandular ulcers which occasionally perforate, and perforating rumenal (nonglandular) ulcers. Ulceration results primarily from acid and pepsin digestion [350]; distention, producing mucosal ischaemia, is not a contributing factor [351]. Ulceration is effectively blocked by vagotomy, antimuscarinic agents, antacids, and antipepsins [45, 350, 352-354], and several drugs now widely used in man were originally found to be effective in the Shay rat preparation [355-357].

The Shay rat preparation is probably second in popularity to the stress-induced ulcer technique, but is unreliable unless adequate numbers of animals are used and strict attention is paid to controlling experimental variables such as animal nutrition, hours of animal fasting before surgery, animal dehydration, room temperature during the experiment, etc.

A survey of the effects of clinically useful drugs on ulcer incidence and gastric secretion using the pylorus-ligated technique suggests that this preparation is probably the best single ulcer test for predicting therapeutic usefulness [61].

B. Stress-Induced Ulcers

The term "stress ulcer" is commonly used, but is, in reality a misnomer, since the lesions rarely penetrate the muscularis mucosae and are therefore strictly erosions. Stress-induced ulcers are produced by subjecting the rat, and occasionally other animals, to various forms of stress, either singly or in combination; restraining the animal in a small cage, third degree burns, electric shocks, a cold environment, and fasting have been the most popular [358-363]. Irrespective of the technique used, ulcer incidence and pathology are remarkably similar [61, 344], indicating that, with the exception of burning, which probably acts via histamine release [364], all other techniques act through a common mechanism. Multiple stresses do not produce perforated ulcers [61].

The cause of stress-induced ulceration is not known, but several factors have been incriminated. Among the most likely components are increased acid concentration and reduced mucosal blood flow[61, 358, 365-367], reduced mucus secretion [368], reduced gastric epithelial cell turnover [369, 370], and activation of the hypothalamic-pituitary-adrenal axis [362, 371-373].

Pathologically, stress-induced ulcers occur in the glandular stomach but not in the rumen, and because they do not penetrate through the muscularis mucosae, healing is accomplished without scar formation [344, 358]. Antimuscarinic drugs and vagotomy offer some protection against stress-induced ulceration [45, 345, 358, 359, 362, 374-376], and several centrally acting

II. GASTROINTESTINAL DISORDERS — PEPTIC ULCER DISEASE

drugs such as the barbiturates and tranquilizers which are not in themselves antiulcer agents inhibit restraint-induced ulcers [358, 359]; in the case of tranquilizers, dose-efficacy relationships are often unpredictable however [362]. Recently, antimuscarinic agents have been shown to not only prevent classical stress-induced ulcers in rats, but to induce a different type of gastric ulcer [377]; the significance of this lesion is not clear.

Restraint-induced stress has achieved great popularity in recent years and complemements the Shay rat preparation. Restraint-induced stress approaches the ideal technique for ulcer production and the testing of antiulcer agents in rats [358]: The lesions are rapidly induced in the acid secreting mucosa; there is a direct relationship between the ulcer incidence and the degree of restraint; no surgical or anesthetic exposure is required, and there is evidence that gastric acid and pepsin are factors in ulcer production. Furthermore, restraint brings the central nervous system into play, and thus is similar to "stress ulcers" and Curling's ulcer in man [59, 364, 378-380]. Unfortunately, the restraint-induced ulcer technique fails, in that perforation never occurs; the lesions rarely penetrate to the submucosa; the test system is species specific (hamsters and rabbits are not affected); duodenal ulcers are never produced in rats although they may develop in guinea pigs [381] and a fall in ulcer incidence occurs with repeated periods of restraint, indicating an adaptative phenomenon.

There has been no good trial comparing the stress-induced ulcer with the Shay rat preparation for effectiveness, but on theoretical grounds it would seem best to use both methods [382] since they complement each other.

C. Drug-Induced Ulceration

Tests have been designed to evaluate the effectiveness of potential antiulcer agents upon acute and chronic drug-induced lesions.

1. Acute Drug-Induced Ulceration

Ulcerogenic drugs most frequently used [78, 365, 383-389] have been acid and pepsin stimulants (histamine and gastrin and their analogs), antiinflammatory agents (adrenal steroids and indomethacin, phenylbutazone, and salicylates), vasoactive amines (5-hydroxytryptophan, 5-hydroxytryptamine, and epinephrine), amine depletors (reserpine and analogs), and mitotic inhibitors (cinchophen). Mechanisms of drug-induced ulceration are unclear, but increased acid and pepsin secretion, decreased mucosal resistance, and vascular factors are all important. Mucosal damage caused by back diffusion of hydrogen ions [95] was discussed in Section II. At present it is not clear if back diffusion is a usual occurrence with drug-induced ulceration [61, 390].

The value of testing one drug's ability to inhibit drug-induced ulceration is limited since no studies have been reported correlating antiulcer activity in any given test system with subsequent clinical effectiveness in man.

2. Chronic Drug-Induced Ulceration

Techniques have been devised for studying the healing properties of compounds on standardized ulcers produced by either burning the gastric mucosa [357, 391] or following stress [392].

In rats with burn-induced gastric ulceration, chronic corticosteroid administration has been shown to induce ulcer chronicity and perforation [384]. Reduced ulcer healing has been attributed to an alteration in the substratum of cells in the ulcer crater and their inability to support adequately new epithelial growth [384].

One further potentially valuable model is gastrin-induced ulceration in guinea pigs [387]: hog gastrin was injected in 16 percent gelatin (to prolong absorption) and 74 percent of the animals developed duodenal ulcers within 2 weeks. Since there are slight species differences among animal gastrins (Table I), the use of autologous gastrin might produce ulceration in 100 percent of the animals.

Methods for evaluation of ulcer-healing tests are cumbersome, and importantly, there is no satisfactory method for quantitating ulcer healing macroscopically [61]. Adaption of the technique of transillumination or use of the staining properties of various dyes such as fluorescine or india-ink for ulcerated areas might yield more rapid and practical methods for quantitative results. The potential usefulness of a test system of this kind makes it an interesting area for future research.

D. Mann-Williamson Ulcers

The diversion of acid-neutralizing alkaline biliary, pancreatic, or duodenal juices from the upper small bowel results in jejunal ulceration. Of the various techniques studied [347], the Mann-Williamson preparation in dogs has been the most popular [393]. This involves producing a gastro-jejunostomy and blind duodenal loop; ulceration occurs in the jejunum due to removal of neutralizing secretions and to acid hypersecretion [394]. The preparation has little to offer as a screening procedure for new therapeutic agents.

E. Miscellaneous

A recent report [395] suggested that the ferret might become a valuable animal for gastric secretory studies in peptic ulcer research since it secretes acid under basal conditions, it is sensitive to histamine, its gastrointestinal morphology is similar to that of man, and it is readily available.

A variety of other surgical and experimental methods are available to produce gastrointestinal ulceration in animals. Techniques range from induction of chronic pantothenate and riboflavin deficiencies [396, 397] to injection of polyethylene microspheres [398], stimulation or destruction of localized areas within the central nervous system [399-401], and portocaval shunting [243], to name a few.

II. GASTROINTESTINAL DISORDERS — PEPTIC ULCER DISEASE

None of these techniques will be discussed here since they all involve complex preparations, apparatus, or experimental design, and therefore are of no value as routine screening procedures for new therapeutic agents.

V. FUTURE DRUGS FOR THE TREATMENT OF PEPTIC ULCER DISEASE

> The Doctor came round and examined his chest,
> And ordered him Nourishment, Tonics, and Rest.
> "How very effective," he said as he shook
> The thermometer, "all these chrysanthemums look!"
>
> . . . .
>
> The Doctor said, "Tut! It's another attack!"
> And ordered him Milk and Massage-of-the-back,
> And Freedom-from-worry and Drives-in-a-car,
> And murmured, "How sweet your chrysanthemums are!"
>
> (Reprinted, with permission, from A. A. Milne, "The Dormouse and the Doctor," verses 9 and 11, from When We Were Very Young (8th ed.) Methuen Publishing Co., London, 1925, pp. 68-69.

The great advances in our understanding of gastric secretion in recent years indicate several intriguing and novel "leads" for treating peptic ulcer disease. In this section an attempt is made to present a summary of recent information and ideas in this area of gastroduodenal physiology as they apply to potential "breakthrough" drug development. The material is grouped into several sections for clarity, and its arrangement is not meant to imply a descending order of usefulness or reliability.

The simple remedies prescribed by the Doctor for A. A. Milne's Dormouse however, remind us in another way of what has been said recently concerning "breakthrough research" in peptic ulcer disease. Grossman has drawn attention to the need for "nonbreakthroughs" in the study of peptic ulcer disease [402]. He believes that the dollar and manpower emphasis on breakthrough research has drawn attention and support away from two fundamentally important sources of new information, namely, the controlled clinical trial and epidemiological studies. In chronic illnesses such as peptic ulcer disease where etiology is not known and treatment is for the most part empirical, continuous reevaluation of therapy is required. Thus, although the development of new agents for treatment of peptic ulcer disease is desirable, such simple and important questions as whether the millions of dollars patients spend annually on antacids and antimuscarinic agents [47] are well invested have not yet been answered [402].

A. Drugs Acting on the Central Nervous System

Since we are just beginning to explore the complex influence of the hypothalamus and other subcortical areas on gastric physiology, we are a long way from suggesting drugs which might profitably modify them! However, as more becomes known about the effects of central nervous system controls [401, 403, 404] on gastric function, the selective use of potent pharmacological agents interfering with, for example, biogenic amines and appropriate enzymes or humoral agents, may become potentially valuable [330].

Sedatives and tranquilizers probably depress gastric acid secretion indirectly by reducing worry and emotional tension. A search for new agents in these series will be difficult, since in some animal species, for example the rat, tranquilizers increase gastric acid secretion by preventing histamine degradation [405, 406].

B. Drugs Acting on the Gastrointestinal Tract

1. Inhibition of Hydrochloric Acid Secretion

a. *Carbonic Anhydrase Inhibitors.* As discussed in Section III, it is theoretically desirable to use carbonic anhydrase inhibitors to reduce hydrochloric acid secretion. However, this area of drug development is not too promising because, even if selective inhibitors for gastric carbonic anhydrase were found their effectiveness would be limited since the enzyme is not essential for acid secretion.

b. *Histamine and Antihistamines.* Histamine is a potent stimulant of gastric acid secretion in animals and man, but none of the available antihistaminic drugs can effectively block this activity [250]. A possible explanation for this, however, has recently been given. Kier [407], using extended Hückel molecular orbital calculations, showed that the histamine cation exists in two significantly different but equally preferred conformations (A, B) neither of which involves intramolecular hydrogen bonding (Table VII). This finding raises the interesting and important question: Can the histamine molecule *in vivo* elicit two types of biological response from two different receptors, one for each specific conformation?

There is experimental evidence to support this concept of two separate receptors, involving smooth muscle stimulation on the one hand and gastric secretory stimulation on the other [408]. Structural requirements for the histamine receptor in a smooth muscle (guinea-pig ileum, H_1 receptor) differ from those for gastric secretion [408], and Kier has designated this latter receptor as H_2 [407].

The question about which histamine conformation is associated with which receptor has been investigated by Kier. He evaluated the more potent antihistamines in an attempt to find one in which the spatial relationships of key atoms could be reasonably well established and then compared these interatomic distances with conformations A and B. Kier proposed [407]

TABLE VII

Histamine, Its Conformations and the Antihistamine Triprolidine

[Structural diagrams showing Histamine with side chain $CH_2-CH_2-NH_2$, Conformation A with $\theta_{cc}=180°$, $\theta_{ring-C}=120°$ and internitrogen distance 4.55 Å; Conformation B with $\theta_{cc}=300°$, $\theta_{ring-C}=120°$ and internitrogen distance 3.60 Å; and Triprolidine with distance 4.80±0.2 Å]

---

that conformation A is the histamine molecule specific for the receptor H_1 based on comparison with the potent antihistaminic triprolidine. As yet no specific H_2-blocking agents are available, so it cannot be stated that conformation B is the prototype of histamine receptor H_2 activity.

Thus, it is possible that the histamine molecule can exist in the biophase in one of two distinctly different but nearly equally preferred conformations and produce two distinct biological responses depending upon the presence of one or the other complementary receptors. Kier postulates that the H_1 receptor is complementary to the internitrogen relationship

$$\text{\textbackslash N} \xleftrightarrow{4.55 \text{ Å}} N^+$$

and that the H_2 receptor is complementary to the internitrogen relationship

$$\text{\textbackslash N} \xleftrightarrow{3.60 \text{ Å}} N^+$$

A search for potent antihistaminic agents acting on H_2 receptors is indicated and not completely without hope. A key feature of such a molecule would be an interatomic separation of two N atoms by a distance < 4 Å.

c. **Histidine Decarboxylase Inhibitors.** Histamine is formed in the gastric mucosa by the intracellular decarboxylation of the precursor amino acid l-histidine. This can be accomplished by at least two types of enzymes, a specific decarboxylase [409] which requires pyridoxal phosphate as a cofactor [410], and a nonspecific, aromatic-l-amino acid decarboxylase [411]. Large concentrations of histamine are present in the mammalian gastric mucosa [411], and histidine decarboxylase activity can be induced by a variety of acid secretagogues, namely, gastrin [412], cholecystokinin-pancreozymin [413], and prednisolone [414].

Several nonspecific inhibitors of histidine decarboxylase are available (Table VIII). However, in spite of the fact that they reduce histamine

TABLE VIII

Some Histidine Decarboxylase Inhibitors

DL-α-methylhistidine

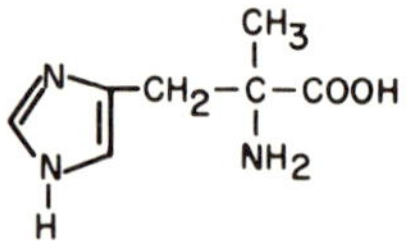

DL-α-methyl-α-hydrazino-3,4-dihydroxyphenylproprionic acid

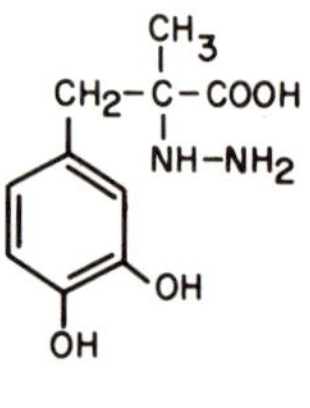

imidazol-4(5H)-ylmethoxyamine

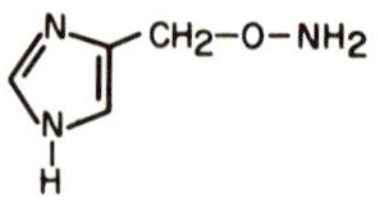

NSD-1024

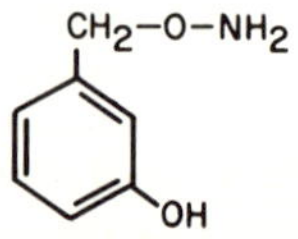

TABLE VIII (cont'd)

Some Histidine Decarboxylase Inhibitors

NSD-1034

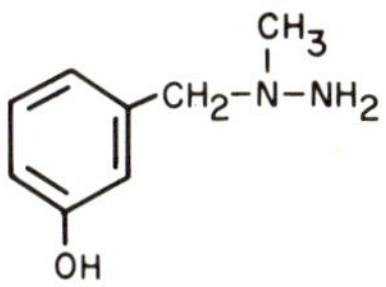

(structure: 3-hydroxybenzyl group with $CH_2-N(CH_3)-NH_2$ side chain)

NSD-1055 (Brocresine)

(structure: bromo, hydroxy-substituted phenyl with CH_2-O-NH_2 side chain)

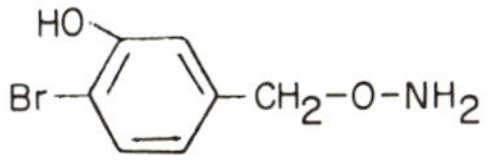

p-toluenesulfonylhydrazine

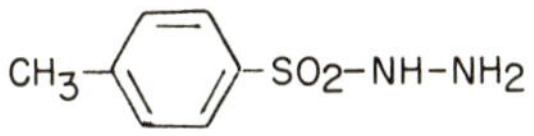

(structure: CH_3-phenyl-$SO_2-NH-NH_2$)

---

formation, gastric acid secretion, and the incidence of restraint-induced ulcers in rats [415-418], their applicability to the treatment of human peptic ulcer disease is not yet clear. This uncertainty arises from two facts: First, none of the histidine decarboxylase inhibitors are selective antagonists of the specific histidine decarboxylase, since they also inhibit the nonspecific aromatic-1-amino acid decarboxylase and possibly other enzymes; and second, the question as to whether histamine plays a role in human gastric acid secretion is still unsettled [2, 419]. Brocresine has been used in two patients with the Zollinger-Ellison syndrome [420]; in the first patient, response was equivocal, whereas in the second patient, significant reduction in acid output was achieved.

There are two theoretical disadvantages however to reducing the tissue histamine level: Histamine has been shown to stimulate wound healing in animals by increasing fibroblast activity [421] and to increase gastrointestinal epithelial cell turnover [45]. The relative importance of these phenomena in the healing of human peptic ulcers is not certain.

d. *Antimuscarinic Drugs.* The lack of selectivity of atropinic drugs for gastric secretion and gastric motility has led to the introduction of many agents with antimuscarinic properties. However, as was pointed out in Section III, atropine is still probably the drug of choice. There is no question that a potent, long-acting antimuscarinic drug with selective action on the stomach would be desirable. Clinical gastroenterologists will eagerly await its discovery.

e. *Gastrin and Gastrin Inhibitors.* Great progress has been made in recent years in the understanding of the hormone gastrin and how it acts[1]. The development of a sensitive immunoassay system has allowed measurement of gastrin levels in several physiological fluids and the identification of the gastrin-containing cell in the gastric mucosa [424, 425]. Gastrins from several species are indicated in Table I. The important discovery that the C-terminal tetrapeptide amide fragment, Try-Met-Asp-Phe-NH_2, common to all gastrins, possessed the complete range of physiological actions of the natural hormones, enabled a detailed investigation of structure-activity relationships [426, 427]. Morley has proposed that at the molecular level the Try-Met- and Phe-portion is concerned with hormone binding at the site of action (Fig. 10) whereas the aspartic amino acid is intimately concerned with hormone activity; the N-terminal tri-decapeptide is probably required for hormonal transport only. On the basis of structure-activity relationships, Morley has proposed development of four types of possible inhibitors of gastrin [426]. To date over 600 congeners of the tetrapeptide-NH_2 have been studied. However, none has been found with greater secretory activity and apart from some minor inhibition of motility, no secretory inhibitors have been identified. Little is known about endogenous gastrin synthesis, plasma protein binding, metabolic degradation, or excretion [428]; however, in the future we may be able to direct and profitably modify each of these steps.

f. *Antibodies to Gastrin.* Antibodies, produced in rabbits to the C-terminal tetrapeptide of gastrin [429] have been shown to reduce the acid response to both endogenous [430] and exogenous [431] gastrin in rats. No information is available however as to the potential duration of antibody inhibition, nor whether the site of inhibition is located at the gastrin-containing cell during transport of the hormone in the plasma or at the gastrin "receptor." Gastrin antibodies crossreact with other polypeptides with a similar terminal amino acid sequence (Table I). Apart from their potential use in ordinary peptic ulcer disease, gastrin antibodies may prove invaluable in treating the severe peptic ulcers occurring in patients with uncontrollable, metastatic Zollinger-Ellison tumors.

g. *Caerulein.* Caerulein is a decapeptide amine which was originally isolated from the skin of the Australian tree frog Hyla caerulea [432]. The five C-terminal amino acid residues are identical with those of gastrin and cholecystokinin-pancreozymin (CCK-PZ) (Table I). The major actions of caerulein are also similar to those of gastrin and CCK-PZ [433], but sulfation of the tyrosine residue is necessary for optimal activity [434]. Several peptide analogs of caerulein have been synthesized [435], but none have shown any inhibitory properties on gastric acid secretion.

II. GASTROINTESTINAL DISORDERS – PEPTIC ULCER DISEASE

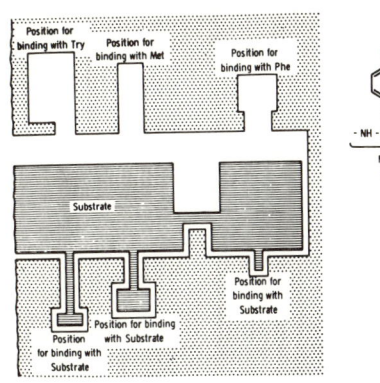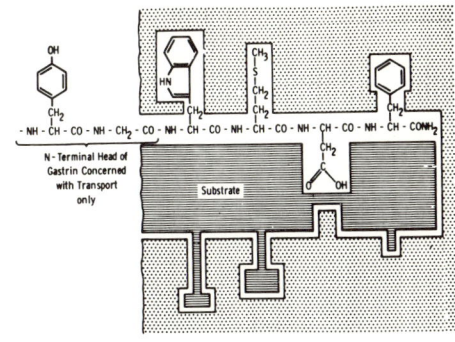

Cell receptor site equipped to receive a substrate but lacking an aspartyl group necessary for its function as an enzyme.

Missing carboxyl group supplied by the C-terminal sequence of a gastrin molecule at exactly the required position. Receptor site can now function as an enzyme.

Fig. 10. Schematic representation of the theory of hormonal action of the gastrins. (Reproduced, with permission, from J. S. Morley, "Structure Activity Relationships," Federation Proc., 27, 1314 (1968), p. 1316, Fig. 3.)

h. Prostaglandins. The prostaglandins (PG) (Fig. 11) are ubiquitous in nature and have been extensively investigated over the past few years [436]. PG have been identified in the gastrointestinal tract of a variety of species and have been shown to possess potent pharmacological actions upon gastric secretion and intestinal motility [436].

In the rat, basal gastric secretion is accompanied by the local release of PGE_1, PGE_2, $PGF_{1\alpha}$, and $PGF_{2\alpha}$ [437-439], and cholinergic stimulation increases this release [440, 441]. Since exogenous PG profoundly inhibit basal and cholinergic-stimulated gastric acid secretion [437], local PG release may be acting to prevent excessive gastric acid production [442].

PGE_1 and analogs are potent inhibitors of basal and stimulated gastric acid secretion in the rat and dog [437, 443-446] and in the bull frog gastric mucosa in vitro [447]. PGE_1 has antiulcer activity against steroid-induced and pylorus ligation-induced ulcers [443, 445].

PGE_1 was ineffective however against gastrin pentapeptide-induced gastric acid secretion in human volunteers [448]. This may have been due to the PG not reaching the appropriate target cell, or from the fact that a relatively ineffective PG was used; PGE_2 is more common in human gastric mucosa [449].

The precise mechanism of PG action is not known, but they may inhibit the formation of cyclic 3', 5'-AMP in gastric mucosa [447] or reduce gastric mucosal blood flow [443]. The synthesis of potent PG inhibitors [450] will

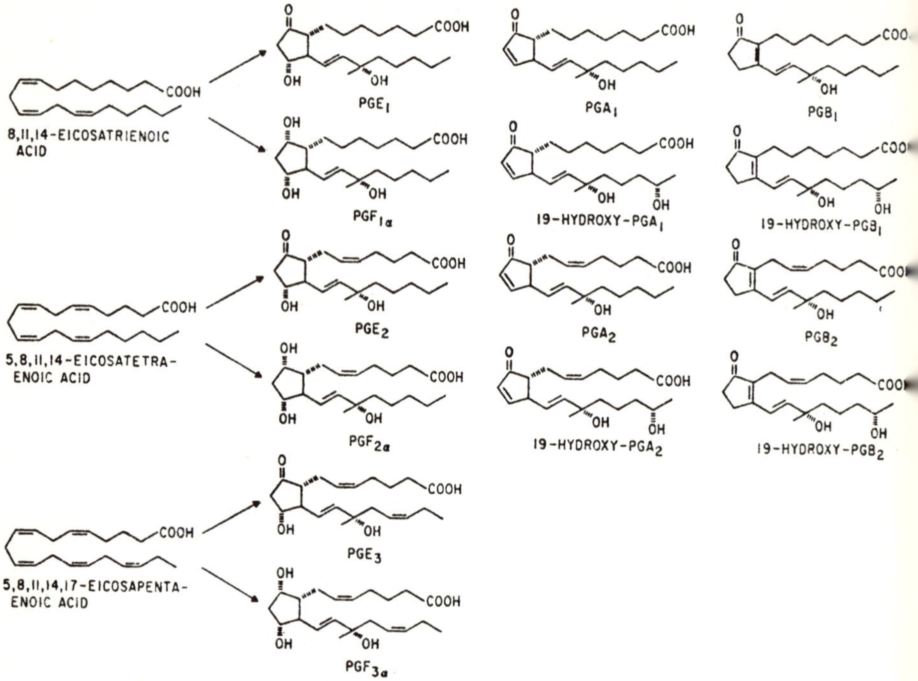

Fig. 11. Structural formulas of the naturally occurring prostaglandins and their precursors. (Reprinted, with permission, from S. Bergström et al., "The Prostaglandins: A Family of Biologically Active Lipids," Pharmacol. Rev., 20, 1 (1968), Fig. 1, p. 3.

hopefully identify more rapidly the precise function of these fatty acid hormones and indicate a rational approach to prostaglandin use in man.

i. Cholecystokinin-Pancreozymin. Until recently, it was believed that two separate hormones, cholecystokinin (stimulating gall bladder contraction) and pancreozymin (stimulating pancreatic enzyme output) were present in intestinal mucosa. However, chemical purification has shown that actions attributed to these two hormones reside in a single polypeptide of 33 amino acids [451, 452]. Cholecystokinin-pancreozymin (CCK-PZ) contains the same C-terminal sequence of amino acids as gastrin for five residues (Table I) and is released from upper intestinal mucosal stores by fatty acids, amino acids, and hydrogen ions. CCK-PZ has been shown to possess a wide spectrum of actions in animal experiments [442, 453], probably resulting from use of impure hormone containing extraneous substances.

One of its most important actions however is strong competitive antagonism of gastrin-induced acid secretion [454]. Determination of CCK-PZ as one of the "enterogastrones"[455] awaits the availability of pure hormone.

II. GASTROINTESTINAL DISORDERS — PEPTIC ULCER DISEASE

In view of its ability to antagonize gastrin-induced acid secretion, CCK-PZ may be as potentially valuable as secretin. See below.

j. Enterogastrone. Fats and fatty acids liberate an "enterogastrone" from the upper small bowel which depresses gastrin-induced acid secretion [9, 24, 25, 464]. Both secretin (see below) and CCK-PZ possess some "enterogastrone" properties [453, 456]; however, they do not account for all enterogastrone activity [456]. Chemical identification of pure enterogastrone will enable the development of a further potentially useful agent for the treatment of gastric acid hypersecretion.

k. SC-15396 [2-phenyl-2-(pyridyl)-thioacetamide]. SC-15396 (Table IX) was initially introduced as a nonantimuscarinic, antigastrin drug possessing antiulcer properties [457, 458]. However, on subsequent investigation it was found to possess a nonspecific inhibitory effect on gastric acid and

TABLE IX

Potential Anti-ulcer Compounds

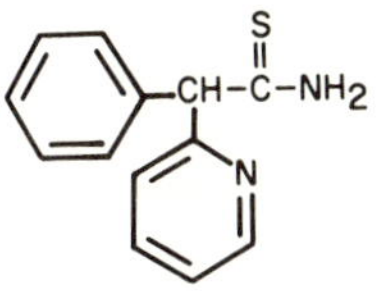

SC-15396

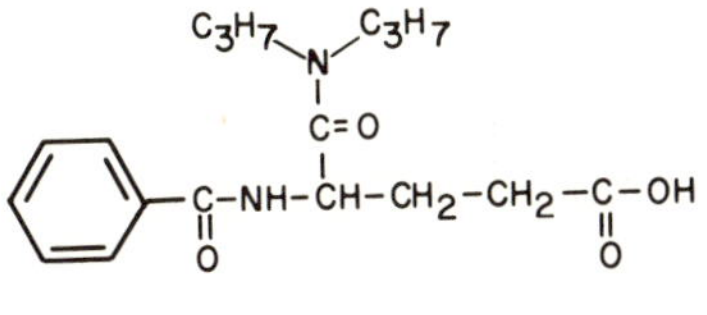

Xylamide

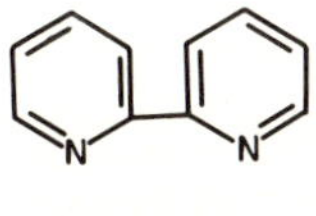

Cl-588

pepsin secretion induced by a variety of different secretagogues and not to block gastrin-induced histamine synthesis in rat gastric mucosa [459-461, 463]. In spite of its nonspecific action, SC-15396 was a promising agent; however, on discovery that it was tumorigenic in female rats, the compound was withdrawn [462]. No analogs are immediately available.

l. Xylamide (N-benzoyl-N, N-di-n-propyl-DL-isoglutamine). Xylamide (Table IX) inhibits gastric acid and pepsin secretion and possesses papaverine-like spasmolytic activity [465]. It is effective against insulin hypoglycemia-induced secretion but apparently has no antimuscarinic activity on the gastric, salivary, or lacrimal glands [466]. Several analogs have been studied [466, 467] and clinical effects in man have been encouraging [442].

m. Miscellaneous Drugs. Several drugs have been found to depress gastric juice volume, or acid output or both in various animal species. The clinical applicability of these studies is small, but a brief note is included.

Cl-588 (2, 2'-bipyridyl) (Table IX) was shown to possess antisecretory antiulcer activity in the rat and antisecretory activity in the dog [468]; it had no antimuscarinic or ganglionic blocking properties. Since Cl-588 possessed chelating activity, a variety of chelating agents were subsequently investigated for antisecretory activity in the rat; none were found [469]. Bass and Patterson studied the relation of rat gastric juice volume changes to a variety of drugs affecting adrenergic mechanisms [470]; in general, catecholamines exerted antisecretory affects independent of vasoactive properties. Pradhan and Wingate found that adrenergic drug-induced gastric secretory depression was due to β-receptor stimulation [471]; however, this was not true in studies in the rat [472]. Lippmann reported the antisecretory effects of a series of chlorinated aralkylamines [473]; antisecretory activity was probably due to reduced uptake of tissue catecholamines.

Cycloheximide which inhibits amino acid incorporation into proteins was found to reduce gastric acid and pepsin output and gastric juice volume in Shay rats in the interprandial state and after several secretagogues [474]. Meyer et al. [475] and Bass et al. [476] have reported on the antisecretory properties of a series of 3-amino-2, 1-benzisothiazoles. Wyllie et al. have reported that bacterial lipopolysaccharides depressed gastric acid secretion in dogs [477]; inhibition paralleled the rise in body temperature produced by the pyrogen. Antiurease compounds are probably obsolete [478].

n. Radiation Therapy. Deep X-irradiation therapy for peptic ulcer disease is not generally suitable, since cellular radiation damage is not selective and reduction in acid and pepsin secretion is transitory [324]. Safer and more specific methods of producing radiation damage to the parietal and chief cells might increase the effectiveness and applicability of this form of therapy. Such a method might involve use of one of the short half-life isotopes of iodine. Iodine is concentrated in gastric mucosa and excreted in gastric juice so that if thyroid iodine uptake were blocked with nonradioactive iodine, the radioactive halogen could be administered safely. Concomitant administration of an antimuscarinic agent to reduce gastric emptying would minimize damage to the small bowel mucosa.

This approach, as far as the author is aware, has never been attempted. Careful gastric secretory analyses in patients receiving I^{131} for thyroid cancer might yield information on the feasibility of this form of therapy.

2. Neutralization of Hydrochloric Acid

a. Antacids. The ideal antacid is still not available, namely, one that is cheap and palatable and a potent acid neutralizer without side effects. Most of the antacids in common use are effective acid neutralizers, but cost and palatability vary and are important insofar as treatment with antacids is a prolonged affair; no antacid is completely without side effects.

Since the rate of gastric emptying is the most important variable factor influencing the efficiency of an antacid, future antacid development should concentrate on the formulation of a "long acting" antacid. Thus, pharmaceutically it may be possible to devise an antacid formulation which coats the mucosa rapidly and by adhering strongly to the mucous coat remains in the stomach for long periods of time. Development of such a formulation will be a difficult task since the mucous coat is constantly being discharged into the gastric lumen and extruded from the stomach.

b. Drugs to Increase Acid Neutralization in the Duodenum. Neutralization of gastric acid in the duodenum is normally accomplished by the bicarbonate secretion from the pancreas and biliary system. In addition, the secretion of Brunner's glands which contains bicarbonate and mucosubstances may provide mucosal protection [479, 480]. Theoretically, an increase in any of these secretions would benefit the patient with high acid output and duodenal ulcer disease.

Secretin. Porcine secretin is a heptacosapeptide (Table I). No analogs or peptide fragments with secretin-like activity have been identified and synthetic secretin has equal potency to natural secretin.

Secretin is liberated from villus cells of the upper small bowel [481] and because of its actions has been dubbed nature's antacid [482]. Both exogenous and endogenous secretin have the following actions: stimulation of pancreatic juice flow and bicarbonate output, stimulation of bile flow and bicarbonate output, inhibition of gastrin-stimulated acid secretion, inhibition of gastric motility, and stimulation of Brunner's gland secretion [483-485]; in addition, secretin causes a sharp rise in pepsin output when combined with histamine or gastrin pentapeptide [486], but the significance of this phenomenon is not clear.

Secretin-induced bicarbonate secretion by the pancreas produces profound alkalinization of the upper duodenum in patients with ordinary duodenal ulcer and duodenal ulcers associated with the Zollinger-Ellison syndrome [482]. Furthermore, secretin-induced bicarbonate secretion prevents gastrin-induced ulcers in Mann-Williamson cats [487]. These results offer hope that commercial preparations of secretin, preferably in a repository, slow release form, might confer benefit in duodenal ulcer disease [482].

Recently, antimuscarinic agents have been shown to block endogenous secretin release [488, 489]; the significance of this finding is not fully clear.

Glucagon. Glucagon is secreted by the α-(A-) cells of the pancreatic islets [228]. It is a 29-amino acid polypeptide very similar to secretin (Table I). Its depressant effects on gastric secretion have been discussed in Section II. The complete 29-amino acid sequence is required for gastric secretory depression [490] whereas only the N-terminal 21-22 amino acids are required for hyperglycemic activity [490, 491]. Glucagon probably has a direct effect on the gastric mucosa rather than acting indirectly via hyperglycemia [199]. Since glucagon is probably secreted maximally during the fasting state (to counteract hypoglycemia), it might prove to be a valuable hormone in preventing acid secretion in patients with peptic ulcer disease. It has an additional advantage over secretin in that it apparently does not stimulate pepsin secretion [492].

3. Inhibition of Pepsin Synthesis and Antipepsins

As more knowledge is accumulated concerning the normal patterns of pepsin formation and secretion, it is not unreasonable to assume that selective inhibitors of pepsin synthesis will be discovered; none are presently available.

Numerous antipepsins have been developed and these have been discussed in Section III. Specific pepsin inhibitors (mucosubstances) may soon be isolated from gastric juice [148, 151, 152, 154] or synthesized [493] (see lignosulfonates below).

4. Stimulation of Mucosubstances

Drugs which would selectively increase the output of mucosubstances and other components of the natural protective barrier and thus reduce the susceptibility of the mucosa to acid and pepsin digestion would be of value. Drugs called "adaptogens" fit into this general class and produce "a state of nonspecifically increased resistance" [494]. Isolation of adaptogens has resulted from the follow-up of "leads" originating in folk medicine.

a. Estrogens. The effectiveness of synthetic estrogens in the treatment of peptic ulcer disease in men was discussed in Section III. Estrogens and progesterones increase "mucous" production in the genital tract and may similarly increase gastric mucosubstance production. Before any synthetic estrogen could assume widespread acceptance however, it would need to display less feminizing activity than stilbestrol; one such compound has recently been reported [495], but it is a moot point whether feminizing activity and "anti-ulcer" activity can be separated. If estrogens increase mucosubstance production through augmentation of mucosal cyclic AMP levels [496], this might help to explain glucocorticosteroid-induced ulcerations, since these drugs inhibit estrogen-induced elevation of cyclic AMP in rat uterus [497].

II. GASTROINTESTINAL DISORDERS — PEPTIC ULCER DISEASE

b. Serotonin. 5-Hydroxytryptamine (serotonin) and its precursor amino acid 1-5-hydroxytryptophan depress gastric acid secretion and stimulate secretion of mucosubstances [41, 42]. Serotonin probably plays a role in normal gastric secretory physiology since serotonin antagonists stimulate gastric secretion in normal and peptic ulcer patients [498]; serotonin may act by release of prostaglandins [499], but because it is so labile it is of no practical value in therapy.

Malhotra has suggested that salivary mucosubstances, by augmenting gastric mucus, may help to protect against peptic ulceration [500]. Development of synthetic or semisynthetic mucosubstances such as lignosulfonates [501] from plant material or mucins from saliva or gastric juice may be feasible. Similarly, urogastrone [501a] is a potentially valuable agent.

c. Carbenoxolone. There seems little doubt now that carbenoxolone is an effective drug for the therapy of gastric ulcer disease, but dosage and mode of administration are not yet optimized in the case of duodenal ulcer. More effective position release forms of Duogastrone® will be required for optimal therapy of duodenal ulcer disease.

Several interesting questions can be asked in this general area: Does the effectiveness of carbenoxolone in aphthous stomatitis [502] and gastric ulceration support the etiological concept that the initial injury in the case of gastric ulcer formation is a virus infection? Since carbenoxolone stimulates mucus production, is drug response directly parallel to the patients' blood group and secretor status, or do those individuals who fail to respond to carbenoxolone, or who relapse on therapy, primarily belong to a single blood and secretor group? Would it be pharmaceutically possible and therapeutically desirable to combine carbenoxolone with irritating drugs normally given orally, such as aspirin, corticosteroids, phenylbutazone? Can derivatives without the troublesome aldosterone-like side effects be developed?

The apparent therapeutic success of deglycyrrhizinated licorice suggests the advisability of screening other licorice derivatives for gastric ulcer disease. Furthermore, the intriguing finding that the ulcer healing properties of carbenoxolone-sodium are blocked by aldosterone antagonists, but not by the thiazide diuretics [286, 287], warrants detailed investigation.

5. Epithelial Cell Kinetics and Ulcer Healing

Very little is known about the healing of peptic ulcers, but many factors must be involved in controlling the local development of granulation tissue, enzyme activity, and epithelial growth, and in the function of fibroblasts in the ulcer crater [195, 503]. It is conceivable that ulcer intractibility may be in part associated with a breakdown in one of these factors; however, as yet no confirming evidence is available although in ascorbic acid deficiency, collagen formation by fibroblasts is defective [504].

One of the important questions central to an understanding of growth and regeneration is: What is it that triggers a growth response in any particular tissue? Are tissue specific growth-promoting factors or inhibitors (chalones) common. Nerve growth factor (NGF) is one such growth promoting agent obtained from salivary glands [505]. Although the chemical basis of NGF action is not known, it does stimulate RNA, protein, and lipid synthesis as well as glucose oxidation. A careful search, particularly in salivary and gastric secretion, for such tissue specific agents which could act either directly or indirectly by inhibition of specific chalones [195] might be rewarding.

a. Zinc Salts. Zinc is an essential metal. In animals and man about 20 percent of the total body zinc is concentrated and stored in epithelial structures where it is necessary for many enzyme systems [506]. In rats, zinc deficiency results in a reduced incorporation of certain amino acids into protein [507].

Recently, zinc sulfate was shown to produce increased healing in various cutaneous wounds in animals and man [508], acceleration of healing being greatest during the stage of epithelialization. The mechanism of this increased healing is not known, but may depend upon stimulation of granulation tissue formation, or on the supply of an essential enzyme cofactor for protein synthesis.

As far as the author is aware, zinc salts have only been used in the treatment of skin ulcers. However, in view of the similarities between the structure and reproduction of skin and gastrointestinal epithelia, a trial of zinc salts in the treatment of peptic ulcer disease is certainly warranted.

Borderline zinc deficiency is common in the U.S., and patients readily go into a negative zinc balance under stress [509]. If zinc is important in wound healing, other gastrointestinal ulcerative conditions may be equally benefited by zinc therapy.

b. Powdered Cartilage. Bovine and shark cartilage contain a substance(s) which, like zinc sulfate, accelerates the healing of experimentally induced skin ulcers following either topical or parenteral administration [510]. The substance of unknown chemical composition may act by supplying a biochemical component necessary to initiate granulation tissue formation since cartilage extracts stimulate mucopolysaccharide synthesis in fibroblasts in vitro [511].

No study is available evaluating the possible healing properties of powdered cartilage in peptic ulcer disease. Such an investigation is certainly warranted.

6. Antifibrinolytic Agents

Fibrinolysin (plasmin) is a proteolytic enzyme present in plasma in an inactive precursor form, plasminogen. Normal plasma contains inhibitors preventing fibrinolysin formation. Fibrinolysin has been shown to possess numerous functions: digestion of fibrin and other clotting factors, formation and inactivation of biologically active polypeptides, activation of several complement fractions, and hydrolysis of γ globulin [512].

The activation of plasminogen to produce fibrinolysin is an important mechanism which guards against inadvertent fibrin formation; however, occasionally it may fail and result in massive bleeding. Cox et al. [178] have reported increased gastric venous free plasmin levels and gastric mucosal plasminogen activator in some peptic ulcer patients. Thus, antifibrinolytic agents may be of some help in therapy if excessive bleeding results in some patients with peptic ulcer disease due to increased fibrinolysin formation.

One potent inhibitor of plasminogen activator is epsilon-aminocaproic acid (EACA) which may also possess some direct antiplasmin activity [513]. EACA has been used in a variety of hemorrhagic conditions, but it is a dangerous agent producing a variety of adverse effects including generalized vascular thrombosis [512]. If significant elevations of plasminogen activator and plasma fibrinolysin are found in cases of peptic ulcer disease, cautious therapy with EACA or its newer derivatives may be of occasional therapeutic value.

7. Antiviral Drugs

No direct evidence is available supporting a viral etiology for peptic ulcer disease. However, Jones et al. [53] suggested that gastric ulcers might arise initially as a superficial ulcer akin to that seen in the oral cavity with herpes simplex-induced aphthous stomatitis. A viral etiology for the initial injury in ulcer formation is attractive, since it would help to explain ulcer recurrence and intractability; stressful situations are known to activate latent virus infections.

It is of interest therefore that carbenoxolone has been found therapeutically successful in treating human aphthous stomatitis [502], suggesting possible "antiviral" activity in this compound; certainly, carbenoxolone inhibits DNA synthesis in isolated cells [514]. It should be relatively simple to test carbenoxolone for additional antiviral activity, and if present it would provide fresh leads in the search for new therapeutic agents.

VI. SUMMARY

"You know," said the Dormouse, "they drew all manner of things — everything that begins with an M_____., such as mouse-traps, and the moon, and memory, and muchness_____, you know you say things are "much of a muchness_____ ".

A Mad Tea-Party, Alice in Wonderland
by Lewis Carroll.

Lewis Carroll's sleepy Dormouse could well have been talking about the plethora of currently available drugs for treating peptic ulcer disease since the two big groups of agents, antacids and antimuscarinics, are in reality "much of a muchness," no single form of therapy being entirely satisfactory.

When attempting to design new drugs for treating peptic ulcer disease, it should be remembered that although hydrochloric acid and possibly pepsin are required for ulcer chronicity, the precise sequence of events leading to ulcer formation is not known. Furthermore, although there are many similarities and associations between gastric and duodenal ulcers, they may be etiologically unrelated phenomena.

A. Inhibition of Hydrochloric Acid Secretion

Since little is known about the controlling influences of the central nervous system, drugs with a selective central action, unless discovered serendipitously, will be a long time coming. This may not apply however to isolation of gastric secretory inhibitors released by cerebral stimulation [521], or the application, in certain cases, of electrosleep.

P. G. Wodehouse would have said, if he had been a physician, that gastroenterologists could be divided into two groups depending upon whether or not they believed histamine played a role in gastric secretory physiology. Some support for the histamine camp has recently been presented by Kier. He has suggested that histamine may exist in the biophase in either of two distinctly different, but nearly equally preferred conformations, and produce two distinct biological responses depending upon the presence of specific receptors, H_1 and H_2 [407]. Kier has further suggested that H_2 receptors may be present in gastric mucosa and anticipates that the action of histamine on these receptors will be blocked by drugs containing

$$N \leftarrow 3.60 \text{Å} \rightarrow N^+.$$

The question of histidine decarboxylase inhibitors is confusing since correlation between <u>in vitro</u> and <u>in vivo</u> activity, and possible effects on other enzymes, have frequently been neglected. For example, NSD-1055, TMA, ATMA, and αHHd (Table V) all have equal <u>in vitro</u> activity. However, TMA, ATMA, and αHHd are more effective inhibitors than NSD-1055 against rat gastric histidine decarboxylase <u>in vivo</u>, whereas NSD-1055 is a stronger inhibitor of nonspecific dopa decarboxylase [423a, 423b]. Slight differences in structure also effect specificity; for example, TMA depletes brain histamine whereas ATMA does not [423a, 423b]. It is thus likely that the question, "Does histamine play a role in the pathophysiology of gastric secretion in man?" may not be answered until we have available a specific selective antagonist of either histamine, or histidine decarboxylase activity, in human gastric mucosa.

The initial excitement engendered following the identification of the structure of gastrin has somewhat waned. Certainly at present, it seems unlikely that a derivative of the C terminal tetrapeptide amide fragment of gastrin possessing "lock and key" type specific inhibition of hormonal activity will be synthesized. On the basis of structure activity relationships Morley has proposed four potential inhibitors of gastrin [426]. However, more than 600 congeners of the tetrapeptide amide fragment have been studied for antisecretory activity to no avail. Greater success may be achieved with caerulein or cholecystokinin-pancreozymin. Development of antibodies to either gastrin or the parietal cell [522] probably have greater potential for success. However, the use of antibodies is not without risk.

The ultimate destiny of the prostaglandins (PG) is difficult to predict. There is no doubt that they are potent gastric secretory inhibitors. However, in view of the fact that they probably act via inhibition of cyclic 3', 5'-AMP

II. GASTROINTESTINAL DISORDERS — PEPTIC ULCER DISEASE

it will certainly be difficult to develop a PG with selective action on the gastric mucosa.

Glucagon has some potential in ulcer treatment for three reasons. First, it would tend to reduce vagal activity caused by hypoglycemia; second, it has a direct depressant effect on gastric acid secretion; and third, it has an additional advantage over secretin in that it apparently does not stimulate pepsin secretion [492].

B. Neutralization of Hydrochloric Acid

Neutralization of hydrochloric acid with alkalis has been the cornerstone of ulcer therapy for years. However, more physiological and attractive ways of accomplishing acid neutralization by the use of secretin or cholecystokinin-pancreozymin are potentially available. Words of caution are warranted, since antimuscarinics commonly employed as adjunct agents in the treatment of peptic ulcer disease have recently been shown to reduce endogenous secretin release [488, 489], and secretin causes, in some instances, a sharp rise in pepsin secretion [486].

C. Pepsin and Mucus Production

Identification of new natural or semisynthetic antipepsins seems likely [148, 152, 493]. The benefit however of a pure "antipepsin" in peptic ulcer disease is at present doubtful. Of greater potential would be substances with additional properties of stimulation of mucus or cell renewal. Synthetic estrogens [495], licorice derivatives and lignosulfonates [501] warrant investigation.

D. Cell Kinetics

Information about factors controlling epithelial cell growth are needed before we can rationally suggest drugs to profitably modify ulcer healing. However, since there is a diurnal variation in such phenomena as cell growth, it is conceivable that drug therapy to achieve optimum results should be restricted to certain times in the day.

In summary, new concepts towards drug design are urgently required since antacids and antimuscarinics have had their day, and as George Eliot observed "Its but little good you'll do a-watering the last years' crop" (Adam Bede, Chapter 18). In this section an attempt has been made to collect some recent information as it applies to the development of novel and unique drugs for peptic ulcer disease. However, many of the suggestions may not either be practical, or found to be useful, but new ideas are an impossibility until they are born. I have attempted to emulate Dr. Watson — "I am inclined to think _____," said I (Dr. Watson). "I should do so," Sherlock Holmes remarked impatiently (The Valley of Fear, Sir Arthur Conan Doyle).

REFERENCES

1. J. C. Thompson, Ann. Rev. Med., 20, 291 (1969).
2. M. I. Grossman, in Handbook of Physiology, Alimentary Canal, Volume II, Section 6, Secretion (C. F. Code, section ed.), American Physiological Society, Washington, D. C., 1967, p. 863.
3. K. G. Wormsley and M. I. Grossman, Gut, 6, 427 (1965).
4. L. Pevsner and M. I. Grossman, Gastroenterology, 28, 493 (1955).
5. P. Thein and B. Schofield, Gastroenterology, 43, 436 (1962).
6. M. I. Grossman, Gastroenterology, 42, 718 (1962).
7. M. I. Grossman, The Physiologist, 6, 349 (1963).
8. C. -E. Elwin and B. Uvnäs, in Gastrin (M. E. Grossman, ed.), U. C. L. A. Forum in Medical Sciences, Number 5. University of California Press, Berkeley and Los Angeles, 1966, pp. 69-82.
9. R. A. Gregory, Secretory Mechanisms of the Gastro-Intestinal Tract, Edward Arnold, London, 1962, p. 248.
10. H. W. Davenport, Physiology of the Digestive Tract, 2nd ed., Year Book Medical Publishers, Chicago, 1966, p. 230.
11. W. W. Nowinski, Amer. J. Surg., 117, 768 (1969).
12. T. Scratcherd and R. M. Case, Gut, 10, 957 (1969).
13. D. P. Mertz, Experientia, 25, 269 (1969).
14. J. B. Harris, K. Nigon, and D. Alonso, Gastroenterology, 57, 377 (1969).
15. I. P. Pavlov, The Work of the Digestive Glands (translated by W. H. Thompson), 2nd ed., Griffin, London, 1910.
16. S. Andersson, in Handbook of Physiology, Alimentary Canal, Volume II, Section 6, Secretion (C. F. Code, section ed.), American Physiological Society, Washington, D. C., 1967, pp. 865-877.
17. E. R. Woodward, E. S. Lyon, J. Landor, and L. R. Dragstedt, Gastroenterology, 27, 766 (1954).
18. H. A. Oberhelman, Jr., E. R. Woodward, J. M. Zubiran, and L. R. Dragstedt, Am. J. Physiol., 169, 738 (1952).
19. R. C. Harrison, W. H. Lakey, and H. A. Hyde, Ann. Surg., 144, 441 (1956).
20. A. Iggo, Quart. J. Exptl. Physiol., 52, 398 (1957).
21. S. Andersson and B. Uvnäs, Gastroenterology, 41, 486 (1961).
22. K. G. Wormsley and M. I. Grossman, Gastroenterology, 47, 72 (1964).

23. I. J. Pincus, M. H. F. Friedman, J. E. Thomas, and M. E. Rehfuss, Am. J. Digest. Diseases, 11, 205 (1944).
24. S. Konturek and M. I. Grossman, Gastroenterology, 49, 481 (1965).
25. W. Sircus, Quart. J. Exptl. Physiol., 43, 114 (1958).
26. I. E. Gillespie and M. I. Grossman, Gut, 5, 342 (1964).
27. D. C. McIlrath and G. A. Hallenbeck, Am. J. Physiol., 206, 1077 (1964).
28. D. Johnston and H. L. Duthie, Gut, 5, 573 (1964).
29. D. Johnston and H. L. Duthie, Lancet, ii, 1032 (1965).
30. K. G. Wormsley, Gut, 10, 1050 (1969), Abstract.
30a. S. J. Rune and K. Viskum, Gut, 10, 569 (1969).
31. B. I. Hirschowitz, in Handbook of Physiology, Alimentary Canal, Volume II, Section 6, Secretion (C. F. Code, section ed.), American Physiological Society, Washington, D. C., 1967, pp. 889-918.
32. J. H. Northrop, M. Kunitz, and R. M. Herriott, Crystalline Enzymes, 2nd ed., Columbia Univ. Press, New York, 1948, p. 352.
33. M. D. Turner, Gut, 9, 134 (1968).
34. D. J. Etherington and W. H. Taylor, Biochem. J., 113, 663 (1969).
35. B. I. Hirschowitz, J. A. London, and H. S. Wiggins, J. Lab. Clin. Med., 53, 577 (1959).
36. K. Meyer, Advan. Protein Chem., 2, 249 (1945).
37. W. A. Sodeman, Jr., N. A. Augur, and H. M. Pollard, Med. Clin. N. Amer., 53, 1379 (1969).
38. M. I. Horowitz, in Handbook of Physiology, Alimentary Canal, Volume II, Section 6, Secretion (C. F. Code, section ed.), American Physiological Society, Washington, D. C., 1967, pp. 1063-1085.
39. R. Menguy and A. E. Thompson, Ann. N. Y. Acad. Sci., 140, 797 (1967).
40. G. B. J. Glass, Ann. N. Y. Acad. Sci., 140, 804 (1967).
41. T. T. White and D. F. Magee, Gastroenterology, 35, 289 (1958).
42. R. Menguy, Am. J. Surg., 117, 806 (1969).
43. M. I. Grossman, Gastroenterology, 53, 821 (1967).
44. I. S. Blumenthal, Gastroenterology, 54, 86 (1968).
45. S. P. Bralow, Am. J. Digest. Diseases, 14, 655 (1969).
46. I. S. Blumenthal, Research and the Ulcer Problem, Report R-336-RC, June 1959, The Rand Corporation, Santa Monica, Calif., 1960.

47. D. Davis, Personal communication, Drug Cosmetic Ind. (1970).
48. L. A. Smith, Peptic Ulcer (A. B. Rivers, ed.), Appleton-Century-Crofts, New York, 1953, pp. 1-10.
49. R. R. Monson and B. MacMahon, New Engl. J. Med., 281, 11 (1969).
50. R. Doll and F. A. Jones (with assistance of M. M. Buckatzsch), Occupational Factors in the Aetiology of Gastric and Duodenal Ulcers with an Estimate of Their Incidence in the General Population, His Majesty's Stationery Office, London, 1951, p. 96.
51. C. A. Clarke, D. A. Price Evans, R. B. McConnell, and P. M. Sheppard, Brit. Med. J., 1, 603 (1959).
52. W. I. Card and I. N. Marks, Clin. Sci., 19, 147 (1960).
53. F. A. Jones, J. W. P. Grummer, and J. E. Leonard-Jones, Clinical Gastroenterology, Blackwell Scientific Pub., Oxford, 1968, pp. 469-547.
54. R. Mangold, Brit. Med. J., 2, 1193 (1958).
55. H. D. Johnson, Lancet, i, 266 (1955).
56. P. Aagaard, M. Andreassen, and L. Kurz, Lancet, i, 1111 (1959).
57. S. C. Truelove and P. C. Reynell, Diseases of the Digestive System, Blackwell Scientific Pub., Oxford, 1963, pp. 148-178.
58. G. Watkinson, Gastroenterology, 18, 377 (1951).
59. B. Eiseman and R. L. Heyman, New Engl. J. Med., 282, 372 (1970).
60. S. F. Townsend, Am. J. Anat., 109, 133 (1961).
61. D. A. Brodie, Gastroenterology, 55, 125 (1968).
62. H. T. Cox, L. Poller, and J. M. Thomson, Gut, 10, 404 (1969).
63. R. I. Russell, J. M. Williamson, A. Goldberg, and E. Wares, Lancet, ii, 603 (1968).
64. B. A. Scobie and R. A. Rovelstad, Gastroenterology, 48, 318 (1965).
65. B. G. A. Moynihan, Duodenal Ulcer, 2nd ed., W. B. Saunders Co., Philadelphia, 1912, pp. 107-157.
66. G. W. Pickering, in Peptic Ulcer (D. J. Sandweiss, ed.), W. B. Saunders Co., Philadelphia, 1951, pp. 90-100.
67. K. G. Lennander, Mitt. Grenzgeb. Med. Chir., 16, 24 (1906).
68. E. C. Texter, Jr., G. R. Vantrappen, H. P. Lazar, E. J. Puletti, and C. J. Barborka, Ann. Internal Med., 51, 1275 (1959).
69. W. L. Palmer, Arch. Internal Med., 38, 694 (1926).
70. W. L. Palmer, Arch. Internal Med., 39, 109 (1927).

71. R. H. Resnick and S. J. Gray, Gastroenterology, 42, 48 (1962).
72. A. F. Hurst, in Gastric and Duodenal Ulcer (A. F. Hurst and M. J. Steward, eds.), Oxford Univ. Press, London, 1929, pp. 1-12.
73. H. Quincke, Deut. Med. Wochschr., 8, 79 (1882).
74. K. Schwarz, Beitr. Klin. Chir., 67, 96 (1910).
75. H. Shay, in Current Gastroenterology (G. McHardy, ed.), Paul B. Hoeber, Medical Division, Harper & Brothers, New York, 1962, pp. 276-296.
76. M. Oi, Y. Ito, F. Kumagai, K. Yoshida, Y. Tanaka, K. Yoshikawa, O. Miho, and M. Kijima, Gastroenterology, 57, 280 (1969).
77. M. I. Grossman, in Peptic Ulcer (D. J. Sandweiss, ed.), W. B. Saunders Co., Philadelphia, 1951, pp. 165-175.
78. S. C. Skoryna, Pathophysiology of Peptic Ulcer, J. B. Lippincott Co., Philadelphia, 1963, p. 497.
79. D. C. H. Sun, Chemistry and Therapy of Peptic Ulcer (I. Newton Kugelmass, ed.), Charles C. Thomas, Springfield, Illinois, 1966, p. 238.
80. M. Susser, J. Chronic Diseases, 20, 435 (1967).
81. F. A. Jones, Brit. Med. J., 1, 719 (1957).
82. G. Garrido-Klinge and L. Peña, Gastroenterology, 37, 390 (1959).
83. J. R. Dogra, Indian J. Med. Res., 28, 145 (1940).
84. I. Aird and H. H. Bentall, Brit. Med. J., 1, 799 (1953).
85. C. N. Pulvertaft, "The Incidence of Peptic Ulcer in Town and Country," in Proc. World Congr. Gastroenterology, Williams and Wilkins, Baltimore, 1958, pp. 364-376.
86. T. L. Cleave, Peptic Ulcer, John Wright & Sons, Bristol, 1962, p. 151.
87. S. L. Malhotra, Gut, 5, 412 (1964).
88. S. L. Malhotra, O. N. Saigal, and G. D. Mody, Brit. Med. J., 1, 1220 (1965).
89. R. Doll, F. Avery Jones, and F. Pygott, Lancet, i, 657 (1958).
90. R. Doll, Scot. Med. J., 9, 183 (1964).
91. J. H. Thompson, Res. Comm. Chem. Pathol. Pharmacol., 1, 230 (1970).
92. J. H. Thompson, Experientia, 26, 615 (1970).
93. H. W. Davenport, Gastroenterology, 56, 439 (1969).

94. R. H. Salter, Am. J. Digest. Diseases, 13, 38 (1968).
95. H. W. Davenport, New Engl. J. Med., 276, 1307 (1967).
96. D. N. Croft and P. H. N. Wood, Brit. Med. J., 1, 137 (1967).
97. P. W. Kent and A. Allen, Biochem. J., 106, 645 (1968).
98. K. D. Rainsford, J. Watkins, and M. J. H. Smith, J. Pharm. Pharmacol., 20, 941 (1968).
99. I. P. T. Häkkinen, R. Johansson, and M. Pantio, Gut, 9, 712 (1968).
100. M. W. Whitehouse, Biochem. Pharmacol., 13, 319 (1964).
101. M. W. Whitehouse and H. Boström, Biochem. Pharmacol., 11, 1175 (1962).
102. D. A. Brodie and B. J. Chase, Gastroenterology, 53, 604 (1967).
103. S. Emås, Am. J. Digest. Diseases, 13, 572 (1968).
104. D. C. H. Sun, Am. J. Digest. Diseases, 14, 107 (1969).
105. B. L. Chapman and J. M. Duggan, Gut, 10, 443 (1969).
106. J. J. Petillo, A. Gulbenkian, and I. I. A. Tabachnick, Biochem. Pharmacol., 18, 1784 (1969).
107. G. Watkinson, Gut, 1, 14 (1960).
108. D. H. Clark, Brit. Med. J., 1, 1254 (1953).
109. R. Doll and J. Buch, Ann. Eugenics, 15, 135 (1950).
110. R. Doll and T. D. Kellock, Ann. Eugenics, 16, 231 (1951).
111. J. J. Dubarry, C. Pisot, and J. Duhamer, in Proc. World Congr. Gastroenterology and 59th Ann. Meeting Am. Gastroenterological Assoc., Washington, D. C., May 25-31, 1958, Vol. 1, Williams and Wilkins, Baltimore, 1959, p. 386.
112. J. R. Kahn, Am. J. Med. Sci., 194, 463 (1937).
113. W. L. Palmer and P. B. Nutter, Arch. Internal Med., 65, 499 (1940).
114. L. R. Dragstedt, Gastroenterology, 30, 208 (1956).
115. A. W. Kay, Brit. Med. J., 2, 77 (1953).
116. A. J. Cox, Arch. Pathol., 54, 407 (1952).
117. J. H. Baron, Gut, 4, 243 (1963).
118. R. M. Zollinger and E. H. Ellison, Ann. Surg., 142, 709 (1955).
119. W. C. Meyers, Gastroenterology, 10, 923 (1948).
120. L. W. Guiss and F. W. Stewart, Arch. Surg. 57, 618 (1948).
121. I. N. Marks and H. Shay, Lancet, i, 1107 (1959).

122. O. H. Wangensteen, R. L. Varco, L. Hay, S. Walpole, and B. Trach, Ann. Surg., 112, 626 (1940).

123. W. Sircus, in Gastric Secretion — Mechanism and Control. Proc. Held at the Faculty of Med., Univ. of Alberta, Edmonton, Canada, Sept. 13-15, 1965. Pergamon, New York, 1967, p. 293.

124. G. P. Crean, D. F. Hogg, and R. D. E. Rumsey, Gastroenterology, 56, 193 (1969).

125. A. J. Cox, Jr., and V. R. Barnes, Proc. Soc. Exptl. Biol. Med., 60, 118 (1945).

126. S. Erasian and J. D. Hardy, J. Surg. Res., 6, 137 (1966).

127. G. P. Crean, M. W. Marshall, and R. D. E. Rumsey, Gastroenterology, 57, 147 (1969).

128. M. D. Kaye, Am. J. Digest. Diseases, 14, 770 (1969).

129. M. D. Kaye, A. Jacobs, M. C. Path, H. Ireson, and D. Trevett, Am. J. Digest. Diseases, 13, 994 (1968).

130. M. D. Kaye, P. Beck, J. Rhodes, and P. M. Sweetnam, Gut, 10, 774 (1969).

131. A. G. Melrose, R. I. Russell, and A. Dick, Gut, 5, 546 (1964).

132. J. Hunter, Phil. Trans. Roy. Soc. (London), 62, 447 (1772).

133. H. Shay, M. Gruenstein, H. Siplet, and S. A. Komarov, Proc. Soc. Exptl. Biol. Med., 69, 369 (1948).

134. B. Holmström, S. Wallensten, and Å. Frisk, Acta Chir. Scand., 117, 215 (1959).

135. G. A. Friedman, J. Med. Res., 32, 95 (1915).

136. M. J. S. Langman, J. H. Hansky, R. A. B. Drury, and F. Avery Jones, Gut, 5, 550 (1964).

137. D. J. du Plessis, Lancet, i, 974 (1965).

138. I. R. Mackay and I. G. Hislop, Gut, 7, 228 (1966).

139. W. M. Capper, G. R. Airth, and J. O. Kilby, Lancet, ii, 621 (1966).

140. J. Rhodes, D. E. Barnardo, S. F. Phillips, R. A. Rovelstad, and A. F. Hofmann, Gastroenterology, 57, 241 (1969).

141. D. Doniach and I. M. Roitt, Seminars in Hematol., 1, 313 (1964).

142. P. A. J. Ball, Lancet, i, 1363 (1961).

143. H. W. Davenport, Gastroenterology, 46, 245 (1964).

144. B. F. Overholt, D. A. Brodie, and B. J. Chase, Gastroenterology, 56, 651 (1969).

145. C. Bernard, Leçons de Physiologie Experimentale Appliqué à la Medicine, Vol. 2, Baillière, Paris, 1856, p. 406.

146. F. Hollander, Arch. Internal Med., 93, 107 (1954).

147. J. B. Kirsner, Gastroenterology, 51, 403 (1966).

148. J. DeGraef and G. B. J. Glass, Gastroenterology, 55, 584 (1968).

149. D. A. P. Evans, R. B. McConnell, W. T. A. Donohoe, W. Sircus, and G. P. Crean, J. Lab. Clin. Med., 61, 660 (1963).

150. C. F. Code, in Gastric Secretion, Mechanisms and Control. Proc. Symp. Held at the Faculty of Med., Univ. of Alberta, Edmonton, Canada, Sept. 13-15, 1965. Pergamon, New York, 1967, p. 405.

151. R. Lambert, F. Martin, C. Andre, L. Descos, and G. Vouillon, Am. J. Digest. Diseases, 13, 941 (1968).

152. J. DeGraef and G. B. J. Glass, Gastroenterology, 55, 594 (1968).

153. N. G. Heatley, Gastroenterology, 37, 313 (1959).

154. F. Martin and R. Lambert, Acta Gastro-Enterol. Belg., 29, 289 (1966).

155. J. Straughn, in The Stomach - Including Related Areas in the Esophagus and Duodenum, The 13th Hahnemann Symp. (C. Thompson, D. Berkowitz, E. Polish, eds., J. H. Moyer, consult. ed.), Grune & Stratton, New York and London, 1967, pp. 141-144.

156. A. Robert, J. P. Phillips, and J. E. Nezamis, Am. J. Digest. Diseases, 11, 546 (1966).

157. R. Fiasse, C. F. Code, and G. B. J. Glass, Gastroenterology, 54, 1018 (1968).

158. W. Anderson, J. Pharm. Pharmacol., 21, 264 (1969).

159. L. C. Hoskins and N. Zamcheck, Gastroenterology, 48, 758 (1965).

160. D. W. Piper, E. M. Griffith, and B. H. Fenton, Am. J. Digest. Diseases, 10, 411 (1965).

161. R. Menguy, Y. F. Masters, and W. Gryboski, Gastroenterology, 46, 32 (1964).

162. J. R. N. Curt and R. Pringle, Gut, 10, 931 (1969).

163. I. Aird, H. H. Bentall, J. A. Mehigan, and J. A. F. Roberts, Brit. Med. J., 2, 315 (1954).

164. C. A. Clarke, W. K. Cowan, J. W. Edwards, A. W. Howel-Evans, R. B. McConnell, J. C. Woodrow, and P. M. Sheppard, Brit. Med. J., 2, 643 (1955).

165. R. Doll, B. F. Swynnerton, and A. C. Newell, Gut, 1, 31 (1960).

166. H. D. Johnson, A. H. G. Love, N. C. Rogers, and A. P. Wyatt, Gut, 5, 402 (1964).
167. H. D. Johnson, Ann. Surg., 162, 996 (1965).
168. I. P. T. Häkkinen, V. Raunio, S. Virtanen, and J. Kohonen, Clin. Exptl. Immunol., 4, 149 (1969).
169. C. A. Clarke, J. W. Edwards, D. R. W. Haddock, A. W. Howel-Evans, R. B. McConnell, and P. M. Sheppard, Brit. Med. J., 2, 725 (1956).
170. R. Doll, H. Drane, and A. C. Newell, Gut, 2, 352 (1961).
171. O. Fodor, S. Vestea, S. Urcan, S. Popescu, L. Sulica, R. Iencica, A. Goia, and V. Ilea, Am. J. Digest. Diseases, 13, 260 (1968).
172. R. B. McConnell, The Genetics of Gastro-Intestinal Disorders, Oxford Univ. Press, London, 1966, p. 282.
173. M. J. S. Langman and R. Doll, Gut, 6, 270 (1965).
174. D. A. P. Evans, L. Horwich, R. B. McConnell, and M. F. Bullen, Gut, 9, 319 (1968).
175. L. Horwich, D. A. P. Evans, R. B. McConnell, and W. T. A. Donohoe, Gut, 7, 680 (1966).
176. L. E. Glynn, E. J. Holborow, and G. D. Johnson, Lancet, ii, 1083 (1957).
177. A. E. Szulman, J. Exptl. Med., 115, 977 (1962).
178. W. M. Watkins, Science, 152, 172 (1966).
179. G. B. J. Glass, A. Ishimori, and J. A. Buckwalter, Gastroenterology, 42, 443 (1962).
180. L. Horwich and D. A. P. Evans, Gut, 7, 525 (1966).
181. M. A. Denborough, Australasian Ann. Med., 15, 314 (1966).
182. G. P. Jori, G. Mazzacca, C. Balestrieri, R. P. Donnorso, B. Gallo, and M. Mansi, Am. J. Digest. Dis., 14, 380 (1969).
183. L. E. Ventzke and M. I. Grossman, Gastroenterology, 42, 292 (1962).
184. R. Virchow, Virchows Arch., 5, 281 (1856).
185. B. J. Haverback and D. F. Bogdanski, Proc. Soc. Exptl. Biol. Med., 95, 392 (1957).
186. R. A. MacDonald, Am. J. Med., 21, 867 (1956).
187. P. H. Guth and P. Hall, Gastroenterology, 50, 562 (1966).
188. H. Necheles, Am. J. Digest. Diseases, 16, 237 (1949).
189. E. D. Palmer and J. L. Sherman, Arch. Internal. Med., 101, 1106 (1958).

190. J. A. Gius, D. E. Boyle, R. H. Congdon, and W. C. Boyd, Arch. Surg., 91, 221 (1965).

191. D. N. Croft, D. J. Pollock, and N. F. Coghill, Gut, 7, 333 (1966).

192. J. D. Thrasher, in Methods in Cell Physiology (D. M. Prescott, ed.), Vol. 11, Academic Press, New York, 1966, pp. 323-357.

193. Y. S. Kim, R. Kerr, and M. Lipkin, Nature, 215, 1180 (1967).

194. C. S. Hooper and M. Blair, Exptl. Cell Res., 14, 175 (1958).

195. W. S. Bullough and E. B. Laurence, Nature, 220, 134 (1968).

196. T. Räsänen, Acta Physiol. Scand., 58, 201 (1963).

197. R. H. Clark and B. L. Baker, Proc. Soc. Exptl. Biol. Med., 111, 311 (1962).

198. H. Teir, Gastroenterology, 44, 536 (1963).

199. J. Kyle, S. D. Clarke, J. T. Ward, A. O. Adesola, and R. B. Welbourn, in Pathophysiology of Peptic Ulcer (S. C. Skoryna, ed.), J. B. Lippincott Co., Philadelphia, 1963, pp. 445-456.

200. J. Orloff and J. S. Handler (A. S. Preston, Tech. Assist.), J. Clin. Invest., 41, 702 (1962).

201. G. A. Robison, R. W. Butcher, and E. W. Sutherland, Ann. Rev. Biochem., 37, 149 (1968).

202. R. C. Haynes, Jr., and L. Berthet, J. Biol. Chem., 225, 115 (1957).

203. E. W. Sutherland and T. W. Rall, Pharmacol. Rev., 12, 265 (1960).

204. J. S. Handler and J. Orloff, Am. J. Physiol., 206, 505 (1964).

205. L. R. Chase and G. D. Aurbach, Science, 159, 545 (1968).

206. R. W. Butcher and E. W. Sutherland, J. Biol. Chem., 237, 1244 (1962).

207. G. Dotevall and H. Westling, Acta Med. Scand., 174, 777 (1963).

208. H. A. Demand, K. Weichmann, and G. Berg, Gastroenterology, 55, 272 (1968).

209. A. R. Cooke, R. M. Preshaw, and M. I. Grossman, Gastroenterology, 50, 761 (1966).

210. A. R. Cooke, Gut, 8, 588 (1967).

211. R. G. Strickland, J. M. Fisher, and K. B. Taylor, Gastroenterology, 56, 675 (1969).

212. S. Z. Sorkin, Medicine, 28, 371 (1949).

213. F. L. Engel, J. Clin. Endocrinol. Metabol., 15, 1300 (1955).

214. J. Kyle, J. S. Logan, D. W. Neill, and R. B. Welbourn, Lancet, i, 664 (1956).
215. B. L. Baker and R. M. Bridgman, Am. J. Anat., 94, 363 (1954).
216. S. P. Bralow, S. A. Komarov, and H. Shay, Am. J. Physiol., 206, 1309 (1964).
217. S. J. Gray, C. Ramsey, R. W. Reifenstein, and J. A. Benson, Jr., Gastroenterology, 25, 156 (1953).
218. A. G. Green and C. N. Pulvertaft, Gut, 3, 327 (1962).
219. B. I. Hirschowitz, D. H. P. Streeten, H. M. Pollard, and H. A. Boldt, Jr., J. Amer. Med. Assoc., 158, 27 (1955).
220. W. T. Wilder, B. Frame, and W. S. Haubrich, Ann. Internal Med., 55, 885 (1961).
221. W. L. Donegan and H. M. Spiro, Gastroenterology, 38, 750 (1960).
222. R. A. Smallwood, Gut, 8, 592 (1967).
223. L. O. Underdahl, L. B. Woolner, and B. M. Black, J. Clin. Endocrinol., 13, 20 (1953).
224. H. S. Ballard, B. Frame, and R. J. Hartsock, Medicine, 43, 481 (1964).
225. R. A. Gregory, H. J. Tracy, J. M. French, and W. Sircus, Lancet, i, 1045 (1960).
226. M. A. Polacek and E. H. Ellison, Surg. Forum, 14, 313 (1963).
227. K. D. Buchanan, M. T. McKiddie, A. C. Lindsay, and W. G. Manderson, Gut, 8, 325 (1967).
228. S. A. Bencosme, E. Liepa, and S. S. Lazarus, Proc. Soc. Exptl. Biol. Med., 90, 387 (1955).
229. D. A. Dreiling and H. D. Janowitz, Gastroenterology, 36, 580 (1959).
230. R. L. von Heimburg and G. A. Hallenbeck, Gastroenterology, 47, 531 (1964).
231. S. D. Clarke, D. W. Neill, and R. B. Welbourn, Gut, 1, 146 (1960).
232. J. Nasio, Prensa Med. Arg., 33, 197 (1946).
233. P. Kelly and A. Robert, Gastroenterology, 56, 24 (1969).
234. C. A. Loehry and B. Creamer, Gut, 10, 112 (1969).
235. S. C. Truelove, Brit. Med. J., 2, 559 (1960).
236. T. D. Kellock, Brit. Med. J., 2, 1117 (1951).
237. A. Norman, Psychophysiology, 5, 673 (1969).

238. H. Shay, D. H. Sun, B. Dlin, and E. Weiss, J. Appl. Physiol., 12, 461 (1958).

239. A. S. Leonard, R. B. Gilsdorf, J. M. Pearl, E. T. Peter, and W. B. Ritchie, in Gastric Secretion, Mechanism and Control, Proc. Symp. Held at the Univ. of Alberta, Edmonton, Canada, Sept. 13-15, 1965, Pergamon, New York, 1967, p. 149.

240. W. H. Hall and G. P. Smith, Gastroenterology, 57, 491 (1969).

241. E. E. Navarret, Rev. A. M. A., 70, 227 (1956).

242. S. Sherlock, Diseases of the Liver and Biliary System, 4th ed., F. A. Davis Co., Philadelphia, 1968, pp. 395-436.

243. J. H. Landor, J. F. Porterfield, and W. S. Wolff, Surg. Gynecol. Obstet., 122, 61 (1966).

244. M. J. Orloff, J. G. Chandler, S. J. Alderman, J. E. Keiter, and H. Rosen, Ann. Surg., 170, 515 (1969).

245. J. B. Kirsner, in Textbook of Medicine (P. B. Beeson and W. McDermott, eds.), 12th ed., W. B. Saunders Co., Philadelphia and London, 1967, pp. 859-880.

246. H. F. West, Brit. Med. J., 2, 680 (1959).

247. "Diet and Duodenal Ulcer," Leading Article, Brit. Med. J., 3, 727 (1969).

248. N. Babouris, J. Fletscher, and J. E. Leonard-Jones, Gut, 6, 118 (1965).

249. L. O. Randall, Diseases Nervous System, 21 (Suppl.), 7 (1960).

250. J. D. B. MacDougall, A. J. Carr, and D. W. Blair, Brit. J. Surg., 51, 937 (1964).

251. F. Hollander, Am. J. Digest. Diseases, 6, 127 (1939).

252. M. I. Grossman, in Current Gastroenterology (G. McHardy, ed.), Paul B. Hoeber, Medical Division, Harper & Brothers, New York, 1962, pp. 303-314.

253. J. Myhill and D. W. Piper, Gut, 5, 581 (1964).

254. E. M. Clarkson, S. J. McDonald, and H. E. de Wardener, Clin. Sci., 30, 425 (1966).

255. E. T. Schroeder, Gastroenterology, 56, 868 (1969).

256. M. Brody and W. H. Bachrach, Am. J. Digest. Diseases, 4, 435 (1959).

257. J. H. Thompson in Essentials of Pharmacology (J. A. Bevan, ed.), Paul B. Hoeber, Medical Division, Harper & Row, New York, 1969, pp. 293-314.

II. GASTROINTESTINAL DISORDERS — PEPTIC ULCER DISEASE

258. P. E. Baume and J. H. Hunt, Australasian Ann. Med., 18, 113 (1969).
259. E. H. Hale and M. I. Grossman, J. Lab. Clin. Med., 34, 228 (1949).
260. E. N. Rowlands, H. H. Wolff, and M. Atkinson, Lancet, ii, 1154 (1952).
261. D. G. Rimer and M. Frankland, J. Am. Med. Assoc., 173, 995 (1960).
262. C. H. Burnett, R. R. Commons, F. Albright, and J. E. Howard, New Engl. J. Med., 240, 787 (1949).
263. J. E. Lennard-Jones, Brit. Med. J., 1, 1071 (1961).
264. E. C. Texter, Jr., C. W. Legerton, Jr., J. M. Ruffin, J. S. Atwater, D. Cayer, F. D. Cheney, R. A. Jackson, B. G. Oren, and J. M. Rumball, Southern Med. J., 46, 1062 (1953).
265. P. H. Friedlander, Lancet, i, 386 (1954).
266. A. G. Melrose and I. W. Pinkerton, Brit. Med. J., 1, 1076 (1961).
267. D. C. H. Sun, Ann. N. Y. Acad. Sci., 99, 104 (1962).
268. D. C. H. Sun, Am. J. Digest. Diseases, 9, 706 (1964).
269. D. G. Friend, Clin. Pharmacol. Therap., 4, 559 (1963).
270. R. D. Mitchell, J. N. Hunt, and M. I. Grossman, Gastroenterology, 43, 400 (1962).
271. I. R. Innes and M. Nickerson, in The Pharmacological Basis of Therapeutics (3rd ed.), (L. S. Goodman and A. Gilman, eds.), Macmillan, New York, 1965, pp. 521-545.
272. J. L. A. Roth, R. L. Wechsler, and H. L. Bockus, Gastroenterology, 31, 493 (1956).
273. F. Steigmann and R. B. Schlesinger, Am. J. Digest. Diseases, 17, 361 (1950).
274. J. E. Berk, in Peptic Ulcer (D. J. Sandwiess, ed.), W. B. Saunders Co., Philadelphia, 1951, pp. 343-371.
275. R. Galloway, in A Symposium on Carbenoxolone Sodium at the Royal Society of Medicine, London, November 20, 1967 (J. M. Robson and F. M. Sullivan, eds.), Butterworths, London, 1968, Session 4, p. 203.
276. G. Watkinson, in A Symposium on Carbenoxolone Sodium at the Royal Society of Medicine, London, November 20, 1967 (J. M. Robson and F. M. Sullivan, eds.), Butterworths, London, 1968, Session 4, p. 245.
277. M. H. Khan and F. M. Sullivan, in A Symposium on Carbenoxolone Sodium at the Royal Society of Medicine, London, November 20, 1967 (J. M. Robson and F. M. Sullivan, eds.), Butterworths, London, 1968, Session 1, p. 5.

278. L. M. Atherden, Biochem. J., 69, 75 (1958).

279. D. V. Parke, in A Symposium on Carbenoxolone Sodium at the Royal Society of Medicine, London, November 20, 1967 (J. M. Robson and F. M. Sullivan, eds.) Butterworths, London, 1968, Session 1, p. 15.

280. L. Horwich and R. Galloway, Brit. Med. J., 2, 1274 (1965).

281. P. D. G. Dean, T. G. Halsall, and M. W. Whitehouse, J. Pharm. Pharmacol., 19, 682 (1967).

282. J. H. Baron, J. D. N. Nabarro, N Guercken, and A. M. Jackson, in A Symposium on Carbenoxolone Sodium at the Royal Society of Medicine, London, November 20, 1967 (J. M. Robson and F. M. Sullivan, eds.), Butterworths, London, 1968, Session 3, p. 127.

283. W. Hausmann and A. L. Tárnoky, in A Symposium on Carbenoxolone Sodium at the Royal Society of Medicine, London, November 20, 1967 (J. M. Robson and F. M. Sullivan, eds.), Butterworths, London, 1968, Session 3, p. 159.

284. V. Wynn, in A Symposium on Carbenoxolone Sodium at the Royal Society of Medicine, London, November 20, 1967 (J. M. Robson and F. M. Sullivan, eds.), Butterworths, London, 1968, Session 3, p. 173.

285. J. H. Baron, J. D. N. Nabarro, J. D. H. Slater, and R. Tuffley, Brit. Med. J., 2, 793 (1969).

286. R. Doll, M. J. S. Langman, and H. H. Shawdon, in A Symposium on Carbenoxolone Sodium at the Royal Society of Medicine, London, November 20, 1967 (J. M. Robson and F. M. Sullivan, eds.), Butterworths, London, 1968, Session 2, p. 51.

287. R. Doll, M. J. S. Langman, and H. H. Shawdon, Gut, 9, 42 (1968).

288. R. M. Baddeley, J. Evans, and J. A. Griffin, Gut, 10, 143 (1969).

289. P. Iveson, D. V. Parke, and R. T. Williams, Biochem. J., 100, 28P (1966).

290. J. B. Cocking and J. N. MacCaig, Gut, 10, 219 (1969).

291. A. M. Connell and R. A. Loane, in A Symposium on Carbenoxolone Sodium at the Royal Society of Medicine, London November 20, 1967 (J. M. Robson and F. M. Sullivan, eds.), Butterworths, London, 1968, Session 1, p. 25.

291a. A. C. B. Dean, in A Symposium on Carbenoxolone Sodium at the Royal Society of Medicine, London, November 20, 1967 (J. M. Robson and F. M. Sullivan, eds.), Butterworths, London, 1968, Session 1, p. 33.

292. M. Lipkin and W. Ludwig, in A Symposium on Carbenoxolone Sodium at the Royal Society of Medicine, London, November 20, 1967 (J. M. Robson and F. M. Sullivan, eds.) Butterworths, London, 1968, Session 1, p. 41.

293. F. R. Johnson, in A Symposium on Carbenoxolone Sodium at the Royal Society of Medicine, London, November 20, 1967 (J. M. Robson and F. M. Sullivan, eds.), Butterworths, London, 1968, Session 3, p. 93.

294. T. E. W. Goodier, L. Horwich, and R. W. Galloway, Gut, 8, 544 (1967).

295. T. E. W. Goodier, in A Symposium on Carbenoxolone Sodium at the Royal Society of Medicine, London, November 20, 1967 (J. M. Robson and F. M. Sullivan, eds.), Butterworths, London, 1968, Session 3, p. 111.

295a. M. J. S. Langman, Postgrad. Med. J., 44, 603 (1968).

296. J. W. Conn, D. R. Rovner, and E. L. Cohan, J. Am. Med. Assoc., 205, 492 (1968).

297. R. D. Montgomery, Gut, 8, 148 (1967).

298. S. Bank, I. N. Marks, P. E. Palmer, A. Gross, and E. van Eldik, S. African Med. J., 41, 297 (1967).

299. T. Hunt, S. African Med. J., 43, 1443 (1969).

300. D. O. Lewis and T. J. Ryan, in A Symposium on Carbenoxolone Sodium at the Royal Society of Medicine, London, November 20, 1967 (J. M. Robson and F. M. Sullivan, eds.), Butterworths, London, 1968, Session 2, p. 83.

301. I. H. Lawrence, D. J. Manton, K. Mendl, and R. D. Montgomery, in A Symposium on Carbenoxolone Sodium at the Royal Society of Medicine, London, November 20, 1967 (J. M. Robson and F. M. Sullivan, eds.), Butterworths, London, 1968, Session 4, p. 217.

302. T. C. Hunt, in A Symposium on Carbenoxolone Sodium at the Royal Society of Medicine, London, November 20, 1967 (J. M. Robson and F. M. Sullivan, eds.), Butterworths, London, 1968, Session 4, p. 195.

303. J. M. Cliff, in A Symposium on Carbenoxolone Sodium at the Royal Society of Medicine, London, November 20, 1967 (J. M. Robson and F. M. Sullivan, eds.), Butterworths, London, 1968, Session 4, p. 239.

304. D. G. Colin-Jones, J. E Lennard-Jones, J. H. Jones, J. J. Misiewicz, and M. J. S. Langman, in A Symposium on Carbenoxolone Sodium at the Royal Society of Medicine, London, November 20, 1967 (J. M. Robson and F. M. Sullivan, eds.), Butterworths, London, 1968, Session 4, p. 209.

305. R. D. Montgomery, I. H. Lawrence, D. J. Manton, K. Mendl, and P. Rowe, Gut, 9, 704 (1968).

306. S. N. Tewari and F. C. Trembalowicz, Gut, 9, 48 (1968).

307. A. G. G. Turpie, J. Runcie, and T. J. Thomson, Gut, 10, 299 (1969).

308. K. Takagi and Y. Ishii, Arzneim.-Forschung, 17, 1544 (1967).

309. T. S. Heineken, Am. J. Gastroenterol., 35, 619 (1961).
310. D. Cayer and J. M. Ruffin, Ann. N. Y. Acad. Sci., 140, 744 (1967).
311. D. C. H. Sun, Ann. N. Y. Acad. Sci., 140, 747 (1967).
312. D. W. Piper and B. Fenton, Am. J. Digest. Diseases, 6, 134 (1961).
313. J. B. Kirsner and R. A. Wolff, Gastroenterology, 2, 93 (1944).
314. D. L. Cook and V. A. Drill, Ann. N. Y. Acad. Sci., 140, 724 (1967).
315. S. Levey and S. Sheinfeld, Gastroenterology, 27, 625 (1954).
316. W. Anderson and J. Watt, J. Pharm. Pharmacol., 11, 318 (1959).
317. D. L. Cook, S. Eich, and P. S. Cammarata, Arch. Intern. Pharmacodyn Therap., 144, 1 (1963).
318. J. Watt, G. B. Eagleton, and R. Marcus, Nature, 211, 989 (1966).
319. J. Watt, G. B. Eagleton, and R. Marcus, J. Pharm. Pharmacol., 18, 615 (1966).
320. D. S. Zimmon, G. Miller, G. Cox, and M. A. Tesler, Gastroenterology, 56, 19 (1969).
321. S. P. Parbhoo and I. D. A. Johnston, Gut, 7, 612 (1966).
322. R. Doll, M. J. S. Langman, and H. H. Shawdon, Gut, 9, 46 (1968).
323. J. B. Kirsner, Am. J. Digest. Diseases, 9, 726 (1964).
324. C. B. Clayman, W. L. Palmer, and J. B. Kirsner, Gastroenterology, 55, 403 (1968).
325. J. M. Ruffin, J. E. Grizzle, N. C. Hightower, G. McHardy, H. Shull, and J. B. Kirsner, New Engl. J. Med., 281, 16 (1969).
326. I. D. A. Johnston, in Recent Advances in Gastroenterology (J. Badenoch and B. N. Brooke, eds.), J. & A. Churchill, London, 1965, pp. 107-115.
327. E. L. Posey, Jr., K. Boler, and L. Posey, III, Am. J. Digest. Diseases, 14, 797 (1969).
328. E. R. Woodward and H. Schapiro, Am. J. Physiol., 192, 479 (1958).
329. J. M. Glassman, G. M. Hudyma, and J. Seifter, J. Pharmacol. Exptl. Therap., 119, 150 (1957).
330. G. McHardy, G. E. Welch, and R. J. McHardy in Current Gastroenterology (G. McHardy, ed.), Paul B. Hoeber, Medical Division, Harper and Brothers, New York, 1962, pp. 643-664.
331. J. W. Baker, Clin. Radiol., 14, 442 (1963).
332. S. Carne, J. Coll. Gen. Practit., 8, 135 (1964).

II. GASTROINTESTINAL DISORDERS — PEPTIC ULCER DISEASE

333. D. W. Piper, F. L. Broderick, B. H. Fenton, and D. Beeston, Am. J. Digest. Diseases, 10, 122 (1965).

334. R. J. Bower and R. M. Myerson, Am. J. Gastroenterol., 42, 515 (1964).

335. M. J. Rheault, L. S. Semb, H. N. Harkins, and L. M. Nyhus, Am. J. Digest. Diseases, 10, 128 (1965).

336. H. D. Janowitz, H. Colcher, and F. Hollander, Am. J. Physiol., 171, 325 (1952).

337. P. Kramer and B. Markarian, Am. J. Digest. Diseases, 4, 130 (1959).

338. A. E. Lindner, N. Cohen, D. A. Dreiling, and H. D. Janowitz, J. Appl. Physiol., 17, 514 (1962).

339. K. N. Ojha and Q. Ahmed, Indian J. Physiol. Pharmacol., 11, 53 (1967).

340. M. L. Kothari, J. C. Doshi, H. G. Desai, A. B. Vaidya, U. K. Sheth, and J. M. Mehta, Gut, 10, 71 (1969).

341. B. A. Muggenburg, S. H. McNutt, and T. Kowalczyk, Am. J. Vet. Res., 25, 1354 (1964).

342. M. Barenfus, J. D. Thrasher, and S. T. Rich, Am. Assoc. Lab. Animal Sci., Oct. 1969, in press.

343. A. W. Williams, J. B. Howie, B. J. Helyer, and L. O. Simpson, Australian J. Exptl. Biol. Med. Sci., 45, 105 (1967).

344. F. C. Mann, in Peptic Ulcer (D. J. Sandweiss, ed.), W. B. Saunders Co., Philadelphia, 1951, pp. 103-113.

345. D. A. Brodie, in Pathophysiology of Peptic Ulcer Disease (S. C. Skoryna, ed.), McGill Univ. Press, Montreal, 1963, pp. 403-411.

346. A. C. Ivy, M. I. Grossman, and W. H. Bachrach, in Peptic Ulcer (A. C. Ivy, M. I. Grossman, and W. H. Bachrach, eds.), Blackiston Co., Philadelphia, 1950, pp. 261-386.

347. M. Berg, Am. J. Digest. Diseases, 16, 35 (1949).

348. H. Shay, S. A. Komarov, S. S. Fels, D. Meranze, M. Gruenstein, and H. Siplet, Gastroenterology, 5, 43 (1945).

349. D. A. Brodie, Am. J. Digest Diseases, 11, 231 (1966).

350. D. C. H. Sun and J. K. Chen, in Pathophysiology of Peptic Ulcer (S. C. Skoryna, ed.), J. B. Lippincott, Philadelphia, 1963, pp. 141-152.

351. J. Madden, H. H. Ramsburg, and J. M. Hundley, Gastroenterology, 18, 119 (1951).

352. S. M. Shea, Brit. J. Pharmacol., 11, 171 (1956).

353. R. G. Bianchi and D. L. Cook, Gastroenterology, 47, 409 (1964).

354. D. M. Brown and D. H. Turner, Arch. Intern. Pharmacodyn. Therap., 145, 489 (1963).

355. W. E. Barrett, R. Rutledge, A. J. Plummer, and F. F. Yonkman, J. Pharmacol. Exptl. Therap., 108, 305 (1953).

356. F. E. Visscher, P. H. Seay, A. P. Tazelaar, Jr., W. Veldkamp, and M. J. Vander Brook, J. Pharmacol. Exptl. Therap., 110, 188 (1954).

357. K. D. Back, R. Kadatz, T. L. Kerley, T. N. Jacobsen, and L. C. Weaver, Toxicol. Appl. Pharmacol., 3, 411 (1961).

358. D. A. Brodie, Gastroenterology, 43, 107 (1962).

359. S. Bonfils, J. P. Ferrier, and C. Caulin, Rev. Franc. Etudes. Clin. Biol., 11, 343 (1966).

360. D. A. Brodie and L. S. Valitski, Proc. Soc. Exptl. Biol. Med., 113, 998 (1963).

361. A. Rosenberg, Am. J. Digest. Diseases, 12, 1140 (1967).

362. S. Bonfils and A. Lambling, in Pathophysiology of Peptic Ulcer (S. C. Skoryna, ed.), J. B. Lippincott, Philadelphia, 1963, pp. 153-171.

363. H. Goldman and C. B. Rosoff, Am. J. Pathol., 52, 227 (1968).

364. C. P. Artz and C. T. Fitts, Surg. Clin. N. Am., 46, 309 (1966).

365. D. M. Nicoloff, E. T. Peter, A. S. Leonard, and O. H. Wangensteen, J. Amer. Med. Assoc., 191, 383 (1965).

366. W. P. Ritchie, Jr., J. J. Breen, D. I. Grigg, and O. H. Wangensteen, Gut, 8, 32 (1967).

367. R. J. Levine and E. C. Senay, Am. J. Physiol., 214, 892 (1968).

368. R. Lambert, C. Andre, and F. Martin, Gastroenterology, 56, 200 (1969).

369. W. M. Ludwig and M. Lipkin, Gastroenterology, 56, 895 (1969).

370. A. R. Imondi, M. E. Balis, and M. Lipkin, Exptl. Mol. Pathol., 9, 339 (1968).

371. M. Simler and J. Schwartz, Rev. Franc. Etudes. Clin. Biol., 7, 962 (1962).

372. G. P. Smith and P. R. McHugh, Am. J. Physiol., 213, 640 (1967).

373. C. B. Rosoff and H. Goldman, Gastroenterology, 55, 212 (1968).

374. R. Menguy, Am. J. Digest. Diseases, 5, 911 (1960).

375. S. Bonfils, M. Dubrasquet, and A. Lambling, J. Appl. Physiol., 17, 299 (1962).

376. D. A. Brodie, H. M. Hanson, J. O. Sines, and R. Adler, J. Neuropsychiat., 4, 388 (1963).

377. K. Takogi and S. Okabe, European J. Pharmacol., 5, 263 (1969).

378. C. R. Grosz and K. T. Wu, Surgery, 61, 853 (1967).

379. D. G. Fletcher and H. N. Karkins, Surgery, 36, 212 (1954).

380. T. B. Curling, Medico-Chirurgical Trans., 25, 260 (1842).

381. D. A. Brodie and H. M. Hanson, Gastroenterology, 38, 353 (1960).

382. B. V. Franko, R. S. Alphin, J. W. Ward, and C. D. Lunsford, Ann. N. Y. Acad. Sci., 99, 131 (1962).

383. J. B. Kirsner, Ann. Internal Med., 47, 666 (1957).

384. D. S. Kahn and M. J. Phillips, in Pathophysiology of Peptic Ulcer (S. C. Skoryna, ed.), J. B. Lippincott, Philadelphia, 1963, pp. 171-181.

385. G. B. Eagleton, J. Watt, and R. Marcus, J. Pharm. Pharmacol., 21, 123 (1969).

386. B. Djahanguiri, J. Haot, and M. Richelle, Arch. Intern. Pharmacodyn. Therap., 153, 300 (1965).

387. W. G. Gobbel, Jr., and R. B. Adkins, Am. J. Surg., 113, 183 (1967).

388. H. L. Segal., Am. J. Med., 29, 780 (1960).

389. S. Emås and M. I. Grossman, Gastroenterology, 52, 959 (1967).

390. D. A. Brodie and B. J. Chase, Gastroenterology, 56, 206 (1969).

391. A. W. Williams, Brit. J. Surg., 48, 564 (1961).

392. H. M. Hanson and D. A. Brodie, J. Appl. Physiol., 15, 291 (1960).

393. F. C. Mann and C. S. Williamson, Ann. Surg., 77, 409 (1923).

394. C. Manzano, C. de la Rosa, E. R. Woodward, and L. R. Dragstedt, Arch. Surg. 93, 492 (1966).

395. C. J. Pfeiffer and C. M. Peters, Gastroenterology, 57, 518 (1969).

396. Y. S. Kim and J. P. Lambooy, J. Nutr., 91, 183 (1967).

397. J. Seronde, Yale J. Biol. Med., 36, 141 (1963).

398. R. Seirafi and L. C. Reid, Surgery, 51, 233 (1962).

399. F. P. Brooks, in The Stomach-Including Related Areas in the Esophagus and Duodenum, The Thirteenth Hahnemann Symposium (C. Thompson, D. Berkowitz, E. Polish, eds., J. H. Moyer, consult. ed.), Grune & Stratton, New York and London, 1967, pp. 119-123.

400. Y. H. Lee, J. H. Thompson and J. J. McNew, Am. J. Physiol., 217, 505 (1969).

401. F. P. Brooks, in Handbook of Physiology, Alimentary Canal, Volume 11, Section 6, Secretion (C. F. Code, sect. ed.), American Physiological Society, Washington, D. C., 1967, pp. 805-826.

402. M. I. Grossman, New Engl. J. Med., 281, 43 (1969).

403. Y. Tomiyama, A. Geisel, N. C. Jefferson, P. Lott, Jr., and H. Necheles, Gaestronterologia, 108, 261 (1967).

404. F. P. Brooks, Gastroenterology, 57, 613 (1969).

405. B. O. Amure and M. Ginsburg, Brit. J. Pharmacol. Chemotherap., 22, 520 (1964).

406. C. R. Merril, S. H. Snyder, and D. F. Bradley, Biochim. Biophys. Acta, 118, 316 (1966).

407. L. B. Kier, J. Med. Chem., 11, 441 (1968).

408. A. S. F. Ash and H. O. Schild, Brit. J. Pharmacol. Chemotherap., 27, 427 (1966).

409. R. W. Schayer, Am. J. Physiol., 189, 533 (1957).

410. S. Ono and P. Hagen, Nature, 184, 1143 (1959).

411. R. Håkanson and C. Owman, Biochem. Pharmacol., 15, 489 (1966).

412. S. H. Snyder and L. Epps, Mol. Pharmacol., 4, 187 (1968).

413. J. F. Caren, D. Aures, and L. R. Johnson, Proc. Soc. Exptl. Biol. Med., 131, 1194 (1969).

414. J. M. Telford and G. B. West, Intern. Arch. Allergy, 22, 11 (1963).

415. J. E. Fischer and S. H. Snyder, Science, 150, 1034 (1965).

416. G. Kahlson, E. Rosengren, D. Svahn, and R. Thunberg, J. Physiol., 174, 400 (1964).

417. R. J. Levine, Federation Proc., 24, 1331 (1965).

418. R. J. Levine, T. L. Sato, and A. Sjoerdsma, Biochem. Pharmacol., 14, 139 (1965).

419. C. F. Code, Federation Proc., 24, 1311 (1965).

420. R. J. Levine, Federation Proc., 27, 1341 (1968).

421. E. R. Trethewie, Pharmacology, 1, 195 (1968).

422. D. Aures and W. G. Clark, Anal. Biochem., 9, 35 (1964).

423. M. A. Reilly and R. W. Schayer, Brit. J. Pharmacol., Chemotherap., 34, 551 (1968).

II. GASTROINTESTINAL DISORDERS — PEPTIC ULCER DISEASE

423a. D. Aures, G. H. Hamor, and W. G. Clark, Fourth Intern. Congr. Pharmacol., Schwabe and Co., Basel, Switzerland, 1969, pp. 179-180.

423b. M. K. Menon, D. Aures, and W. G. Clark, Pharmacologist, 12, 205 (1970).

424. R. S. Yalow and S. A. Berson, Gastroenterology, 58, 1 (1970).

425. J. E. McGuigan and W. L. Trudeau, Gastroenterology, 58, 139 (1970).

426. J. S. Morley, Federation Proc., 27, 1314 (1968).

427. J. S. Morley, Proc. Roy. Soc. (London), Ser. B, 170, 97 (1968).

428. L. Laster and J. H. Walsh, Federation Proc., 27, 1328 (1968).

429. J. E. McGuigan, Gastroenterology, 53, 697 (1967).

430. B. M. Jaffe, W. T. Newton, and J. E. McGuigan, Surgery, 65, 633 (1969).

431. B. M. Jaffe, W. T. Newton, and J. E. McGuigan, Gastroenterology, 58, 151 (1970).

432. A. Anastasi, V. Erspamer, and R. Endean, Experientia, 23, 699 (1967).

433. G. Bertaccini, R. Endean, V. Erspamer, and M. Impicciatore, Brit. J. Pharmacol., Chemotherap., 34, 311 (1968).

434. L. R. Johnson, G. F. Stening, and M. I. Grossman, Gastroenterology, 58, 208 (1970).

435. A. Anastasi, L. Bernardi, G. Bertaccini, G. Bosisio, R. de Castiglione, V. Erspamer, O. Goffredo, and M. Impicciatore, Experientia, 24, 771 (1968).

436. S. Bergstrom, L. A. Carlson, and J. R. Weeks, Pharmacol. Rev., 20, 1 (1968).

437. P. W. Ramwell and J. E. Shaw, J. Physiol., 195, 34P (1968).

438. J. E. Shaw and P. W. Ramwell, in Prostaglandin Symp. of the Worcester Foundation for Experimental Biology (P. W. Ramwell and J. E. Shaw, eds.), Interscience (John Wiley & Sons), New York, 1967, pp. 55-66.

439. A. Bennett, C. A. Friedmann, and J. R. Vane, Nature, 216, 873 (1967).

440. F. Coceani, C. Pace-Asciak, F. Volta, and L. S. Wolfe, Am. J. Physiol., 213, 1056 (1967).

441. F. Coceani, C. Pace-Asciak, and L. S. Wolfe, in Prostaglandin Symp. of the Worcester Foundation for Experimental Biology (P. W. Ramwell and J. E. Shaw, eds.), Interscience (John Wiley & Sons), New York, 1967, pp. 39-45.

442. H. J. Hess, in Ann. Rept. Med. Chem, 1968 (C. K. Cain, ed.), Academic Press, 1969, pp. 56-66.

443. A. Robert, J. E. Nezamis, and J. P. Phillips, Gastroenterology, 55, 481 (1968).

444. A. Robert, J. E. Nezamis, and J. P. Phillips, Am. J. Digest. Diseases, 12, 1073 (1967).

445. A. Robert, in Prostaglandin Symp. of the Worcester Foundation for Experimental Biology (P. W. Ramwell and J. E. Shaw, eds.), Interscience (John Wiley & Sons), New York, 1967, pp. 47-54.

446. W. Lippmann, J. Pharm. Pharmacol., 21, 335 (1969).

447. L. Way and R. P. Durbin, Nature, 221, 874 (1969).

448. E. W. Horton, I. H. M. Main, C. J. Thompson, and P. M. Wright, Gut, 9, 655 (1968).

449. A. Bennett, J. G. Murray, and J. H. Wyllie, Brit. J. Pharmacol. Chemotherap., 32, 339 (1968).

450. J. Fried, T. S. Santhanakrishnan, J. Himizu, C. H. Lin, S. H. Ford, B. Rubin, and E. O. Grigas, Nature, 223, 208 (1969).

451. V. Mutt and J. E. Jorpes, Biochem. Biophys. Res. Commun., 26, 392 (1967).

452. J. E. Jorpes, Gastroenterology, 55, 157 (1968).

453. M. I. Grossman, Med. Clin. N. Amer., 52, 1297 (1968).

454. G. F. Stening, L. R. Johnson, and M. I. Grossman, Gastroenterology, 57, 44 (1969).

455. D. F. Magee and S. Nakijima, Experientia, 25, 1051 (1969).

456. L. R. Johnson and M. I. Grossman, Am. J. Physiol., 216, 1176 (1969).

457. R. G. Bianchi and D. L. Cook, Federation Proc., 27, 1331 (1968).

458. B. S. Bedi, G. Gillespie, and I. E. Gillespie, Lancet, i, 1240 (1967).

459. A. M. Connell, R. A. Hill, I. B. Macleod, W. Sircus, and C. G. Thomson, Gut, 9, 641 (1968).

460. G. Kahlson, E. Rosengren, and S. E. Svensson, Brit. J. Pharmacol. Chemotherap., 33, 493 (1968).

461. G. Gillespie, V. I. McCusker, B. S. Bedi, H. T. Debas, and I. E. Gillespie, Gastroenterology, 55, 81 (1968).

462. D. L. Cook, personal communication, 1969.

463. K.-F. Sewing, P. D. Gorinsky and F. Lembeck, Arch. Pharmakol. Exptl. Pathol., 261, 89 (1968).

II. GASTROINTESTINAL DISORDERS — PEPTIC ULCER DISEASE 197

464. R. A. Gregory, in Gastric Secretion, Mechanisms and Control (T. A. Shnitka, J. A. L. Gilbert, and R. C. Harrison, eds.), Pergamon Press, London, 1967, p. 469.

465. A. L. Rovati, Brit. J. Pharmacol. Chemotherap., 34, 677P (1968).

466. A. L. Rovati, P. L. Casula, L. Lepori, and G. Da Re, Minerva Med., 58, 3653 (1967).

467. A. L. Rovati, P. L. Casula, and G. Da Re, Minerva Med., 58, 3651 (1967).

468. P. Bass, R. A. Purdon, M. A. Patterson, and D. E. Butler, J. Pharmacol. Exptl. Therap., 152, 104 (1966).

469. P. Bass, D. E. Butler, M. A. Patterson, and R. A. Purdon, Arch. Intern. Pharmacodyn. Therap., 169, 131 (1967).

470. P. Bass and M. A. Patterson, J. Pharmacol. Exptl. Therap., 156, 142 (1967).

471. S. N. Pradhan and H. W. Wingate, Arch. Intern. Pharmacodyn. Therap., 162, 303 (1966).

472. A. Misher, R. G. Pendleton, and R. Staples, Gastroenterology, 57, 294 (1969).

473. W. Lippmann, Experientia, 24, 1151 (1968).

474. S. D. J. Yeh and M. E. Shils, Proc. Soc. Exptl. Biol. Med., 130, 807 (1969).

475. R. F. Meyer, B. L. Cummings, P. Bass, and H. O. J. Collier, J. Med. Chem., 8, 515 (1965).

476. P. Bass, R. A. Purdon, and M. A. Patterson, J. Pharmacol. Exptl. Therap., 153, 292 (1966).

477. J. H. Wyllie, J. M. Limbosch, and L. M. Nyhus, Nature, 215, 879 (1967).

478. F. D. Mann and F. C. Mann, Am. J. Digest. Diseases, 6, 322 (1939).

479. K. Hartiala, A. C. Ivy, and M. I. Grossman, Am. J. Physiol., 162, 110 (1950).

480. A. R. Cooke, in Handbook of Physiology, Alimentary Canal, Volume 11, Section 6, Secretion (C. F. Code, sect. ed.), American Physiological Society, Washington, D. C., 1967, pp. 1087-1095.

481. E. L. Krawitt, G. R. Zimmerman, and J. A. Clifton, Am. J. Physiol., 211, 935 (1966).

482. M. I. Grossman, Gastroenterology, 50, 912 (1966).

483. M. Vagne, G. F. Stening, F. P. Brooks, and M. I. Grossman, Gastroenterology, 55, 260 (1968).

484. G. F. Stening and M. I. Grossman, Gastroenterology, 56, 1047 (1969).
485. J. P. Pascal, N. Vaysse, D. Augier, and A. Ribet, Scand. J. Gastroenterol., 3, 444 (1968).
486. S. Nakajima, M. Nakamura, and D. F. Magee, Am. J. Physiol., 216, 87 (1969).
487. S. J. Konturek, Am. J. Digest. Diseases, 13, 874 (1968).
488. H. Schapiro, L. D. Wruble, J. W. Estes, R. Sherman, and L. G. Britt, Am. J. Digest. Diseases, 13, 608 (1968).
489. H. Schapiro and L. D. Wruble, Gastroenterology, 56, 640 (1969).
490. T. M. Lin and G. F. Spray, Gastroenterology, 54, 1254 (1968).
491. J. W. Singleton, Gastroenterology, 56, 342 (1969).
492. A. M. Brooks, J. Isenberg, and M. I. Grossman, Gastroenterology, 57, 159 (1969).
493. T. P. Almy, Gastroenterology, 58, 270 (1970).
494. I. I. Brekhman and I. V. Dardymov, Ann. Rev. Pharmacol., 9, 419 (1969).
495. M. Siurala, K. Varis, O. Gorbatow, P. Kause, M. Laulajainen, and L. O. Nyberg, Scand. J. Gastroenterol., 4, 469 (1969).
496. D. M. Griffin and C. M. Szego, Life Sci., 7, 1017 (1968).
497. C. M. Szego and J. S. Davis, Life Sci., 8, 1109 (1969).
498. R. H. Resnick, C. F. Adelardi, and S. J. Gray, Gastroenterology, 42, 22 (1962).
499. J. H. Thompson and M. Angulo, Experientia, 25, 721 (1969).
500. S. L. Malhotra, Gut, 8, 548 (1967).
501. J. A. Vocac and R. S. Alphin, Arch. Intern. Pharmacodyn. Therap., 177, 150 (1969).
501a. E. L. Gerring, Gut, 10, 1053 (1969).
502. O. W. Samuel, The Practitioner, 199, 220 (1967).
503. J. E. Dunphy, New Engl. J. Med., 268, 1367 (1963).
504. I. Gore, Y. Tanaka, T. Fujinami, and M. L. Goodman, J. Nutr., 87, 311 (1965).
505. R. Levi-Montalcini and P. U. Angeletti, Physiol. Rev., 48, 534 (1968).
506. E. J. Underwood, Trace Elements in Human and Animal Nutrition, 2nd ed., Academic Press, New York, 1962, p. 429.

II. GASTROINTESTINAL DISORDERS — PEPTIC ULCER DISEASE

507. J. M. Hsu, W. L. Anthony, and P. J. Buchanan, J. Nutr., 99, 425 (1969).
508. W. J. Pories, J. H. Henzel, C. G. Rob, and W. H. Strain, Lancet, i, 121 (1967).
509. U. S. Department Health Education and Welfare, Drinking Water Standards, 1962, Gov't Printing Office, Washington, D. C.
510. J. F. Prudden, Arch. Surg., 89, 1046 (1964).
511. K. Karzel, D. A. Kalbhen, and R. Domenjoz, Med. Pharmacol. Expt., 14, 332 (1966).
512. O. D. Ratnoff, New Engl. J. Med., 280, 1124 (1969).
513. F. B. Ablondi and E. C. DeRenzo, Proc. Soc. Exptl. Biol. Med., 102, 717 (1959).
514. M. W. Whitehouse and R. W. Doskotch, Biochem. Pharmacol., 18, 1790 (1969).
515. P. H. Bentley, G. W. Kenner, and R. C. Sheppard, Nature, 209, 583 (1966).
516. H. Gregory, P. M. Hardy, D. S. Jones, G. W. Kenner, and R. C. Sheppard, Nature, 204, 931 (1964).
517. R. A. Gregory, Gastroenterology, 51, 953 (1966).
518. R. A. Gregory, Proc. Intern. Union Physiol. Sci. (24th Intern. Congr., Washington, D. C., 1968), 6, 188 and discussion.
519. J. S. Morley, H. J. Tracy, and R. A. Gregory, Nature, 207, 1356 (1965).
520. V. Mutt and J. E. Jorpes, Proc. Intern. Union Physiol. Sci., 24th Intern. Congr., Washington, D. C., 1968, 6, 193 and discussion.
521. D. H. Reigel, S. J. Larson, and A. Sances, Jr., Surgery, 68, 217 (1970).
522. N. Tanaka and G. B. Jerzy Glass, Gastroenterology, 58, 482 (1970).

Chapter III

PSYCHOACTIVE DRUG EVALUATION:
PHILOSOPHY AND METHODS

Samuel Irwin

Department of Psychiatry
University of Oregon Medical School
Portland, Oregon

I.	INTRODUCTION	201
II.	APPROACHES TO BEHAVIORAL ANALYSIS	202
	A. Normal versus Abnormal	202
	B. Target Diagnosis, Symptom or Function	204
III.	PRINCIPLES OF EXCLUSION AND INCLUSION	212
IV.	OBSERVATION AND INSTRUMENTATION	212
V.	PREDICTION FROM NORMAL SUBJECTS	213
	A. The Animal Model	213
	B. Strategy and Tactics	214
	C. Comprehensive Observational Assessment Procedures	215
VI.	ANIMAL DRUG SCREENING AND EVALUATION	217
	A. Abbreviated Observational Procedures	217
	B. Nonobservational Procedures	218
	C. Predictability	218
VII.	DRUG ASSESSMENT IN HUMANS	221
	A. Adaptation of Animal Observational Procedures	221
	B. Discrete versus Global Behavior Modification	229
VIII.	SUMMARY	230
	REFERENCES	231

I. INTRODUCTION

There is no simple, one-method approach for new psychoactive drug development, evaluation, and use — only a multiplicity of strategies and tactics reflecting the biases and whims of the individual investigator. The underlying attitudes and assumptions upon which they are based are rarely examined, openly discussed, validated or invalidated. Few approaches to drug assessment and the interpretation of data have appeared so compellingly useful as to encourage widespread adherence. Most procedures are empirically based, with preclinical laboratories often inadequately distinguishing between the different information requirements for drug screening and for drug evaluation [1-3].

The situation has not been aided by psychiatrists who fail to specify the most important behavioral characteristics of patients of varying diagnostic type or to ask for specific actions in a therapeutically useful drug beyond the usual request for one that "makes the patient well." The problem becomes further confused when some apply the medical disease model to certain psychiatric diagnostic states while others seem less willing to make such generalizations. Those that accept the disease model for schizophrenia, for example, conclude that drugs affecting and controlling the behavior must do so by mechanisms that could not be studied in normal subjects. Many investigators question not only the value of animal studies for predicting the behavioral effects of drugs on humans, but also the value of studies on normal human subjects for predicting the behavioral effects of drugs on even maladapted individuals.

The recognized purpose of preclinical drug evaluation in animals and normal humans is to establish the probable usefulness of a drug and to specify or predict (1) the nature and magnitude of the actions of therapeutic value, (2) the patient population, (3) the therapeutic dose range, (4) the time-course of drug action, (5) dose-response relationships and steepness of the dose-response slope, (6) the nature of any untoward side effects or toxicity, (7) the doses at which they occur, (8) the occurrence of tolerance or cumulative effects with repeated administration, and (9) any psychological or physical dependence liability. The appropriate questions, I feel, are not whether it is possible or not possible to make such predictions, but rather to what extent and under what circumstances can such predictions be made from animal and normal human studies for patients of varying type. The comparative animal and human studies required for establishing these criteria have yet to be done.

The time is long overdue to reorient and redirect psychopharmacology from its present trial-and-error empiricism toward a more rational approach. The purpose of this chapter is to suggest a course of action, starting with a discussion of what we mean by the terms normal and abnormal when referring to subjects or patients.

II. APPROACHES TO BEHAVIORAL ANALYSIS

A. Normal versus Abnormal

If I examine my own past behavior and that of my associates, I find that our "normal" daily lives do not always proceed with equanimity, without swings from feelings of well-being to depression, without tension or fear, without occasional suicidal thoughts, or without unusual or strange perceptions and inappropriate behavior. I thus conclude that there exists a broad range and scope of behavior that must enter our definition of normal.

Perhaps it would be simpler to start with a definition of abnormal. Clearly there are certain behaviors that most would agree are abnormal, so that by the process of exclusion we might arrive at a definition of normal. What comes most immediately to mind as abnormal are the schizophrenias, severe depression, or extreme obsessive-compulsive behavior. But one finds that schizophrenic-like behavior (for which a genetic, inherited component can be shown) and severe depression can result from unusual distress or loss, and that obsessive-compulsive behavior can be developed experimentally with suitable training [4]. Are these abnormal states actually disease entities? Are they distinct from normal modes by which the behavior of an individual is expressed under certain conditions? Does the concept of abnormal imply an underlying etiological process largely independent of environmental shaping, or is the dichotomy between normal and abnormal as mythical as the dichotomy once accepted between the body and mind?

In their consideration of normal and abnormal behavior, Ullman and Krasner [5] have noted that in a stimulus-response situation, a person must perceive and attend to the stimulus, have the skill or capacity to make the appropriate response, and emit the response at the right time and the right place. Moreover, he must be reinforced for it and receive accurate feedback about the consequences of his act. The failure to do this is called deviance; behavior for which intervention by the medical profession has been sanctioned is called abnormal. They conclude that professionals could at present more effectively understand and modify behaviors called abnormal without excessively lingering on the concept of abnormality. I am in agreement with that conclusion, without necessarily excluding the disease model as a possibility.

If a disease-induced state really exists, it is more easily identified by a broad specification of the individual's behavioral, physiological, and biochemical state than by our present diagnostic categories. A psychiatric diagnosis is little more than an abstract label of convenience, often loosely applied. To regard it as real and of etiological significance masks differences between individuals so categorized and interferes with the progress of investigational studies. Similar adverse consequences have resulted, I feel, from calling drugs antipsychotics or antidepressants because of their favorable effects on states so labeled.

Language seems a mixed blessing providing on the one hand a means of symbolizing experience for description, analysis, evaluation, and communication and, on the other, a potential barrier to direct experience. According to Bower [6], "one of the important notions in man's use of symbols is that the symbol X does not equal anything in man's external world. As a symbol it contains n degrees of individual interpreting, organizing, experiencing, and meaning. ... Often we find it easier or more satisfying to substitute the symbol for the reality without knowing either one well.... The insidious outcome of this process for man is that meaning comes to reside not in things and events but primarily in the symbol concept." Accordingly, when our word symbols or beliefs are not tested and validated against direct experience, they become mere cliches that block thinking, perpetuate delusional beliefs, and often lead to nonrelevant or inappropriate behavior.

The study of drug effects in normal subjects who are adaptive and functioning without undue distress or discomfort has considerable value. If a drug produces increased or decreased wakefulness, relaxation, behavioral arousal, or locomotor activity under normal conditions, similar effects may appear in disturbed states as well. Although extrapolation of drug effects observed in normal subjects is likely to be relevant, it is nevertheless important to evaluate drugs under the actual conditions of concern. This is particularly cogent for drugs having such specificity of action as to exhibit no observable biologic effects except in the presence of the disturbed condition, e.g., lithium in the treatment of manic disorders.

Perhaps it would be less misleading and more useful to describe individuals as variously functional or dysfunctional rather than as normal or abnormal. It is my feeling that the ability to make predictions will increase as we substitute an adequate description of the subject for abstract labels, develop a better understanding of the correlates and antecedents of the differing states of psychosocial functioning, and learn how initial baseline levels and psychosocial states affect the response to drugs.

B. Target Diagnosis, Symptom or Function

The medical disease model has led to the use of target-diagnosis and target-symptom approaches for modifying disturbed or disordered behavior. Drugs have been classified and assessed largely from the framework of how they affect these states. Predictability from diagnosis alone has been improved by Klein and his associates [7,8] by constructing diagnostic configurational states based entirely upon responsiveness to certain classes of drugs - that is, by more clearly defining those behavioral states and sets which on a trial-and-error basis have been shown to most favorably respond to drug treatment.

When using a target-diagnosis approach, however, one excludes from measurement most of the prevailing behavior of the individual and learns little else about what drugs do. The target-symptom approach recommended and used by Freyhan and Merkel [9] has provided a broader baseline of information for discrete symptom modification — a dimension of information that would seem to enhance prediction over that of the target-diagnosis approach, but a major problem has been that the indicated target-symptoms are represented by ambiguous terms that require qualification to be appropriately understood. Moreover, these qualifications and distinctions are rarely made. For example, the symptom <u>depression</u> and its response to treatment varies considerably depending upon a variety of configurational factors. These may either result from or give rise to the subjective feeling

III. PSYCHOACTIVE DRUG EVALUATION

of depression, or indicate whether the depression was associated with hostility or agitation, activation, or retardation. The symptom <u>hostility</u> also has little meaning apart from the mode by which it may be expressed, i.e., offensively, defensively, or through negativism or resistance. All reflect modes of operant responding (active approach and active and passive avoidance behaviors) which may be affected differently by drugs.

The target-symptom approach also has lacked an adequate framework for discrete symptom modification, depending too heavily on trial-and-error techniques. Although this approach has increased the range of observation of the subject over the target-diagnosis approach, it still excludes large components of information.

My own inclination is to favor a target-function approach [10] predicated on an unambiguous quantitative specification of as much of the elemental components of behavior as one can identify and describe — elements that collectively express the state of the organism and its ability to function and cope. With this broader information, I feel, one can more clearly and unambiguously define the psychosocial-physiological state of functioning of the individual, the qualitative and quantitative actions of the various types of psychoactive drugs on them, and the correlates and antecedents of the various distress and disordered states of concern. This information coupled with the rational framework I propose below can then be used for more predictably and discretely modifying the behavior of an individual as desired. This, however, is not to suggest that the target-symptom and target-diagnosis approaches are without value, but only that their value and meaning would be enhanced by a more complete and accurate description of the patient's behavior.

Moreover, certain drugs are used by individuals for such extra-therapeutic purposes as modifying perceptual states or activity levels. To be preoccupied with drug effects on symptoms or diagnostic states alone is to ignore certain larger components of information, from which may appear a more rational approach to drug use for pleasure, social purposes, or therapy.

The most economical approach I have been able to conceive for comprehensively specifying the psychosocial-physiological state and behavior of an organism is shown in Tables I and II. Listed are the target-functions or elemental building blocks of behavior that seem at present the most valid and usefully descriptive for mammalia, whether applied to an individual or a group. Certain of the items, more important to individual functioning and treatment than others, are so indicated. To use this target-function approach appropriately for behavioral analysis and for discrete behavior modification, I think it necessary to consider certain key concepts described below.

1. Freedom and Control

Perhaps most important to the individual is a state of freedom, a condition where he is in complete control over his action and choice (e.g., for

TABLE I

Framework for Individual or Group Assessment of Physiological State and Behavior

A. Physical Appearance
   1. Age-Sex
   2. Weight-Height
      a. Short-Tall
      b. Thin-Obese
      c. Frail-Muscular
   3. Normal-Disabled
      a. Healthy-Ill
   4. Clean-Dirty
      a. Neat-Sloppy
   5. Seductive-Repulsive
   6. Conventional-Unconventional

B. Environmental Setting
   1. Controlled-Free
   2. Supportive-Depriving
      a. Enhancing-Violating
   3. Isolated-Group

C. Stimulus
   1. Sensation-Perception
      a. Internal-External
      b. Strong-Weak
      c. Reality-Illusion
      d. Dream-Hallucination

D. Stimulus Significance
   1. Pleasure-Distress
      a. Reward-No Reward
      b. Punishment-No Punishment

E. Interactional Object
   1. Self-Other
      a. Animate-Inanimate
      b. Responsive-Indifferent

F. Interactional Role
   1. Participant-Observer
      a. Initiator-Responder

G. Physiological State
   1. Neuromuscular-Autonomic Arousal
      a. Sympathetic-Parasympathetic
   2. Balance-Imbalance
      a. Active-Sluggish
      b. Strong-Weak
      c. Rigid-Flaccid
   3. Rhythmic-Arrhythmic
   4. Coordinate-Incoordinate
   5. Voluntary-Involuntary Movements
   6. Functional-Dysfunctional

relaxation, enjoyment, self-discovery, or goal-fulfillment) without constraint or restraint from forces inside or outside of himself, but there is a very narrow zone of conditions in which a mammal (human or nonhuman) can really be free. He is thrown out of balance and control by relatively minor deviations of atmospheric, climatic, dietary, environmental, or physiological conditions that dull, relax, excite, or promote distress, e.g., as with changes of altitude, oxygenation, temperature, or humidity. His freedom of choice and action also is altered or impaired when he becomes increasingly detached or involved, joyous or depressed, weak or tense, neurologically impaired or cognitively disorganized.

III. PSYCHOACTIVE DRUG EVALUATION

TABLE II

Framework for Individual or Group Assessment of
Psychosocial State

A. Conscious-Unconscious

B. Awake-Asleep
   1. Light-Deep
   2. Insomnia-Narcolepsy

C. Aroused-Dulled
   1. Perceptual-Cognitive Arousal
   2. Excitement-Distress Arousal

D. Pleasure-Distress Affect
   1. Somatic-Mental
   2. Relaxed-Tense
   3. Joyful-Gloomy
   4. Stable-Labile

E. Energetic-Weak

F. In-Out of Control
   1. Optimistic-Pessimistic
   2. Adequate-Inadequate
   3. Confident-Fearful
   4. Trusting-Suspicious
   5. Friendly-Hostile
   6. Content-Grieving
   7. Flexible-Rigid
   8. Pride-Shame
   9. Reality-Delusions

G. Attentive-Inattentive
   1. Easy-Difficult Concentration
   2. Stimulus Involvement-Detachment
   3. Interest-Disinterest

H. Focused-Distorted Perception
   1. Increased-Decreased Threshold
   2. Time Faster-Slower
   3. Heightened-Dulled Perception
   4. Bigger-Smaller
   5. Closer-Farther
   6. Detached-Dreamlike
   7. Derealized-Depersonalized

I. Accurate-Inaccurate Cognition
   1. Rapid-Slow
   2. Short-Long Term Memory
   3. Oriented-Confused
   4. Reality-Delusion

J. Goal Directed-Aimless Activity
   1. Rapid-Slow Movement
   2. Spontaneous-Inhibited
   3. Playful-Serious
   4. Respondent-Operant
      a. Stay-Escape
      b. Approach-Avoidance
      c. Active-Passive
      d. Skilled-Unskilled

Each of these factors, whether drug-induced or not, shift the probabilities for choice and action and make it more or less difficult to maintain some required performance. The more deviant or intense the change of state, the more effort and energy is required to perform even the most routine, simple task. At some point of dulling, excitement, distress, or impairment — usually of moderate to marked grade — the individual loses virtually all possibility for control and is then in the grip of his own internal state, a prisoner.

This relationship conceived between an individual's sense of freedom or control in relation to his level of behavioral arousal or distress is illustrated in Fig. 1. The correlation is that of an inverted U-shaped function, with optimal freedom and control achieved during the early phase of excitement arousal when the individual is alert, attentive, and only mildly animated. Control is then considered to be reduced as one becomes more relaxed or dulled (shift to the left) or enters a state of excitement or distress-arousal (shift to the right). The distress arousal may be precipitated by feelings of discomfort, pain, depression, tension, or by any of the other distress-affect items listed in Tables I and II, all of which tend to interfere with sleep. As already mentioned, at some moderate to marked point of dulling, excitement, or distress arousal, the individual finds it difficult or impossible to mobilize his energy. An important object of therapy, I feel, is to restore the sense of freedom and control required for optimal functioning.

2. Excitement and Distress Arousal

When an individual's state of excitement or distress affect and arousal becomes excessive, he tends to go out of control, with all the consequences shown in Table II, e.g., increased pessimism, feelings of inadequacy, fearfulness, suspiciousness, hostility, or social withdrawal. Also he becomes increasingly involved with his internal state of distress and increasingly detached from the external environment. Under extreme conditions, perception and cognition can be distorted to the point of derealization and depersonalization or hallucinations and delusional modes of thinking (as more commonly experienced during sleep). The behavior also can become increasingly disorganized or shift to aimless, stereotyped, or bizarre mannerisms or posturing (as seen after amphetamine-induced excitement). Such extreme deviancy of perception and function is usually labeled schizophrenia, but this seems merely one of several modes by which an individual may respond to states of extreme excitement or distress.

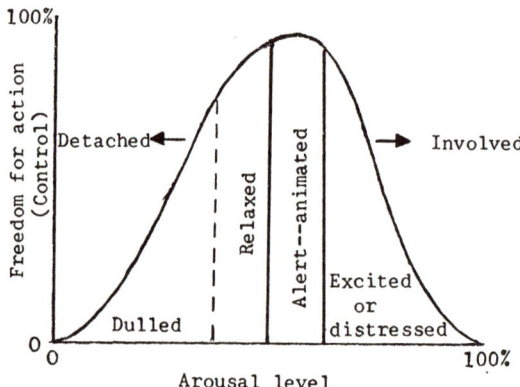

Fig. 3-1. Correlation between arousal level and freedom.

III. PSYCHOACTIVE DRUG EVALUATION

Not surprisingly, all the drugs labeled antipsychotics have the capacity to reduce the level of excitement arousal (and presumably in part distress arousal) to levels compatible with more optimal perception, cognition, and functioning. Similarly, one might expect that drugs with the capacity to reduce distress arousal, a property perhaps most characteristic of the narcotic analgesics, can be expected to have an ameliorating effect on virtually all components of distress affect where excitement is not a significant factor.

Seemingly correlated with the level of behavioral arousal as an inverted U-shaped function are the levels of awareness, attention, spatial locomotor activity, and social interaction, there being an optimum level of arousal for maximum function of each of these, with decrement of function as the level of arousal is increased or decreased from the optimum [11,12]. Positively correlated and evolving with increasing levels of arousal are increased wakefulness, increased responses to stimuli, apprehension, irritability, agitation, and delirium. Parenthetically, amphetamine-type drugs increase arousal mechanisms [13-15] and, with increasing dosage, can produce all the above concomitants of increasing states of arousal; chlorpromazine-type agents reduce arousal mechanisms [15,16] and can produce such concomitant effects as reduced responses to stimuli, reduced locomotor activity, stupor, and coma.

The level of arousal of an individual can be shown to greatly influence the qualitative and quantitative (dose-requirement) responses to drugs. Even the noise level of a room can reduce the effectiveness of a phenothiazine-type tranquilizer for controlling behavior. An important concept to consider in treatment, therefore, is the "arousal-provoking quality" of the environment. It should be minimized when attempting to reduce the patient's state of arousal and augmented when attempting to increase it [15,17].

3. Stimulus Detachment or Involvement

Another important mode by which drugs may modify the feeling and functioning state of a distressed individual is by producing a perceptual detachment from his internal distress stimuli (perhaps another property of the narcotic analgesics). In such instances, the distress may seem too distant or remote to be concerned about. I feel that the tricyclic antidepressants may in part produce their effects through this mechanism. A sense of detachment, also, can be produced by drugs that cause dulling, or which impair memory storage and recall of past or present distress experiences.

4. Desired Subjective State

Each individual defines for himself how he most prefers to be or feel at a particular time and may select or prefer drugs for use that enable him to approximate that desired state. Drug effects that alter or diminish it are viewed negatively or with concern; those that promote the desired state are viewed positively.

Certain drug effects are considered adverse whenever they occur; others must be judged in relation to the state of the subject and what he most desires. For example, vomiting, excessive sweating, or dizziness are likely to be disturbing to all subjects, but excessive sedation, clouded thinking, greater detachment, or even impaired memory might be considered a boon to some. Potentially negative drug effects may be considered desirable when they provide relief from greater distress or otherwise improve functioning.

5. Mode of Operant Response

The individual's pattern of response to provoking stimuli ("defense mechanism") is another target function area of importance. When stimulated or provoked, the individual can respond in only a limited number of ways, but with many permutations of each. I think it most useful to assess these interactional patterns of response from the framework of operant psychology. From present concepts, one can consider that there are only one of four contingencies or expectations that exist in any stimulus situation, i.e., reward, no reward, and a combination of these with punishment or no punishment. From these there are only six possibilities for response, both active and passive forms of approach (contact-seeking), avoidance (contact-avoidance), and escape (contact-escape) behavior, each of which can be differentially affected by drugs. The discrete mode and character by which the operant response is then expressed is determined by whether the individual expects reward or punishment, is optimistic or pessimistic in outlook, and is of friendly, fearful, or angry disposition. An attitude of optimism and expectation of reward predisposes one toward active approach behavior; that of pessimism and fear of punishment, toward avoidance and active escape behavior; that of pessimism and expectation of no reward, from active to more passive modes of responding, primarily passive escape.

Almost all individual and group behavior can be distinguished and classified from this simple framework, e.g., the hippie (with a pessimistic, no reward-punishment outlook), responding with active escape from the established system and active or passive approach toward his new one; the militant activist (with an optimistic, angry, reward-punishment outlook), exhibiting active approach (confronting) behavior with anger superimposed. The subcategories of "schizophrenia" and certain oscillatory "psychotic" behaviors, I feel, can be similarly distinguished and better understood from this framework. One can presuppose that, even under the rules of "psychotic logic," the operant mode of response is likely to parallel the prior adaptive patterns of response and behavioral oscillations of the individual. Also, the response may shift from active to more passive modes as the person's state changes with chronicity toward an increasingly pessimistic, depressive outlook.

For example, as shown in Fig. 2, the manic-depressive may be viewed as a primarily successful (reward-no punishment) individual with poorly developed avoidance modes of responding (e.g., defense mechanisms). He thus tends to oscillate between the extremes of an optimistic reward (active approach) and pessimistic-no reward (passive escape) mode of response. His framework is not one of fear of punishment, but mainly of reward and absence of reward.

III. PSYCHOACTIVE DRUG EVALUATION 211

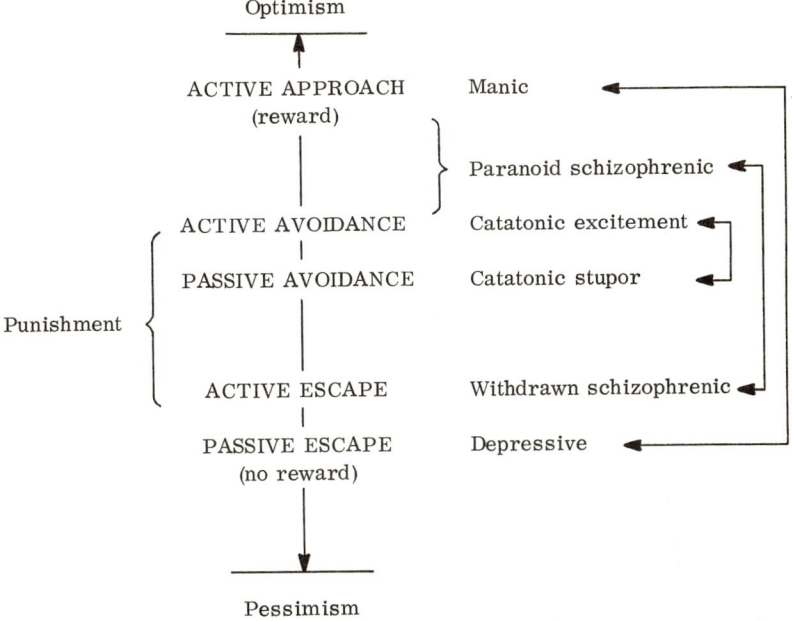

Fig. 3-2. Operant modes of response.

The catatonic schizophrenic, on the other hand, may be a primarily fearful, punishment-no reward oriented individual with actively developed avoidance rather than approach modes of responding. He thus tends to oscillate between a punishment-no reward framework of catatonic excitement (active avoidance) and catatonic stupor (passive avoidance, i.e., suppressed behavior) with shifts to and from a more pessimistic outlook. Similarly, the paranoid schizophrenic may be a primarily successful, often punished (hence fearful and angry) individual with actively developed reward-punishment (approach-avoidance) modes of responding. He thus tends to exhibit these features of active approach-avoidance behavior with fear and anger superimposed when "psychotic," and to shift later to a withdrawn schizophrenic state (active escape) with further change to a more depressed, pessimistic outlook in response to sustained punishment-no reward.

Using this approach together with the one suggested by Kornetsky and Mirsky [18] that schizophrenia might be a response to a "hyperaroused" state, one can more readily understand why major tranquilizers favorably affect both agitated and withdrawn patients. These drugs significantly reduce the state of arousal and abolish all active modes of operant responding (approach, avoidance, and escape). Conversely, amphetamine-like stimulants, which produce psychosocial effects opposite in direction to those of the major tranquilizers rapidly produce in humans a state indistinguishable from paranoid schizophrenia replete with auditory hallucinations and a well-developed paranoid delusional system.

Moreover, drugs that abolish passive avoidance modes of response, such as the minor tranquilizers and hypnotics, eliminate catatonic stupor (passive avoidance). Frequently such treatment causes a shift into catatonic excitement (active avoidance), a state which is more rapidly controlled by major tranquilizers. Observations such as these tend to support the speculative framework I have presented.

III. PRINCIPLES OF EXCLUSION AND INCLUSION

The principle of exclusion seems to me to be common to present modes of conducting research; that is, whenever an isolated belief, preoccupation, or role is accepted and responded to, it becomes a "belief-system" with a tendency to exclude, disregard, or resist all other belief-systems and modes of responding. The prevailing "belief-systems" in psychoactive drug research tend to exclude the possibility for any meaningful prediction of drug effects on disturbed behavior from the study of normal subjects (animal or human), or the possibility for predicting drug effects on many components of human behavior from animal studies.

Such exclusionary attitudes have resulted in the following errors of omission and commission: (1) an information vacuum derived from the exclusion of potentially important information; (2) a failure to develop information required to validate or invalidate the prevailing belief-systems; (3) a failure to develop information that might provide a more rational basis for drug development, evaluation, and therapeutic use; (4) a failure to develop information from which better predictions might be made, and (5) an overaccumulation of relatively inappropriate or useless information.

The prediction of drug effects from animals to man or from functional to dysfunctional states has in the past been inadequate because only a small portion of the total information required was ever collected and appropriately applied. Furthermore, that small portion was usually a cumulative total derived across species rather than from any single species or individual. In order to enhance predictiveness, the principle of inclusion should be incorporated into research philosophy. This principle simply calls for a unified systems approach [3], involving the accumulation of maximal information from each individual. Its advantages are apparent by comparison with some of the current approaches of selecting separate components of information from different individuals and species.

IV. OBSERVATION AND INSTRUMENTATION

When the scientist investigates drug effects on the electrophysiological or biochemical state of an organism, he has no recourse but to employ nonhuman instrumental measurement. An observer is unable to perceive and

III. PSYCHOACTIVE DRUG EVALUATION

quantify these events without some instrumental extension of his abilities. This limitation does not apply to the description and quantification of psychosocial behavior and functioning, where the situation tends to be the reverse, i.e., the inanimate instrument is unable to identify and record much of the pertinent information. Using instrumental techniques under these circumstances, the large body of information required for drug assessment must be derived from different subjects at different times and under different experimental conditions.

Since the response to a drug is dependent as much on the system of measurement and experimental conditions as upon the type of drug and dose used, the reliance on instrumentation in effect requires the use of multiple systems of measurement. Accordingly, the variety of drug effects produced in any one individual are often unobtainable. Further, the process of measurement itself alters that which is measured. While instrumentation provides added reliability of measurement, it sometimes results in decreased validity due to incompleteness, artifacts of measurement, and restrictions on response imposed by the mere presence of a measuring device.

In my experience there is little that can be measured instrumentally within the framework of psychosocial behavior that cannot be carried out with sufficient reliability using systematic, careful, quality-controlled human observation. Instrumental psychosocial measurement can provide more objective data when only limited information on discrete models of behavioral function and dysfunction is required.

V. PREDICTION FROM NORMAL SUBJECTS

A. The Animal Model

Studies of animal behavior suggest that the higher animals and man are far more alike than dissimilar in structure, biochemical organization, and psychosocial-physiological functioning [19, 20]. As shown in Tables I and II, it is hard to find any primary human behaviors that are not present in other mammalia. Such characteristics as wakefulness, arousal, attention, motor activity, memory, mood and affect, cognitive functioning, operant behavior, and psychological and physical drug dependence seem as present and available for study in animals as in man. My experience indicates that a positive correlation often exists between the qualitative and quantitative responses of animal and human to drugs influencing behavior. The problem is to find that species or model of behavior most intrinsically like that of the human in its attributes and responses to treatment. As with the normal-abnormal issue, I think it more useful to proceed experimentally in animal studies with a concept of anthropomorphism than without it provided that one is aware of the tenuous nature of such a supposition. In time, it will be empirically validated or invalidated.

With respect to models, if one insists on defining schizophrenia as primarily a thinking disturbance requiring language as a substrate, one can conveniently rule out other mammalia from study. If one is prepared to forego the language factor, there is no question but that behavior that would be diagnosed as schizophrenic in the human also occurs in nonhuman mammalia. All that language offers is additional modes for aberrant or operant responding and for communicating how one thinks and feels. Within the range and scope of daily behavior, all mammalia probably experience the extremes of discomfort and distress; detachment and involvement; tension, fear, gloom, illusions, and delusions; and inappropriate and maladaptive behavior. These do not seem attributes of man alone as attested by numerous animal behaviorists.

Just as no two humans or members of other species are exactly alike, neither are they totally dissimilar. The differences between some humans in response to drugs are known to be greater than the variance in the responses of other species. Appreciable variability also occurs when one individual is observed at different times. There is no standard human, mouse, cat, or monkey, and no individual unvarying with time and experience. A human is unquestionably a better general model of another human than are members of another species, and vice versa. But the ability to predict a particular drug effect requires a suitable model for study, regardless of the species. The most predictive effect of a drug is one that is independent of species, environmental contingencies, or behavioral state. The problem is to undertake the studies necessary to establish or eliminate any such possible relationships. From such studies, the most suitable animal model for human prediction could be identified.

My own experience suggests that the various classes of psychoactive drugs can be most easily distinguished or classified from studies with the mouse; estimation of human oral doses predicted from the cat; assessment of the time-course of drug action in humans from the Squirrel monkey (Saimiri sciurea); overall qualitative effects of drugs from the Squirrel or Cebus apella monkeys; tolerance, cumulative effects, or physical dependence development from Rhesus monkeys (the only monkey species adequately studied for this); and most adverse drug side effects from the cat.

B. Strategy and Tactics

If the response of nonhumans is to be meaningfully correlated with the response of humans to drugs, a uniform methodology must be used that is applicable across mammalian species regardless of baseline state or condition. In addition, appropriate animal models of dysfunctional states should be used. Because we cannot verbally communicate with nonhumans, it is obviously more difficult to derive information based on subjective or perceptual changes.

The necessary framework for psychopharmacology and drug therapy provides that the psychosocial-physiological effects of drugs on normal, functional individuals and on suitable experimental models of behavioral functions and dysfunctions are relevant to the therapeutic use of drugs. The accrual of

III. PSYCHOACTIVE DRUG EVALUATION

this information is the first step for rational drug therapy. It follows that there are effects of drugs independent of state or diagnoses that are shared by functional and dysfunctional individuals alike, so that it is important to rational prediction for therapy to establish the extent of this comparability. Once predictable psychosocial and physiological effects have been defined and quantified, it should be possible to induce discrete modification of behavior with drugs. It is further inferred that optimizing the functional apparatus of a patient so as to enhance his ability to cope with the environment causes a shift in the probability for a more favorable "therapeutic outcome." The latter is then determined primarily by the adaptive resources of the patient, the facilitating or destructive features of his environment (or "therapeutic milieu"), and his desire to "get well" [3].

The necessary strategy for drug assessment and evaluation, I feel, demands as a minimum the most comprehensive, simultaneous, quantitative measurement of the psychosocial-physiological state and effects of drugs in each individual as is possible (including time-dose-response effects on a mg/kg basis). Unless this is undertaken, the information otherwise obtained is incomplete and discernment of relationships between different items of measurement extremely difficult.

The necessary tactics involve a highly structured situation based on nonverbal communication between a well-trained observer and the subject, i.e., incorporating a rating system of behavior and evoked responses without regard to the content of verbal exchange. In addition, suitable models of relevant functional states are required as well as different experimental conditions of provocation. Instrumental procedures of scheduling and measuring are also advantageous, when assessing drug effects on perceptual and cognitive functioning or on psychological dependence development.

C. Comprehensive Observational Assessment Procedures

The evaluation of a patient's condition requires examination and differential diagnosis. The physician relies heavily on subjective observation, the pharmacologist on special *in vitro* and *in vivo* laboratory procedures. The two approaches — those of subjective observation and objective recording — are complementary and furnish different kinds of information. The physician views the total patient, notes significant behavioral, neurological, or autonomic changes, integrates the information and often completes a diagnosis in minutes. The pharmacologist performs a series of laboratory tests at different times, under different conditions, in different species, and by different routes of administration. He then integrates this information and may complete his analysis in weeks or months. The physician observes symptomatic changes within a direct, clinical context; the pharmacologist is more often concerned with measures and preparations far removed from the clinical situation. Nevertheless, both the physician and the pharmacologist may make an incorrect diagnosis because of excessive reliance on either the subjective or objective approach. The physician has turned more and more to the laboratory for confirmation of a diagnosis. Conversely, the pharmacologist would obtain additional pertinent information by incorporating aspects of the physician's subjective approach. Both sources of information are required for drug evaluation, due attention being paid to the differences in the nature of the derived information.

The use of observational techniques has several major weaknesses, but these are not intrinsic and they are not insurmountable. It would be pointless to deny that individuals differ in their ability to rate behavioral events. Observation requires attentiveness and a high degree of training. However, in order to minimize differences between observers, the procedures and rating scales developed must depend as little as possible on skill and experience. This is best achieved by describing behavior where possible in terms of duration or frequency of occurrence per unit of time or trial. Where intensity is to be measured, observed behavior can be quantified on the basis of an all-or-none rating scale of events. Thus, for example, the depth of ether anesthesia has been operationally described on the basis of a rating scale of eight progressive steps. It is similarly possible to establish techniques for grading the degree of impairment of the righting reflex, the struggle behavior of animals placed in a series of unusual postures, a visual placing reaction, and many other attributes of behavior or performance [21]. Once such techniques have been established, observer and interobserver reliability can be readily subjected to statistical analysis and validation. My own experience and study indicate that a high level of reliability is possible.

Certain measures, however, such as malaise, stupor, or fearfulness, are more difficult to define and quantify and will remain a challenge for some time. For measures such as these, which involve a complexity of attributes, a sequence of pictures or a film may serve as a standard of reference. The point at issue, however, is that rigid criteria such as we apply for the acceptance of objective techniques of measurement can also be applied to observational techniques. The establishment of such criteria merely awaits serious consideration and development.

Other weaknesses in the use of observational techniques are (1) a tendency toward subjective bias, (2) the possibility that rating scales may be nonlinear and therefore nonadditive, and (3) a tendency to have an insufficient number of steps in the rating scale. In the latter case, one tends to lose information, whereas excessive subdivision does little harm. How many steps are appropriate in a rating scale, however, and whether the scale is linear or nonlinear can be determined through statistical analysis of the acquired data. Subjective bias can be minimized through the use of blind procedures. The weaknesses attributed to observation are therefore not intrinsic. They arise primarily from the use of procedures which have not been standardized, validated, and systematically carried out, and the objections would apply equally to objective procedures carried out in similar fashion.

My own approach has been [1] to develop comprehensive observational procedures for systematically assessing and quantifying drug effects on

III. PSYCHOACTIVE DRUG EVALUATION

psychosocial-physiological behavior and functioning across species (mouse, rat, cat, monkey, and man), using sufficient operational description and quality control to assure reliability [22], (2) to accumulate time-dose-response data for representatives of all classes of psychoactive drugs across species (11 strains of mice, 6 strains of rats, cats, 12 species of monkeys, and humans with and without psychiatric disturbance), and (3) to develop the target-function framework discussed above for discrete behavior modification and for interpreting drug-response data [10]. These studies have revealed widespread strain and species differences in quantitative and qualitative responses to drugs; as widespread seemingly as between the responses of normal human subjects and patients of varying diagnostic type.

VI. ANIMAL DRUG SCREENING AND EVALUATION

A. Abbreviated Observational Procedures

The observational assessment procedure described by me for use with the mouse was first developed for drug screening and classification and only later developed as a quantitative procedure for comprehensively assessing the psychosocial and physiological state of the organism for drug evaluation [22]. Although more information was generated than needed for drug screening and although an adequate description of the procedure was not published until 1968, its popular application as a general screening procedure was derived from the Gordon Research Conference on Medicinal Chemistry, 1959.

In most laboratories the procedure is carried out coarsely with minimal quantification. Yet, even with such coarse measurement, most investigators in the field find observational assessment a useful tool for identifying and classifying new drugs of potential interest. Unfortunately, however, compounds of interest are rarely evaluated in an appropriately systematic manner. My recommendation is to provide additional training as required to carry out the procedure systematically and quantitatively for promising compounds and to use an abbreviated form for screening purposes.

For drug screening, the procedure can be reduced to the following measures (which are unlikely to miss any significant drug actions): locomotor activity and bizarre behavior; transfer arousal; touch-escape and grasp-irritability; positional passivity and visual placing; tail-pinch, corneal, and pinna responses; tail evaluation, body-abdominal tone, and grip strength; righting reflex and gait incapacity (ataxic or hypotonic); tremors, twitches, and convulsions; pupil size, palpebral closure, and exophthalmos; salivation and diarrhea; piloerection, hypothermia, skin color, and respiratory rate; acute and delayed death.

The procedures for quantitatively assessing the different components of behavior in mice can also be applied to obtain more limited information; as from animal models used for assessing drug effects under specialized conditions of environmental stimulation or scheduling or with drug-drug interaction studies. With most of our special procedures, for example, we assess the following items to define the general state of awareness and functioning of the animal just prior to testing: transfer arousal, spatial locomotion, body tone, gait incapacity, pupil size, and ptosis. Such information enables one to better interpret the significance of the experimental results obtained. In drug-drug interaction studies, several components of information can be derived to provide new information and to enhance interpretation of the data, e.g., in morphine interaction studies, effects on positional passivity, abdominal tone, tail elevation, tail-pinch response, gait incapacity, and pupil size should be assessed.

B. Nonobservational Procedures

The operant bar-press technique is among the most useful instrumental procedures for drug screening and evaluation because it is reliable and applicable across species. It can be applied to a wide range of measurement and is most useful in assessing drug effects on approach, avoidance, and escape behavior; on information processing including perception thresholds and acquisition and extinction curves of learning; on latency, rates, and efficiency of responding including errors of omission and commission; and in assessing the aversive or appetitive characteristics of reinforcement such as electroshock (self) stimulation of portions of the brain.

One can identify and classify the effects of drugs on a screening basis with operant techniques or with electroencephalographic measurement. Experience has shown, however, that the bar-press operant and electrophysiological approaches are generally less efficient and more costly for drug screening than other available approaches, so that they have either been discontinued or more appropriately used on a discriminant basis for research and drug evaluation. The most useful and commonly applied of these are the Sidman Avoidance procedure [23], and some analog of the Geller-Conflict procedure [24], techniques used for assessing drug effects on active and passive (punishment suppressed) avoidance behavior, respectively. The value of the Sidman procedure is that it provides information not only on avoidance responding, but also on latency, rate, and efficiency of responding from which different classes of drugs can be distinguished. The Geller-Conflict procedure has been useful for measuring disinhibitive effects of drugs on punishment suppressed behavior, thereby characterizing minor tranquilizers and hypnotics. Recently developed, however, are the promising "one-trial" conflict procedures [25]. These enable one to obtain relevant information from naive animals in a single day, as contrasted with the months of training and difficulties of sustaining the behavior with the original procedure.

C. Predictability

The prediction of drug effects from animals to man could be enhanced if suitable models of the conditions of interest were available for study. If there was a known etiological, target-biochemical substrate basis for a

III. PSYCHOACTIVE DRUG EVALUATION

particular diagnostic state, for example, one might be able to find an animal species in which the whole human configuration of the disturbance could be duplicated and the effects completely reversed with an appropriate agent. Under such circumstances, the predictability of drug effects from animals to man could have a high degree of certainty. The agent might be corrective for a deficiency state, as with thiamine in thiamine deficiency states, or dopamine in Parkinsonism; or it might counteract the effects of an accumulated substrate, as with the competitive antagonism of histamine by antihistamines or the antagonism of amphetamine-like drugs or dopamine by major tranquilizers with opposing biological effects.

Biochemical screening through drug-drug interaction studies with known agonists or antagonists can provide a useful means for identifying drugs with unique interactional properties. The merit of such procedures is in uncovering new agents of possible interest unlikely to be detected by other screening techniques. The chief disadvantage, however, is that too little is known about the molecular basis of behavior and central nervous system functioning to establish predictive expectations from such drug effects. Unless concomitant effects can be demonstrated at a functional level in normal animals or test models, there is a low probability for such agents proving of value in psychiatric or neurological dysfunctional states. The "drug in search of a disease" problem involves too high a cost for most pharmaceutical companies to consider unless some rational basis of expectation can be defined.

Nonetheless, a number of drug-drug interaction studies have been of considerable empirical value, e.g., the blockade of apomorphine-induced effects for identifying narcotic antagonists and the antiamphetamine test for characterizing major tranquilizers [26,27]. Parenthetically, the blockade of apomorphine-induced emesis is as highly correlated with the relative potency of the major tranquilizers as is their ability to produce catalepsy, reduce motor activity, or abolish active avoidance behavior. Anticonvulsant testing with subcutaneously administered metrazol is of value for revealing seizure related effects. It is also highly correlated with the relative potency of minor tranquilizers. For new drug evaluation, drug-drug interaction studies should be undertaken with agents to which patients are likely to be exposed during therapy, i.e., alcohol, hypnotics, narcotics, and stimulants, in particular.

Other drug-drug interaction models such as antagonism of strychnine and tetrabenazine are of questionable value. What they predictably reveal is the ability of a drug to partially or completely reverse or potentiate the effects of another drug. They may also provide insights regarding possible mechanisms of drug action, but other inferences from such studies have proven to be unreliable. There are many mechanisms by which drugs interact with one another. Accordingly, models of behavior that are not dependent upon chemical induction (behavior either naturally present in certain species or strains or evoked by environmental change or stimulation) should be given priority.

Although it would be desirable to have a model of the entire configurational state of human disturbance available for study, it may not be essential. In the absence of information on etiology, predictiveness can be enhanced by identifying the principal target function or symptom components of a disturbance and developing useful models of each for assessment. For example, conditions of intense sensory provocation (foot shock) may provide models of excitement, distress arousal, fear-suppressed behavior, or increased aggressiveness. The survival-stress contingency of swimming tests may represent a model of hopelessness and powerlessness.

An analysis of the retarded depressive state further suggests that isolation of the following factors (models) for separate study could be a productive means of evaluating new drugs:

(1) depressed mood (with pessimism of outlook and its consequences as a by-product, Table II),

(2) high distress arousal (with anorexia and insomnia as by-products),

(3) intense involvement with the distress state and its implications (leading to continuous, disturbing, ruminative preoccupations),

(4) extreme passivity (unresponsiveness) and slowness of movement and speech, and

(5) weakness and fatigue (with great effort and expenditure of energy when attempting even the simplest tasks).

Assuming the above analysis of the primary dysfunctions to be valid, I am aware of no drug with a spectrum of activity sufficient to affect all factors. A narcotic analgesic might be found to reverse items (1), (2), and (3) and promote sleep; the tricyclic antidepressants, to improve items (2), (3), and (4), leading to indirect improvement of items (1) and (5) over time; the minor tranquilizers, to partially improve items (2) and (3); the major tranquilizers, to partially improve (2) and (3) and worsen (4) and possibly (5); psychomotor stimulants, to improve (1), (4), and (5) and worsen (2) and (3). I would expect from such an analysis that the combination of a narcotic analgesic and a psychomotor stimulant might be more effective in the "retarded depressions" than tricyclic antidepressants alone. However, the addition of a tricyclic antidepressant and a minor tranquilizer to this combination could make an even more effective "antidepressant cocktail."

An analysis of the effects of orally administered marijuana suggests that it could be an important drug for the lonely, unhappy, irritable, geriatric patient who has no interest in food or his environment. Marijuana could potentially affect all of these factors and provide relaxation, contentment, and sleep. It could rekindle an interest in the environment and transform the process of eating into one of anticipatory pleasure.

III. PSYCHOACTIVE DRUG EVALUATION 221

VII. DRUG ASSESSMENT IN HUMANS

A. Adaptation of Animal Observational Procedures

The procedure we have developed for drug assessment in paid "normal" human volunteers is one modeled after our animal procedures (particularly that of the cat), so that direct comparisons can be made between various animal and human responses to drugs. In addition, other components of information are obtained by means of a subjective state questionnaire and cognitive performance tests. The procedure has been designed for comprehensive assessment of the state of the individual, whether normal or abnormal (functional or dysfunctional) and for the effects of drugs upon that state. This total information can be derived within 55 min of testing on two subjects, each simultaneously.

The baseline state of each subject is assessed before treatment and at 20, 80, 160, 220, and 280 min after treatment. This observational assessment procedure includes the quantitative determination of 60 items of psychosocial and physiological behavior and an additional 61 items (primarily scored on a 0-8 rating scale) derived from the subjective state questionnaire (SSQ). The SSQ also includes information on 24 of the most commonly reported drug side effects. The cognitive tests include a repeat-digit procedure described by Hebb, in which 15 ten-digit numbers are presented to the subject for purposes of recall. Of these numbers, 10 are random and 5 are replicated, so that the procedure reveals drug effects on both short-term recall and short-term learning. An arithmetic test, digit symbol substitution test, and Minnesota Clerical Test also are employed for information on total performance and errors of omission and commission in performance. The only items omitted from this procedure are those that relate to approach, avoidance, and escape behavior, since paid volunteers are unlikely to exhibit significant variance in these.

Figures 3, 4, and 5 show representative samples of the data obtained from the same subject on two occasions, one with placebo and the other with 0.6 mg/kg of amitriptyline hydrochloride administered orally. Except where otherwise indicated, most of the information obtained was on a 0-8 rating scale; the two assessments were five weeks apart.

Figure 3 shows the information systematically derived by a trained observer. The time-response data for placebo were relatively constant over the five hours of testing, except for a very slight reduction in light-pupil response, slowed heart rate, and increased blood pressure and pupil size.

Amitriptyline had an approximately 30-min onset of action with peak effects occurring at $2\frac{1}{2}$ to 3 hours. Pertinent observations include increased sleep and palpebral closure (ptosis); reduced frequencies of motor activity, smiling, and self-play; diminished speed and vigor of movement; and decreased alerting, attentiveness, and approach-arousal. The subject was dull and detached, less friendly and cooperative, but also less restless and

Species	Kg. Wt.	Sex	Route	Time of Drug Admin.	Base Factor	Temp. (°F)	Observer	Date
Human #32	84.1	M	Oral	0930	1.13	78	R. G. Kinohi	1/31/70 3/7/70

	Placebo						Amitriptyline (0.6 mg/kg)					
	Minutes						Minutes					
	-60	20	80	160	220	280	-60	20	80	160	220	280
Sleep(+)	0	0	0	0	0	0	0	0	0	0	+	0
Palpebral Closure	2.0	2.5	2.0	2.0	2.0	2.0	2.5	2.0	2.0	3.5	4.0	2.5
Eyes Alert Open (f)	48	45	48	48	36	48	43	39	27	0	0	38
Eyes Closed	0	0	0	0	0	0	0	0	15	46	45	0
Lying (f)	0	0	0	0	0	0	0	0	0	0	0	0
Standing (f)	0	0	0	0	0	0	0	0	0	0	0	0
Complete Rest (f)	0	0	0	0	12	0	0	3	21	46	45	10
Spatial Activity (f)	0	0	0	0	0	0	0	0	0	0	0	0
Speed Movement	5.0	6.0	6.0	6.0	6.0	6.0	5.0	5.5	3.0	2.0	3.0	4.0
Strength Movement	4.5	5.0	5.0	5.0	5.0	4.5	5.0	5.0	4.0	3.0	3.0	3.5
Vocalizing (f)	0	0	0	0	0	5	0	2	1	0	0	2
Smiling (f)	8	6	11	13	0	5	5	0	0	0	0	4
Crying (f)	0	0	0	0	0	0	0	0	0	0	0	0
Grimacing (f)	0	0	0	0	0	0	0	0	0	0	0	0
Grooming (f)	0	0	0	0	0	0	0	1	0	0	0	0
Self-Play (f)	12	23	13	16	29	7	26	28	9	0	0	26
Bizarre Behavior (f;0-8)	0	0	0	0	0	0	0	0	0	0	0	0
Alerting Response	8.0	8.0	8.0	8.0	8.0	8.0	8.0	8.0	8.0	4.0	6.0	8.0
Attentiveness	7.5	7.5	7.0	7.0	6.5	7.0	6.5	6.0	5.5	3.0	3.5	6.0
Eye Staring (f)	7	0	6	0	0	10	6.6	6.6	0	0	0	0
Eye Scanning (f)	3	0	2	10	0	3	0	0	0	0	0	0
Approach Arousal	4.5	4.0	4.5	4.5	4.0	4.0	4.0	4.0	3.0	2.5	2.5	3.5
Dulled-Excited	4.5	4.5	4.5	4.0	4.0	4.0	4.0	4.0	4.0	2.5	3.0	4.0
Detached-Involved	5.5	6.5	6.5	6.0	6.0	6.0	5.5	5.5	3.0	3.0	3.0	5.0
Friendly-Angry	2.0	2.0	2.0	2.0	2.0	2.0	2.0	2.0	3.0	4.0	4.0	3.0
Cooperative-Negative	2.0	2.0	2.0	2.0	2.0	2.0	2.0	2.0	2.5	3.0	3.5	2.5
Relaxed-Tense	3.0	3.0	3.0	3.0	2.5	2.5	3.0	3.0	2.0	1.0	1.0	2.5
Calm-Anxious	3.0	3.0	3.0	3.0	3.0	3.0	4.0	4.0	4.0	2.0	2.0	4.0
Restless (4-8)	4.5	5.0	5.0	5.0	5.0	4.5	5.5	5.0	4.5	4.0	4.0	5.0

Fig. 3-3. Test sheet for comprehensive observational assessment in man.

III. PSYCHOACTIVE DRUG EVALUATION

Item	Placebo Minutes						Amitriptyline (0.6 mg/kg) Minutes					
	-60	20	80	160	220	280	-60	20	80	160	220	280
Confident-Fearful	3.0	2.5	2.5	2.5	2.5	2.5	3.0	3.0	3.5	4.0	4.0	3.0
Trusting-Suspicious	3.0	3.0	2.5	2.0	2.0	2.0	3.0	3.0	4.0	4.0	4.0	4.0
Joyful-Depressed	3.0	3.0	2.0	2.0	2.0	2.0	3.0	2.5	4.0	4.0	4.0	3.0
Grief-Anguish (4-8)	4.0	4.0	4.0	4.0	4.0	4.0	4.0	4.0	4.0	4.0	4.0	4.0
Talk-Time Est. (15 sec)	13	15	14	14	15	17	14	12	14	15	15	14
Reading Time (sec)	28	26	26	25	27	25	24	24	26	25	25	26
Light-Pupil Response	6.0	6.0	5.0	5.0	5.0	6.0	6.0	6.5	6.0	4.0	4.0	5.5
Wink Response (+)		+	+	+	+	+	+	+	+	+	+	++
Dysequilibrium (cm)	4	5	6	5	6	6	6	5	6	8	10	7
Ataxia	0	0	0	0	0	0	0	0	0	1.0	1.0	0.5
Speech Slurring	0	0	0	0	0	0	0	0	0.5	2.5	2.0	1.0
Nystagmus (+)	0	0	0	0	0	0	0	0	0	0	0	0
Lower Limb Weakness	0	0	0	0	0	0	0	0	0	0.5	0.5	0
Grip Strength (kg)	58.0	58.0	59.5	61.0	57.5	55.0	55.5	56.0	60.0	58.0	56.0	58.0
Upper Limb Tone	5.0	5.0	5.0	5.0	4.5	4.5	5.5	5.0	4.5	3.5	3.5	4.5
Tremors	0	0	0	0	0	0	0	0	0	0	0	0
Twitches	0	0	0	0	0	0	0	0	0	0	0	0
Oral Temperature (°F)	98.0	97.8	97.8	97.8	97.6	97.6	98.0	97.8	98.2	97.8	97.6	97.6
Respir. Rate/Min.	18	20	20	20	18	18	18	18	16	12	12	18
Heart Rate/Min.	72	68	60	60	60	60	72	64	68	60	60	60
Blood Pressure (Sit/Std)	120	118	130	128	130	130	124	118	124	122	120	118
	122	118	124	124	126	130	124	120	124	120	118	118
Palmar Skin Color	5.0	5.5	5.5	5.0	4.5	5.0	5.0	4.0	4.0	3.0	2.5	4.5
Conjunctival Congestion	1.5	1.5	2.0	2.0	2.0	2.0	2.0	2.0	3.0	2.0	3.0	2.0
Pupil Size	2.5	3.0	4.0	4.0	3.5	4.0	2.0	2.5	3.0	4.5	2.0	2.5
Visual Blurring (+)	0	0	0	0	0	0	0	0	0	0	0	0
Exophthalmos (+)	0	0	0	0	0	0	0	0	0	0	0	0
Lacrimation (+)	0	0	0	0	0	0	0	0	0	0	+	0
Salivation	1.5	1.0	1.0	1.5	1.5	2.0	2.0	1.0	2.0	2.0	1.0	1.5
Palmar Sweating (+)	0	0	0	0	0	0	+	0	+	0	0	0
Goose Flesh (+)	0	0	0	0	0	0	0	0	0	0	0	0
Liquid Food (Cups)	0	0	2	2	1	1	0	0	2	2	2	2

Fig. 3-3. Test sheet for comprehensive observational assessment in man. (Cont'd)

more relaxed and calm. Light-pupil and wink responses were slightly reduced. Neurological impairment was evidenced by slight ataxia, impaired equilibrium, and slurred speech. Autonomic changes included increased blanching, conjunctival congestion, and pupil size, but the latter two did not differ significantly from the placebo control. Other subjects have revealed lesser and greater overall effects, including mydriasis, nystagmus, conjunctival congestion, visual blurring, lacrimation, and lower limb weakness. Similar effects were produced by imipramine hydrochloride in doses three times greater than amitriptyline. On an equal dose basis, imipramine was significantly less sedative and more mydriatic than amitriptyline.

The data in Fig. 4 show the time-response effects of placebo and amitriptyline obtained through use of a subjective state questionnaire of 61 items, scored on a 0-8 rating scale. For items 1 to 25 and 61, increasing values denote a shift toward intensification and decreasing values, a shift toward attenuation. For items 26 to 60, values of 4.0 denote a midpoint between polar opposites — a neither/nor state. Values below 4.0 indicate the degree of improvement and those above the degree of impairment or untoward symptomatology. Several items, as shown, were assessed on a 4-8 scale only.

The placebo time-response data were fairly constant over the five hours of testing, except for a tendency to feel slightly less "good, hopeful, proud, confident and calm" with the passage of time. The response to the drug revealed significant effects at 105 min post-drug and peak effects at 3 to 4 hours as shown by the diminished values for wakefulness, attentiveness, energy, and ease of coping as well as for activity, initiative, and talk drives. The subject also indicated feeling less "good, joyful, hopeful, confident, friendly, cooperative, and trusting," perhaps because of the significant loss reported for behavioral control, decisiveness, and increased difficulty of concentration, reading, speaking, and remembering.

In Fig. 5 are summarized the results of various performance tasks and a weighted summary of the observed frequency data on eye opening, body position, and locomotor activity, expressed on a 0-8 scale. The data for the placebo again is remarkable for its uniformity with time, save for some increase in errors of commission on the digit-symbol substitution and Minnesota Clerical tests. Amitriptyline produced a significant reduction of eye opening (tendency toward increased sleep) and motor activity. Handwriting length also was diminished, as was the number of correct repeat-digits (possibly due to reduced attentiveness) and completed items in the arithmetic, digit-symbol substitution, and Minnesota Clerical tests. A tendency towards increased errors of omission was observed after amitriptyline but errors of commission were not significantly different from placebo controls. This subject had no untoward side effects.

In future studies we will apply the same procedures to patients of varying type to determine the extent to which "normal" subjects and patients may differ in their qualitative and quantitative responses and how these differences may relate to therapeutic outcome.

III. PSYCHOACTIVE DRUG EVALUATION

Item	Placebo						Amitriptyline (0.6 mg/kg)					
	Minutes						Minutes					
	-20	45	105	185	245	305	-20	45	105	185	245	305
1. Wakefulness	5.1	5.5	4.8	4.8	4.4	4.3	4.7	4.3	2.9	1.2	0.8	3.6
2. Interest	4.0	4.5	4.4	4.1	4.3	4.0	4.3	4.4	4.0	4.0	4.0	4.0
3. Attentiveness	5.2	5.6	5.5	5.4	4.1	4.0	5.6	4.4	3.7	4.0	2.8	4.0
4. Energy	4.9	5.0	5.2	5.4	4.5	4.7	4.5	5.5	3.7	2.3	1.9	4.0
5. Ease of Coping	4.9	5.1	4.9	4.6	4.2	4.4	5.0	5.3	3.6	1.7	2.6	3.7
6. Health	6.2	6.2	5.7	5.7	5.9	5.8	6.4	6.3	6.2	5.9	6.3	5.9
7. Excitement	4.0	4.1	4.0	4.0	4.0	4.0	4.3	4.3	4.0	3.6	4.0	4.0
8. Speed Movement	4.0	4.0	4.0	4.0	4.0	4.0	4.1	4.0	4.0	4.0	4.0	4.0
9. Speed Thoughts	4.0	4.0	4.0	4.0	4.0	4.0	4.0	4.0	4.0	4.0	4.0	4.0
10. Activity Drive	4.0	4.0	4.0	4.0	4.0	4.0	5.4	4.4	4.0	2.4	3.0	4.0
11. Initiative Drive	4.0	4.0	4.0	4.0	4.0	4.0	5.1	5.0	4.0	4.0	3.9	4.0
12. Talk Drive	4.0	4.0	4.0	4.0	4.0	4.0	4.2	4.3	4.0	3.3	3.4	4.0
13. Social Drive	4.0	4.0	4.0	4.0	4.0	4.0	4.8	4.4	4.0	4.0	4.0	4.0
14. Attention Seeking	4.0	4.0	4.0	4.0	4.0	4.0	4.0	4.0	4.0	4.0	4.0	4.0
15. Sex Drive	4.0	4.0	4.0	4.0	4.0	4.0	4.0	4.0	4.0	4.0	4.0	4.0
16. Punishment Seeking	4.0	4.0	4.0	4.0	4.0	4.0	4.0	4.0	4.0	4.0	4.0	4.0
17. Survival Drive	8.0	7.9	8.0	8.0	8.0	8.0	8.0	8.0	8.0	8.0	8.0	8.0
18. Self-Involvement	4.0	4.0	4.0	4.0	4.0	4.0	4.0	4.0	4.0	4.0	4.0	4.0
19. External Involvement	4.0	4.0	4.0	4.0	4.0	4.0	4.0	4.0	4.0	4.0	4.0	4.0
20. Intensity Emotions	4.0	4.0	4.0	4.0	4.0	4.0	4.0	4.0	4.0	4.0	4.0	4.0
21. Sensory Acuity	4.0	4.0	4.0	4.0	4.0	4.0	4.0	4.0	4.0	4.0	4.0	4.0
22. Brightness Objects	4.0	4.0	4.0	4.0	4.0	4.0	4.0	4.0	4.0	4.0	4.0	4.0
23. Closeness Objects	4.0	4.0	4.0	4.0	4.0	4.0	4.0	4.0	4.0	4.0	4.0	4.0
24. Feel Big	4.0	4.0	4.0	4.0	4.0	4.0	4.0	4.0	4.0	4.0	4.0	4.0
25. Speed Time	4.0	4.0	4.0	4.0	3.4	4.0	4.0	3.8	3.5	3.4	4.0	3.8
26. Good-Miserable	2.1	2.5	2.2	2.6	2.4	3.4	3.0	3.4	3.2	4.0	4.0	3.5
27. Lonely (4-8)	4.0	4.0	4.0	4.0	4.0	4.0	4.0	4.0	4.0	4.0	4.0	4.0
28. Playful-Serious	4.0	4.0	4.0	4.0	4.0	4.0	4.0	4.0	4.0	4.0	4.0	4.0
29. Joyful-Depressed	2.9	2.8	4.0	4.0	4.0	4.0	3.3	3.5	4.0	4.0	4.0	4.0
30. Grieving (4-8)	4.0	4.0	4.0	4.0	4.0	4.0	4.0	4.0	4.0	4.0	4.0	4.0

Fig. 3-4. Summary of subjective state questionnaire.

Item	Placebo Minutes						Amitriptyline (0.6 mg/kg) Minutes					
	-20	45	105	185	245	305	-20	45	105	185	245	305
31. Hopeful-Hopeless	1.9	2.3	2.4	2.6	3.0	2.5	2.1	3.2	2.9	3.4	3.0	3.5
32. Proud-Worthless	1.8	2.1	2.4	2.4	2.3	2.1	2.2	2.4	2.5	2.6	2.1	2.1
33. Guilt (4-8)	4.0	4.0	4.0	4.0	4.0	4.0	4.0	4.0	4.0	4.0	4.0	4.0
34. Confident-Fearful	2.5	2.0	4.0	3.0	4.0	4.0	1.8	2.7	4.0	4.0	4.0	2.4
35. Somatic Concern (4-8)	4.0	4.0	4.0	4.0	4.0	4.0	4.0	4.0	4.0	4.0	4.1	4.0
36. Spontaneous-Inhibited	4.0	4.0	2.9	2.4	2.3	4.0	3.7	3.2	3.9	4.0	4.0	2.7
37. Relaxed-Tense	2.5	2.4	3.0	2.6	2.2	2.0	2.1	2.7	2.0	1.7	2.3	2.4
38. Calm-Anxious	2.1	2.5	3.2	2.5	2.2	3.1	1.9	2.4	2.0	1.6	1.4	2.4
39. Patient-Restless	3.2	2.7	2.5	2.1	3.6	3.4	3.8	3.3	3.7	2.6	3.1	4.0
40. Friendly-Angry	2.1	2.0	2.5	2.1	2.3	2.1	1.7	2.0	3.0	3.7	2.1	2.4
41. Cooperative-Rebellious	2.4	2.2	2.5	2.0	2.1	2.2	1.9	2.0	2.5	3.8	2.4	2.9
42. Affectionate-Aloof	3.2	2.4	2.5	2.0	2.4	2.9	4.0	3.2	3.0	4.0	4.0	3.5
43. Trusting-Suspicious	2.0	2.0	2.4	1.8	2.1	1.9	1.6	1.9	2.2	2.6	4.0	2.0
44. Paranoia (4-8)	4.0	4.0	4.0	4.0	4.0	4.0	4.0	4.0	4.0	4.0	4.0	4.0
45. Constructive-Destructive	2.4	2.1	2.6	2.1	2.6	2.5	4.0	4.0	4.0	4.0	4.0	3.0
46. Loss Behavior Control	1.9	1.8	1.5	1.4	2.1	2.1	1.4	1.4	5.0	3.7	4.0	2.6
47. Difficult Concentration	3.1	3.3	2.9	2.8	3.4	3.5	2.2	2.6	4.0	4.0	4.0	3.7
48. Difficult Read-Speak	1.8	2.7	2.6	2.2	2.5	2.6	1.8	1.8	4.0	4.1	4.0	1.8
49. Difficult Remembering	3.5	3.5	3.2	3.6	3.6	3.4	2.4	2.6	4.6	5.8	4.0	4.0
50. Decisive-Confused	2.8	2.1	2.1	2.1	2.6	2.6	1.4	1.7	2.3	4.0	4.0	2.7
51. Self-Power-Outside Control	4.0	4.0	4.0	4.0	4.0	4.0	4.0	4.0	4.0	4.0	4.0	4.0
52. Unusual Thoughts (4-8)	4.0	4.0	4.0	4.0	4.0	4.0	4.0	4.0	4.0	4.0	4.0	4.0
53. Obsessions (4-8)	4.0	4.0	4.0	4.0	4.0	4.0	4.0	4.0	4.0	4.0	4.0	4.0
54. Mind Working (4-8)	4.0	4.0	4.0	4.0	4.0	4.0	4.0	4.0	4.0	4.0	4.0	4.0
55. Uncertainty Self-Image	0	0	0	0	0	0	0	0	0	0	0	0
56. Unusual Body Sensations	4.0	4.0	4.0	4.0	4.0	4.0	4.0	4.0	4.0	4.0	4.0	4.0
57. Unusual Sense Perception	4.0	4.0	4.0	4.0	4.0	4.0	4.0	4.0	4.0	4.0	4.0	4.0
58. Detached/Dreamlike (4-8)	4.0	4.0	4.0	4.0	4.0	4.0	4.0	4.0	4.0	4.0	4.0	4.0
59. Body Distortion (4-8)	4.0	4.0	4.0	4.0	4.0	4.0	4.0	4.0	4.0	4.0	4.0	4.0
60. Hallucinations (4-8)	4.0	4.0	4.0	4.0	4.0	4.0	4.0	4.0	4.0	4.0	4.0	4.0
61. Accuracy Answers (4-8)	7.0	7.0	7.2	7.2	6.9	6.6	6.9	6.9	6.0	5.9	5.1	6.8

Fig. 3-4. Summary of subjective state questionnaire. (Cont'd)

III. PSYCHOACTIVE DRUG EVALUATION

Item	Placebo Minutes						Amitriptyline (0.6 mg/kg) Minutes					
	-20	45	105	185	245	305	-20	45	105	185	245	305
Eye Opening	8.0	7.8	8.0	8.0	7.0	8.0	7.6	7.3	5.0	0.2	0.3	7.2
Body Position	4.0	4.0	4.0	4.0	4.0	4.0	4.0	4.0	4.0	4.0	4.0	4.0
Motor Activity	1.6	1.6	1.6	1.6	1.2	1.6	1.6	1.5	0.9	0.1	0.1	1.3
Performance Tests												
Handwriting (mm)	129	130	127	148	129	138	139	127	116	117	128	127
Reading Time (sec)	28	26	26	25	27	25	24	24	26	25	25	26
Talk-Time Est. (15 sec)	13	15	14	14	15	17	14	12	14	15	15	14
Repeat-Digit												
Correct: Random	96	100	93	93	87	91	90	98	76	68	63	93
Repeat	50	46	50	50	50	50	50	37	47	35	47	44
Arithmetic Test												
Completed	40	40	32	37	38	39	37	35	25	14	23	30
Errors Commission	0	0	2	0	0	0	1	0	4	2	2	0
Digit Symbol Subst.												
Completed	63	57	62	52	55	53	60	53	52	45	51	46
Errors Commission	0	3	2	1	0	0	0	0	0	0	0	0
Minnesota Clerical												
Completed	184	200	191	200	197	200	179	186	113	20*	114	160
Errors Omission	2	0	0	3	2	2	2	1	5	1	8	3
Errors Commission	7	10	7	12	11	12	5	9	5	1	2	6
Side Effects (+)												
Stuffy Nose												
Stuffy Head												
Light Headed												
Heavy Headed												
Headache												
Dizzy												
Faint												

Fig. 3-5. Summary of various performance tasks and side effects.

Item	Placebo Minutes					Amitriptyline (0.6 mg/kg) Minutes					
	-20	45	105	185	245	305	-20	45	105	185	245	305
Numb												
Blurred Vision												
Ringing Ears												
Hot or Cold Spells												
Itchy												
Sweating												
Salivating												
Dry Mouth												
Diarrhea												
Stomach Ache												
Heartburn												
Nausea												
Vomiting												
Hard Swallowing												
Hard Breathing												
Heart Racing												
Tremors												

Comments:
Bizarre Behavior:

Other:
Amitriptyline Effects
105 - "Drowsy"
185 - "Very sleepy, cold - Put on my jacket". *Tendency to fall asleep.
245 - "Very sleepy"
305 - "Effects nearly gone"

Fig. 3-5. Summary of various performance tasks and side effects (Cont'd)

III. PSYCHOACTIVE DRUG EVALUATION

B. Discrete versus Global Behavior Modification

The object of drug therapy, as I view it, is to so modify the functional state or disposition of the individual as to reverse the direction of responses toward normal. Whether a patient is labeled "normal," "neurotic," or "psychotic," nonspecific drugs such as those in use are likely to affect behavior in two steps: (1) an immediate <u>direct effect</u> on the target functions of behavior, altering them in a predictable way; and (2) a slowly evolving <u>indirect effect</u> resulting from the interaction of the individual with his environment as he is better able to cope with it. The indirect effects are influenced mainly by the adaptive resources of the patient and the milieu (including other treatment modalities); the early direct effects, mainly by the drugs. Accordingly, the greater the early target-function response to a drug and the greater the adaptive resources of the patient, the more rapid and complete the therapeutic response is likely to be. Thus, so long as tolerance to the drug does not develop with continued use, it is possible to predict the probable therapeutic outcome from relatively short-term studies, i.e., to the extent that the target-function effects of drugs are known and can be used.

The potential of a drug for therapy seems best revealed early in the course of therapy, before the interactional effects from the environment have too greatly influenced the patient's behavior. Yet emphasis in most studies has been the reverse, with greater attention to the later effects of drugs. But the placebo response also occurs early in therapy; unless adequately controlled, it too can obscure the results.

As a basis for drug selection and use, I believe it necessary to view and assess the patient in terms of the disruptive target-function components of his behavior. Where drug treatment is indicated, the tactical problem is to select that agent or combination of agents with "target-function" actions best suited to produce the desired changes. Also, dosage is increased, consonant with safety, until the expected results are obtained. When drugs are applied rationally in this manner, with specific target areas of expected change defined and predicted in advance, each patient can serve as a test of the validity and usefulness of one's concepts regarding patient assessment and the specific actions of a drug. Also, one need not get into the present logistic difficulties of finding a homogeneous diagnostic group of patients for assessment studies. Using this approach, the treatment of disordered behavior becomes similar in principle to the treatment of somatic disorders, where discrete drug-induced changes are usually sought.

A patient, however, is not in a static state but undergoes continuous change. This means that the drugs and dose of choice must be adjusted as required to meet the changing state and needs of the patient. The object of drug therapy is to optimize the patient's functioning to achieve some stated goal. This criterion is not met by a static concept of continuing medication, or by the uninterrupted administration of drugs when this no longer seems needed. A corollary is that it is not always in the patient's interest to conduct prolonged studies of "therapeutic efficacy" with a single drug.

In my judgment, "therapeutic outcome" should not be the overwhelming focus in drug evaluation studies that it has been. It tends to obscure the main issue of such studies — defining the measurable target-function effects of drugs so that they may be used more effectively to enhance the therapeutic course. May and Wittenborn [28] have noted that the great bulk of published results on controlled studies does not identify the response itself but rather presents a value judgment (usually of global response) regarding "improvement." They suggest that it might be clinically more meaningful if discrete manifestations of change (improvement in a particular aspect) were determined in a sophisticated manner without resorting to value judgments. This coincides with my own view.

VIII. SUMMARY

Several approaches to psychoactive drug evaluation and prediction have been reviewed, some of which are based upon beliefs and assumptions that have not been validated. A tendency exists to exclude from investigation a wide range of information required for rational drug development, evaluation, prediction, and use. Consequently, self-defeating errors of omission and commission are not uncommon.

An alternative framework, strategy, and tactics based upon a systems approach that is not exclusionary is presented which offers at least a rational approach for drug evaluation and prediction. To it can be appended the presently available diagnostic modes of approach, which contribute important dimensions of information and insight. Also presented is a list of terms specifying behavioral and physiological information required for an economical and yet comprehensive assessment of the state of an individual and his response to drugs.

Current therapeutic approaches have been severely hampered by a failure to use normal subjects (animal or human) and experimental modes of behavioral dysfunction to define the limitations and possibilities for predicting drug effects in patients. My past and present research efforts with animals and humans have focused on this aspect of systematic prediction, using a common experimental (multifactor observational) procedure. The goals have been to determine (1) which of the animal species is most predictive of drug effects in normal humans and (2) the relationship between drug effects in normal humans and in patients. It is anticipated that incorporation of these principles into present experimental and clinical approaches may enhance discrimination, efficiency, and reliability in drug evaluation and predictiveness.

ACKNOWLEDGMENT

Research was supported by Public Health Service grants MH-10990 and MH-12214 from the National Institute of Mental Health.

REFERENCES

1. S. Irwin, Science, **136**, 123 (1962).
2. S. Irwin, Psychopharmacologia, **9**, 259 (1966).
3. S. Irwin, Perspectives Biol. Med., **11**, 654 (1968).
4. J. H. Masserman, Behavior and Neurosis, An Experimental Psychoanalytic Approach to Psychobiologic Principles, Univ. of Chicago Press, Chicago, 1943, pp. 168-170.
5. L. P. Ullman and L. Krasner, A Psychological Approach to Abnormal Behavior, Prentice-Hall, Englewood Cliffs, New Jersey, 1969, pp. 92-105.
6. E. M. Bower, Natl. Educ. Assoc. J., January 1968.
7. D. F. Klein, Psychopharmacologia, **13**, 359 (1968).
8. D. F. Klein and J. M. Davis, Diagnosis and Drug Treatment of Psychiatric Disorders, Williams & Wilkins, Baltimore, 1969, pp. 1-16 and 436-454.
9. F. A. Freyhan and J. Merkel, in Mental Patients in Transition (M. Greenblatt, D. J. Levinson and G. L. Klerman, eds.), Thomas, Springfield, Illinois, 1961, p. 302.
10. S. Irwin, Am. J. Psychiat. Suppl., **124**, 1 (1968).
11. D. Bindra, Psychol. Rev., **66**, 96 (1959).
12. R. B. Malmo, Psychol. Rev., **66**, 367 (1959).
13. P. B. Bradley, in Reticular Formation of the Brain (H. H. Jasper, L. D. Proctor, R. S. Knighton, W. D. Noshay, and R. T. Costello, eds.), Little, Brown, Boston, 1958, pp. 123-149.
14. J. Elkes, in The Physiology of Emotions (A. Simon, ed.), Thomas, Springfield, Illinois, 1961, p. 95.
15. S. Irwin, in The Dynamics of Psychiatric Drug Therapy (G. J. Sarwer-Foner, ed.), Thomas, Springfield, Illinois, 1960, pp. 1-22.
16. S. Courvoisier, J. Clin. Exptl. Psychopathol., **17**, 25 (1956).
17. S. Irwin, Arch. Intern. Pharmacodyn., **142**, 152 (1963).
18. C. Kornetsky and A. F. Mirsky, Psychopharmacologia, **8**, 309 (1966).
19. S. Irwin, in Psychopharmacology Frontiers (Nathan S. Kline, ed.), Little, Brown, Boston, 1959, pp. 251-258.
20. S. Irwin, in Research Conference on Therapeutic Community (H. C. B. Denber, ed.), Thomas, Springfield, Illinois, 1959, pp. 29-42.
21. S. Norton and E. J. DeBeer, Ann. N. Y. Acad. Sci., **65**, 249 (1956).

22. S. Irwin, Psychopharmacologia, 13, 222 (1968).
23. M. Sidman, Science, 118, 157 (1953).
24. I. Geller and J. Seifter, Psychopharmacologia, 1, 482 (1960).
25. J. R. Vogel, B. Beer, and D. E. Clody, The Pharmacologist, 11, 246 (1969).
26. P. A. J. Janssen, C. J. E. Niemegeers, and K. H. L. Schellekens, Arzneimittel-Forsch., 15, 104 (1965).
27. C. J. E. Niemegeers, F. J. Verbruggen, and P. A. J. Janssen, Psychopharmacologia, 16, 161 (1969).
28. P. R. A. May and J. R. Wittenborn, in Psychotropic Drug Response (P. R. A. May and J. R. Wittenborn, eds.), Thomas, Springfield, Illinois, 1969, pp. 3-11.

Chapter IV

SELECTIVE BETA RECEPTOR DRUG INTERACTIONS

Bernard Levy

Department of Pharmacology
University of Texas Medical Branch
Galveston, Texas

I.	INTRODUCTION	233
II.	SELECTIVE BETA RECEPTOR ANTAGONISM	237
III.	SELECTIVE BETA RECEPTOR ACTIVATION	253
IV.	CONCLUSIONS	256
	REFERENCES	257

I. INTRODUCTION

The ability of drugs to interact with receptors has been and continues to be a tool which pharmacologists have attacked with great relish. The fact that most receptors have not been identified as specific chemical or physical entities has in no way dampened the ardor of the curious investigator. The concept of a receptor mechanism, at least in relation to drug actions, was originally conceived by Langley [1,2] to explain the action of curare on skeletal muscle. Dale [3] was probably the first to apply the receptor concept in relation to drugs acting on the sympathetic nervous system. This classical study by Dale demonstrated that the cardiac stimulant effects of epinephrine were not reduced by doses of ergot extracts which reversed its pressor response. Table I represents Dale's classification of sympathetic effects according to their response before and after ergot (alpha receptor blockade) treatment.

In 1948, Ahlquist [4] formulated the presently accepted concept of two fundamental types of adrenergic receptors. This classification was based upon relative orders of potencies of a series of racemic sympathomimetic amines most closely related structurally to epinephrine.

Table II represents Ahlquist's original classification of structures and functions associated with each of the two types of adrenergic receptors. The alpha adrenergic receptor subserves primarily excitatory responses with one

TABLE I

Classification of Sympathetic Effects [a] [b]

Organ	Effects of stimulating sympathetic nerve-supply, or injecting adrenaline intravenously	
	Before ergot	After ergot
Arteries (cat, dog, ferret)	M	I
Arteries (rabbit)1	M	Nil or weak M
Cardiac muscle	M	Nil or weak M
Spleen (cat)	M	I
Stomach (cat)	I	I
Small intestine (cat, dog, monkey)	I	I
Large intestine (cat)	I	I
Ileocolic sphincter (cat)	M	Nil
Internal anal sphincter (cat)	M	I
Gall bladder	I	I
Fundus of urinary bladder (cat)	I	I
Fundus of urinary bladder (ferret)	M	I
Base of bladder and urethra (cat)	M	Nil
Pilomotor muscles	M	Nil
Dilator iridis	M	Nil with adrenaline Weak M with cervical sympathetic
Uterus (cat, nonpregnant)	I or M and I	I
Uterus (cat, pregnant)	M	I
Uterus (rabbit)	M	I (slight)
Uterus (monkey)	M	I
Retractor penis (dog)	M	Nil

[a] Reprinted from Ref. [3], p. 29, by courtesy of Pergamon Press, London.

[b] M = motor effect, i.e., increase of tone, augmentation or acceleration of rhythm. I = inhibition, i.e., relaxation of tone, cessation, weakening, or slowing of rhythm.

important inhibitory function, intestinal relaxation. The beta adrenergic receptor subserves primarily inhibitory responses with one important excitatory function, cardiac stimulation. The only important modification of

TABLE II

Structures of Functions Containing or Associated with Each of the Two Types of Adrenotropic Receptors [a,b]

Alpha receptor	Beta receptor
Vasoconstriction	Vasodilation
Viscera	Skeletal muscle
Skin	Coronary
Nictitating membrane	Viscera (few)
Uterus (excitatory)	Myocardium
Rabbit	Uterus (inhibitory)
Dog	Rat
Human	Cat
Intestine	Dog
Ureter	Human
Dilator pupillae	Bronchi [20]

[a] The following structures or functions have not as yet been completely tested: spleen, erectores pilorum, urinary bladder, glands, and glycogenolysis.

[b] Reprinted from Ref. [4], p. 596, by courtesy of Williams and Wilkins Co., Baltimore, Md.

Ahlquist's original classification of adrenergic receptors was the observation that intestinal smooth muscle possessed both alpha and beta receptors, both subserving inhibition of motility [5-7].

The classification by Ahlquist of two adrenergic receptor types, alpha and beta, was based almost exclusively upon qualitative differences in orders of potency of the catecholamines that he used. He did make the rather casual observation that those responses classified as alpha receptor responses could be blocked by the adrenergic blocking agents then available, while responses to beta receptor activation were relatively unaffected. The adrenergic blocking agents then available were all alpha receptor antagonists and included such drugs as phenoxybenzamine, phentolamine, dibenamine, and piperoxan. This receptor classification proposed by Ahlquist did not achieve universal acceptance by skeptical members of the scientific community until Powell and Slater in 1958 [8] described the beta receptor blocking properties of dichloroisoproterenol (DCI). DCI selectively blocked those responses due to beta receptor activation while alpha receptor responses were relatively unaffected. The ranks of beta receptor blocking agents were soon increased by the addition of such agents as MJ 1999 (sotalol) [9], pronethalol [10], propranolol [11], and a number of others that, like DCI, were derivatives of isoproterenol (Fig. 1) [12]. Aside from differences in potency and the presence or absence of intrinsic or nonadrenergic activity, all of these beta receptor blocking agents are qualitatively similar in that they will block beta receptors to a significant extent in all tissues in a dose range that is characteristic for each agent.

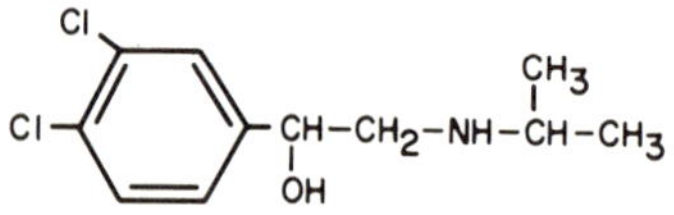

Dichloroisoproterenol (DCI)

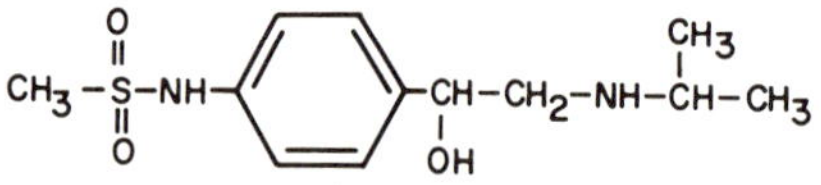

Sotalol (MJ-1999)

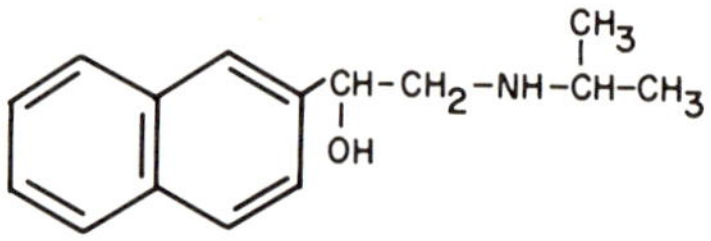

Pronethalol

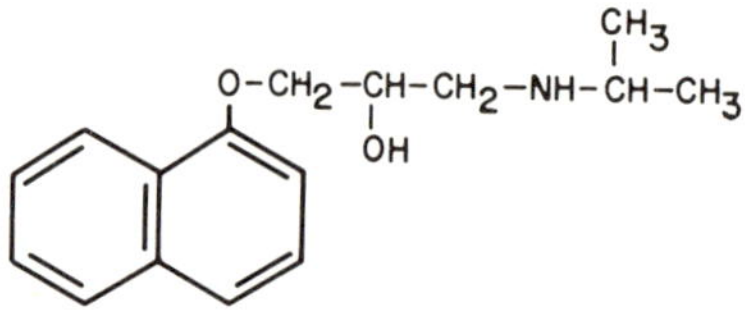

Propranolol

Fig. 1. Dichloroisoproterenol (DCI), sotalol (MJ 1999), pronethalol, propranalol.

IV. SELECTIVE BETA RECEPTOR DRUG INTERACTIONS

It is not the purpose of this chapter to simply review the area of beta receptor blockade. The pharmacology and clinical effectiveness of beta receptor antagonists has been the subject of a number of recent and excellent reviews [13-18]. Propranolol (Inderal) is the first beta receptor antagonist to be introduced into clinical medicine. Since its introduction in 1969, propranolol has proved itself to be effective in the treatment of a variety of cardiovascular disorders. The significance of propranolol is not so much its effectiveness but rather the fact that it represents a "new" type of drug mechanism. The title of this book, "Search for New Drugs," could read "Search for New Drug Mechanisms" insofar as the content of this chapter is concerned. It is the purpose of this chapter to look beyond propranolol and to examine the hypothesis that highly selective beta receptor drug interactions are a reality and will result in the development of clinically useful agents that will be as effective as propranolol, for example, but much more selective in their ability to block the beta adrenergic receptor. What follows is the authors appraisal of this area of pharmacology; hopefully, an objective viewpoint.

II. SELECTIVE BETA RECEPTOR ANTAGONISM

The hypothesis that drugs may selectively interact with beta receptors in specific tissues has been most clearly demonstrated with beta receptor antagonists. Before describing those studies supporting the hypothesis of selective beta receptor blockade certain guidelines and criteria must be rigidly established. Beta receptor blocking agents as a class might be classified as selective adrenergic blocking agents if one compares their beta receptor blocking properties to their alpha receptor blocking properties, which are essentially negligible. What we are saying is that there are beta receptor blocking agents that have a relatively greater beta receptor blocking effect in certain tissues than in others. These agents are quantitatively and possibly even qualitatively different from DCI, MJ 1999, pronethalol, propranolol, and the host of other agents that are loosely referred to as beta receptor antagonists. Powell and Slater [8] originally described DCI as an agent capable of blocking the vasodepressor response and bronchodilator response as well as the intestinal inhibitory response to isoproterenol. These findings were obtained in a variety of species and were further complicated by the fact that DCI had the ability to initially stimulate beta receptors. Moran and Perkins [19] demonstrated the ability of DCI to block the positive inotropic, positive chronotropic, and vasodepressor responses to isoproterenol in the same dose range. This showed that the vascular and cardiac responses to isoproterenol were both blocked by DCI and that DCI was not selective according to its ability to block beta receptors in the same species.

Figure 2 demonstrates the ability of DCI to reduce the positive chronotropic, vasodepressor, and intestinal inhibitory responses to isoproterenol in the anesthetized dog. The specificity of this blocking action is indicated by the fact that these same responses to epinephrine were essentially unaffected [12]. Since propranolol is the only beta receptor antagonist presently used, at least in this country, it is appropriate to consider propranolol as

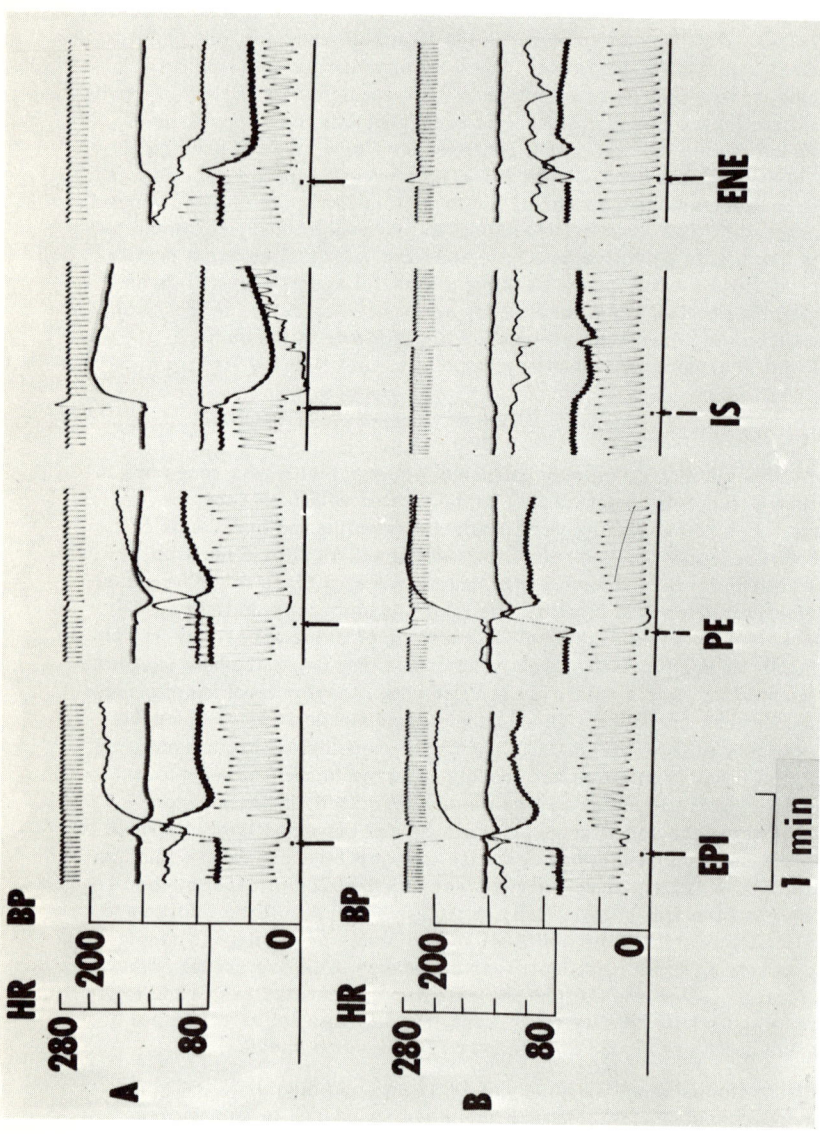

Fig. 2. Blockade of beta adrenergic receptors by dichloroisoproterenol (DCI) in a dog anesthetized with morphine-pentobarbital and given atropine. From above, downward, in each panel: respiration; heart rate (calibration in beats/min); retractor penis; mean arterial pressure (calibration in mm Hg); intestine. (A) Control responses to intravenous doses of epinephrine (EPI), phenylephrine (PE), isoproterenol (IS), and ethylnorepinephrine (ENE). (B) Responses to amines after DCI, 2 mg/kg, intravenously. Reprinted from Ref. [40], p. 203, by courtesy of Williams and Wilkings

IV. SELECTIVE BETA RECEPTOR DRUG INTERACTIONS

the prototype of those beta receptor antagonists that are not selective in their beta receptor blocking actions. This lack of beta receptor blocking selectivity for propranolol has been well demonstrated in the anesthetized dog [20,21].

Methoxamine, like phenylephrine, is an example of an adrenergic agonist that is a relatively pure alpha receptor agonist. This does not imply that methoxamine cannot stimulate beta receptors. All adrenergic agonists will stimulate both alpha and beta receptors and these effects can be shown under the proper experimental conditions. Certainly, one would agree that all of the clinically useful actions of methoxamine reflect its ability to stimulate only alpha receptors. Figure 3 shows the effects of beta receptor blockade (DCI 2 mg/kg, panel B) and alpha receptor blockade (Dibozane 2 mg/kg, panel C) on the intestinal inhibitory and pressor responses to methoxamine. Since both of these responses were due to alpha receptor activation, they were unaffected by beta receptor blockade but were reduced by alpha receptor blockade.

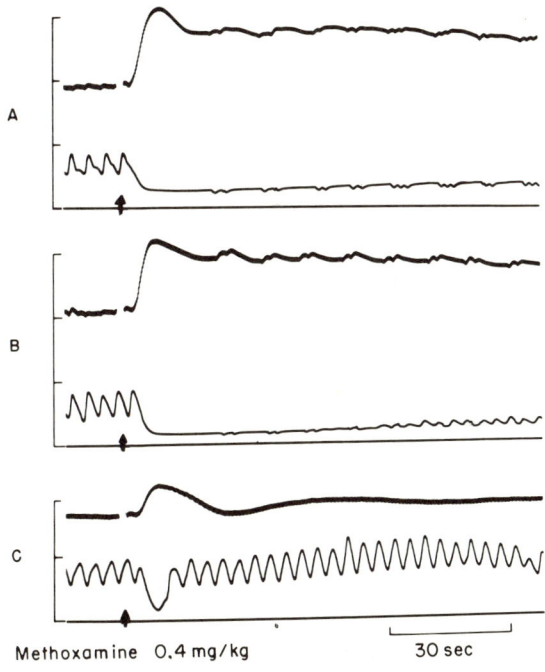

Fig. 3. Methoxamine response as modified by DCI and dibozane in the atropine treated, anesthetized dog. A — control; B — after DCI, 2 mg/kg; C — after Dibozane, 1 mg/kg. In each section from above: mean arterial pressure (scale graduated at 30 mm Hg intervals); intestinal activity: "zero" baseline for arterial pressure. Reprinted from Ref. [5], p. 155, by courtesy of Williams and Wilkins Co., Baltimore, Md.

In a series of publications [22-24] methoxamine and its N-isopropyl analog, isopropylmethoxamine (IMA), were reported to be capable of blocking, in both anesthetized and unanesthetized dogs, the rise in plasma free fatty acids and glucose produced by injected epinephrine. The adrenergic receptor mediating these responses in the dog has been classified as a beta receptor based upon the ability of DCI to completely block these responses [25].

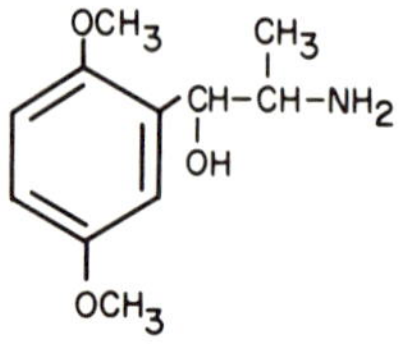

Methoxamine

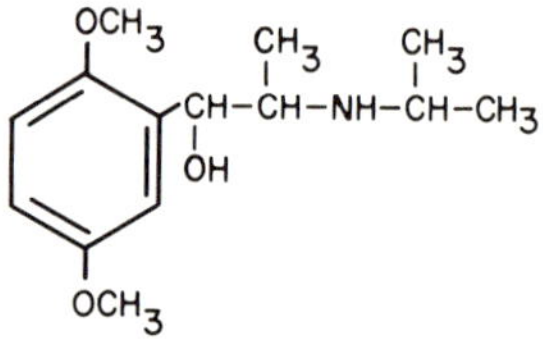

N-Isopropylmethoxamine

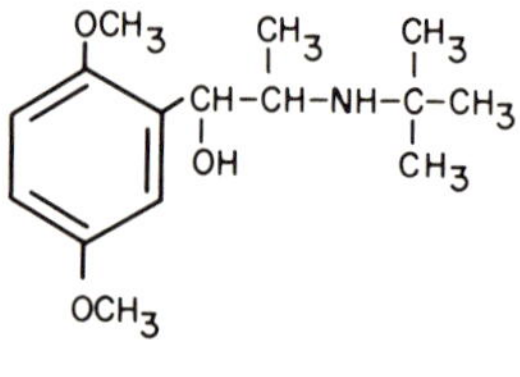

Butoxamine

Fig. 4. Methoxamine, N-isopropylmethoxamine (IMA), butoxamine.

IV. SELECTIVE BETA RECEPTOR DRUG INTERACTIONS 241

Similar studies in man have shown that the rise in free fatty acids in response to epinephrine could be abolished by pronethalol but not by phenoxybenzamine [26]. Epinephrine-induced hyperglycemia in man was abolished by neither pronethalol nor phenoxybenzamine. Despite the obvious differences due to species variation, it would appear that in man at least only the epinephrine-induced mobilization of free fatty acid was mediated by the beta adrenergic receptor. The conclusions that we drew from these results suggested the possibility that in addition to its alpha receptor activating properties methoxamine might possibly also block beta receptors. Any attempt to determine the adrenergic blocking properties of methoxamine on the cardiovascular system in the dog is complicated by the potent vasopressor responses evoked by methoxamine. This was less evident but was still a problem with the isopropyl analog of methoxamine, isopropylmethoxamine (IMA), since this agent slowly released methoxamine in vivo. However, in the rat uterus, a tissue which possesses a predominance of beta receptors [27], both methoxamine and IMA were able to produce a blockade of rat uterine beta receptors as is shown in Fig. 5. This blocking action resembled that produced by typical beta receptor antagonists such as propranolol. In the dog, neither agent blocked the positive chronotropic, intestinal inhibitory, or the femoral vascular flow responses to isoproterenol. Another methoxamine analog, N-tert-butylmethoxamine (butoxamine), exhibited the same metabolic blocking properties as those of IMA and methoxamine [28, 29], but was not metabolized to methoxamine in vivo.

Butoxamine, in the anesthetized dog, blocked the vasodilator response to isoproterenol without significant inhibition of the positive inotropic, positive chronotropic, or intestinal inhibitory responses to isoproterenol [30]. Figure 6 demonstrates the ability of butoxamine (TMA) to selectively block the vasodilator but not the positive chronotropic responses to isoproterenol. Like IMA, butoxamine produced a blockade of beta receptors in the rat uterus resembling the blockade produced by propranolol or DCI. As a result of these studies, particularly with butoxamine, but first proposed for IMA [31], two possible explanations were presented. First, IMA and methoxamine as well as butoxamine might be considered to be more specific beta adrenergic receptor blocking agents than DCI or pronethalol in that they selectively block beta receptors only in certain tissues in the same species. Second, the beta receptor of the rat uterus as well as that in vascular smooth muscle are different types of beta receptors from those in the heart. In retrospect, it is probable that both explanations are true. The same type of selective blockade of vascular rather than cardiac beta receptors occurred with other agents closely related chemically to butoxamine, including α-[1-(isopropylamino)ethyl]-2,4-dimethylbenzyl alcohol (DIMA) [32] and α-[1-(isopropylamino)ethyl]-p-methylbenzyl alcohol(H35/25)[33]. Their chemical structures are shown in Fig. 7. The alpha methyl analog of DCI has been reported to exert a selective blocking effect on vascular beta receptors qualitatively similar to the agents cited above [34]. Butoxamine and H 35/25 have been compared to the general beta receptor antagonists MJ 1999 and propranolol, respectively, in the anesthetized dog [35, 33].

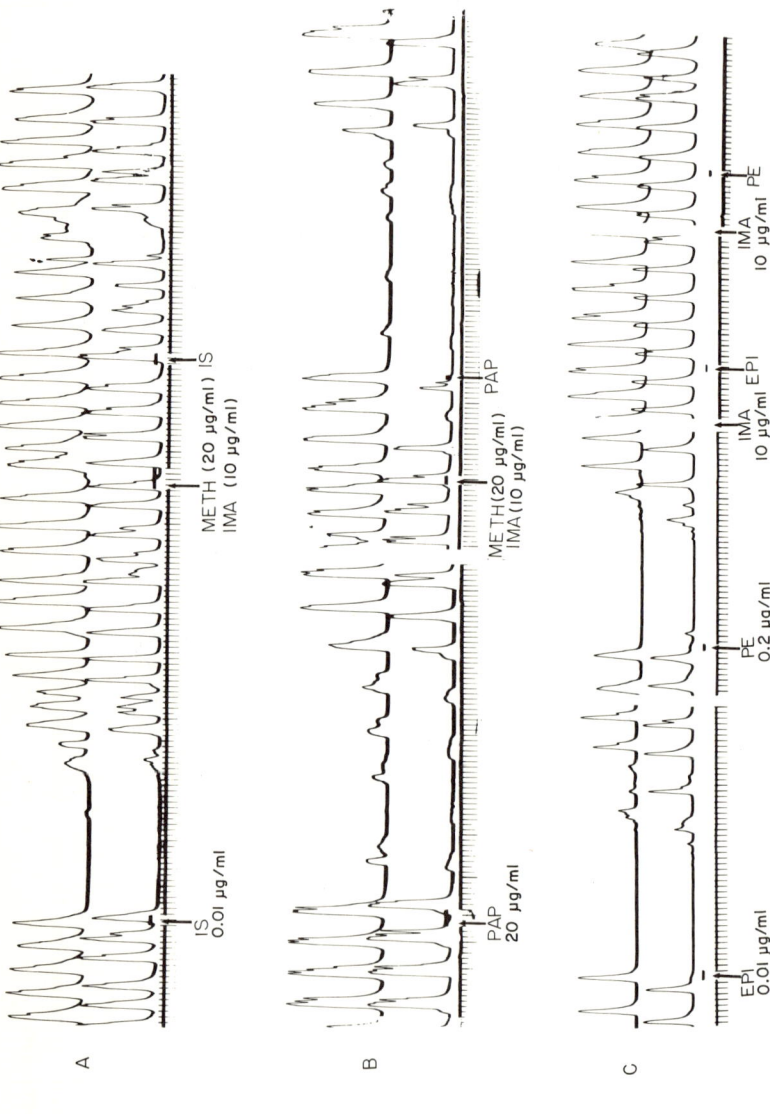

Fig. 5. Effects of N-isopropylmethoxamine (IMA) and methoxamine on isometric contractions of the isolated rat uterus. (A) Responses to isoproterenol (IS) before and after methoxamine (upper trace 20 μg/ml) and IMA (lower trace, 10 μg/ml). (B) Responses to papaverine (PAP, 20 μg/ml) before and after methoxamine and IMA. (C) Responses to EPI (0.01 μg/ml) and PE (0.2 μg/ml) before and after IMA. Time marks, 10 sec.

IV. SELECTIVE BETA RECEPTOR DRUG INTERACTIONS 243

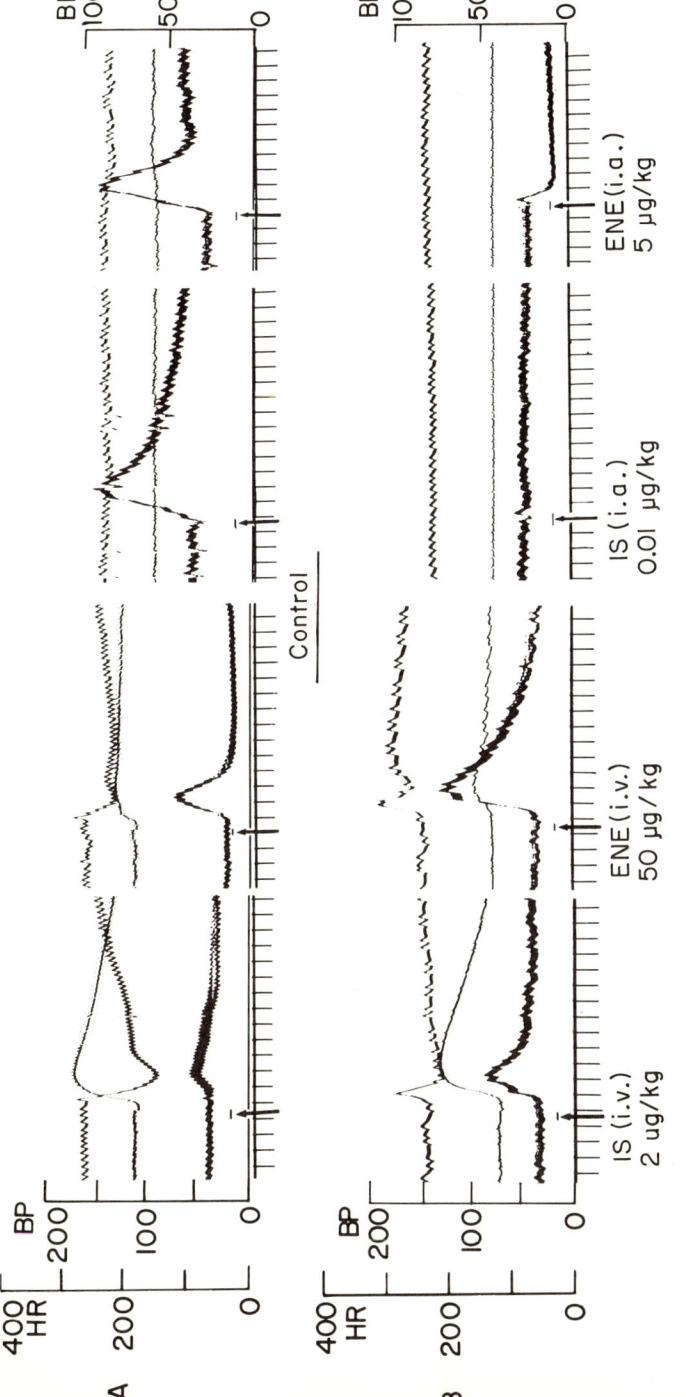

Fig. 6. Effect of N-tert-butyl methoxamine (TMA) on responses to isoproterenol (IS) and ethylnorepinephrine (ENE) in a dog anesthetized with pentobarbital. From top down in each panel: mean arterial pressure (BP, calibration in mm Hg); heart rate (HR, calibration in beats/min); and blood flow (BF, calibration in ml/min). (A) Control responses to IS (2 μg/kg, i.v.; 0.01 μg/kg, i.a.) and ENE (50 μg/kg, i.v.; 5 μg/kg, i.a.) (B) Responses to control agents after TMA (5 mg/kg, i.v.). Time marks, 10 sec. Reprinted from Reference [30], p. 420, by courtesy of Williams and Wilkins Co., Baltimore, Md.

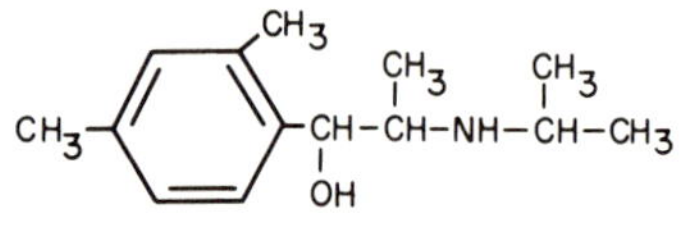

α-[1-(Isopropylamino)ethyl]-2,4-dimethylbenzyl alcohol (DIMA)

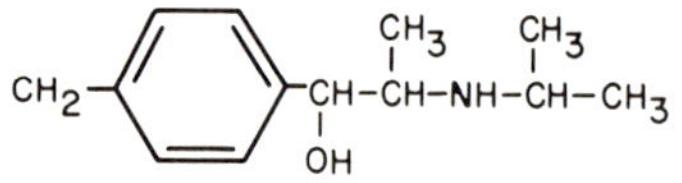

α-[1-(Isopropylamino)ethyl]-p-methylbenzyl alcohol (H 35/25)

Fig. 7. α-[1-(Isopropylamino)ethyl]-2,4-dimethylbenzyl alcohol (DIMA), α-[1-(Isopropylamino)ethyl]-p-methylbenzyl alcohol (H35/25).

Figures 8, 9, and 10 demonstrate the selective beta receptor blocking action of butoxamine which unlike MJ 1999 did not produce a significant blockade of cardiac beta receptors while producing a marked blockade of vascular beta receptors. In a recent study [36] the threo and erythro forms of α-[1-(isopropylamino)ethyl]-p-nitrobenzyl alcohol (α-methyl-INPEA) produced a similar selective blockade of vascular but not cardiac beta receptors. The parent compound INPEA is a general beta receptor antagonist qualitatively similar to propranolol but much weaker. All of the blocking agents that appear to be selective for vascular beta receptors have the methyl group substitution in the alpha carbon position of the ethanolamine side chain.

Dunlop and Shanks [37] found 4'-[2-hydroxy-3-(isopropylamino)propoxy]-acetanilide (ICI 50172, practolol) to be a beta receptor antagonist that selectively blocked cardiac but not vascular beta receptors. Wale et al. [38] have obtained similar results with practolol and have compared its beta receptor blocking action to propranolol and other similar blocking agents. A comparative study in the anesthetized dog of the beta receptor blocking properties of practolol, α-[(isopropylamino)methyl]-p-methylbenzyl alcohol

IV. SELECTIVE BETA RECEPTOR DRUG INTERACTIONS 245

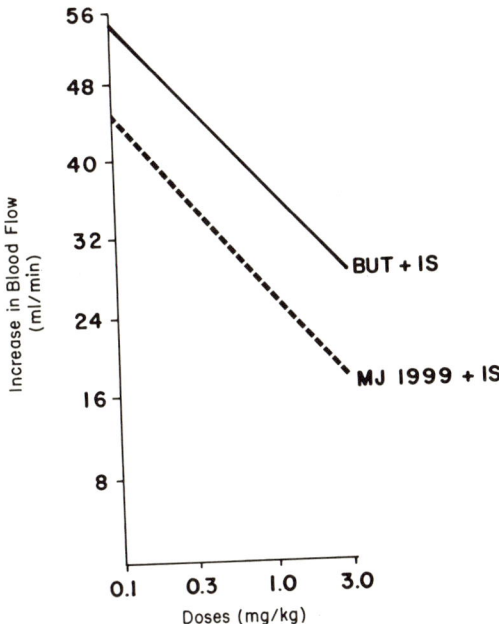

Fig. 8. Comparison of the adrenergic blocking actions of MJ 1999 and butoxamine (BUT) on the femoral flow response to isoproterenol (IS) in anesthetized dogs.

(─────) Calculated regression line of femoral flow responses to isoproterenol on the log doses of butoxamine in seven dogs; (---------) calculated regression line of femoral flow responses to isoproterenol on the log doses of MJ 1999 in seven dogs. Femoral flow response is indicated as the increase in femoral flow (ml/min) after the injection of 0.01 μg/kg of isoproterenol (injected i.a.), above preinjection levels. Reprinted from Ref. [44], p. 221, by courtesy of St. Catherine Press, Tempelhof 37, Brugge, Belgium.

(H29/50) and H35/25 (see Fig. 11 for chemical structures) on the positive chronotropic, vasodepressor, and intestinal inhibitory responses to isoproterenol yielded some interesting but predictable results [39].

H29/50 was included in this study because it differed from H35/25 in that it did not possess an alpha methyl group on the ethanolamine side chain. We predicted that H29/50 would behave like a weaker version of propranolol. Indeed H29/50 blocked all three parameters in the same dose range as is shown in Fig. 12. Figure 13 demonstrates the ability of H35/25 to block the vasodepressor but not the cardiac responses to isoproterenol and Fig. 14

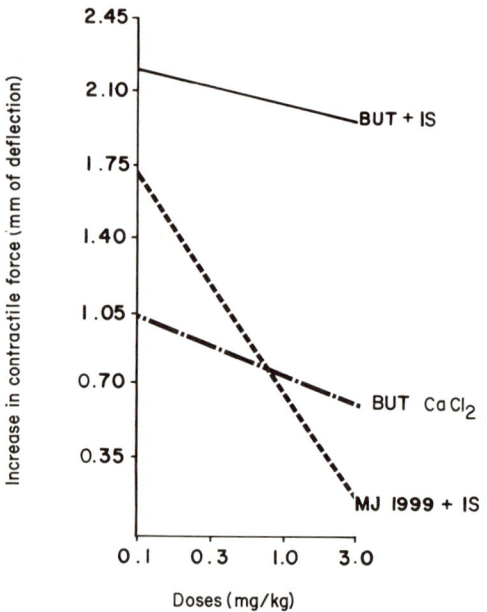

Fig. 9. Comparison of the adrenergic blocking actions of MJ 1999 and butoxamine (BUT) on the positive inotropic response to isoproterenol (IS) in anesthetized dogs.

(―――――) Calculated regression line of the positive inotropic responses to isoproterenol (IS) on the log dose of butoxamine (BUT) in six dogs; (‐‐‐‐‐‐‐‐‐) calculated regression line of the positive inotropic responses to isoproterenol (IS) on the log doses of MJ 1999 in 5 dogs; (_._._._.) calculated regression line of the positive inotropic responses to $CaCl_2$ on the log doses of butoxamine (BUT) in six dogs. Positive inotropic response is indicated as increase in contractile force (mm of deflection) after the injection of 1 μg/kg of isoproterenol (i.v.) or $CaCl_2$, 20 mg/kg (i.v.), above preinjection levels. Reprinted from Ref. [44], p. 222, by courtesy of St. Catherine Press, Tempelhof 37, Brugge, Belgium.

demonstrates the reverse effect for practolol. The intestinal inhibitory response to isoproterenol was only blocked by those agents that were able to block cardiac beta receptors, specifically practolol and H29/50.

On the basis of the results cited above we have proposed that there are at least three types of beta receptor blocking agents. One type is capable of blocking vascular but not myocardial beta receptors and includes butoxamine, H35/25, and all of the other alpha methyl analogs of methoxamine. The second type is capable of blocking myocardial but not vascular beta receptors and includes practolol (ICI 50172). The third type is capable of blocking beta receptors in all tissues and includes in addition to H29/50, all of the classical

IV. SELECTIVE BETA RECEPTOR DRUG INTERACTIONS   247

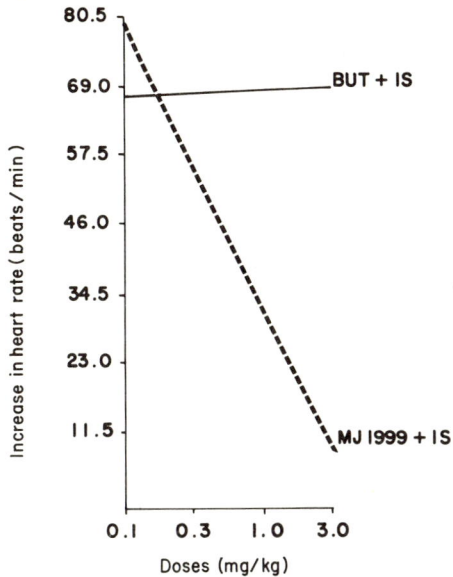

Fig. 10. Comparison of the adrenergic blocking activity of MJ 1999 and butoxamine (BUT) on the positive chronotropic response to isoproterenol (IS) in anesthetized dogs.

(——————) Calculated regression line of the positive chronotropic responses to isoproterenol (IS) on the log doses of butoxamine (BUT) in 10 dogs; (----------) calculated regression line of the positive chronotropic responses to isoproterenol (IS) on the log doses of MJ 1999 in 10 dogs. Positive chronotropic response is indicated as the increase in heart rate (beats/min) after the injection of 1 µg/kg of isoproterenol (i.v.), above preinjection levels. Reprinted from Reference [44], p. 223, by courtesy of St. Catherine Press, Tempelhof 37, Brugge, Belgium.

beta receptor blocking agents such as DCI, pronethalol, MJ 1999, and propranolol. These results also support the possibility of several different subtypes of beta receptors. It would certainly appear that cardiac and vascular beta receptors are different subtypes of beta adrenergic receptors.

Isolated organ studies are of great value in that they may yield quantitative data that may further demonstrate and extend the phenomenon of selective beta receptor antagonism. A comparison of the beta receptor blocking properties of propranolol and butoxamine on the rat uterus and duodenum demonstrated the ability of propranolol to block the beta adrenergic receptors in both tissues simultaneously (Fig. 15). Butoxamine was capable of blocking the beta adrenergic receptors in the uterus but not in the duodenum [40].

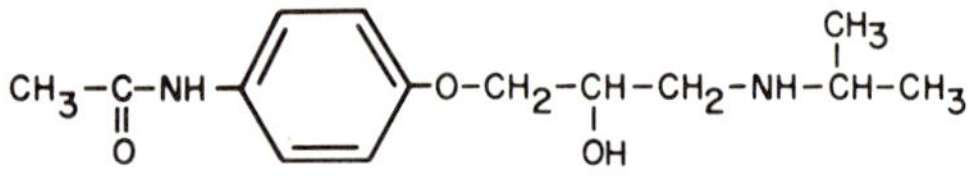

Practolol (ICI 50172)

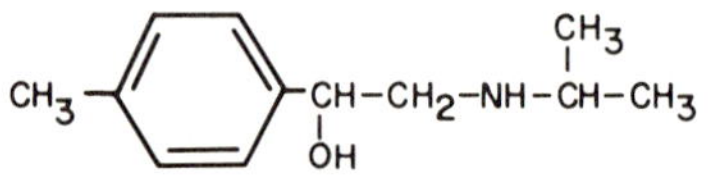

α- [(Isopropylamino) methyl] -p-methylbenzyl alcohol (H 29/50)

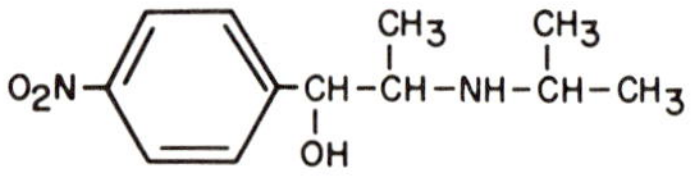

α- [1- (Isopropylamino) ethyl] -p-nitrobenzyl alcohol (α-methyl-INPEA)

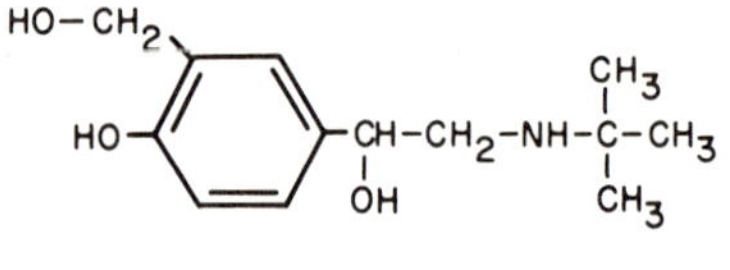

Salbutamol

Fig. 11. Practolol (ICI 50172), α-[(Isopropylamino) methyl)]-p-methylbenzyl alcohol (H 29/50), α-[1-(Isopropylamino) ethyl]-p-nitrobenzyl alcohol (α-methyl-INPEA), Salbutamol.

These preliminary results obtained with rat uterus and duodenum have been extended in a more quantitative manner. Butoxamine, practolol, and propranolol have been compared according to their ability to shift the concentration response curves for isoproterenol in isolated rat uterus,

IV. SELECTIVE BETA RECEPTOR DRUG INTERACTIONS

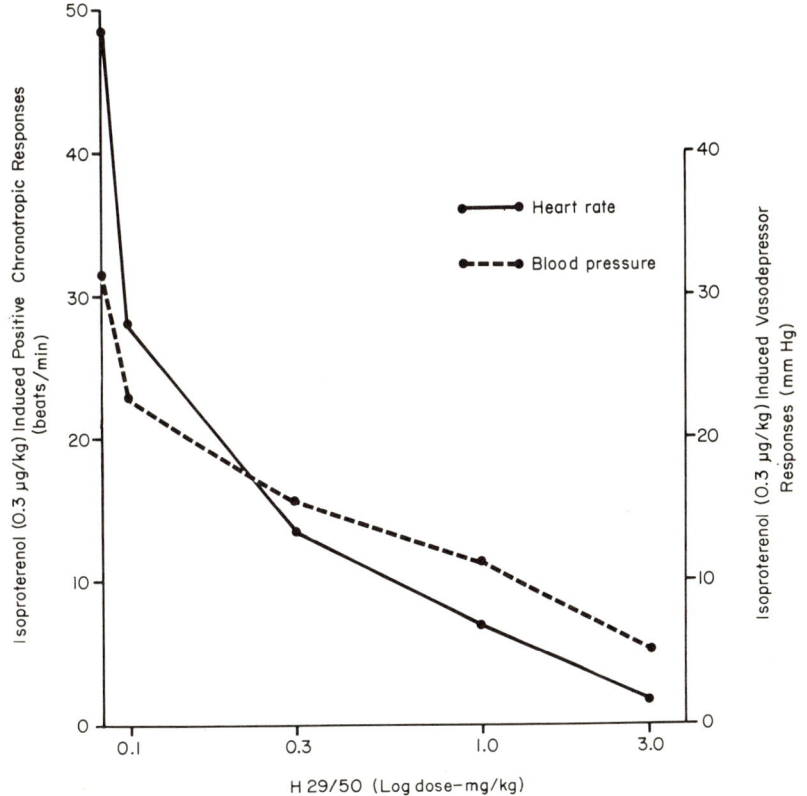

Fig. 12. Effects of H 29/50 on the positive chronotropic (beats per min) and vasodepressor (mm Hg) responses to isoproterenol (IS, 0.3 μg/kg, i.v.) in the anesthetized dog. All points are mean responses obtained from five dogs. H 29/50 was given in increasing doses (mg/kg on log scale, abscissa) at approximately 20-30 min intervals. Doses of H 29/50 represent individual rather than cumulative doses. Reprinted from Reference [27], p. 229, by courtesy of North-Holland Publishing Co., Amsterdam, Holland.

fundus, and atria [41]. Determinations of the pA_2 values for each antagonist in each tissue plus the slopes of the regression lines obtained by plotting the negative log of the concentrations of the antagonist ($-pA_x$) against the logs of the ratio of the concentrations of isoproterenol in the presence of antagonist versus its concentration in the absence of antagonist minus 1 (log x - 1) were made [42, 43]. The pA_2 value is a measure of the affinity of an antagonist and may be defined as the negative logarithm of the molar concentration of a competitive antagonist which reduces the response to a double dose of an agonist to that of a single dose. Measuring pA_2 values is a rational method

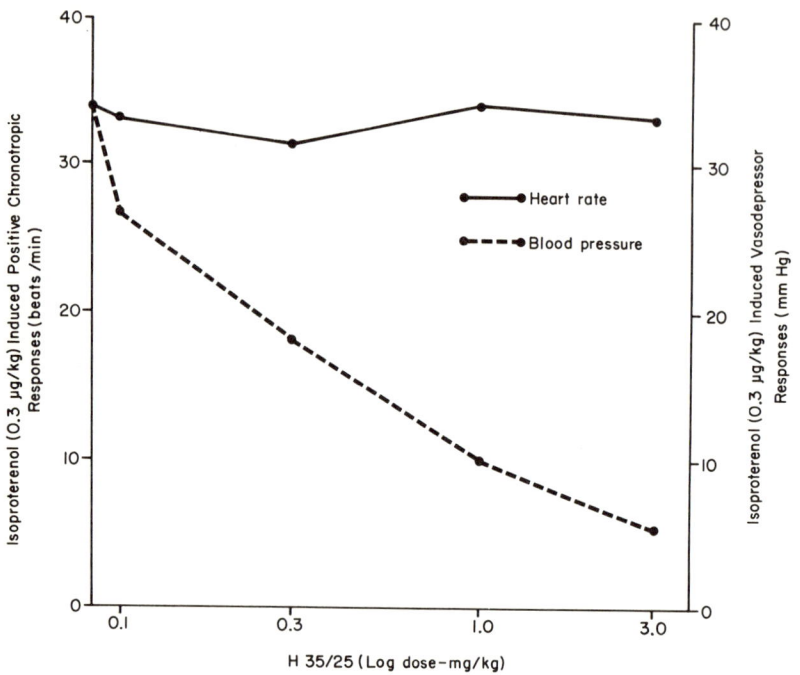

Fig. 13. Effects of H 35/25 on the positive chronotropic (beats/min) and vasodepressor responses (mm Hg) to isoproterenol (IS, 0.3 µg/kg, i.v.) in the anesthetized dog. All points are mean responses from five dogs. H 35/25 was given in increasing doses (mg/kg on log scale, abscissa) rather than cumulative doses. Reprinted from Ref. [27], p. 231, by courtesy of North-Holland Publishing Co., Amsterdam, Holland.

for classifying drugs as well as receptors. If an antagonist is acting upon the same receptor in a variety of tissues, the pA_2 values should be equivalent. This determination is also independent of the potency of the agonist used as long as the given agonists activate the same receptor in the same qualitative manner. In the case of a simple competitive antagonism, a plot of $\log(x - 1)$ versus $\log(-pA_x)$ will yield a straight line with a slope of 1. The results of this study are summarized in Table III. A comparison of pA_2 values for each antagonist allows one to draw certain basic conclusions. Practolol is relatively selective for blocking beta receptors in atria and fundus but not in the uterus. Butoxamine is relatively selective for blocking beta receptors in the uterus but not in the atria or fundus. Propranolol is relatively nonselective in that it blocks beta receptors well in all three tissues. However, propranolol has a relatively lower pA_2 value in the rat fundus (8.11) than it has in the rat atria and uterus, with values of 9.59 and 9.93, respectively. This additional observation lends further support to the

IV. SELECTIVE BETA RECEPTOR DRUG INTERACTIONS

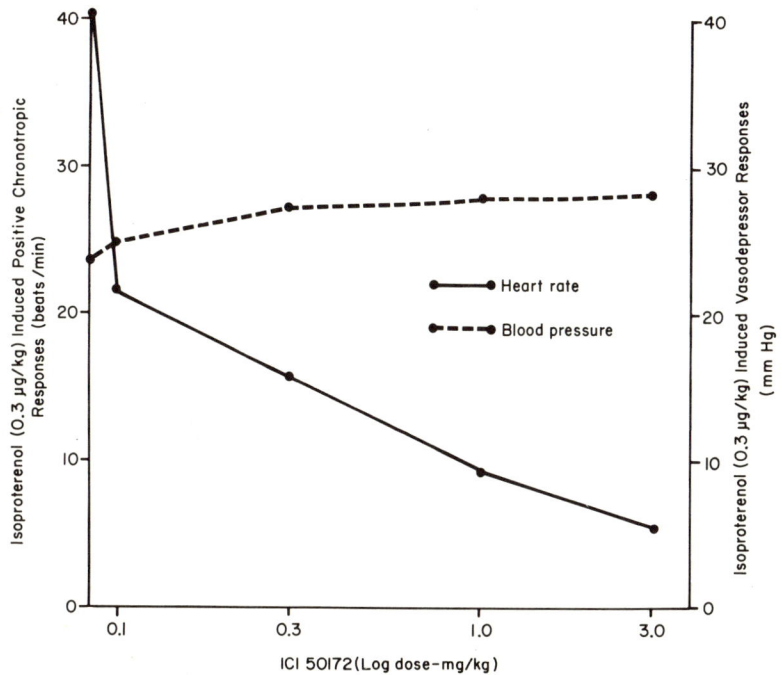

Fig. 14. Effects of ICI 50172 (practolol) on the positive chronotropic (beats/min) and vasodepressor (mm Hg) responses to isoproterenol (IS, 0.3 μg/kg, i.v.) in the anesthetized dog. All points are mean responses obtained from five dogs. ICI 50172 was given in increasing doses (mg/kg on log scale, abscissa) at approximately 20-30 min intervals. Doses of ICI 50172 represent individual rather than cumulative doses. Reprinted from Ref. [27], p. 232, by courtesy of North-Holland Publishing Co., Amsterdam, Holland.

TABLE III

pA_2 and Slope Values for Beta Receptor Antagonists in Isolated Rat Organs

Isolated organ	Drug		
	Propranolol	Practolol	Butoxamine
Rat uterus	pA_2 = 9.93 slope = 0.91	No significant blockade	pA_2 = 6.82 slope = 0.71
Rat fundus	pA_2 = 8.11 slope = 0.65	pA_2 = 6.85 slope = 0.50	No significant blockade
Rat atria	pA_2 = 9.59 slope = 0.81	pA_2 = 7.33 slope = 0.78	No significant blockade

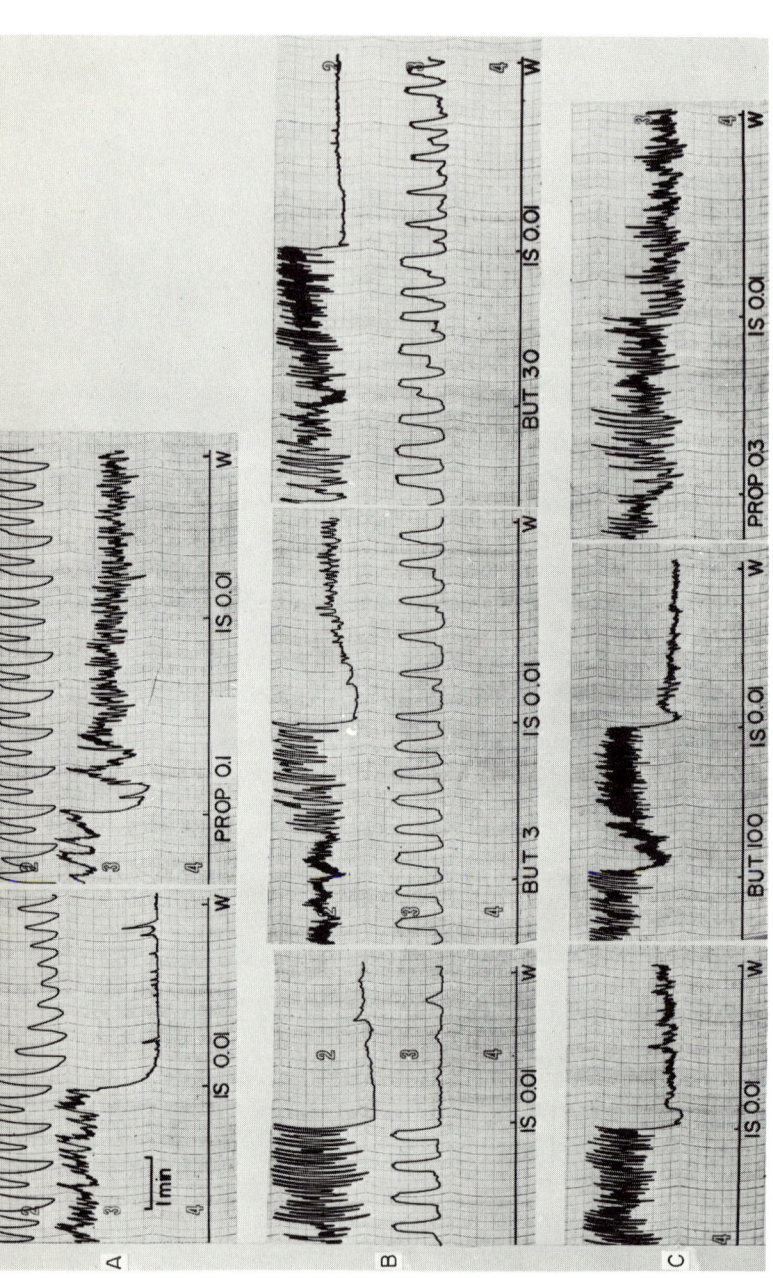

Fig. 15. Effects of propranolol (PROP) and butoxamine (BUT) on the responses to isoprenaline (IS) of the isolated rat uterus and the isolated rat duodenum (isometric contractions). (A) Responses to IS (0.01 μg/ml) before and after PROP (0.1 μg/ml). Upper trace represents uterine motility, lower trace represents duodenal motility. (B) Responses to IS (0.01 μg/ml) before and after BUT (3 and 30 μg/ml). Upper trace represents duodenal motility, lower trace represents uterine motility. (C) Responses to IS (0.01 μg/ml) before and after BUT (100 μg/ml) and PROP (0.3 μg/ml) on rat duodenum. Reprinted from Ref. [23], p. 423, by courtesy of St. Catherine Press, Tempelhof 37, Brugge,

IV. SELECTIVE BETA RECEPTOR DRUG INTERACTIONS

concept that in addition to differences in antagonists we may also have fundamental differences between the beta receptors in the rat fundus versus those in the uterus and atria. We are unable to explain the fact that the majority of slope values were less than 1. The marked differences in slope cannot be explained by diffusion barriers since the pA_2 values for the antagonists studied were essentially the same following 1 and 2 h exposure periods. It is possible that some of these agents are binding to sites other than the beta receptor. Wenke et al. [44] and Goldstein et al. [45] have proposed that agonists and antagonists may react with receptors in a trimolecular (one molecule of drug with two receptor sites) as well as the usual bimolecular (one molecule of drug with one receptor) manner. However, since there were large differences in slopes, other ratios of drug combinations (e.g., 5 molecules + 4 receptors and 5 molecules + 2 receptors) might also be considered. Bristow et al. [46] have recently completed a similar study using isolated rabbit atria, aorta, stomach, and trachea. They attempted to detect differences in beta receptor antagonists by determining apparent dissociation constant (K_B) values for practolol, H35/25, and propranolol. The K_B values for H35/25 were similar in aorta and atrium. Propranolol, a "nonselective" beta receptor antagonist, was considerably less potent in the stomach than in the aorta or atria. Practolol was approximately 660 times more potent in atria than in aorta but only 15 times more potent in the atria than in trachea. One interesting observation that they made was the fact that quinterenol [47], an agent reported to selectively stimulate beta receptors in smooth muscle, was found to be a beta receptor antagonist in atrium with little effect on beta receptors in aorta, stomach, or trachea. This demonstrates a very serious problem and that is the possibility of ascribing selective beta receptor stimulating properties to a compound which in reality may simply be a partial agonist. The beta receptor blocking properties of such compounds are difficult to demonstrate in isolated organ studies because of their predominant stimulating properties. A comparison of pA_2 and slope values in isolated guinea pig tracheal spiral strips has yielded additional confusing results [48]. These results are shown in Table IV. Propranolol, pronethalol, and MJ 1999 appear to differ only in potency from each other since their slopes were essentially equivalent. Practolol and butoxamine had equivalent pA_2 values, indicating beta receptor blockade. However, their slope values of 0.48 and 0.40 were considerably lower than those of the propranolol group (0.70 to 0.82). Does this indicate that the difference is in the receptor or the antagonist? We will next consider the possibility that in addition to selective beta receptor antagonists, selective beta receptor agonists might also exist.

III. SELECTIVE BETA RECEPTOR ACTIVATION

The concept that drugs may stimulate certain beta receptors more than others has been suggested in the literature. The experimental evidence supporting this concept to date consists of demonstrating differences in the order of relative potencies of adrenergic agonists for activity on various tissues. Furchgott [49] has probably presented the most convincing

TABLE IV

Slopes and pA_2 Values for β-Receptor Antagonists in the Guinea Pig Trachea[a]

	Propranolol	MJ 1999	Pronethalol	Practolol	Butoxamine
pA_2	9.76	6.89	8.43	7.26	6.92
Slope	0.82	0.73	0.70	0.48	0.40
	(8)	(8)	(6)	(8)	(6)

[a] Numbers in parentheses indicate the number of tissues used. pA_2 is defined as the negative logarithm of the concentration of the antagonist that doubles the concentration of the agonist required to achieve a given effect. pA_2 values and slopes were obtained from regression lines plotted from the pooled results of six to eight experiments. Reprinted from Ref. [48], by courtesy of North-Holland Publishing Co., Amsterdam, Holland.

evidence that beta receptors in different tissues and in different species may in some instances respond quantitatively differently. Relative potencies of norepinephrine, epinephrine, phenylephrine, and isoproterenol on responses mediated by both alpha and beta receptors were determined in isolated tissues from rabbits and guinea pigs under carefully controlled experimental conditions. Alpha receptors appeared to be of the same type in the rabbit thoracic aorta, stomach, and duodenum based upon both similar dissociation constants (K_B values) for phentolamine and similar orders of potency of sympathomimetic amines. Van Rossum [50] has suggested that different types of alpha receptors may exist in the rabbit intestine and rat vas deferens because of the differences in pA_2 values observed with a number of alpha adrenergic receptor antagonists. These latter results might be criticized because of the failure of the investigator to prevent uptake of catecholamines by cocaine pretreatment or to allow the antagonists to act for a sufficiently long period of time. These factors may account for wide variations in results if they are not taken into consideration.

Furchgott [49] suggested that beta receptors appeared to consist of at least three types. The beta receptors in both rabbit aorta and guinea pig trachea were different from those in rabbit and guinea pig atria and guinea pig duodenum, which were in turn different from those beta receptors in rabbit duodenum and rabbit stomach muscle. These apparent differences in beta receptors may simply reflect differences in the surrounding molecular structures, the biophase. These "silent" receptors may in some way interfere with the agonist receptor interaction even though the beta receptors may be identical molecules within the same species.

IV. SELECTIVE BETA RECEPTOR DRUG INTERACTIONS

Lands et al. [51] have proposed the subdivision of the beta receptor into beta-1 and beta-2 subtypes based upon results somewhat similar to those described by Furchgott [49]. They have proposed that the beta-1 receptor subserves lipolysis and cardiac stimulation and the beta-2 receptor subserves bronchodilation and vasodepression. In my opinion, such a classification at this time is not appropriate and is not entirely supported by all experimental data. While it is true that one can pick isolated studies out of the literature that would tend to support this hypothesis [39], other studies particularly in isolated tissues do not support this hypothesis [46]. We have been determining dose response curves for isoproterenol before and after treatment with a variety of beta receptor antagonists in the isolated guinea pig tracheal strip. One observation worthy of mention at this time is that propranolol shifts the dose-response curve of isoproterenol to the right in the typical competitive reversible manner. A 10-fold increase in the dose of propranolol results in a 10-fold (1 log unit) shift to the right of the dose-response curve and this same degree of shift occurs with pronethalol (the "classical" type of beta receptor antagonist). Butoxamine and practolol also cause a parallel shift to the right of the dose-response curve of isoproterenol so that the antagonism appears to be competitive and reversible. However, a ten-fold increase in the dose of either of these agents results in only a 2- or 3-fold (0.2 - 0.3 log units) shift of the dose response curve for isoproterenol. Do these differences indicate a difference in beta receptor types within tracheal smooth muscle or do they reflect the ability of these antagonists to react with the same receptor in a different manner? I do not deny that selective beta receptor interactions do occur; they certainly do. However, to postulate a rigid classification of beta receptor subtypes at the present time is not warranted by the experimental evidence available. The original classification by Ahlquist of two receptors served and continues to serve a very important purpose as a teaching tool. It now appears that the presentation of adrenergic pharmacology must be qualified to include apparent exceptions.

A compound that is supposed to exert a selective beta adrenergic stimulant effect has been reported in the literature and is undergoing clinical trials as a possible brochodilator. This agent is supposedly longer acting than isoproterenol and its selectivity involves a potent bronchodilating action with a relatively weak cardiac stimulating effect. This compound, salbutamol, α^1-[(tert-butylamino)methyl]-4-hydroxy-m-xylene-a,a'-diol, was only slightly less active than isoproterenol as a bronchodilator in anesthetized dogs and conscious guinea pigs, but considerably less potent as a cardiac and vasodepressor agent. Data also indicated that salbutamol was about 1/10 as potent as isoproterenol on the isolated guinea pig atria [52]; such data utilized to support these imposing activity ratios is open to some question. The slopes of the dose response curves for salbutamol were much flatter than were those of isoproterenol. This might indicate that salbutamol is acting as a partial agonist and may ultimately exert beta receptor blocking properties. Salbutamol in this respect might be compared to dichlorisoproterenol (DCI) since DCI does exert a prominent beta receptor stimulant effect prior to its beta receptor blocking properties. This latter effect is difficult to demonstrate in vitro, but it can be done. Whether salbutamol is truly a selective beta receptor stimulant or simply a drug like DCI remains to be proved. One should also consider another basic difference between salbutamol and isoproterenol and that is the fact that while isoproterenol is metabolized by catechol-0-methyl transferase, salbutamol is not. It is indeed important to determine the specific mechanisms of drug action of these selective acting agonists and there are certainly differences of opinion in this area. However, there is no question that drugs can exert end organ effects that imply selective beta receptor interactions and this point must not be overlooked.

Finally, quinterenol, 8-hydroxy-α-[(isopropylamino)methyl]-5-quinolinemethanol, exerted all of the properties of isoproterenol with the exception that it did not produce any significant positive chronotropic effect in most species tested [47]. However, Bristow et al. [46] have described quinterenol as a beta receptor antagonist in atrium with little or no effect on beta receptors in aorta, stomach, or rabbit trachea.

IV. CONCLUSIONS

Since our initial observation in 1964 that a drug, butoxamine, appeared to produce a selective blockade of beta adrenergic receptors, much has happened. The classification of beta receptor antagonists and indeed even beta receptor mechanisms was dependent on the "classical" beta receptor antagonists' ability to block beta receptors nonselectively in all tissues. On the basis of what has been done and what has been cited in this chapter, I would conclude that the ability of drugs to produce selective beta receptor blockade is indeed a reality. Whether this effect is due to a difference in beta receptors, thus implying beta receptor subtypes, or to physicochemical differences in the antagonists still remains to be determined. The case for selective beta receptor activation at this writing still remains in doubt. However, from a philosophical point of view, one would expect either both or neither to occur. I would prefer to think that both selective activation and blockade of beta adrenergic receptors is possible.

If we consider the possible clinical implications of these selective beta receptor interactions a few new drug types are presently possible. Practolol, a beta receptor antagonist with more selective actions on the heart than on bronchial smooth muscle, is a potentially useful type of agent. Unlike propranolol, practolol would not be contraindicated in patients with bronchial asthma. This would probably be the only advantage of practolol over propranolol. Practolol is probably less of a cardiac depressant than.is propranolol, but it is less potent as well. Butoxamine, as a prototype of agents with metabolic blocking properties similar to propranolol but relatively devoid of cardiac beta receptor blocking activity, might be of clinical value in hyperlipidemia, hyperthyroidism, thiazide hyperglycemia, and possibly diabetes mellitus. It might also be an effective antiarrhythmic drug. At this point it might be appropriate to suggest the use of some of the dextro isomers of propranolol and other beta receptor antagonists also as possible antiarrhythmic drugs, since all of the antiarrhythmic actions of propranolol are not due to beta receptor blockade.

There are presently two agents tentatively but shakily classified as selective beta receptor agonists and they are quinterenol [47] and salbutamol [52]. Quinterenol has recently been described as a beta receptor antagonist [46] and salbutamol shows some indication of also being a partial agonist. In any case, any agent with selective bronchial beta receptor stimulant properties would be a clinically useful bronchodilator.

These speculations, relating to new clinical agents, are based upon experiments that have been described in the recent literature. While they are indeed only speculation, this author would hope to see a greater research effort expended towards the development of selectively acting beta receptor drugs.

ACKNOWLEDGMENTS

The author is grateful to Byron Wilkenfeld and Martin Wasserman, two graduate students, who contributed greatly to much of the work cited from this department. I and the two individuals cited above are collectively grateful to Miss Margaret Elizabeth Gregory who in her capacity as research technician was responsible for much of the experimental data, particularly in the isolated organ studies. I am also grateful to the National Heart Institute (N.I.H.) for supporting much of this work (HE 12989-01, the most recent grant number). Finally, I must recognize the role of Dr. R. P. Ahlquist who really started this whole area of research.

REFERENCES

1. J. N. Langley, Proc. Roy. Soc., Ser. B, 78, 170 (1906).
2. J. N. Langley, J. Physiol., 33, 374 (1915).
3. H. H. Dale, J. Physiol., 34, 163 (1906).
4. R. P. Ahlquist, Am. J. Physiol., 153, 586 (1948).
5. B. Levy, J. Pharmacol., 127, 150 (1959).
6. R. P. Ahlquist and B. Levy, J. Pharmacol. Exptl. Therap., 127, 146 (1959).
7. B. Levy and R. P. Ahlquist, Ann. N.Y. Acad. Sci., 139, 781 (1967).
8. C. E. Powell and I. H. Slater, J. Pharmacol. Exptl. Therap., 122, 480 (1958).
9. H. C. Stanton, T. Kirchgessner, and K. Parmenter, J. Pharmacol. Exptl. Therap., 149, 174 (1965).

10. J. W. Black and J. S. Stephenson, Lancet, ii, 311 (1962).
11. J. W. Black, A. F. Crowther, R. G. Shanks, and A. C. Dornhorst, Lancet, ii, 1080 (1964).
12. B. Levy and R. P. Ahlquist, J. Pharmacol. Exptl. Therap., 133, 202 (1961).
13. E. Braunwald, Am. J. Cardiol., 18, 303 (1966).
14. N. C. Moran, Ann. N. Y. Acad. Sci., 139, 545 (1967).
15. C. T. Dollery, J. W. Paterson, and M. E. Conolly, Clin. Pharmacol. Therap., 10, 765 (1969).
16. S. E. Epstein and E. Braunwald, New Engl. J. Med., 275, 1106 (1966).
17. S. E. Epstein and E. Braunwald, New Engl. J. Med., 275, 1175 (1966).
18. J. D. Fitzgerald, J. Clin. Pharmacol., 10, 292 (1969).
19. N. C. Moran and M. E. Perkins, J. Pharmacol. Exptl. Therap., 124, 223 (1958).
20. R. G. Shanks, Am. J. Cardiol., 18, 308 (1960).
21. R. G. Shanks, Brit. J. Pharmacol., 26, 322 (1966).
22. J. J. Burns and K. I. Colville, Pharmacologist, 4, 178 (1962).
23. K. I. Colville, L. A. Lindsay, R. A. Salvador, and J. J. Burns, Federation Proc., 23, 542 (1964).
24. R. A. Salvador, K. I. Colville, L. A. Lindsay, and J. J. Burns, Federation Proc., 22, 508 (1963).
25. S. Mayer, N. C. Moran, and J. Fain, J. Pharmacol. Exptl. Therap., 134, 18 (1961).
26. T. R. E. Pilkington, R. D. Lowe, B. F. Robinson, and E. Titterington, Lancet, ii, 316 (1962).
27. B. Levy and S. Tozzi, J. Pharmacol. Exptl. Therap., 142, 178 (1963).
28. J. J. Burns and L. Lemberger, Federation Proc., 24, 299 (1965).
29. R. A. Salvador and S. A. April, Federation Proc., 24, 298 (1965).
30. B. Levy, J. Pharmacol. Exptl. Therap., 151, 413 (1966).
31. B. Levy, J. Pharmacol. Exptl. Therap., 146, 129 (1964).
32. B. Levy, Brit. J. Pharmacol., 27, 277 (1966).
33. B. Levy, J. Pharmacol. Exptl. Therap., 156, 452 (1967).
34. D. R. Van Deripe and N. C. Moran, Federation Proc., 24, 712 (1965).

35. B. E. Wilkenfeld and B. Levy, Arch. Intern. Pharmacodyn. Therap., 176, 218 (1968).
36. P. Somani, Brit. J. Pharmacol., 37, 609 (1969).
37. D. Dunlop and R. G. Shanks, Brit. J. Pharmacol., 32, 201 (1968).
38. J. Wale, L. Pur, and M. J. Rand, Europ. J. Pharmacol., 8, 25 (1969).
39. B. Levy and B. E. Wilkenfeld, Europ. J. Pharmacol., 5, 227 (1969).
40. B. Levy, Arch. Intern. Pharmacodyn. Therap., 170, 418 (1967).
41. M. Wasserman and B. Levy, Federation Proc., 29, 478 (1970).
42. H. O. Schild, Brit. J. Pharmacol., 2, 189 (1947).
43. O. Arunlakshana and H. O. Schild, Brit. J. Pharmacol., 14, 48 (1950).
44. M. Wenke, J. Lincová, J. Capelik, and S. Hynie, Ann. N.Y. Acad. Sci., 139, 860 (1967).
45. A. Goldstein, L. Aranow, and S. M. Kalman, Principles of Drug Action, Hoeber, New York, 1968, pp. 77-88.
46. M. Bristow, T. R. Sherrod, and R. D. Green, J. Pharmacol. Exptl. Therap., 171, 52 (1970).
47. A. Scriabine, P. F. Moore, I. C. Iorio, I. M. Goldman, W. K. McShane, and K. O. Booner, J. Pharmacol. Exptl. Therap., 162, 60 (1968).
48. B. Levy and B. E. Wilkenfeld, Europ. J. Pharmacol., in press.
49. R. F. Furchgott, Ann. N. Y. Acad. Sci., 139, 553 (1967).
50. J. M. Van Rossum, J. Pharm. Pharmacol., 17, 202 (1965).
51. A. M. Lands, A. Arnold, J. P. McAuliff, F. P. Luduena, and T. G. Brown, Jr., Nature, 214, 597 (1967).
52. V. A. Cullum, J. B. Farmer, D. Jack, and G. P. Levy, Brit. J. Pharmacol., 35, 141 (1969).

Chapter V

DRUGS AFFECTING ATHEROSCLEROSIS *

David Kritchevsky[†]

The Wistar Institute of Anatomy and Biology
Philadelphia, Pennsylvania

I.	INTRODUCTION		261
II.	SERUM CHOLESTEROL LOWERING AGENTS		265
	A.	Inhibitors of Cholesterol Absorption	266
	B.	Hormones	269
	C.	Aryloxy-Substituted Aliphatic Acids	270
	D.	Heparin	271
	E.	Nicotinic Acid	272
	F.	Other Compounds	273
III.	CURRENT STATUS		274
	A.	Methodology	275
	B.	Research Strategy	277
IV.	SUMMARY		279
	REFERENCES		279

I. INTRODUCTION

Vascular disease in one form or another is the principal cause of death in the western world. Among the various vascular diseases, the leading cause of death is coronary heart disease. In the United States in 1966 [1] there were more deaths from coronary heart disease (573,191) alone than there were from cancer (303,736). In fact, almost as many persons under 65 years of age (253,684) died from cardiovascular disease as did people of

---

* This work was supported, in part, by Public Health Service Research Grant HE-03299 and a research career award (K06-HE-0734) from the National Heart Institute.

[†] Author is Wistar Professor of Biochemistry, Division of Animal Biology, School of Veterinary Medicine, University of Pennsylvania

Copyright © 1972 by Marcel Dekker, Inc. **NO PART of this work may be reproduced or utilized in any form or by any means**, electronic or mechanical, including Xeroxing, photocopying, microfilm, and recording, or by any information storage and retrieval system, without permission in writing from the publisher.

all ages from cancer. These figures reflect the fact that, in the western world, the advent of drugs and greater vigilance in regard to public health have almost eradicated infectious disease as a cause of death. In 1966 in the United States there were 60,785 deaths from pneumonia compared with 113,563 from accidents and 34,597 from sequelae of diabetes [1]. The matter of importance here is not the prevention of death (a theological matter which is not within the purview of this presentation) but the prevention of unnecessarily early death from heart disease.

Heart disease is the result of the interaction of a number of factors. These include aortic structure and metabolism and the chemical composition of the blood in contact with which the aorta exists. The metabolic relationship between these two factors can be modified by several internal and external forces, such as genetic and hormonal influences, stress, and diet. The longer adverse aspects of these factors coexist, the more severe is the product of their interaction. Thus, longevity becomes an important contributor to the complex metabolic equation which is responsible for the development of heart disease.

The descriptions of coronary heart disease, or arteriosclerosis, date back over a century, as several reviews have pointed out [2, 3]. Focus on the lipid component of the arterial deposit [4] dates to Virchow's [5] hypothesis that the disease was initiated by intimal imbibition of lipids from the plasma. This is known as the "filtration" theory. Rokitansky [6] had also recognized the presence of lipids but had attributed the initial injury to deposition of fibrin.

The term "atherosclerosis" was coined by Marchand [7] in an effort to describe the hyperplastic and degenerative changes which are found simultaneously within arterial lesions. "Athero" is the Greek word for gruel and the early fat-rich lesions (atheromata) resemble porridge in color and consistency. A more inclusive definition of atherosclerosis was arrived at in 1957 by a study group of the World Health Organization [8]:

> Atherosclerosis is a variable combination of changes of the intima of arteries (as distinct from arterioles) consisting of focal accumulation of lipids, complex carbohydrates, blood and blood products, fibrous tissue, and calcium deposits, and associated with medial changes.

Manipulation of the diet has been the approach most consistently used to establish atherosclerosis in experimental animals. This work began with the successful production by Ignatowski [9] of lesions in rabbits by feeding them meat, milk, and eggs. Ignatowski, however, believed the lesions were due to toxic protein. Saltykow [10] and Stuckey [11] carried out experiments in which lipid-rich diets were administered to rabbits together with toxins, but they finally concluded that the atheromatous lesions observed in the rabbits were due to the fat in the diet. In 1913 two groups of investigators, Anitschkow and Chalatow [12] and Wacker and Hueck [13], independently observed that atherosclerosis could be established in rabbits by feeding them cholesterol in

V. DRUGS AFFECTING ATHEROSCLEROSIS

sunflower seed oil. These observations led to establishment of the first animal model for the study of the pathogenesis of atherosclerosis.

Research into a disease requires a specific etiological agent and a suitable model. A role for cholesterol in the pathogenesis of arterial disease is generally acknowledged but there are other views that range from the belief that cholesterol is a minor component [14] to the assignment of initial important contributions to local (arterial) factors [15, 16].

The choice of a suitable model is no less complicated. The two most commonly used experimental animals, the rabbit and the cockerel, have been criticized as not being a carnivore or a mammal, respectively. Other animals which might be used, the rat and the dog, are generally immune to cholesterol-induced atherosclerosis unless the thyroid is ablated and, in the case of the rat, unless cholic acid is present in the diet. Atherosclerosis can be induced in the rat on an essential fatty acid-deficient diet [17] and in the dog after a long-term regimen on a cholesterol-rich, semisynthetic diet [18]; consequently, these species may yet be useful, albeit the dietary modalities are severe and of long duration. Recently there has been considerable interest in subhuman primates as experimental animals. Monkey species exhibit variable susceptibility to the dietary regimens used, ranging from ease of establishment of atheromata in the squirrel monkey to difficulty in the cebus monkey [19-22]. The expense of procuring, maintaining, and handling primates, however, argues against their suitability for large-scale dietary or screening experiments.

The evidence in man, based upon a wealth of epidemiological data, is that a relationship exists between blood cholesterol levels and susceptibility to heart disease. In the absence of an unequivocal antemortem test to predict a coronary attack, we have only the statistical assurance that more men with elevated blood cholesterol levels will be susceptible to coronary disease than those with low cholesterol levels. The thrust of most investigations, then, is to find an agent which will lower cholesterol levels.

The lipids of the blood circulate as part of a series of lipid-protein complexes of varying composition, size, and density. These lipoproteins may be subfractionated by precipitation methods using charged polysaccharides, such as heparin or dextran sulfate, by electrophoresis, or by ultracentrifugation.

Ultracentrifugation in media of specific densities [23] permits separation of the α-lipoprotein (also referred to as high-density lipoprotein or HDL), the β-lipoprotein (low density lipoprotein or LDL), the very light β-lipoproteins (VLDL), and chylomicrons. Within the β-lipoproteins, the triglyceride content falls and the cholesterol content rises with increasing density. Table I lists the chemical composition of the various lipoproteins.

The elevation of serum β-lipoproteins is most closely correlated with the establishment of atherosclerosis in animals. In general, elevation of serum β-lipoproteins is a <u>sine qua non</u> for production of atheromata.

TABLE I

Chemical Composition of Lipoproteins

Type	Average Concentration (mg/100 ml)	d [a]	S_f [b]	Cholesterol Free	Cholesterol Ester	Triglyceride	Phospholipid	Non-esterified Fatty Acid	Protein
Chylomicron	0.50	<0.96	$10^4 - 10^5$	1	3	87	8	—	1
β-Lipoprotein	150	0.96–1.006	20–400	7	14	52	19	1	7
	50	1.006–1.019	12–20	8	31	26	23	1	11
	350	1.019–1.063	0–12	8	38	10	22	1	21
α-Lipoprotein	50	1.063–1.125	HDL 2	6	21	11	29	—	33
	300	1.125–1.210	HDL 3	3	12	5	20	3	57

[a] Density.
[b] Ultracentrifugal rates of flotation after Gofman et al. [23].

V. DRUGS AFFECTING ATHEROSCLEROSIS

Cholesterol-free diets which cause atherosclerosis in rabbits [24, 25] cause moderate elevations in cholesterol levels, but marked elevations in β-lipoproteins [26]. Examination of normal serum cholesterol and β-lipoprotein levels in animals [27] shows that regardless of the cholesterol level, those animals with a high β-lipoprotein level are most susceptible to experimental atherosclerosis.

In man, the Framingham study has revealed a close correlation between serum cholesterol levels and the risk of coronary disease, especially in the case of men under age 50 [28, 29]. The serum triglycerides have also been implicated as predictors of high risk [30-33]. The Framingham study has shown that the degree of discrimination between high- and low-risk patients is only slightly stronger for the total cholesterol or S_f 0-20 lipoproteins than for S_f 20-100 or S_f 100-400 lipoproteins [34]. These findings demonstrate that the serum cholesterol level is a strong enough predictor of the risk of coronary heart disease to warrant focal attention when studying agents which may affect the course of this disease.

II. SERUM CHOLESTEROL LOWERING AGENTS

There are several mechanisms by which the levels of circulating cholesterol can be reduced. Interference with lipoprotein synthesis or release would seem to be the critical point of attack but, as yet, not enough is known about normal lipoprotein metabolism to make this possible.

The next best approach would appear to be reducing availability of the components of the β-lipoprotein. A logical step would involve interference with cholesterol synthesis or acceleration of cholesterol catabolism. The inhibition of cholesterol synthesis entails certain inherent dangers. Cholesterol is a very necessary component of the biochemical economy, being required for the synthesis of bile acids, sex hormones, and adrenocortical hormones. The critical physiological site of inhibition of cholesterogenesis is at the step involving the conversion of β-hydroxy-β-methylglutaryl CoA (HMG-CoA) to mevalonic acid [35]. Compounds which interfere with later stages of cholesterol synthesis may cause a buildup of other unsaponifiable products. The steroidal products may be atherogenic per se. Compounds that cause accumulation of 24-dehydrocholesterol [36] or 7-dehydrocholesterol [37] have been the subject of extensive research but they may cause deleterious side effects [39, 40]. There is no direct evidence that the accumulation of sterols other than cholesterol is the cause of the observed side effects, but the possibility is enough to kill interest in these compounds. Compounds that inhibit cholesterol synthesis at stages earlier than HMG-CoA may also exhibit toxic manifestations [40-42] and for one of them (2-phenylbutyric acid) the suggested regimen in man is not one of continuous dosage [43].

Inhibition of cholesterol absorption offers an interesting approach and the inhibition of bile acid reabsorption (which inhibits cholesterol absorption) is of corollary interest. Dietary cholesterol is known to be deposited in the aortas of animals or man [44, 45]. Squalene feeding will result in accumulation of liver cholesterol but not formation of atheromata in rabbits [46]. Recent work by Buchwald [47] has shown that surgical interference with cholesterol absorption results in hypocholesteremia.

One other modality under study does not involve cholesterol metabolism directly but rather inhibition of lipolysis or release of free fatty acids (FFA). Nicotinic acid, which has a hypocholesteremic action, has been shown to inhibit lipolysis and to lower serum FFA in man [48].

The mechanism by which inhibition of FFA release affects cholesterol levels is not clear and the two effects may prove to be unrelated. It is known that reductions in FFA levels precede triglyceride lowering and that this is followed by hypocholesteremia. A possible effect on lipoprotein synthesis may be adduced but has not yet been proven [49]. These findings, however, have stimulated a search for FFA-lowering agents.

The usual progression of drug investigation in the area of atherosclerosis starts with the discovery of a drug which lowers cholesterol in a test animal; actual studies of its effects in atherosclerosis are usually limited to rabbits or chickens and clinical studies are limited to serum cholesterol or lipoprotein determinations. This is understandable since the animal models are far from ideal and studies of prevention of heart disease in man are prolonged and difficult to carry out.

This discussion, then, will concern itself with drugs affecting serum lipid levels with data on atherosclerosis given when available. It is of no purpose to discuss all of the compounds which have been tested against experimental atherosclerosis in the past few decades: They are tabulated in several older reviews [2,3,50-52]. An excellent and thorough review on hypolipemic agents by Bencze et al. [53] has appeared recently. This discussion will, instead, concern itself with compounds of current interest.

At this writing there are seven pharmaceutical agents available for use as hypolipemic agents. An eighth is available, but not specifically as a lipid-lowering drug. A number of other compounds of interest are being tested in the laboratory or in clinical trial and some of these will also be discussed.

A. Inhibitors of Cholesterol Absorption

Sperry and Bergmann [54] first reported in 1937 that when mice were fed sitosterol, their liver cholesterol concentrations were reduced. Many years later Peterson and his co-workers [55, 56] found that when chicks were fed an atherogenic diet to which mixed soybean sterols had been added,

V. DRUGS AFFECTING ATHEROSCLEROSIS

they exhibited neither hypercholesteremia nor atherosclerosis. Peterson showed further [57] that pure β-sitosterol (1), ergosterol, and stigmasterol

were equally effective in preventing atherosclerosis in chicks. The plant sterols inhibit cholesterol absorption [58] by competing for intestinal sites of esterification [59]. Soy sterols or β-sitosterol have been clinically effective in lowering serum cholesterol and β-lipoprotein levels [60, 61]. The minimum effective dose is 10 g daily taken in divided doses between meals and before snacks. The usual daily dose is 12-25 g. Serum cholesterol levels fall about 15% within a few weeks after institution of therapy. The side effects most usually seen are anorexia, cramps, and diarrhea. The greatest limitations of this drug are the large dose needed and the requirement for therapy before every meal.

Cholesterol absorption also appears to be inhibited by cholestane-3β, 5α, 6β-triol (CT) (2) and several substituted amides of linoleic acid. When fed

to rabbits at a level of 0.5%, CT almost completely inhibits atherosclerosis [62]. This compound has been shown to compete for sites of cholesterol esterification [63] and will cause a large increase in sterol excretion when fed to rats [64]. However, Cook and MacDougall [65] have found that when CT is fed to rabbits in small doses (30 mg/kg/day) over long periods of time, lesions which closely resemble human lesions appear in the aorta.

The cyclohexylamine amide of linoleic acid is effective in inhibiting atherosclerosis in cholesterol-fed rabbits when fed at a dose of 200-600 mg/

day [65, 66]. Two other active derivatives are now available. The α-methylbenzylamine amide (AC223) (3) will significantly reduce atheromata

$$CH_3(CH_2)_4CH=CH-CH_2-CH=CH-(CH_2)_7-\overset{O}{\underset{\|}{C}}-\overset{H}{\underset{}{N}}-\overset{CH_3}{\underset{H}{C}}-\bigcirc$$

(3)

(26%) and serum cholesterol levels (49%) at a dose of 50 mg/day [67]. The α-phenyl-β-(p-tolyl)ethylamine amide (AC485) (4) will inhibit atheromata by

$$CH_3(CH_2)_4CH=CH-CH_2-CH=CH-(CH_2)_7-\overset{O}{\underset{\|}{C}}-\overset{H}{\underset{}{N}}-\overset{H}{\underset{}{C}}-\overset{H}{\underset{H}{C}}-\bigcirc-CH_3$$

(4)

93% and cholesterol levels by 76% when fed at a level of 25 mg/day [68]. Clinical data on the use of AC223 are available [68] and show a marked (20-25%) reduction of cholesterol levels in man when fed at a dose of 2.25 g/day. These compounds inhibit absorption of cholesterol in the rat [69, 70] as evidenced by reduced recovery of label from plasma, lymph, and liver when $4-^{14}C$-cholesterol is administered to rats.

The obligatory function of bile and bile acids in the absorption of cholesterol is well known [71, 72]. The hypothesis that precipitation of bile acids would inhibit cholesterol absorption was first tested by Siperstein et al. [73] who fed ferric chloride to chicks and found that the compound was effective but toxic. Tennent et al. [74] found that cholestyramine, an insoluble, polystyrene-based, anion-exchange resin would bind bile acids in vitro and in vivo and was an effective hypocholesteremic agent in dogs and chicks. At levels of 13-15 g/day this material lowers cholesterol levels in man [75, 76]. In some cases disappearance of xanthomas has been observed [76]. At a level of 15 g/day this drug causes intestinal distress, nausea, and constipation. Cholestyramine is not yet available for prescription as a cholesterol-lowering drug, but another preparation of this compound can be used for relief from biliary pruritis.

The antibiotic, neomycin, administered at a level of 1.5-2.0 g/day reduces cholesterol levels in man [77, 78]. This drug by virtue of its basicity increases excretion of bile acids in man [79]. N-methylneomycin, which is basic, but not an antibiotic, lowers cholesterol levels in chickens, whereas N-acetylneomycin, which is an antibiotic, but is not basic, has no effect [80]. The principal side effect of neomycin therapy is diarrhea which occurs in nearly one-third of the patients [77].

B. Hormones

1. Estrogens

It is generally acknowledged that premenopausal women are relatively immune to coronary disease. One biochemical manifestation of circulating estrogens is a tendency for more of the serum cholesterol to be transported via the α-lipoproteins. Young women may have 34% of their cholesterol in the α-lipoprotein fraction, whereas in young men or in older men and women this fraction carries only about 22-25% of the cholesterol [81]. Administration of estrogen usually increases α-lipoprotein concentration and reduces the serum cholesterol/phospholipid ratio rather than affecting cholesterol levels directly [82]. Synthetic estrogens do not appear to affect mortality or morbidity in men [83, 84], but mixed conjugated equine estrogens (Premarin) have been reported to increase survival rates in survivors of heart attacks [84, 85]. Whatever the benefits of estrogen therapy, it also induces loss of libido, gynecomastia, and aspermogenesis. It is doubtful whether the average male would submit to this formidable array of side effects.

2. Thyroid

Hyperthyroidism and hypothyroidism are generally associated with hypocholesteremia and hypercholesteremia, respectively. It has been well documented that thyroid hormone or thyroid powder will protect susceptible animals from cholesterol-induced atherosclerosis, whereas ablation of the thyroid will render usually resistant species susceptible to dietary atherogenesis [86, 87].

There is a reluctance to use the active thyroid hormones L-thyroxine and L-triiodothyronine because of their side effects, such as tachycardia, angina, diarrhea, and weight loss.

One approach to the synthesis of a thyroid derivative which would retain the hypocholesteremic activity without any concomitant calorigenic effect centered upon derivatives in which either the iodination pattern of the ring system or the structure of the side chain was altered. The effect of a number of such compounds has been reviewed [50], but none of these is in current use. Another approach, the use of the dextrarotatory isomer of the natural hormones (D-thyroxine, DT_4, or D-triiodothyronine, DT_3) has been more fruitful. DT_4 has been investigated extensively since the initial report by Starr and his co-workers [88] that this compound was non-calorigenic and was an effective hypocholesteremic agent. There exists a large literature concerning the effectiveness of DT_4 in lowering cholesterol and β-lipoprotein levels in man. Cohen [89] has reported a high level of success over a six-year period in treating patients with 2-8 mg/day of DT_4. A review of over 6000 cases also attests to the effectiveness of DT_4 as a cholesteropenic agent [90]. The compound is as effective as LT_4 in reducing atherosclerosis in cholesterol-fed rabbits [91].

The mechanism of action of thyroid hormones has been the subject of several fairly recent reviews [92, 93]. Thyroid hormone appears to stimulate cholesterol biosynthesis (possibly an acute phenomenon). While it does not affect synthesis of bile acids, it does alter the bile acid spectrum; principally it alters the cholic-acid/chenodeoxycholic acid ratio from 3:1 to 1:3 [94, 95]. In a study conducted in myxedematous patients, Miettinen observed a definite increase in neutral sterol excretion, but a questionable increase in bile acid excretion [96]. Hyperthyroid animals have a higher total body cholesterol content than do eu- or hypothyroid animals due to redistribution of cholesterol from serum and liver into muscle and skin [97].

C. Aryloxy-Substituted Aliphatic Acids

Presently one of the most widely used hypocholesteremic agents is the ethyl ester of α-(p-chlorophenoxy) isobutyric acid (5). This compound, which

$$CH_3-\underset{\underset{O}{|}}{\overset{\overset{CH_3}{|}}{C}}-C\overset{\nearrow O}{\underset{}{-}}OC_2H_5$$

(structure with p-chlorophenyl attached via O)

(5)

is also referred to as CPIB, clofibrate, or Atromid-S, was found by Thorp and Waring [98] to be the most active and least toxic of a series of aryloxy-isobutyric acids. Administered in daily doses of 1.5-3.0 g, this compound has been found to be an effective lipid-lowering agent [99, 100]. The major side effect is weight gain in some patients. On rare occasions a transient rise in serum transaminase [101] or creatine phosphokinase is observed [102]. Reduced anticoagulant therapy is usually required [103].

Because this compound is principally effective in lowering serum triglycerides [104], Strisower has suggested that it be administered together with a more potent hypocholesteremic agent, such as DT_4 [105].

In the rat, clofibrate induces hepatomegaly with an increase in the number and size of peroxisomes or microbodies [106, 107] and a marked increase in mitochondrial glycerol-1-phosphate dehydrogenase activity [108]. Mitochondrial cholesterol oxidase activity is also increased [109]. Clofibrate reduces atherogenesis in cholesterol-fed rabbits [110].

The mechanism of action of clofibrate is unclear. Experiments carried out in rats and in man suggest one or another of the following: inhibition of cholesterol synthesis; reduced synthesis of lipoproteins; inhibition of release of lipoproteins; and increase of cholesterol turnover [111-113]. Maragoudakis has found that compounds of the general structure of clofibrate inhibit hepatic acetyl CoA carboxylase [114].

V. DRUGS AFFECTING ATHEROSCLEROSIS

A compound related structurally to clofibrate and reported equally effective is 2-methyl-(p-1,2,3,4-tetrahydro-1-naphthylphenoxy) propionic acid (SU-13,437 or nafenopin) (6). This compound is an effective hypolipemic

agent in rats [115, 116]. It is primarily effective in lowering triglyceride and, like clofibrate, causes hepatomegaly. In man, SU-13,437 affects reductions of about 25% in serum cholesterol levels and 50-70% in triglyceride levels [117, 118].

Another aryloxy acid being tested is 1-methyl-4-piperidyl bis (p-chlorophenoxy) acetate (SaH 42-348) (7). SaH 42-348 reduces all classes of serum

lipids in rats but does not influence cholesterol synthesis [119]. Like clofibrate and nafenopin, it also causes hepatomegaly and increases in liver triglyceride levels. At present its mode of action is thought to involve increased cholesterol catabolism [120].

To date there has been little work on attempts to explain the mechanism(s) by which aryloxy derivatives of aliphatic acids cause hepatomegaly in rats.

D. Heparin

Heparin stimulates release of lipoprotein lipase, an enzyme which catalyzes the hydrolysis of triglycerides, thus causing lipemic serum to clear [121, 122]. Heparin treatment has been reported to reduce levels of LDL and to decrease mortality in cardiac patients [123]. The disadvantages of heparin therapy include hematomas at the site of injection, lumbar pain, and allergic reactions [123]. The greatest drawback is the need for biweekly injection.

E. Nicotinic Acid

Since the first report of the hypocholesteremic action by Altschul et al. [124], this compound has been used successfully by a large number of clinicians. Parsons [125, 126] has accumulated the widest experience with this compound. Nicotinic acid (8) treatment will result in reductions in

$$\underset{N}{\underset{\|}{\bigcirc}}\text{-COOH} \quad (8)$$

serum β-lipoproteins, cholesterol, triglyceride, and phospholipid [127].

The mechanism of action of nicotinic acid is not yet clear. A number of hypotheses have been proposed and discarded. These have included a vitamin effect, cutaneous vasodilation, heparin release, and anorexia. The influence on cholesterol synthesis in animals is variable but usually inhibition is observed [49]. Studies by Miettinen [128] and Sodhi et al. [129] suggest that the principal effect of nicotinic acid on cholesterol metabolism in man is mobilization and excretion rather than inhibition of synthesis. With the administration of nicotinic acid, increased oxidation of cholesterol by rat liver mitochondria [130] or by intact rats [131] has been observed, but there is no increase of bile acid excretion in man [128, 129, 132].

It has been suggested that the antilipolytic action of nicotinic acid [133, 134] may cause the reductions in FFA observed in man [48] and might be the first step in the chain which leads to reductions in plasma cholesterol levels. The course of events following administration of nicotinic acid to rats [135] or to man [127] is lowering of FFA levels, then, triglyceride levels, and finally, cholesterol levels. In the absence of continued therapy a rebound to starting levels may be observed.

The major side effects of nicotinic acid therapy are cutaneous flushing and itching. These are said to disappear after several weeks of treatment and can be further controlled by the use of aluminum [136] or potassium [137] nicotinate. The impaired glucose tolerance and symptomatic diabetes observed in some patients during nicotinic acid therapy [126, 138] are reversed when treatment is stopped.

Nicotinic acid will inhibit cholesterol-induced atherosclerosis in rabbits [139], but not in cockerels [140] or pigeons [141].

A number of esters of nicotinic acid, such as the fructose [142] or pentaerythritol [143] tetranicotinoates and the sorbitol [144] or inositol [145] hexanicotinoates, have been found to be effective cholesterol-lowering agents.

1. Compounds Resembling Nicotinic Acid in Action

The effectiveness of nicotinic acid has led to the investigation of compounds with similar structure as hypocholesteremic agents or as inhibitors

V. DRUGS AFFECTING ATHEROSCLEROSIS

of lipolysis. Of a large series of nicotinic acid homologs only 3-pyridylacetic acid (9) has a marked cholesterol-lowering effect [146]. Nicotinyl alcohol (10)

also lowers cholesterol levels [147, 148] in man.

Among nicotinic acid derivatives which lower plasma FFA in man are the 5- and 6-fluoro-, 5-chloro-, 5- and 6-amino-, and 5-hydroxy compounds [127]. Nicotinyl alcohol also has an antilipolytic effect [135, 149]. Other active inhibitors of lipolysis are 3,5-dimethylpyrazole (11) [150], 5-methyl-

pyrazole-3-carboxylic acid (12) [151], and 5(3-pyridyl)tetrazole (13) [152].

F. Other Compounds

Pyridinolcarbamate (14) has been reported to prevent atheromatous

changes in rabbits fed cholesterol without affecting their serum cholesterol levels [153]. This compound was found ineffective in monkeys maintained on an atherogenic diet [154]. The proceedings of a recently held conference on pyridinolcarbamate have been published [155] and give in detail the effects of this compound upon many aspects of vascular disease in man as well as upon atherosclerosis in chickens and rabbits. Pyridinolcarbamate has been reported to exhibit antianginal activity in man [156] and also to have a definitely curative effect in atherosclerosis obliterans [157]. In the rat, pyridinolcarbamate will inhibit cholesterol synthesis from acetate, but not from mevalonate [158].

A large number of hydroxylamine derivatives have been synthesized and shown to be hypocholesteremic [159]. One of these, N-α-phenylpropyl-N-benzyloxy acetamide (W-1372) (<u>15</u>) has been reported to inhibit atherosclero-

$$\text{C}_6\text{H}_5\text{-CH}_2\text{-ON(COCH}_3)\text{-CH}_2\text{CH}_2\text{CH}_2\text{-C}_6\text{H}_5$$

(15)

sis in rabbits and squirrel monkeys [160]. This compound, when fed at a level of 0.25-0.30% to rats, will cause increases in liver size and liver lipids [161, 162]. At the 2% level, W-1372 will significantly reduce atherogenesis and liver cholesterol levels in cholesterol-fed rabbits, but will not affect serum cholesterol levels [163]. The mechanism of action of W-1372 has not been elucidated, but experiments with a somewhat similar compound (benzyl N-benzylcarbethoxyhydroxamate) indicate that it acts via inhibition of cholesterol reabsorption [164].

The list of compounds reported to possess hypocholesteremic activity increases yearly. Many of the newer compounds have been discussed in recent reviews [53, 165]. If yet another hypocholesteremic meteor flashes across the lipemic skies before this review appears in print, it will not be unexpected.

III. CURRENT STATUS

Although cardiovascular disease is of multiple etiology, the focus of most of the experimental pharmacology has been on only one important factor, hyperlipidemia. This has not been due to oversight, but rather to the fact that hyperlipidemia lends itself to easy analysis. The possibility that lipid deposition in the arterial wall is simply due to hypercholesteremia [166] or to affluent living [167] is certainly not a new concept. The importance of cholesterolemia as a risk factor has been amply demonstrated by the Framingham study [28, 29]. Using the Framingham data, Cornfield [168] has derived a regression equation which suggests that incidence of the disease is proportional to the 2.66th power of serum cholesterol level. Thus a 15% reduction in serum cholesterol should result in a 35% reduction in risk. All of the findings in this area are statistically valid. But there are a number of deaths in persons with relatively low cholesterol levels; and high serum cholesterol, while significantly associated with the risk of coronary disease, is not a certain indicator of a future coronary attack. Before the advent of insulin, a statistical study of blood glucose levels might have given similar results in a study of diabetics.

The intelligent application of hypolipemic therapy requires a more accurate assessment of the lipemia to be treated than may be offered by simple analysis of blood lipids, although these are certainly an important initial indicator. Such a method may lie in the electrophoretic classification of hyperlipemias which has been devised by Fredrickson and his co-workers

V. DRUGS AFFECTING ATHEROSCLEROSIS

[169, 170]. The five types of lipoproteinemia are summarized in Table II. With a clue to the origin of the lipemia it is possible to determine whether the course of the treatment should be diet, a particular drug, or both. Levy and Fredrickson [171-173] have presented several excellent discussions of the different approaches to diagnosis and treatment.

A. Methodology

The screening of drugs still depends upon finding compounds which safely and effectively reduce lipid levels in experimental animals. The choices of animal and screening method to use are still difficult to make.

For ease and economy, the rat would be most useful, but production of lipemia in this species is difficult. Weanling rats, who are somewhat hypercholesteremic, usually return to normal levels rapidly and it is hard to determine what portion of the decline of serum lipid levels can be attributed to a drug. Lipemia induced by surface-active agents has been used [174], but this type of lipemia is not atherogenic [175] and thus may not be representative of the condition to be treated. Perhaps the rat should be used at some stage in testing since a compound must be potent to be hypolipemic in this species.

The cholesterol-fed rabbit is used for studies of antiatherogenic drugs and in this species one can get answers concerning atherosclerosis, as well as lipemia. We may not have made the most efficient use of this animal. The rabbit has a low normal cholesterol level, but a high level of endogenous β-lipoprotein.

Possibly screening experiments should be carried out in normal rabbits. Marked reductions in serum cholesterol and β-lipoprotein levels might provide better clues than could studies in hypercholesteremic rabbits, since this animal is remarkably sensitive to dietary cholesterol.

Other animals offer even fewer advantages because of resistance (dog), size (pig), or expense (primate). A unique screening method has been devised by Chevillard and his colleagues [176] who measure inhibition of cholesterol-dependent growth of <u>Blatella germanica</u> larvae. Little use has been made of tissue culture or other <u>in vitro</u> techniques; the use of such techniques is complicated by the insolubility of most hypolipemic agents.

Determining whether to screen simply for hypolipemia or for other parameters as well is important. Although we know that cholesterol is as good a prognosticator of coronary disease as any of the other lipid components of the serum, we also have data which show that young women are less susceptible because of their high levels of α-lipoprotein cholesterol. Estrogens appear to shift cholesterol from serum β- to α-lipoprotein [177].

Methodology, such as dextran sulfate precipitation [178, 179], makes it relatively easy to screen for "lipid shifting" rather than for hypocholesteremia alone.

TABLE II

Classification of Hyperlipoproteinemias [a]

Type	Prevalence	Electrophoretic characteristics	Appearance of plasma	Cholesterol	Triglyceride
I Exogenous hypertriglyceridemia or hyperchylomicronemia	Rare	Strong chylomicron band	Creamy top layer on standing. Clear infranatant	N or +	+++
II Hyperbeta-lipoproteinemia	Common	Strong β band	Clear or faintly opalescent	+++	N
III Broad beta disease	Relatively uncommon	Strong β and pre-β bands	Clear, cloudy, or milky	++	+
IV Endogenous hypertriglyceridemia	Common	Strong pre-β band	Lactescent	N or +	++
V Mixed hyperlipoproteinemia	Uncommon	Marked chylomicron, β, and pre-β band	Creamy top layer over milky infranatant	++	++ or +++

[a] After Fredrickson et al. [170].

V. DRUGS AFFECTING ATHEROSCLEROSIS

Probably the most difficult aspect of screening is that the site of the action — the arterial wall — is not accessible for testing or observation. Relatively rapid induction of atherosclerosis in rabbits (6-8 weeks) may not be rapid enough for an extensive screening program. Recent experiments by Rothblat and his co-workers [180-182] on the uptake of cholesterol by cells in culture suggest a possible screening method. Although direct tests might be difficult because of insolubility of the drugs used, the influence of sera obtained from treated animals may provide useful data.

Cholesterol uptake by cells is a function of the chemistry of the medium [182] and a tissue culture screening method may provide a sensitive method for detecting changes in serum, which cannot be determined by current methods.

B. Research Strategy

Research in atherosclerosis has followed observations concerning conditions influencing susceptibility in man. Thus the relative immunity of women and of hyperthyroid patients has stimulated research on estrogens and thyroactive compounds. The observation that the biliary glycocholanic-/taurocholanic acid ratio is generally high in susceptible species [183] has stimulated experiments in which taurine has been fed to animals or man [184, 185]. Unfortunately, dietary taurine is ineffective. However, it has been found [186] that taurocholic acid enhances hydrolysis of cholesteryl oleate by aorta homogenates. This finding impinges upon another observation — namely, the increase in aortic cholesteryl ester observed with aging in man and in experimental atherosclerosis in animals. An increase in cholesteryl ester has been found by many investigators and their results have been summarized [187]. The importance of this finding lies in the increase in cholesteryl ester and in the large proportion of cholesteryl oleate found in the aorta. The latter can be explained by a combination of cholesteryl ester deposition from the serum (in which cholesteryl linoleate predominates) and local synthesis of cholesteryl oleate from serum free cholesterol and newly synthesized oleic acid. Zemplenyi [188] has shown that a resistant species, such as the rat, exhibits greater endogenous aortic lipolytic activity than do the rabbit or chicken. A study of the spectrum of enzyme activity in the aorta has been published by him [189]. Kirk [190] has also summarized knowledge on arterial enzymes. It is known that there is a flux of free cholesterol in the plaque [191, 192] and that cholesteryl ester accumulation within a cell is due to lack of hydrolytic activity rather than excess of esterifying activity or ester imbibition [193]. Whether the reduction of aortic cholesteryl ester will lead to lessening of atherosclerosis is an open question. There is no way, yet, to test for reduction of plaque size and severity, short of autopsy. How can one screen for a compound of known hydrolytic activity if some indicator is not found in the blood?

This leads to the crux of the argument — namely, can plaques regress and can they regress readily? In other words, we can easily cause atherogenesis but what is known of atheroexodus? Regression of preestablished plaques (as opposed to inhibition of formation of plaques) has been observed in rabbits who have been taken off an atherogenic regimen for a long period of time [194, 195]. Spontaneous atherosclerosis disappears from aortas of rabbits after weaning [196] and phosphatide infusions [197], thyroid, and estrogens [198, 199] have been found to exert a similar effect. In dogs, time and removal of stimulus will also lead to plaque regression [200]. Estrogens will cause regression of coronary atherosclerosis in cockerels [201]. Cholesterol deposits in tissue cultures of aortic cells will disappear upon removal of this sterol from the tissue culture medium [202]. The reduction in size or disappearance of xanthomata has been noted in some cases of drug or dietary treatment. Since xanthomata are not universally seen in hypercholesteremic patients, a study of their regression cannot be used generally, but it may be indicative of efficacy in causing regression of lipid deposits. Taylor et al. [203] have marshalled arguments to support the view that human plaques are resorbable.

Proof of the efficacy of hypocholesteremic therapy depends upon demonstration that such a regimen will reduce the incidence of the first coronary attack in man (primary prevention) or will delay the onset of a second coronary attack in men who have survived the first (secondary prevention). Human trials are difficult for many reasons not the least of which is that alterations may occur in the mode of living, behavior, or dietary pattern in the populations under study. This is especially true for studies in free-living populations.

In several dietary primary prevention trials, there has been evidence of reduction of cardiovascular disease but not total mortality [204-206]. A secondary prevention trial using diet as the hypocholesteremic agent gave significant positive results in Norway [207] but a very similarly designed diet study carried out in London [208] yielded no differences between test and control groups. The differences in results point up the possibility that other factors such as serum electrolytes, coagulability, aortic anoxia, and dietary components other than the lipids play more or less of a determining role in different populations.

Several drug studies are in progress or in preparation throughout the world. The U.S. Veterans Administration has conducted a secondary prevention study using conjugated equine estrogens (Premarin), DT_4, and nicotinic acid as the drugs. An interim report based on five years' experience [209] indicated improvement in survival time in patients on DT_4 and nicotinic acid. This study involves about 600 patients. The National Heart and Lung Institute is carrying out a larger secondary prevention study with a starting cohort of over 8000 men. The drugs being studied are clofibrate, DT_4, nicotinic acid, and Premarin. The study has been under way for about 5 years but no data are available at this writing. Oliver [210] has described the design for a large primary prevention study with clofibrate which is being conducted in Europe, but data are not yet available.

IV. SUMMARY

Cardiovascular disease, the principal cause of death in much of the western world, is a disease of multiple etiology for which there is no unequivocal ante mortem diagnosis. Of the many known contributing factors, the serum lipids are most easily amenable to manipulation by diet or drugs. Newer screening methods now indicate that not all hyperlipoproteinemias are identical and that each type requires its specific therapeutic measures. The screening of hypolipemic drugs is made difficult by the absence of uniform methods for establishing hyperlipemia in animals and the variability of the different animal species. A truly valid animal model has not yet been found.

The emergence of several safe, effective hypolipemic drugs has made possible a number of primary and secondary prevention trials which will further our knowledge of hyperlipemia and coronary disease. The refinement of methods for screening populations will identify those persons at whom this therapy should be aimed.

There are still a number of questions that are not, and perhaps cannot be, resolved. Very little is known about the factors which trigger the acute event and so we know almost nothing about how lipemia affects the onset of a coronary attack. Social interactions have been shown to affect the severity of atherosclerosis in zoo animals [211, 212] in a setting where diet and environment have been kept constant. This adds yet another variable to a complex equation. Work in the field of atherosclerosis has proceeded at a brisk pace in the face of a number of uncertainties. This has been due to the identification of one potential contributing agent — the serum lipids — and concentration upon it. There is little doubt that this is an important factor but it is not the only determining factor.

There are many other factors, dietary as well as physiological and psychological that are emerging. It behooves the scientist to scan the rest of the playing field while keeping his eye on the ball that is currently in play.

REFERENCES

1. National Vital Statistics Division, U. S. Public Health Service, 1966.
2. D. Kritchevsky, Cholesterol, Wiley, New York, 1958, p. 139.
3. C. Moses, Atherosclerosis, Lea and Febiger, Philadelphia, 1963, p. 27.
4. J. Vogel, The Pathological Anatomy of the Human Body, Lea and Blanchard, Philadelphia, 1847.
5. R. Virchow, Phlogore und Thrombose in Gefäss-system, Ges. Abh. Med., 1856.
6. C. Rokitansky, Lehrbuch der Pathologische Anatomie, Sydenham Soc., London, 1852.

7. F. Marchand, Verhandl. Kongr. Med., 21, 23 (1904).
8. World Health Organization, Tech. Reports, Ser. 143, 4 (1957).
9. A. Ignatowski, Arch. Pathol. Anat. Physiol., 198, 248 (1909).
10. S. Saltykow, Verhandl. Deut. Apth. Ges., 14, 119 (1910).
11. N. W. Stuckey, Zentr. Allgem. Pathol. Pathol. Anat., 21, 668 (1910).
12. N. Anitschkow and S. Chalatow, Zentr. Allgem. Pathol. Pathol. Anat., 24, 1 (1913).
13. L. Wacker and W. Hueck, Muench. Med. Wochschr., 60, 2097 (1913).
14. S. Clarkson and L. H. Newburgh, J. Exptl. Med., 43, 595 (1926).
15. L. Aschoff, Arteriosklerose. Beihefte 2, Med. Klin., Vol. X, 1914, p. 16.
16. G. L. Duff, Arch. Pathol., 20, 81, 259 (1935).
17. R. J. Morin, S. Bernick, and R. B. Alfin-Slater, J. Atherosclerosis Res., 4, 387 (1964).
18. H. Malmros and N. H. Sternby, in Progr. Biochem. Pharmacol. (C. J. Miras, A. N. Howard, and R. Paoletti, eds.), Vol. 4, S. Karger, Basel, 1968, p. 482.
19. O. W. Portman and S. B. Andrus, J. Nutr., 87, 429 (1965).
20. T. B. Clarkson, H. B. Lofland, B. C. Bullock, N. D. M. Lehner, R. St. Clair, and R. W. Prichard, Ann. N. Y. Acad. Sci., 162, 103 (1969).
21. D. A. Eggen, J. P. Strong, and W. P. Newman, III, Ann. N.Y. Acad. Sci., 162, 110 (1969).
22. C. B. Taylor, G. E. Cox, P. Manalo-Estrella, and J. Southworth, Arch. Pathol., 66, 32 (1958).
23. J. W. Gofman, F. Lindgren, H. Elliott, W. Mantz, J. Hewitt, B. Strisower, V. Herring, and T. P. Lyon, Science, 111, 166 (1950).
24. G. F. Lambert, J. P. Miller, R. T. Olsen, and D. V. Frost, Proc. Soc. Exptl. Biol. Med., 97, 544 (1958).
25. H. Malmros and G. Wigand, Lancet, ii, 749 (1959).
26. D. Kritchevsky and S. A. Tepper, J. Atherosclerosis Res., 8, 357 (1968).
27. R. E. Olson, Perspectives Biol. Med., 2, 84 (1958).
28. A. Kagan, W. B. Kannel, T. R. Dawber, and N. Revotskie, Ann. N. Y. Acad. Sci., 97, 883 (1963).
29. W. B. Kannel, T. R. Dawber, A. Kagan, N. Revotskie, and J. Stokes, III, Ann. Intern. Med., 55, 33 (1961).

30. M. J. Albrink, Arch. Internal Med., 109, 345 (1962).

31. L. A. Carlson, Acta Med. Scand., 167, 399 (1960).

32. D. F. Brown, Am. J. Med., 46, 691 (1969).

33. D. F. Brown, S. H. Kinch, and J. T. Doyle, New Eng. J. Med., 273, 947 (1965).

34. W. B. Kannel, T. R. Dawber, G. D. Friedman, W. E. Glennon, and P. M. McNamara, Ann. Internal Med., 61, 881 (1964).

35. M. D. Siperstein and M. J. Guest, J. Clin. Invest., 39, 642 (1960).

36. J. Avigan, D. Steinberg, H. E. Vroman, M. J. Thompson, and E. Mosettig, J. Biol. Chem., 235, 3123 (1960).

37. D. Dvornik, M. Kramel, J. Dubuc, M. Givner, and R. Gaudry, J. Am. Chem. Soc., 85, 3309 (1963).

38. R. W. P. Achor, R. K. Winkelmann, and H. O. Perry, Proc. Staff Meetings Mayo Clinic, 36, 217 (1961).

39. R. C. Laughlin and T. F. Carey, J Am. Med. Assoc., 181, 339 (1962).

40. D. Kritchevsky, A. W. Moyer, W. C. Tesar, R. F. J. McCandless, J. B. Logan, R. A. Brown and M. E. Englert, Angiology, 7, 156 (1956).

41. J. S. King, Jr., T. B. Clarkson, and N. H. Warnock, Circulation Res., 4, 162 (1956).

42. D. S. Fredrickson and D. Steinberg, Circulation, 15, 391 (1957).

43. J. Cottet and A. Mathivat, Presse Med., 63, 1005 (1955).

44. M. W. Biggs and D. Kritchevsky, Circulation, 4, 34 (1951).

45. M. W. Biggs, D. Kritchevsky, D. Colman, J. W. Gofman, H. B. Jones, F. T. Lindgren, G. Hyde, and T. P. Lyon, Circulation, 6, 359 (1952).

46. D. Kritchevsky, A. W. Moyer, W. C. Tesar, J. B. Logan, R. A. Brown, and G. Richmond, Circulation Res., 2, 340 (1954).

47. H. Buchwald, Diseases Chest, 51, 459 (1967).

48. L. A. Carlson and L. Orö, Acta Med. Scand., 172, 641 (1962).

49. D. Kritchevsky, in Nicotinic Acid Workshop (K. F. Gey and L. A. Carlson, eds.), Huber, Berne, in press.

50. D. Kritchevsky, in Drill's Pharmacology in Medicine, 4th ed. (J. R. DiPalma, ed.), McGraw-Hill, New York, in press.

51. A. Studer and K. Reber, Ergeb. Allgem. Pathol. Pathol. Anat., 43, 1 (1963).

52. R. Hess, in Adv. Lipid Res. (R. Paoletti and D. Kritchevsky, eds.), Vol. 2, Academic Press, New York, 1964, p. 296.

53. W. L. Bencze, R. Hess, and G. de Stevens, in Progr. Drug Res. (E. Jucker, ed.), Vol. 13, Birkhäuser, Basel, 1969, p. 217.

54. W. M. Sperry and W. Bergmann, J. Biol. Chem., 119, 171 (1937).

55. D. W. Peterson, Proc. Soc. Exptl. Biol. Med., 78, 143 (1951).

56. D. W. Peterson, C. W. Nichols, Jr., and E. A. Shneour, J. Nutr., 47, 57 (1952).

57. D. W. Peterson, E. A. Shneour, N. F. Peek, and H. W. Gaffey, J. Nutrition, 50, 191 (1953).

58. H. H. Hernandez and I. L. Chaikoff, Proc. Soc. Exptl. Biol. Med., 87, 541 (1954).

59. L. Swell, E. C. Trout, Jr., H. Field, Jr., and C. R. Treadwell, J. Biol. Chem., 234, 2286 (1959).

60. C. Joyner, Jr., and P. T. Kuo, Am. J. Med. Sci., 230, 636 (1955).

61. J. W. Farquhar, R. E. Smith, and M. E. Dempsey, Circulation, 14, 77 (1956).

62. Y. Aramaki, T. Kobayashi, Y. Imai, S. Kikuchi, T. Matsukawa, and K. Kanazawa, J. Atherosclerosis Res., 7, 653 (1967).

63. M. Ito, W. E. Connor, E. J. Blanchette, C. R. Treadwell, and G. V. Vahouny, J. Lipid Res., 10, 694 (1969).

64. Y. Imai, S. Kikuchi, T. Matsuo, Z. Suzuoki, and K. Nishikawa, J. Atherosclerosis Res., 7, 671 (1967).

65. K. Toki and H. Nakatani, in Progr. Biochem. Pharmacol. (D. Kritchevsky, R. Paoletti, and D. Steinberg, eds.), Vol. 2, S. Karger, Basel, 1967, p. 203.

66. D. Kritchevsky and S. A. Tepper, J. Atherosclerosis Res., 7, 527 (1967).

67. H. Fukushima, K. Toki, and H. Nakatani, J. Atherosclerosis Res., 9, 57 (1969).

68. K. Toki, personal communication.

69. H. Nakatani, H. Fukushima, A. Wakimura, and M. Endo, Science, 153, 1267 (1966).

70. H. Fukushima, S. Aono, Y. Nakamura, M. Endo, and T. Imai, J. Atherosclerosis Res., 10, 403 (1969).

71. J. H. Mueller, J. Biol. Chem., 27, 463 (1916).

72. M. D. Siperstein, I. L. Chaikoff, and W. O. Reinhardt, J. Biol. Chem., 198, 111 (1952).

V. DRUGS AFFECTING ATHEROSCLEROSIS

73. M. D. Siperstein, C. W. Nichols, Jr., and I. L. Chaikoff, Science, 117, 386 (1953).
74. D. M. Tennent, H. Siegel, M. E. Zanetti, G. W. Kuron, W. H. Ott, and F. J. Wolf, J. Lipid Res., 1, 469 (1960).
75. S. S. Bergen, T. B. Van Itallie, D. M. Tennent, and W. H. Sebrell, Proc. Soc. Exptl. Biol. Med., 102, 676 (1959).
76. S. A. Hashim and T. B. Van Itallie, J. Am. Med. Assoc., 192, 289 (1965).
77. P. Samuel and A. Steiner, Proc. Soc. Exptl. Biol. Med., 100, 193 (1959).
78. P. Samuel, Proc. Soc. Exptl. Biol. Med., 102, 194 (1959).
79. G. A. Goldsmith, J. G. Hamilton, and O. N. Miller, Arch. Internal Med., 105, 512 (1960).
80. H. Eyssen, E. Evrard, and H. Vanderhaeghe, J. Lab. Clin. Med., 68, 753 (1966).
81. D. P. Barr, Circulation, 8, 641 (1953).
82. D. P. Barr, J. Chronic Diseases, 1, 63 (1955).
83. M. F. Oliver and G. S. Boyd, Lancet, ii, 499 (1961).
84. J. Marmorston, F. J. Moore, C. E. Hopkins, O. T. Kuzma, and J. Weiner, Proc. Soc. Exptl. Biol. Med., 110, 400 (1962).
85. J. Stamler, R. Pick, L. N. Katz, A. Pick, B. M. Kaplan, D. M. Berkson, and D. Century, J. Am. Med. Assoc., 183, 632 (1963).
86. L. N. Katz and J. Stamler, Experimental Atherosclerosis, Thomas, Springfield, Illinois, 1953.
87. D. Kritchevsky, in Lipid Pharmacology (R. Paoletti, ed.), Academic Press, New York, 1964, p. 63.
88. P. Starr, P. Roen, J. L. Freibrun, and L. A. Schleissner, Arch. Internal Med., 105, 830 (1960).
89. B. M. Cohen, Current Therap. Res., 9, 618 (1967).
90. L. D. Bechtol and W. L. Warner, Angiology, 20, 565 (1969).
91. D. Kritchevsky, J. L. Moynihan, J. Langan, S. A Tepper, and M. L. Sachs, J. Atherosclerosis Res., 1, 211 (1961).
92. N. B. Myant, in Lipid Pharmacology (R. Paoletti, ed.), Academic Press, New York, 1964, p. 299.
93. D. Kritchevsky, Giorn. Arteriosclerosi, 5, 175 (1967).
94. S. Eriksson, Proc. Soc. Exptl. Biol. Med., 94, 582 (1957).

95. R. B. Failey, Jr., E. Brown, and M. E. Hodes, Am. J. Clin. Nutr., 11, 4 (1962).

96. T. A. Miettinen, J. Lab. Clin. Med., 71, 537 (1968).

97. C. H. Duncan, M. M. Best, and R. J. Lubbe, Metabolism, 13, 1 (1964).

98. J. M. Thorp and W. S. Waring, Nature, 194, 948 (1962).

99. K. G. Green and G. Margetts, in Progr. Biochem. Pharmacol. (D. Kritchevsky, R. Paoletti, and D. Steinberg, eds.), Vol. 2, S. Karger, Basel, 1967, p. 378.

100. G. G. Duncan, F. A. Elliott, T. G. Duncan, and J. Schatanoff, Metabolism, 17, 457 (1968).

101. A. Konttinen and J. Paloheimo, J. Atherosclerosis Res., 3, 525 (1963).

102. R. I. Levy, S. H. Quarfordt, W. V. Brown, H. R. Sloan, and D. S. Fredrickson, in Advan. Exptl. Med. Biol. (W. L. Holmes, L. A. Carlson, and R. Paoletti, eds.), Vol. 4, Plenum, New York, 1969, p. 377.

103. G. E. Owen Williams, M. J. Meynell, and R. Gaddie, J. Atherosclerosis Res., 3, 658 (1963).

104. E. H. Strisower, J. Atherosclerosis Res., 3, 445 (1963).

105. E. H. Strisower, Circulation, 33, 291 (1966).

106. R. Hess, W. Staübli, and W. Riess, Nature, 208, 856 (1965).

107. D. Svoboda, H. Grady, and D. Azarnoff, J. Cell. Biol., 35, 127 (1967).

108. R. Hess, W. Riess, and W. Staübli, in Progr. Biochem. Pharmacol. (D. Kritchevsky, R. Paoletti, and D. Steinberg, eds.), Vol. 2, S. Karger, Basel, 1967, p. 325.

109. D. Kritchevsky, S. A. Tepper, P. Sallata, J. R. Kabakjian, and V. J. Cristofalo, Proc. Soc. Exptl. Biol. Med., 132, 76 (1969).

110. D. Kritchevsky, P. Sallata, and S. A. Tepper, J. Atherosclerosis Res., 8, 755 (1968).

111. D. R. Avoy, E. A. Swyryd, and R. G. Gould, J. Lipid Res., 6, 369 (1965).

112. D. L. Azarnoff, D. R. Tucker, and G. A. Barr, Metabolism, 14, 959 (1965).

113. P. J. Nestel, E. Z. Hirsch, and E. A. Couzens, J. Clin. Invest., 44, 891 (1965).

114. M. E. Maragoudakis, Biochemistry, 9, 413 (1970).

115. R. Hess and W. L. Bencze, Experientia, 24, 418 (1968).
116. D. Kritchevsky and S. A. Tepper, Experientia, 25, 699 (1969).
117. G. Hartmann and G. Forster, J. Atherosclerosis Res., 10, 235 (1969).
118. P. Weiss, C. A. Dujovne, S. Margolis, L. Lasagna, and J. L. Bianchine, Clin. Pharmacol. Therap., 11, 90 (1970).
119. A. R. Timms, L. A. Kelly, R. S. Ho, and J. H. Trapold, Biochem. Pharmacol., 18, 1861 (1969).
120. L. A. Kelly and R. S. Ho, Federation Proc., 27, 242 (1968).
121. P. F. Hahn, Science, 98, 19 (1943).
122. E. D. Korn, J. Biol. Chem., 215, 1 (1955).
123. H. Engelberg, R. Kühn, and M. Steinman, Circulation, 13, 489 (1956).
124. R. Altschul, A. Hoffer, and J. D. Stephen, Arch. Biochem. Biophys., 54, 558 (1955).
125. W. B. Parsons, Jr., Arch. Internal Med., 107, 639 (1961).
126. W. B. Parsons, Jr., Arch. Internal Med., 107, 653 (1961).
127. L. A. Carlson, in Advan. Exptl. Med. Biol. (W. L. Holmes, L. A. Carlson, and R. Paoletti, eds.), Vol. 4, Plenum, New York, 1969, p. 327.
128. T. A. Miettinen, Clin. Chim. Acta, 20, 43 (1968).
129. H. S. Sodhi, L. Horlick, and B. Kudchodkar, Clin. Res., 17, 395, 663 (1969).
130. D. Kritchevsky, M. W. Whitehouse, and E. Staple, J. Lipid Res., 1, 154 (1960).
131. H. Lengsfeld, in Nicotinic Acid Workshop (K. F. Gey and L. A. Carlson, eds.), Huber, Berne, in press.
132. O. N. Miller, J. G. Hamilton, and G. A. Goldsmith, Am. J. Clin. Nutr., 8, 480 (1960).
133. J. N. Fain, D. J. Galton, and V. P. Kovacev, Mol. Pharmacol., 2, 237 (1966).
134. D. Steinberg, Ann. N. Y. Acad. Sci., 139, 897 (1967).
135. C. Dalton, C. Kowalski, J. Mallon, and C. Marschhaus, J. Atherosclerosis Res., 8, 265 (1968).
136. W. B. Parsons, Jr., Current Therap. Res., 2, 137 (1960).
137. E. J. Boyle, J. Am. Geriat. Soc., 10, 822 (1962).

138. H. Gurian and D. Adlersberg, Am. J. Med. Sci., 237, 12 (1959).
139. R. Altschul, Z. Kreislaufforsch., 45, 573 (1956).
140. J. D. Hunter and L. C. Wong, Arch. Pathol., 72, 465 (1961).
141. B. A. Kottke, J. L. Bollman and J. L. Juergens, Circulation Res., 11, 108 (1962).
142. P. Siegenthaler, Praxis, 25, 616 (1960).
143. R. Brattsand and L. Lundholm, Abstracts, 3rd Intern. Symp. Drugs Affecting Lipid Metabolism, Milan, Italy, 1968, p. 95.
144. G. Dell'Omodarme and F. Brunori, Boll. Chim. Farm., 100, 732 (1961).
145. H. Hammerl, C. Kränzl, O. Pichler, and M. Studlar, Wien. Klin. Wochschr., 80, 269 (1968).
146. G. Ratti and E. DeFina, Lancet, ii, 917 (1959).
147. W. Zeller, Klin. Wochschr., 44, 1022 (1966).
148. Z. N. Gaut and W. J. R. Taylor, J. Clin. Pharmacol., 8, 370 (1968).
149. E. R. Nye and P. A. McCaw, J. Pharmacol. Exptl. Therap., 167, 374 (1969).
150. J. J. Barboriak, R. C. Meade, J. Owenby, and R. A. Stiglitz, Arch. Intern. Pharmacodyn. Therap., 176, 249 (1968).
151. F. Kupiecki and N. B. Marshall, J. Pharmacol. Exptl. Therap., 160, 166 (1968).
152. J. N. Pereira, G. F. Holland, F. A. Hochstein, S. Gilgore, S. Defelice, and R. Pinson, J. Pharmacol. Exptl. Therap., 162, 142 (1968).
153. T. Shimamoto, F. Numano, and T. Fujita, Am. Heart J., 71, 216 (1966).
154. M. R. Malinow, A. Perley, and P. McLaughlin, J. Atherosclerosis Res., 8, 455 (1968).
155. T. Shimamoto and F. Numano, Atherogenesis, Excerpta Med. Found., Amsterdam, 1969.
156. T. Shimamoto, H. Maezawa, H. Yamazaki, T. Atsumi, T. Fujita, I. Ishioka, and T. Sunaga, Am. Heart J., 71, 297 (1966).
157. T. Shimamoto, T. Atsumi, S. Yamashita, T. Motomiya, N. Isokane, T. Ishioka, and A. Sakuma, Am. Heart J., 79, 5 (1970).
158. D. Kritchevsky and S. A. Tepper, Experientia, 23, 1006 (1967).
159. B. J. Ludwig, F. Duersch, M. Auerbach, K. Tomeczek, and F. M. Berger, J. Med. Chem., 10, 556 (1967).

160. F. M. Berger, B. J. Ludwig, J. F. Douglas, and S. Margolin, Abstracts, 3rd Intern. Symp. Drugs Affecting Lipid Metabolism, Milan, Italy, 1968, p. 88.

161. F. M. Berger, J. F. Douglas, G. G. Lu, and B. J. Ludwig, Proc. Soc. Exptl. Biol. Med., 132, 293 (1969).

162. D. Kritchevsky and S. A. Tepper, Arzneimittel Forsch., 20, 584 (1970).

163. D. Kritchevsky, P. Sallata, and S. A. Tepper, Proc. Soc. Exptl. Biol. Med., 132, 303 (1969).

164. J. F. Douglas, B. J. Ludwig, S. Margolin, and F. M. Berger, J. Atherosclerosis Res., 6, 90 (1966).

165. D. Kritchevsky, Federation Proc., 30, 825 (1971).

166. G. Lemoine, Bull. Soc. Med. Hop. Paris, 33, 227 (1912).

167. S. R. Rosenthal, Arch. Pathol., 18, 473 (1934).

168. J. Cornfield, Federation Proc., 21 (4) Part 2, 58 (1962).

169. D. S. Fredrickson and R. S. Lees, Circulation, 31, 321 (1965).

170. D. S. Fredrickson, R. I. Levy, and R. S. Lees, New Engl. J. Med., 276, 32, 94, 148, 215, 273 (1967).

171. R. I. Levy and D. S. Fredrickson, Am. J. Cardiol., 22, 576 (1968).

172. R. I. Levy, Modern Treatment, 6, 1313 (1969).

173. R. I. Levy and D. S. Fredrickson, Postgrad. Med., 47, 130 (1970).

174. R. Paoletti, Am. J. Clin. Nutr., 10, 277 (1962).

175. A. Kellner, J. W. Correll, and A. T. Ladd, J. Exptl. Med., 93, 373 (1951).

176. I. Chevillard, C. Bournique, H. Kagan, and R. Portet, Therapie, 20, 371 (1965).

177. R. H. Furman, R. P. Howard, M. R. Shetlar, E. C. Keaty, and R. Imagawa, Circulation, 17, 1076 (1958).

178. A. Castaigne and A. Amselem, Ann. Biol. Clin., 17, 336 (1959).

179. D. Kritchevsky, S. A. Tepper, P. Alaupovic, and R. H. Furman, Proc. Soc. Exptl. Biol. Med., 112, 259 (1963).

180. G. H. Rothblat, R. W. Hartzell, Jr., H. Mailhe, and D. Kritchevsky, Biochim. Biophys. Acta, 116, 133 (1966).

181. G. H. Rothblat and D. Kritchevsky, Biochim. Biophys. Acta, 144, 423 (1967).

182. G. H. Rothblat, M. Buchko, and D. Kritchevsky, Biochim. Biophys. Acta, 164, 327 (1968).

183. D. Kritchevsky, Cholesterol, Wiley, New York, 1958, p. 188.
184. J. Sjövall, Proc. Soc. Exptl. Biol. Med., 100, 676 (1959).
185. R. G. Herrmann, Circulation Res., 7, 224 (1959).
186. D. Kritchevsky, S. A. Tepper, and G. H. Rothblat, Lipids, 3, 454 (1968).
187. D. Kritchevsky, in Atherosclerotic Vascular Disease (A. N. Brest and J. H. Moyer, eds.), Appleton-Century-Crofts, New York, 1967, p. 1.
188. T. Zemplenyi, Z. Lojda, and O. Mrhová, in Atherosclerosis and Its Origin (M. Sandler and G. H. Bourne, eds.), Academic Press, New York, 1963, p. 459.
189. T. Zemplenyi, Enzyme Biochemistry of the Arterial Wall, Lloyd-Luke Ltd., London, 1968.
190. J. E. Kirk, Enzymes of the Arterial Wall, Academic Press, New York, 1969.
191. H. Field, Jr., L. Swell, P. E. Schools, Jr., and C. R. Treadwell, Circulation, 22, 547 (1960).
192. R. G. Gould, R. W. Wissler, and R. J. Jones, in Evolution of the Atherosclerotic Plaque (R. J. Jones, ed.), Univ. of Chicago Press, Chicago, 1963, p. 205.
193. G. H. Rothblat, R. Hartzell, Jr., H. Mailhe, and D. Kritchevsky, in Lipid Metabolism in Tissue Culture Cells (G. H. Rothblat and D. Kritchevsky, eds.), Wistar Inst. Symp., No. 6, Wistar Press, Philadelphia, 1967, p. 129.
194. N. Anitschkow, Verhandl. Deut. Ges. Pathol., 23, 473 (1928).
195. T. Leary, Arch. Pathol., 17, 453 (1934).
196. J. H. Bragdon, Circulation, 5, 641 (1952).
197. M. Friedman and S. O. Byers, Circulation, 16, 883 (1957).
198. R. N. Chakravarti, V. N. De, and B. Mukerji, Indian J. Med. Res., 44, 683 (1956).
199. P. Constantinides and N. Gutmann-Auersperg, Arch. Pathol., 70, 35 (1960).
200. M. Bevans, J. D. Davidson, and F. E. Kendall, Arch. Pathol., 51, 288 (1951).
201. R. Pick, J. Stamler, S. Rodbard, and L. N. Katz, Circulation, 6, 858 (1952).
202. D. D. Rutstein, E. F. Ingenito, J. M. Craig, and M. Martinelli, Lancet, i, 545 (1958).

V. DRUGS AFFECTING ATHEROSCLEROSIS

203. C. B. Taylor, G. E. Cox, and R. E. Trueheart, Ill. Med. J., 119, 80, (1961).
204. S. Dayton, M. L. Pearce, S. Hashimoto, W. J. Dixon, and U. Tomiyasu, Am. Heart Assoc. Monograph No. 25 (1969).
205. S. H. Rinzler, Bull. N.Y. Acad. Med., 44, 936 (1968).
206. O. Turpeinen, M. Miettinen, M. J. Karvonen, P. Roine, M. Pekkarinen, E. J. Lehtosuo, and P. Alivirta, Am. J. Clin. Nutr., 21, 255 (1968).
207. P. Leren, Acta Med. Scand., Suppl., 466 (1966).
208. A Research Committee Report, Lancet, ii, 693 (1968).
209. H. K. Schoch, in Advan. Exptl. Med. Biol. (W. L. Holmes, L. A. Carlson, and R. Paoletti, eds.), Vol. 4, Plenum, New York, 1969, p. 405.
210. M. F. Oliver, in Advan. Exptl. Biol. Med. (W. L. Holmes, L. A. Carlson, and R. Paoletti, eds.), Vol. 4, Plenum, New York, 1969, p. 339.
211. H. L. Ratcliffe, T. G. Yerasimides, and G. A. Elliott, Circulation, 21, 730 (1960).
212. H. L. Ratcliffe and R. L. Snyder, Circulation, 26, 1352 (1962).

Chapter VI

THE INTERFERON SYSTEM

Richard H. Adamson, Hilton B. Levy, and Samuel Baron

Laboratory of Chemical Pharmacology
National Cancer Institute and Laboratory of Viral Diseases
National Institute of Allergy and Infectious Diseases
National Institutes of Health
Bethesda, Maryland

I.	INTRODUCTION	292
II.	BIOMEDICAL ASPECTS OF THE INTERFERON SYSTEM	292
	A. Resistance to and Recovery from Viral Infection	292
	B. Antibody as a Defense against Viral Infection	293
	C. Nonimmunological Factors in Recovery from Established Viral Infections	293
III.	BIOCHEMICAL ASPECTS OF THE INTERFERON SYSTEM	295
	A. General Considerations	295
	B. Synthesis of the Interferon Protein — Control by Host Cell Genome	296
	C. Biological Properties	296
	D. The Molecular Basis of Interferon's Antiviral Activity	297
IV.	PHARMACOLOGICAL ASPECTS OF THE INTERFERON SYSTEM	299
	A. General Considerations	299
	B. Pharmacological Properties of Interferon	299
	C. Pharmacological Properties of Inducers of Interferon	300
	D. The Antitumor Effect of Interferons and Inducers of Interferon	303
V.	INTERFERON AND INTERFERON INDUCERS IN MAN	305
	A. Interferon	305
	B. Live Viruses	306
	C. Killed Viruses	306
	D. Pyran Copolymer	307
	E. Poly I · Poly C	307
VI.	CONCLUSIONS	310
	REFERENCES	311

Copyright © 1972 by Marcel Dekker, Inc. **NO PART** of this work may be reproduced or utilized in **any form or by any means**, electronic or mechanical, including Xeroxing, photocopying, microfilm, and recording, or by any information storage and retrieval system, without permission in writing from the publisher.

I. INTRODUCTION

It is surprising that most viral infections are self-limited when it is recognized that many hundreds of lethal doses of virus are ultimately produced in the infected tissues during infections initiated by sublethal amounts of virus. This observation has led to the recognition that potent host defenses are activated during virus multiplication.

The interferon defense system was discovered in 1957 by Isaacs and Lindenmann [1]. During the first decade after its recognition, most of the work on the interferon mechanism has been in relation to both its role during natural viral infections and its mechanism of action at the cellular and subcellular levels [2-8]. The fundamental information gained in these studies has recently begun to be applied to prevention and therapy of viral diseases of animals and man.

This chapter will consider biomedical, biochemical, and pharmacological aspects of the interferon system as well as clinical applications and the potential usefulness of the interferon system.

II. BIOMEDICAL ASPECTS OF THE INTERFERON SYSTEM

A. Resistance to and Recovery from Viral Infection

A schematic representation of the natural course of many viral diseases of susceptible animals or human beings is illustrated in Fig. 1. When virus is first implanted in a susceptible animal, it can be stated that the resistance to infection is low because the virus multiplies to high titers and frequently spreads through the body via the bloodstream. It then reaches target organs like the brain in the case of encephalitis and the skin during rash diseases. By multiplying there to high titers it causes the disease process. However,

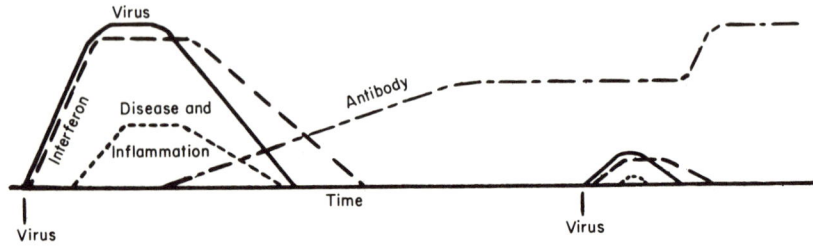

Fig. 1. A schematic representation of the natural course of many viral diseases and the host reaction to the viral infections.

VI. THE INTERFERON SYSTEM

most viral infections are self-limited. The limitation of the viral infection is first heralded by a decrease in the rate of viral growth and is followed by a declining titer of virus within the infected animal. Virus is eventually eliminated and the disease manifestations subside. The process by which virus growth is slowed and the virus is eventually eliminated may be termed the "recovery process," and it represents recovery from the already established viral infection. If the animal which has recovered from the viral infection is reexposed to the same antigenic type of virus then at most only a limited, local, and asymptomatic reinfection usually occurs. This is referred to as high resistance to infection. Thus, the susceptible host may initially have low resistance to infection and the recovered host may have high resistance to infection. By these criteria the resistance to reinfection can be distinguished from the ability of the animal to recover from a fully established infection.

B. Antibody as a Defense against Viral Infection

Over many years much evidence has accumulated to support the causal correlation of antibody with the high resistance to reinfection in the recovered animal [3-6, 9]. Although the causal correlation of antibody and resistance to reinfection seems to be secure, the causal correlation of antibody and recovery from a fully established viral infection has not been established and is in doubt. Recent evidence has reopened the possibility that cellular immunity may play a partial role in recovery but more studies are needed [10].

C. Nonimmunological Factors in Recovery from Established Viral Infections

There have been a number of studies of the role of nonimmunological factors in recovery from the already established viral infection. These nonimmunological mechanisms include the interferon system, the febrile response, local acidity, and local hypoxia at the site of infection [4]. Interferon has been the most carefully studied of these mechanisms and it will be considered in some detail.

Figure 2 schematizes two cells; the first is a cell infected by the virus and in which the virus replicates. During infection an unknown mechanism (possibly the viral RNA) is believed to signal the nucleus of the cell to derepress the normally repressed gene site which carries the information for interferon. Alternatively, preformed interferon may be activated and released from cells (see Sec. III. B). As a result, interferon is rapidly produced by the infected cell. The interferon itself does not inhibit the virus and so the infected cell may produce both virus and interferon. The interferon is rapidly released from the cell into the extracellular fluids where it comes in contact with surrounding and as yet uninfected cells. The available evidence indicates that reaction of the interferon with these cells results in the derepression of a second and distinct gene site within the cell [11]. This

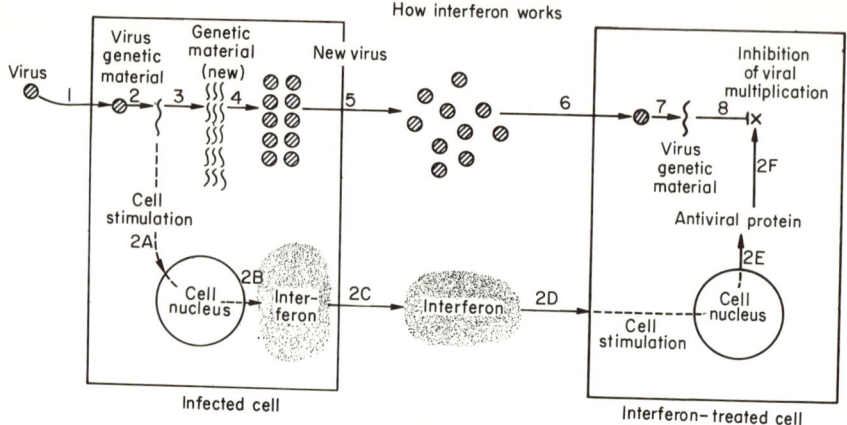

Fig. 2. Beginning at the left of the figure (1), virus comes in contact with the cell and penetrates the cell membrane. The virus then releases its genetic material (2), which organizes the cell to make many copies of the genetic material (3). The new genetic material (4) is coated with viral protein to form completed new virus, and (5) the new virus is released into the fluid around the cells where it can now spread to other cells. During the early stages of infection the process of viral multiplication within the cell stimulates the cell (2a) to utilize the stored information for interferon synthesis. Through a series of complex procedures, the interferon protein is made (2b) and released rapidly (2c) into the extracellular fluid. In some cases there may exist in cells a preformed but inactive interferon protein which can be activated by certain stimuli. In many instances, the interferon precedes new virus to surrounding cells. The interferon stimulates the surrounding cells (2d) to utilize another set of stored information to produce an intracellular antiviral protein (2e). The antiviral protein (2f) acts to change the cell's protein-synthesizing machinery so that it cannot be used by viral genetic material subsequently encountered. Therefore, any infection by new virus of the interferon-protected cell (6) still leads to release of the viral genetic material (7), but that viral genetic material is discriminated against by the cell synthesizing machinery (8) and essential viral materials fail to be produced. Thus, viral multiplication is inhibited and the cell is protected.

second gene site appears to code for a protein which is antiviral and remains intracellular. Details will be considered in the section on biochemistry.

The functioning of the interferon system to inhibit the replication of viruses intracellularly makes the interferon mechanism a likely candidate as an important factor in recovery from viral infection. Studies examining the causal relationship of interferon to recovery indicate a positive correlation [2-7, 10]. Interferon has been shown in many systems to be produced within the infected tissue within a few hours of virus infection.

VI. THE INTERFERON SYSTEM   295

Interferon and the antiviral state which it induces is present not only before but during the recovery process from virus infection. Systems in which the interferon mechanism has been rendered inactive demonstrate an impaired ability to recover with the expected increased mortality. Studies involving the transfer of interferon have demonstrated that interferon can prevent viral infection and in a few instances enhance recovery from certain established viral infections [12-14]. Finally, interferon induces a nonspecific resistance to many types of viruses — a property which coincides with the nonspecific resistance to viruses manifested by naturally recovering organs.

Taken together the available evidence strongly supports the idea that antibody which prevents spread of virus normally functions to prevent reinfection by viruses which have previously infected that organism. Antibody may also terminate viremia during the primary infection and thereby protect target organs from severe infection [15]. On the other hand, interferon and other nonimmunological mechanisms are strongly implicated in recovery from the already established viral infection.

III. BIOCHEMICAL ASPECTS OF THE INTERFERON SYSTEM

A. General Considerations

Interferon is a protein elaborated by most cells as a response to infection by most viruses [3]. The amount of interferon synthesized varies greatly with the cells synthesizing the interferon and with the virus used to stimulate its induction. When solutions containing this protein are incubated with other cells for several hours, under conditions which allow the cells to synthesize RNA and protein, these cells develop resistance to subsequent virus infection; that is to say, they synthesize less virus when infected than do cells not previously exposed to interferon. The amount of resistance developed varies greatly, both with the type of cell and the virus used to test the resistance. The requirement for RNA and protein synthesis is interpreted to mean that the antiviral activity requires the mediation of a new interferon-induced protein. Interferon shows a high degree of specificity for the animal species — that is, chicken interferon does not protect mouse cells, etc. It shows no specificity for the virus; for example, interferon produced by stimulation with influenza virus is indistinguishable from that produced upon stimulation by Newcastle disease virus in its ability to inhibit the replication of a broad range of viruses. Isaacs originally predicted that the foreign nucleic acid was the essential stimulus for induction of interferon [3,16]. However, technical problems prevented the firm establishment of this concept for a number of years. Recent findings have reawakened interest in nucleic acid as the stimulus for induction of interferon.

Evidence bearing on the nature of the viral inducer of interferon comes from the findings that double-stranded RNA derived from MS2 phage, other phages, reovirus, or even several synthetic double-stranded RNAs can induce interferon [17-21]. More recently it has been shown that single-stranded RNAs and DNA can induce interferon [22,24].

The concept of a single type of inducer substance or a single inducer mechanism for interferon is appealing for its simplicity and may hold true for most cell types. However, the variety of inducers under certain conditions suggests that the derepression mechanism may vary with the cell being induced. There is increasing evidence to suggest that a few cell types (lymphoid-type cells) are capable of being induced by stimuli which are insufficient to induce most cell types [8]. Examples include phytohemagglutinin stimulation of leukocytes, polkweed mitogen stimulation of leukocytes, endotoxin stimulation of explanted macrophages, antigen stimulation of sensitized lymphocytes, mannan stimulation of macrophages, and spontaneous production of interferon by macrophages and leukocytes. It is not yet clear whether pyran copolymers induced cell types other than leukocytes and macrophages.

B. Synthesis of the Interferon Protein — Control by Host Cell Genome

Five observations suggest the information for the synthesis of interferon resides in host cell DNA: (1) the high degree of cell specificity of the antiviral action of interferon, (2) the similarity of the interferon produced regardless of the inducing virus, and (3) the lack of immunological relationship between viral proteins and interferon. (4) Antibody against interferon is species specific. (5) Evidence of a more biochemical nature has been obtained through the use of actinomycin D, which inhibits DNA dependent RNA synthesis. This inhibitor blocks the synthesis of interferon both in tissue culture and in vivo even when the inducing virus is insensitive to actinomycin D. Also, studies using the protein inhibitors puromycin and fluorophenylalanine showed that active synthesis of protein was needed to produce interferon. However, host DNA synthesis is not needed for interferon production [7,8].

C. Biological Properties

The word interferon was conceived originally because of the viral interfering activity of a substance in fluids that had been in contact with virus infected cells. It soon became apparent that the responsible factor was proteinaceous. It later developed that this biological activity was associated with entities of different molecular weights, ranging between 30,000 and over 100,000.

Several properties are shared by all of the substances which have been called interferon: (1) Interferons do not directly inactivate virus but induce cellular metabolic alterations which inhibit viral replication. (2) There is relative species specificity, in that an interferon produced by cells of a given animal species is most active in cells of the same species. Diminished antiviral activity is frequently found in the cells of closely related species. (3) Antiviral activity is exerted against a wide variety of viruses. (4) There is no antigenic relationship between interferon, which is a product of a cell gene, and the virus or any virus specified product (see Ref. [3,7,25]).

Many of the early appearing interferons, which tend to have higher molecular weights may be "preformed." That is, their production is not inhibited under conditions of strong inhibition of cell RNA and protein synthesis in vivo and in vitro [26]. Virus stimulation of animals leads to early appearance of this high molecular weight interferon and to later appearance of much larger amounts of low (30,000) or intermediate (68,000) molecular weight interferons the synthesis of which, in contrast, is blocked by inhibition of RNA and protein synthesis [27]. These observations have been interpreted as indicating that the early appearing high molecular weight interferon was already present in some cells and can be released into the serum. The light interferon was newly synthesized after stimulation.

Most interferons have been found to be stable over a wide pH range. In general, exposure of interferon to pH 2-10 has no effect upon biological activity [28]. This stability makes it possible to destroy most residual viruses by acidifying interferon preparations to pH 2. Most species of interferon studied seem to retain this pH stability even after extensive purification. Some forms of human interferon, however, have been reported to be unstable at pH 3 or less.

Several factors have been observed to effect the development of cellular resistance to viruses during exposure to interferon. This section will utilize the working interpretation that resistance which is induced by interferon is a reflection of the intracellular production and accumulation of an antiviral protein [11]. It was generally agreed that metabolic activity was needed for development of interferon's antiviral action. Taylor [11] noted that actinomycin D blocked the development of antiviral activity in cells treated with interferon and concluded that DNA directed RNA synthesis was needed. It was shown that fluorophenylalanine (FPA), an inhibitor of functional protein synthesis, also prevented the antiviral action of interferon [29,30].

The need for protein synthesis to induce antiviral activity is related to the synthesis of modified ribosomal subunits and ribosomes (interferon-type ribosomes) in which reside the ability to block viral replication (see Sec. III. D). Using the concept that modified ribosomal subunits and ribosomes account for interferon's antiviral action, the available evidence is probably best explained by the interpretation that the finally established level of viral resistance is maintained by a continual induction by interferon of modified subunits and ribosomes which serve to replace decaying subunits and ribosomes.

D. The Molecular Basis of Interferon's Antiviral Activity

The locus of action of interferon has been shown to be on a step in virus replication that occurs after the penetration and uncoating of virus, since interferon exerts its antiviral action even when infectious viral RNA (or DNA) is used as the challenge. Also, the synthesis of new viral RNA is inhibited in cells treated with interferon. The synthesis of replicative forms of viral RNA has been shown to be blocked in interferon treated cells.

These as well as other consequences of interferon on virus specified events, such as synthesis of infectious RNA, virus induced enzymes, and proteins, may be explained by the fact that interferon has an effect on the earliest interaction of the RNA of the infecting particle with a cellular component (see Refs. [7,24]). During the course of a normal infection of L cells with Mengo virus, the earliest detected event involving the viral genome is its association with a small cell component, probably the 40S ribosomal subunit. This association is detectable 30 min after infection. As virus replication proceeds, the RNA of the parental virus is found on the viral polysome where viral proteins are made. Some viral RNA synthetase is found in association with this polysome. In cells pretreated with interferon, the association of the viral RNA with the 40S subunit is greatly inhibited. Some virus polysome-like material is found late in infection in these interferone treated cells, but it is not functional in that it does not synthesize viral proteins. As would be expected, the viral RNA synthetase is found in greatly decreased amounts in interferon treated cells [31-34].

Interferon treatment of vaccinia virus infected L cells also prevents the incorporation of virus mRNA into a virus polysome [35]. Analysis of this reaction is complicated by the fact that initial association of the mRNA with the 40S subunit is not always measurable in L cells. To examine the effects of interferon on vaccinia virus mRNA-40S subunit association, it would be necessary to utilize HeLa cells in which this association is more readily observable. These observations, made in whole cells, are supported and amplified by experiments made with isolated ribosomes from interferon treated and control cells. Interferon type and control ribosomes from mouse L cells and chick cells bind cell RNA and bind and translate synthetic polynucleotides equally well, but only the control ribosomes bind and translate viral RNA [34,36]. A short treatment of the interferon type chick ribosomes with trypsin augments somewhat its ability to bind and translate the viral RNA, suggesting that the interferon type ribosomes contains additional proteins that enable it to distinguish between cell and viral RNA [36].

The in vivo and in vitro data indicate that the action of interferon is to cause the modification of the 40S ribosomal subunits and the ribosomes. These modified structures are able to carry out the synthesis of normal cell proteins, and so support normal cell growth. They are able to reject viral RNA to a large extent, and so virus growth is inhibited. Closely related to the RNA recognition mechanisms is the observation that the RNA for the oncogenic virus T antigen is inhibited in interferon treated cells during acute infection but not in transformed cells where the viral genome is somehow integrated with the host genome [37].

Also of interest are observations that interferon inhibits the growth of Toxoplasma in tissue culture and may inhibit the growth of Plasmodium berghei in animals [38-40]. Both of these organisms are obligate intracellular parasites. Their sensitivity to the action of interferon may indicate that they need host cell ribosomes for their replications or that their ribosome may become modified by the host's antiviral protein.

It is apparent that the basic effect of interferon is on normal cells, and not on the infecting virus. It will be recalled that the establishment of the

VI. THE INTERFERON SYSTEM

virus resistant state in interferon treated cells requires the synthesis of cellular RNA and protein subsequent to the exposure to interferon and prior to exposure to the challenge virus.

Future research with interferon may prove useful in understanding a wide range of biochemical and biological problems, some of which have been suggested by topics considered in this chapter. Studies of the two derepression steps involved in the interferon system may improve understanding the activation of gene function. Also, since the action of interferon involves the ability of ribosomes to make distinctions among different RNAs, future investigations should throw light on the control of protein synthesis at the ribosomal level.

IV. PHARMACOLOGICAL ASPECTS OF THE INTERFERON SYSTEM

A. General Considerations

As has been mentioned previously, a number of substances other than viruses can lead to the production of interferon. These substances include microorganisms, bacterial endotoxins, rickettsiae, mold products such as helenine and statolon, various polyanions such as the pyran copolymers, the recently described synthetic RNAs such as polyinosinic·polycytidylic acid and the orally active bis-DEAE-fluorenone (3, 7-bis[2-(diethylamino) ethoxy] fluorene-9-1-dihydrochloride) [17,41-45]. All of these agents lead to the production of interferon in vivo, but only a few of these agents are active in tissue culture. Current evidence suggests that some of these agents such as bacterial endotoxins release preformed interferon from cells whereas other agents and viruses lead to the synthesis of interferon.

B. Pharmacological Properties of Interferon

Four pharmacological properties of interferon have been described in detail in Sec. II and III. These include the broad antiviral spectrum of interferon, the necessity of time for activity, the requirement for cellular metabolic response, and the relative species specificity. Three other properties of interferon will be described here; its apparent low antigenicity, its toxicity, and its physiological disposition.

Although interferons are proteins, they seem to be poor antigens. The poor antigenicity of interferon may only be apparent since even very active preparations contain very small amounts of interferon protein. In particular, homologous interferons have not been shown to be antigenic and preparations of heterologous interferon evoked a relatively weak antibody response [46]. If interferons play an important role in the defense of the individual against viruses, it seems unlikely that they would be antigenic in the homologous species.

The protection of mice against systemic virus infections by intraperitoneal, intramuscular, or subcutaneous injections of interferon indicates that the agent must be absorbed from these sites of injection. Interferons injected intravenously into mice or rabbits disappear rapidly from the blood. The serum half-time of virus-induced interferon in the rabbit is 11 min. After intravenous injection of interferon in mice, 40% could be detected in the serum, kidney, and liver 5-13 min later, provided these tissues were promptly frozen when harvested. Less interferon was found in the liver if it was held at room temperature for 30 min before freezing [47-49]. Various workers have shown that blood does not break down interferon, but that it may be broken down by the liver or gut. However, isolated perfused rabbit liver did not inactivate exogenous interferon even though these liver preparations were functional with regard to breakdown of other proteins [50]. Only small amounts of injected interferon, 0.2-2.0%, appear in the urine [49]. Also no interferon could be detected in urines collected from 30 children in the acute stages of measles, mumps, or chicken-pox, even though some of the urine samples were concentrated by pressure dialysis before assay [51]. No interferon has been found in the bile of rabbits inoculated with Newcastle disease virus and interferon induced in pregnant rabbits by this virus apparently crosses the placenta to a slight extent one week before term [49,52]. Studies of this type have also demonstrated blood-brain and blood-eye barriers to the diffusion of interferon.

Although studies to date indicate that interferon has little or no toxicity, these studies are mitigated by the fact that the amounts of interferon needed for clinical effects in man have not been definitively assessed. The lack of antigenicity to homologous interferon has previously been mentioned. Thus, a child 6 years old who received over 3 liters of fluid containing interferon during 440 days did not develop antibodies to the interferon. Up to 30 ml per day of crude leukocyte interferon have been given intravenously to newborn humans with various viral diseases without evidence of toxicity other than shivering and slight malaise [53]. Human leukocyte interferon sprayed into the nose of volunteer patients produced no untoward reactions [54]. Likewise animal interferon preparations have little toxicity in vivo or in vitro [55-58].

C. Pharmacological Properties of Inducers of Interferon

The Pharmacological properties of three inducers of interferon which have been or are of promise for clinical trial will be considered. These three inducers are pyran copolymers, poly I· poly C (polyriboinosinic · polyribocytidylic acid complex) and bis-DEAE-fluorenone (BDF).

Pyran copolymer fractions of molecular weight of 17,000 to 450,000 induce interferon production after intraperitoneal administration to mice. The interferon levels induced by pyran copolymers are between 159 and 246 units. A molecular weight of 17,000 may be required to prevent urinary excretion. A required structure for interferon induction by pyran copolymers appears to be a saturated linear polymer with carboxylate groups on 2 of every 4 or 5 carbons in either alternate or adjacent positions. The interferon inducing capacity appears to be altered by bulky modifying groups which sterically hinder the carboxylate groups in their interaction with the cell. Thus, when the anionic groups are completely substituted or are not present, the polymers lack activity [41,59]. One pyran copolymer (copolymer of divinyl ether and maleic anhydride) of molecular weight 17,000 has been tested in mice and man and induces interferon in both species. Pyran copolymer produced moderate splenic enlargement in normal mice and in man produced a thrombocytopenia which was dose limiting. In addition this compound (NSC-46015) deposited in white cells and in the reticuloendothelial cells [60] (see Sect. V). Some of the toxicity of this compound may be due to its slow breakdown in the body.

Polyriboinosinic · polyribocytidylic acid (poly I·poly C) is an effective inducer of interferon and is active against viral infection in vivo and in vitro [14,18,61]. In investigations of a series of naturally occurring RNA's and various complexed polynucleotides, homopolymers, copolymers, oligonucleotides, nucleotides, nucleosides, and bases of nucleic acids, the essential feature for very high biological activity seemed to be complex formation (double strandedness) and polymer length [18]. Not only poly I·poly C, but also poly A·poly U, and mixtures of polyinosinic acid and cytidylylcytidine (poly I + CpC) were active in microgram amounts in inducing interferon in rabbits. A variety of homopolymers and copolymers tested singly and in combination were inactive, as were a large number of oligonucleotides, dinucleotides, nucleotides, nucleosides, and free bases. A requirement of double strandedness was also shown for the RNA (HeI-RNA) isolated from extracts of Penicillium funiculosum and for the double stranded RNA from type 3 reovirus virions [17,21]. However, as previously mentioned, recent reports indicate that synthetic single stranded RNA's can induce amounts of interferon in quantities of 1/10 to 1/100 of that induced by the double stranded molecule under certain conditions [22].

The high activity of poly I·poly C against experimental viral infections in vivo and in vitro has lead to a study of its toxicologic properties prior to clinical trial [62]. The acute LD_{50} dose of poly I·poly C administered i.p. to $CD_2 F_1$ mice was 34.7 mg/kg (95% confidence interval of 30.1 to 39.9; slope of 1.34). Beagle dogs tolerated 28 daily i.v. injections of poly I·poly C at doses of 0.03 to 1 mg/kg. Injections of 3, 5 or 10 mg/kg i.v. resulted in lethality after 1 to 4 doses. Autopsy of dogs at death revealed congestion of several organs and engorgement of the cerebral vasculature. Signs of toxicity preceding death from single i.v. doses were reminiscent of anaphylactic or endotoxin shock except for the relative slowness of the response. Typically, the dog vomited repeatedly and passed loose watery stools. The extremities became cold to the touch although the rectal temperature rose 2-3° F. The dog then became ataxic, the blood pressure fell to 35-50 mm Hg, the animal lost its ability to stand, and finally lost consciousness. Three hours after dosing, the animal died by respiratory failure. Two hours after dosing, the blood did not coagulate and prothrombin activity was indetectable. Serum transaminase and alkaline phosphatase activities had increased four- to ten-fold at this time. The most consistent biochemical response observed in dogs at all dose levels were abnormally high serum glutamic oxaloacetic transaminase (SGOT), serum glutamic pyruvic transaminase (SGPT), and alkaline phosphatase. Prolonged increases in prothrombin time and decreased hemoglobin and hematocrit were also seen. Recovery of hematocrit and hemoglobin values required 1-3 weeks after the last dose. Rhesus monkeys also tolerated doses greater than 1 mg/kg for only a few days but were able to survive 28 daily doses of 0.1, 0.3, or 1 mg/kg. Animals dying at high doses exhibited salivation, emesis, and depression, and upon autopsy showed myocardial infarction and engorgement of a variety of organs including heart, liver, lung, and kidney. Frequent hematological and biochemical changes seen at all dose levels included anemia and elevated SGOT and lactic dehydrogenase activities [62]. The various lesions seen in dogs and monkeys together with the marked thrombocytopenia and prolonged prothrombin time are compatible with the concept that high doses of poly I· poly C given intravenously caused intravascular clotting which resulted in a consumptive coagulopathy and secondary hemorrhagic lesions, shock, and death. This concept would account for the marked decrease in toxicity when poly I· poly C is given by routes other than i.v. and lack of severe toxicity with topical use.

Poly I· poly C was also found to be embryotoxic when given to pregnant rabbits. Thus poly I· poly C produced 100% resorptions when given s.c. on days 8 and 9 to pregnant rabbits at 2 mg/kg. Similar effects were obtained using 1 mg/kg since 80% of the implantations underwent resorption. The compound was also embryotoxic when given on days 11 and 12. Poly I· poly C did not seem to possess significant teratogenic activity under these experimental conditions since only three fetuses were grossly malformed as compared to two controls. It is of interest that poly I· poly C treatment of pregnant rats at 8 mg/kg on days 7 and 8 of pregnancy did not produce any resorptions or malformations [62, 63]. Because of its potential usefulness as an interferon inducer and its embryotoxic effects, poly I· poly C was tested in newborn mice for possible carcinogenic properties. The compound did not possess significant carcinogenic activity when evaluated on a variety of doses and schedules. Thus only two pulmonary tumors were observed out of 55 mice which were treated. This incidence of pulmonary tumors was comparable to that of untreated mice in the colony. No other tumors could be detected in other organs or tissues [64]. Consideration of this and other data on toxicity of poly I· poly C in animals led to the conclusions that safe dosage levels of poly I · poly C could be used in carefully monitored studies in man. Intravenous use of the compound was therefore planned in the treatment of malignant tumors or severe viral illness for which there was no adequate therapy.

Few toxicity studies have thus far been done on bis-DEAE-fluorenone. Oral and intraperitoneal acute LD_{50} doses for mice are 959 mg/kg and 145 mg/kg. The minimum effective single oral dose is 10 to 25 mg/kg varying with the type of infecting virus [44, 45]. Further antiviral, pharmacological, and toxicity studies are needed on this compound and its congeners before its role in human therapy can be established.

D. The Antitumor Effect of Interferons and Inducers of Interferon

Various murine leukemias such as those induced by the Friend virus are inhibited by exogenous interferon [13]. In addition, the growth of a dimethylbenzanthracene induced tumor is also inhibited by interferon. Statolon, an inducer of interferon, also inhibits leukemia induced by Friend virus [65,66]. Pyran copolymer also has an antitumor effect and reduces the gross splenic enlargement normally seen with Friend leukemia virus [41].

The interferon inducer poly I · poly C also exerts a potent inhibitory effect against experimental tumors in mice and rats [62, 67-71]. Results presented in Table I summarize the activity of poly I · poly C against several experimental tumors. Generally the optimal antitumor dose was 10 mg/kg/day or 20 mg/kg every other day given intraperitoneally. As can be seen, the reticulum cell sarcomas J96132 and A-RCS are the most responsive mouse tumors to poly I · poly C. Comparable antitumor effect is also shown against the rat Walker 256 carcinosarcoma. Poly I · poly C was generally less active against the experimental plasma cell tumor YPC-1 and the mouse leukemias. In a study of factors affecting the antitumor activity of poly I · poly C, it was demonstrated that the compound was effective when given subcutaneously or intraperitoneally but without effect when given orally [69]. Poly I · poly C gave the same degree of response in mice of either sex, but better antitumor activity was generally seen when poly I · poly C was given every other day or every third day than when administered daily. In addition, the homopolymers poly I and poly C manifest lower antitumor activity [70]. Since poly I · poly C is a potent inducer of interferon in mice, it is likely that at least a part of the antitumor action of the double-stranded RNA is through the interferon system.

A second aspect of the activity of poly I · poly C may be as a direct chemotherapeutic agent. Poly I · poly C is a double-stranded RNA, the homopolymers of which can code for the synthesis of polypeptides in a suitable cell-free test system. Poly C, for example should code for the synthesis of polyproline. If the poly C component of the poly I · poly C were responsible for the synthesis of polyproline in the cell, one might imagine any number of cellular reactions to the presence of this "nonsense" protein. Poly I · poly C does stimulate the incorporation of proline into the proteins of L-cells but it also stimulates incorporation of a number of other amino acids for which it should not code. Further, polyadenylic-polyurydilic acid also stimulates proline incorporation, for which it does not code and it does not stimulate phenylalanine incorporation for which the poly U would code. One can conclude that the double-stranded RNA's do stimulate amino acid incorporation into proteins, but are not acting intracellularly as synthetic messenger RNA's.

Altered macromolecular metabolism is also seen in animals. Experiments were done with C57 black Kaplan strain of mice bearing the J96132

TABLE I

Effect of Poly I · Poly C on Various Tumors

Tumor[a]	Percent Increase in Median Survival over Control
Leukemia L1210	35
Plasma cell YPC-1	39
Ehrlich Ascites	70
Carcinosarcoma Walker 256	100
Reticulum cell sarcoma A-RCS	89
Reticulum cell sarcoma J96132	130
Reticulum cell sarcoma ovarian	20
Leukemia P388	16
Leukemia K1964	12

[a] All experimental tumors are carried in the mouse with the exception of the Walker 256 carcinosarcoma which is carried in Sprague-Dawley rats.

reticulum cell sarcoma, the tumor most sensitive to poly I·poly C. The animals received poly I·poly C overnight and ^{14}C-proline and ^{3}H-uridine in the morning. Poly I·poly C treatment caused marked inhibition of protein and RNA synthesis in the tumor. This inhibition ranged from 60 to 95% in different experiments. It appears reasonable to think that this inhibition of protein synthesis would be inhibitory to tumor growth. It is possible however that the tumors had been damaged by some other mechanism and that the decreased protein synthesis was a reflection of this, rather than a cause of the tumor inhibition [71].

A third facet of the antitumor action of poly I·poly C is its ability to enhance cell mediated defense mechanisms against foreign antigens such as those in tumor cells. If spleen cells from adult mice are injected into newborn F_1 hybrids, one of whose parents is the strain of the donor mice, the donor cells develop a graft versus host reaction which affects the recipient animals in a number of ways. One of these is the establishment of a splenomegaly in the recipient. The degree of spleen enlargement is a function of the activity and the logarithm of the number of donor cells. This test is useful in evaluating immune suppressive drugs and antilymphocytic serum. The depressed reactivity of the spleen cells from treated donor animals results in less of a splenomegaly in the recipient than do spleen cells from untreated donors. When donor mice are given poly I · poly C their subsequently removed spleen cells show enhanced immunological reactivity against the foreign antigens in the recipient and result in increased splenomegaly [71].

It is reasonable to think that enhancement by poly I · poly C of such cell mediated rejections of foreign antigens could effectively act against the foreign antigens of the tumor, facilitating the rejection of the tumors. Indeed, the inhibition of macromolecular synthesis discussed earlier may be a manifestation of such cellular immunological activity. Such enhancement of immunological reactivity by polynucleotides has been observed previously [72].

V. INTERFERON AND INTERFERON INDUCERS IN MAN

A. Interferon

Interferons made from tissue cultures of monkey cells can inhibit the growth of viruses in human cells and interferons made from this source have been used in a few volunteer experiments and clinical trials. In the first volunteer study, 38 volunteers were vaccinated at two sites in the arm 5 cm apart. At one site, 0.1 ml of monkey interferon had been injected on the previous day and at the other site "dummy" control material. Interferon treatment led to a statistically significant reduction in the incidence of vaccinia virus infection [73]. In addition the same preparation of interferon gave encouraging clinical results in the treatment of six cases of eye infection with vaccinia virus [74]. In another study, large quantities of interferon prepared from human leukocytes or amnion cells were injected into patients with acute leukemia and into three babies with cytomegalic viral disease. The three babies infected with cytomegalic virus, normally a fatal disease, survived and there was a generally favorable clinical impression in most of the patients. However, the authors drew no definite conclusions from the study [53]. In another study human leukocyte interferon gave a marked protective effect against influenza viral infections especially when applied intranasally 2 h or preferably 24 h and 2 h before infection [54].

These studies suggest that interferon per se may be useful in humans and a number of systems for the large scale manufacture of interferon have been suggested. One of the most promising methods is the use of human leukocytes obtained as by-products from blood transfusion centers. Optimal conditions for the production of such interferon have been described [53, 75]. Another system has been described which involves the mass production of interferon from intact amniotic membranes in organ culture [76]. If interferon itself could be mass produced, it might be of considerable use in clinical medicine for control of viral infections and perhaps as an antineoplastic agent. It is within the range of possibility that the interferon polypeptide could be produced synthetically in the not too distant future. This synthetic production would require prior purification and determination of its amino acid sequence.

B. Live Viruses

The basis for studies of induction of interferon in man has come from prior studies in animals. When it was recognized that many instances of viral interference in animals were mediated at least in part by the interferon system, it was logical to conclude that similar manifestations of viral interference in man could be mediated by the same system. The search for interferon during natural viral infections of man quickly confirmed this hypothesis. In this way interferon has been detected in human tissue and body fluid samples from diverse virus infections of the upper and lower respiratory tract, the alimentary tract, the nervous system, the skin, and the vascular system [77-85].

Analogously, live virus vaccines and non-attenuated viruses have been observed to induce interferon in man and to interfere with challenge viruses [86-89]. For example, live polio vaccine virus interferes with other strains of live polio virus vaccine, measles vaccine virus inhibits vaccination at the time interferon is maximal in the circulation, vaccinia virus interferes with local infection with yellow fever virus vaccine, and yellow fever vaccine virus interferes with live measles vaccine virus [90-94].

Live virus vaccines also have been observed to protect against natural infection by wild viruses; e.g., live polio virus vaccine inhibits antigenically unrelated types of enteroviruses in the human alimentary tract [90,95], yellow fever vaccine virus inhibits natural dengue virus infection [96], measles virus vaccine inhibits natural influenza B virus infection even as late as three days after natural infection has begun [97,98].

The recent observations that inducers of interferon as well as interferon itself can inhibit a wide range of animal tumors of apparent spontaneous, carcinogen and virus-etiology suggests that the antitumor effect of experimental viral infections in some cases may be associated with the induction or action of interferon [99-101]. In one such instance apparent virus-induced remissions during human leukemia were accompanied by interferon production [100].

C. Killed Viruses

Experiments in animals have demonstrated that many types of inactivated viruses protect against subsequent infection by means of induction of the interferon system. This principle has been applied to man in the form of ultraviolet light inactivated influenza virus or heat inactivated arbovirus group A, Semliki forest virus strain. Protection in man against naturally occurring influenza or against live influenza vaccine virus has been reported to occur following intranasal instillation of ultraviolet light irradiated influenza virus [102]. Similarly the heat inactivated Semliki forest virus inducer of interferon has been employed to prevent and to treat several different types of virus infections in man [103]. Some of these human trials were reported to be carefully controlled. In this way protection from eye infections has been related to herpes simplex virus, and from adenovirus, trachoma, and skin infections to herpes simplex virus and herpes zoster virus.

D. Pyran Copolymer

The observation that the antitumor agent, pyran copolymer, is capable of inducing interferon *in vivo* has led to a study of its ability to induce interferon in human cancer patients [41,42]. The circulating interferon response was found to depend on the dose of pyran copolymer in that 12 mg/kg of body weight produced antiviral activity in the serum of only 1 of 4 patients but 15 to 16 mg/kg of body weight was consistently effective in 3 patients. These levels of circulating interferon previously had been shown to be capable of prophylactically protecting against several viral infections, both in animals and in man [73]. Pyran copolymer has been found to be broken down slowly within the body and therefore exerts a prolonged inducing effect. However, this slow breakdown may account for some of the observed toxicity which includes thrombocytopenia and granules within leukocytes [42]. The pyran copolymers do exert an antitumor effect which may be related to their ability to induce interferon [104].

E. Poly I· Poly C

The finding that poly I· poly C is among the most potent synthetic inducers of interferon, its availability, and its acceptable toxicity at doses that induce interferon has lead to a number of experimental applications in animals and to clinical trial of poly I· poly C.

1. Herpes Simplex Encephalitis

The first patient treated intravenously with poly I· poly C was a four and one-half month old white male with herpes simplex encephalitis. The child was comatose and had frequent generalized convulsions for 3 days before treatment was begun [105]. During this time both a brain biopsy and lumbar puncture yielded specimens with characteristic findings for herpes simplex encephalitis; virus was recovered from both brain tissue and cerebrospinal fluid. This patient was treated with 0.1 mg/kg/day of poly I· poly C for 11 days. The drug was given in a single daily dose by slow intravenous injection with the exception of the first day when the drug was given in two equally divided doses. Within 12 hours of the first dose the convulsions stopped and his high fever began to decrease. The patient improved but he was left with residual mental retardation and motor spasticity. He developed a seizure disorder which responded well to anticonvulsant therapy. Eight months after the patient was discharged he died of overwhelming bacterial sepsis secondary to otitis media. An autopsy showed the brain to be grossly normal and there was no microscopic evidence of residual brain damage. Virus isolation attempts from several sections of the brain including the temporal lobe were negative.

This patient had high levels of interferon before administration of poly I·poly C, 700 units in cerebrospinal fluid and 300 in serum. Initiation of poly I·poly C treatment in this patient was not associated with a significant increase in the interferon levels. Interferon remained present until the treatment was stopped. However, interferon titers in the cerebrospinal fluid were higher than in serum, suggesting viral induction. The titers decreased after the fifth day of treatment and were no longer detectable after poly I·poly C treatment was terminated. It was not possible to definitely conclude that the drug either induced interferon or that it enhanced recovery.

2. Administration to Children with SSPE

Two children with subacute sclerosing panencephalitis (SSPE) with marked neurological and mental deterioration were given a trial of poly I·poly C therapy [106]. These children both had serologic evidence of rubeola infection. One was a 4 3/4 year old girl, the other an $8\frac{1}{2}$ year old boy. Poly I·poly C was administered in a dose of 0.1 mg/kg/day intravenously in a daily slow injection for 10 days. In both patients the condition was stable after drug treatment was begun, although the existing deficits showed no regression. Both patients did not have detectable serum interferon when treatment began, but both reached peak titers of 100 units per ml, 12 hours after the first dose. By 48 hours after the initiation of treatment, the titers fell to 7 units and < 5 units per ml and remained at these low levels throughout the treatment period, despite continued administration of the drug. Interferon was not detected in CSF taken 6 h and 10 days after initiation of treatment.

In these two cases of SSPE no significant improvement occurred, but the patients' conditions appeared to remain stable for several months. More treated cases will be necessary to assess the effect of poly I·poly C on SSPE.

The interferon response of the two children with SSPE showed that the interferon inducing property of poly I·poly C which has been extensively studied in animals could be exploited to induce serum interferon in man. The appearance of the highest levels of interferon only during the early part of the treatment period indicates that when given in the dose employed in these patients, a hyporeactive period lasting at least 8 days developed with continued treatment. In the patient with herpes simplex encephalitis, the high titers of interferon induced by the virus infection precluded determining whether or not any of the interferon detected subsequently was produced in response to poly I·poly C treatment.

All of the patients given poly I·poly C were observed closely for signs of drug toxicity during and immediately after treatment. The patients with SSPE developed a fever which reached a maximum of 40.5° and 40.6° C 24 h after the drug was initiated; however, the temperature returned to normal by the fifth day of treatment. In the patient with herpes simplex encephalitis the high fever which was due to the infection fell rapidly after poly I·poly C was started; this patient was afebrile after the first day of treatment. A mild anemia with a reticulocytosis occurred in the infant with herpes simplex encephalitis; this was attributed to frequent phlebotomy rather than drug toxicity. Serum enzyme, blood chemistry, and hematological studies in the three pediatric patients were normal except for transient elevations in the SGPT, LDH, and alkaline phosphatase which occurred coincident with stopping the drug (after the eleventh daily dose) in the child with herpes simplex encephalitis.

Another study using poly I· poly C in man is going on at the University of Siena, Italy [107]. Here the effect of the drug on herpes simplex eye infection in man is being studied in a double-blind experiment. Preliminary decoding and evaluation has indicated a significant therapeutic effect during the acute phase of the infection. Studies comparing the usefulness of poly I· poly C and other interferon inducers with the efficacy of IDU in herpes simplex eye infections are necessary. It may be that a suitable combination of an interferon inducer and IDU would be most efficacious, particularly for prevention of recurrences of herpetic keratoconjunctivitis.

3. Administration to Cancer Patients

Because of its antitumor activity against viral and nonviral animal tumors, clinical trials of poly I· poly C were initiated in patients with various tumors [108]. Thus far, fourteen patients with advanced malignancies have been evaluated at four dose levels, 0.3, 1.0, 2.5, and 4 mg/square meter of body surface area (0.008, 0.03, 0.07, 0.1 mg/kg). Significant interferon levels have been noted at three of the four dose levels tested. Figure 3 shows the interferon titers in units/ml plotted against the dose. A trend toward increasing titers of interferon was noted with increasing doses. At the lowest dose, interferon levels were not measurable. Significant levels were found in two of four patients at the next dose level and the highest interferon titer thus far noted was in one patient at the highest dose. Measurable interferon has not been found in cerebrospinal fluid. Figure 4 illustrates

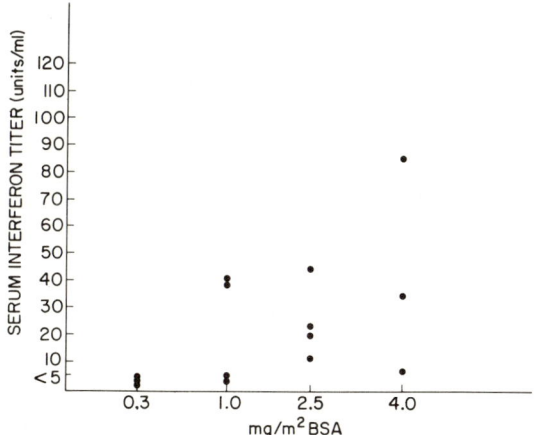

Fig. 3. Induction of interferon in man with poly I· poly C at doses of 0.3, 1.0, 2.5, and 4 mg/m^2 of body surface area.

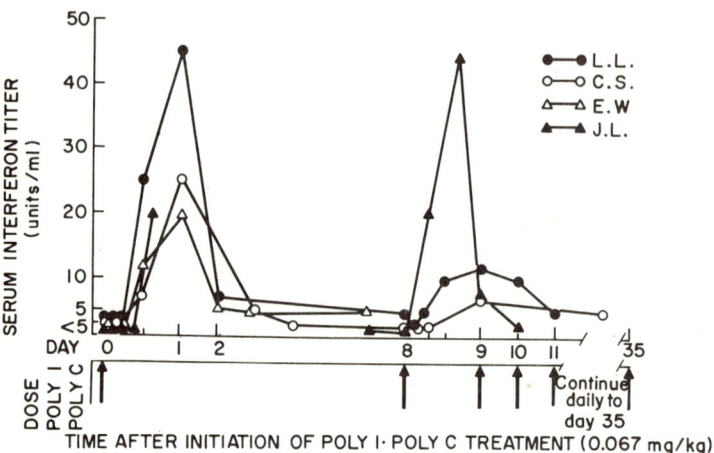

Fig. 4. Time course of serum interferon following a single dose and repeated administration of intravenous poly I·poly C at doses of 2.5 mg/m^2 in 4 patients.

representative data on the time course of interferon following a single dose and repeated administration of poly I·poly C in 4 patients at the 2.5 mg/m^2 dose levels. There are three points of interest in this figure: (1) The time to the peak level of interferon, following a single dose, is longer than in mice with a peak being noted at 24 h in all cases with adequate data points. In mice, peak levels after a single dose are reached before 12 h. Interferon levels rapidly fall to insignificant levels by 48 h. (2) After the second injection one week later, a second but lower response is noted in two-thirds of the patients with the same dose. (3) With repeated administration a hyporesponsive period is noted in spite of continued administration at the same dose. This same hyporesponsive phenomenon has been noted in animals and, in general, has not compromised the antiviral or antitumor activity. Clinical toxicity was similar to that produced by poly I·poly C in animals and consisted of occasional fever, allergic reactions, mild liver function abnormalities, mild anemia, and evidence of mildly accelerated intravascular coagulation. Antitumor activity has not yet been demonstrated at doses that induce interferon with acceptable toxicity.

VI. CONCLUSIONS

The discovery of interferon has led in a brief thirteen years to much new knowledge concerning the body defense mechanisms against viruses, concerning the pathogenesis of viral disease, and concerning unsuspected mechanisms of control of protein synthesis within the cell. Application of the interferon defense mechanism has brought us to the verge of practical usefulness in man. It is hoped that problems associated with mass production of human interferon can be overcome. Alternatively, it is hoped that an inducer of interferon suitable for widespread use in man will soon be found. Among the characteristics for an ideal drug which induces interferon would be (1) rapid induction of interferon, (2) little or no hyporesponsiveness to interferon induction, (3) oral effectiveness, (4) wide margin of therapeutic safety, (5) few side effects, and (6) low cost to the patient.

REFERENCES

1. A. Isaacs and J. Lindenmann, Proc. Roy. Soc. (London), Ser. B, 147, 258 (1957).
2. S. Baron and A. Isaacs, New Scientist, 11, 81 (1961).
3. A. Isaacs, Advan. Virus Res., 10, 1 (1963).
4. S. Baron, Advan. Virus Res., 10, 39 (1963).
5. S. Baron and H. B. Levy, Ann. Rev. Microbiol., 20, 291 (1966).
6. S. Baron, in Modern Trends in Medical Virology, Butterworths, London, 1967, pp. 77-110.
7. H. B. Levy, S. Baron, and C. E. Buckler, in Biochemistry of Viruses, (H. B. Levy, ed.), Dekker, New York, 1969, p. 579.
8. N. B. Finter, ed., Interferons, North-Holland Publ., Amsterdam, 1966, 1970.
9. R. M. Friedman and S. Baron, J. Immunol., 87, 379 (1961).
10. S. Baron, in Interferons (N. B. Finter, ed.), North-Holland Publ., Amsterdam, 1970.
11. J. Taylor, Biochem. Biophys. Res. Commun., 14, 447 (1964).
12. S. Baron, C. E. Buckler, R. M. Friedman, and R. V. McClosky, J. Immunol., 96, 17 (1966).
13. I. Gresser, J. Coppey, D. Fontaine-Brouty-Boye, R. Falcoff, E. Falcoff, and A. Zajdela, Nature, 215, 174 (1967).
14. J. H. Park and S. Baron, Science, 162, 811 (1968).
15. B. R. Murphy and L. A. Glasgow, Antimicrobiol Agents and Chemotherapy, 661-667 (1967).
16. A. Isaacs, S. Baron, and A. C. Allison, Sci. Am., 204, 51 (1961).
17. G. P. Lampson, A. A. Tytell, A. K. Field, M. M. Newes, and M. R. Hilleman, Proc. Natl. Acad. Sci. U. S., 58, 782 (1967).
18. A. K. Field, A. A. Tytell, G. P. Lampson, and M. R. Hilleman, Proc. Natl. Acad. Sci. U. S., 58, 1004 (1967).
19. A. K. Field, G. P. Lampson, A. A. Tytell, M. M. Newes, and M. R. Hilleman, Proc. Natl. Acad. Sci. U. S., 58, 2102 (1967).

20. W. J. Kleinschmidt, L. F. Ellis, R. M. Van Frank, and E. B. Murphy, Nature, 220, 167 (1968).
21. A. A. Tytell, G. P. Lampson, A. K. Field, and M. R. Hilleman, Proc. Natl. Acad. Sci. U. S., 58, 1719 (1967).
22. S. Baron, N. Bogomolova, H. B. Levy, A. Billiau, C. E. Buckler, R. Stern, and R. Naylor, Proc. Nat. Acad. Sci. U. S., 64, 67 (1969).
23. A. Billiau, C. E. Buckler, F. Dianzani, C. Uhlendorf, and S. Baron, Proc. 2nd Symp. Antiviral Substances N. Y. Acad. Sci., 173, 657 (1970).
24. W. J. Kleinschmidt, R. J. Douthard, and E. B. Murphy, Federation Proc., 29, 635 (1970).
25. D. A. J. Tyrrell, Nature, 184, 452 (1959).
26. J. S. Youngner, and W. R. Stinebring, Virology, 29, 310 (1966).
27. J. V. Hallum, J. S. Youngner, and T. C. Merigan, Virology, 34, 802 (1968).
28. J. Lindenmann, D. Burke, and A. Isaacs, Brit. J. Exptl. Pathol., 38, 551 (1957).
29. R. M. Friedman and J. A. Sonnabend, Nature, 203, 366 (1964).
30. R. Z. Lockart, Biochem. Biophys. Res. Commun., 15, 513 (1964).
31. H. B. Levy and W. A. Carter, Abstracts 1st Intern. Symp. Interferon, NIH, December 1966. Interferon Information Exchange, January, 1965.
32. N. Miner, W. J. Ray, Jr., and E. H. Simon, Biochem. Biophys. Res. Commun., 24, 264 (1966).
33. J. A. Sonnabend, E. M. Martin, E. Mecs, and K. H. Fantes, J. Gen. Virol., 1, 41 (1967).
34. H. B. Levy and W. A. Carter, J. Mol. Biol., 31, 561 (1968).
35. W. K. Joklik and T. C. Merigan, Proc. Natl. Acad. Sci. U. S., 56, 558 (1966).
36. P. I. Marcus and J. M. Salb, in The Interferons (G. Rita, ed.), Academic Press, New York, 1968.
37. M. N. Oxman, W. P. Rowe, and P. H. Black, Proc. Natl. Acad. Sci., U. S., 57, 941 (1967).
38. R. I. Jahiel, J. Vilcek, R. Nussenzweig, and J. Vanderberg, Science, 161, 802 (1968).
39. J. S. Remington and T. C. Merigan, Science, 161, 804 (1968).
40. W. W. Schultz, K. Y. Huang, and F. B. Gordon, Nature, 220, 709 (1968).

41. W. Regelson, Proc. Intern. Symp. Atherosclerosis and Reticuloendothelial Systems, Como, Italy, Plenum Press, New York, 1967.
42. T. C. Merigan and W. Regelson, New Engl. J. Med., 277, 1283 (1967).
43. W. J. Kleinschmidt and G. W. Probst, Antibiot. Chemotherapy, 12, 298 (1962).
44. G. D. Mayer and B. A. Fink, Federation Proc., 29, 635 (1970).
45. R. F. Krueger and S. Yoshimura, Federation Proc., 29, 635 (1970).
46. K. Paucker, J. Immunol., 94, 371 (1965).
47. I. Gresser, D. Fontaine, J. Coppey, R. Falcoff, and E. Falcoff, Proc. Soc. Exptl. Biol. Med., 124, 91 (1967).
48. T. P. Subrahmanyan and C. A. Mims, Brit. J. Exptl. Pathol., 47, 168 (1966).
49. M. Ho and B. Postic, in 1st Intern. Conf. Vaccines Against Viral and Rickettsial Diseases of Man, PAHO/WHO Scientific Publication 147, 1967.
50. V. Bocci, M. Russi-Sorce, G. Cirri, and G. Rita, Proc. Soc. Exptl. Biol. Med., 129, 62 (1968).
51. N. B. Finter, in Interferon (G. E. W. Wolstenholme and M. O'Connor, ed.), Little, Brown, Boston, 1967.
52. V. Bocci, M. Russi-Sorce, G. Cirri, G. Rita, and P. Cantagalli, in The Interferons (G. Rita, ed.), Academic Press, New York, 1968.
53. E. Falcoff, R. Falcoff, F. Fournier, and C. Chany, Ann. Inst. Pasteur, Paris, 111, 562 (1966).
54. V. D. Soloviev, in The Interferons (G. Rita, ed.), Academic Press, New York, 1968.
55. G. P. Lampson, A. A. Tytell, M. M. Nemes, and M. R. Hilleman, Proc. Soc. Exptl. Biol. Med., 112, 468 (1963).
56. H. B. Levy and T. C. Merigan, Proc. Soc. Exptl. Biol. Med., 121, 53 (1966).
57. I. Gresser, J. Coppey, E. Falcoff, and D. Fontaine, Proc. Soc. Exptl. Biol. Med., 124, 84 (1967).
58. K. Cantell and V. Tommila, Lancet, ii, 682 (1960).
59. T. C. Merigan, Nature, 214, 416 (1967).
60. W. Regelson, Advan. Chemother., 3, 303 (1968).
61. M. R. Hilleman, J. Cell. Physiol., 71, 43 (1968).
62. R. H. Adamson, S. Fabro, E. R. Homan, R. W. O'Gara, and R. P. Zendzian, Antimicrobial Agents and Chemotherapy-1969-148-152(1970).

63. R. H. Adamson and S. Fabro, Nature, 223, 718 (1969).
64. R. H. Adamson, unpublished observations, 1969.
65. E. F. Wheelock and R. P. B. Larke, Proc. Soc. Exptl. Biol. Med., 127, 230 (1968).
66. E. F. Wheelock, N. L. Caroline, and R. D. Moore, J. Virol., 4, 1 (1969).
67. H. B. Levy, L. W. Law, and A. S. Rabson, Proc. Natl. Acad. Sci. U. S., 62, 357 (1969).
68. L. D. Zeleznick and B. K. Bhayan, Proc. Soc. Exptl. Biol. Med., 130, 126 (1969).
69. R. H. Adamson, Federation Proc., 29, 682 (1970).
70. S. Baron, H. duBuy, C. E. Buckler, M. L. Johnson, J. Park, A. Billau, P. Sarma, and P. J. Huebner, Proc. 2nd Symp. Antiviral Substances N. Y. Acad. Sci., in press.
71. H. B. Levy, R. Asofsky, F. Riley, A. Garapin, H. Cantor, and R. Adamson, Ann. N. Y. Acad. Sci., in press.
72. W. Braun, M. Nakano, L. Jaraskova, Y. Yajima, and L. Jiminez, in Nucleic Acids in Immunology, Springer-Verlag, New York, 1968.
73. Scientific Committee on Interferon, Lancet, i, 873 (1962).
74. B. R. Jones, J. E. K. Galbraith, and M. K. Al-Hussaini, Lancet, i, 875 (1962).
75. H. Strander and K. Cantell, Ann. Med. Exptl. Biol. Fennlae (Helsinki), 44, 265 (1966).
76. C. Chany, F. Fournier, and E. Falcoff, in Interferon (G. E. W. Wolstenholme and M. O'Connor, eds.), Little, Brown, Boston, 1967.
77. R. Jao, E. F. Wheelock, and G. G. Jackson, J. Clin. Invest., 44, 1062 (1965).
78. E. F. Wheelock, in Vaccines against Viral and Rickettsial Diseases of Man, Pan Am. Health Organ. Sci. Pub. No. 147, 1967.
79. I. Gresser and H. B. Dull, Proc. Soc. Exptl. Biol. Med., 115, 192 (1964).
80. M. K. Voroshilova, personal communication, 1969.
81. R. Kono, M. Hoshino, and M. Hinobara, in Interferon (Y. Nagano and H. B. Levy, eds.) Igaku Shoin Ltd., Tokyo, 1970.
82. I. Gresser and K. Naficy, Proc. Soc. Exptl. Biol. Med., 117, 285 (1964).
83. R. P. B. Larke, Can. Med. Assoc. J., 96, 21 (1967).

84. V. Knight, W. F. Fleet, and D. J. Lang, J. Am. Med. Assoc., 188, 690 (1964).

85. D. Waddell, T. C. Merigan, J. Wilbur, and S. Walker, Clin. Res., 15, 312 (1967).

86. E. F. Wheelock, Proc. Soc. Exptl. Biol. Med., 117, 650 (1964).

87. E. F. Wheelock and J. H. Dingle, New Engl. J. Med., 271, 645 (1964).

88. J. K. Petralli, T. C. Merigan, and J. R. Wilbur, New Engl. J. Med., 273, 198 (1965).

89. V. D. Soloviev, T. A. Bektemirov, and L. J. Neklyudova, Vopr. Virusol., 13, 146 (1968).

90. A. B. Sabin, M. Ramos-Alvarez, J. Alvarez-Amezquita, W. Pelon, R. H. Michaels, I. Spigland, M. A. Koch, J. M. Barnes, and J. S. Rhim, J. Am. Med. Assoc., 173, 1521 (1960).

91. A. B. Sabin, Roy. Soc. Health J., 82, 51 (1962).

92. J. K. Petralli, T. C. Merigan, and J. R. Wilbur, Lancet, ii, 401 (1965).

93. G. W. A. Dick and E. S. Horgan, J. Hyg., 50, 376 (1952).

94. H. M. Meyer, Jr., D. D. Hostetler, Jr., B. C. Bernheim, N. G. Rogers, P. Lambin, A. Chassary, R. Labusquiere, and J. E. Smadel, Bull. World Health Organ., 30, 783 (1964).

95. J. P. Fox, D. R. LeBlanc, H. M. Gelfand, D. J. Clemmer, and L. Potash, Pan Am. Health Organ. Sci. Pub. No. 50, 144, 1960.

96. A. B. Sabin, Am. J. Trop. Med. Hyg., 1, 30 (1952).

97. G. I. Watson, Brit. Med. J., i, 860 (1963).

98. E. B. Byrne, B. J. Rosenstein, A. A. Jaworski, and R. A. Jaworski, J. Am. Med. Assoc., 199, 619 (1967).

99. C. M. Southam and A. E. Moore, Cancer, 5, 1025 (1952).

100. E. F. Wheelock, R. P. B. Larke, and N. L. Caroline, Prog. Med. Virol., 10, 286, 1968. (Also see Ref. [87].)

101. W. A. Cassel and R. E. Garrett, Cancer, 18, 863 (1965).

102. T. Balenzina, Yu. V. Borisov, Z. V. Ermolieva, E. S. Zalmanzon, N. I. Korabelnikova, and E. P. Pilatskata, Vopr. Virusol., 2, 235 (1966).

103. N. A. Zeitlenok, in Interferon and Interferonogens (N. A. Zeitlenok, ed.). Vol. 10, Institute of Poliomyelitis and Viral Encephalitides, Moscow, 1967.

104. W. Regelson and J. F. Holland, Clin. Pharmacol. Therap., 3, 730 (1962).

105. J. Bellanti and L. Catalano, J. Ped., 78, 136 (1971).

106. M. A. Guggenheim and S. Baron, personal communication, 1970.

107. R. Guerra, R. Frezzotti, R. Bonanni, F. Dianzani, and G. Rita, in Proc. 2nd Conf. Antiviral Substances, N.Y. Acad. Sci., 173, 823 (1970).

108. V. DeVita, G. Canellos, P. Carbone, S. Baron, H. Levy, and H. Gralnick, Proc. Am. Assoc. Cancer Res., 11, 21 (1970).

Chapter VII

ANTITHROMBOTIC AND THROMBOLYTIC DRUGS

Kenneth M. Moser

Department of Medicine
University of California
San Diego, California

I.	INTRODUCTION	317
II.	THROMBOSIS	318
	A. Semantic Considerations	318
	B. The Process of Thrombogenesis	319
	C. Other Variations in Thrombus Composition	321
III.	THE NATURAL HISTORY OF THROMBOEMBOLIC DISEASE	322
	A. The Growth Phase	322
	B. The Resolution Phase	322
	C. Other Factors Which Determine the Consequences of Thromboembolism	325
	D. Special Considerations	327
IV.	THE DIAGNOSTIC DILEMMA	328
V.	THE GOALS OF THROMBOLYTIC THERAPY AND APPROACHES TO ACHIEVING THEM	330
	A. Prophylaxis	330
	B. Treatment	334
VI.	LESSONS OF HISTORY AND THE SEARCH FOR THROMBOLYTIC DRUGS	338
VII.	CONCLUSIONS	340
	REFERENCES	340

I. INTRODUCTION

Each year for the last several, the National Institutes of Health has issued a bibliographic compilation dealing with Fibrinolysis, Thrombolysis and Blood Clotting [1]. The compilation has grown in size annually. The year 1969 is represented by two thick volumes containing some 2000 pages of fine print. Through these pages march thousands of references, arrayed in impeccably computerized ranks. The visual effect of scanning these well-ordered pages is like the review of some massive international army mobilized to deal with a formidable threat to the survival of mankind. Indeed, this simile is not so farfetched. The foe which has generated this awesome display of investigative power is thromboembolism, an enemy which does pose a major threat to the peoples of the earth.

Like any fearsome enemy, thromboembolic disease has multiple weapons in its arsenal. Some of them compromise the victim's function in subtle ways; some maim; some kill. When summed, the toll extracted in terms of death and disability is staggering. And no one is exempt from danger. The counter-attack launched by science has been broad and intensive. Yet it is just beginning to slow the enemy's advance. Perhaps the central reason for this slow progress has been our inability to identify with precision either the enemy or his weaponry. An unidentifiable foe armed with secret weapons cannot be turned back. Therefore, it is appropriate to begin this review of thrombolytic therapy by characterizing the enemy and the tactics he employs.

II. THROMBOSIS

A. Semantic Considerations

The adequacy of a definition depends upon how and by whom the definition is to be used. To a visitor from another planet, the dictionary definition of an automobile as "a usually 4-wheeled automotive vehicle designed for passenger transportation and commonly propelled by an internal combustion engine using a volatile fuel" would be totally inadequate [2]. The multiple shapes, sizes, and colors of objects called automobiles by those "in the know" would confuse the visitor. And what of the fact that these objects also are referred to as "cars"? Is "car" synonymous with "automobile"?. Even more distressing would be an attempt by the visitor to determine how an automobile works. He would soon learn that, covered by the broad definition, "automobiles" are multitudes of engines, suspension systems, gear shifts (or lack of them), electrical systems, etc., which vary so widely that familiarity with one does not assure operational familiarity with another.

These lessons for the stranger to "automobiles" are similar to those encountered by the stranger to the world of thrombosis. The same dictionary quoted previously tells us that thrombosis is "the formation or presence of a blood clot within a blood vessel during life," and that a thrombus is "a clot of blood within a blood vessel and remaining attached to its place of origin" [2]. These general definitions, like the definition of "automobile," hide the complexities which must be understood if one wishes to start, stop, or otherwise manipulate the thrombotic process. For example, is "clot" synonymous with "thrombus"? The debate on this semantic point is often long, loud, and emotional. At the heart of the debate is the differentiation between a "clot" as an in vitro entity and a "thrombus" as an in vivo entity. Yet, even this gross distinction will not stand close scrutiny. Rather than pursuing this semantic point, we can dispose of it at this juncture by agreeing to use the terms henceforth as synonyms — while agreeing that those who are opposed to this may substitute the word they feel most appropriate.

VII. ANTITHROMBOTIC AND THROMBOLYTIC DRUGS

Whatever our semantic choice, we are dealing with a mass composed of blood components which has formed on the wall of a vascular structure in the body. And whether we use "clot" or "thrombus" to describe such masses, there can be no disagreement with two critical points: (1) that all thrombi are not equivalent in terms of structure and composition and (2) that all thrombi are not equivalent in terms of pathogenesis. These are vital points of differentiation because they markedly condition any effort to develop pharmacological approaches that may influence thrombus formation and removal.

B. The Process of Thrombogenesis

It has long been recognized that three major factors promoted the development of intravascular thrombosis, regardless of its site of occurrence; namely, vascular injury, stasis of blood flow, and alterations in the blood coagulation system. The validity of this triad as the point of departure in our understanding of the thrombotic process remains unchanged. What has changed is our understanding of how each factor participates in the sequence of thrombosis in different vessels, and our recognition that we must direct our therapeutic attention to this sequence rather than to its final result, the thrombus itself.

The major distinction which should be made among thrombi is whether they occur on the venous or arterial side of the circulation. It is now clear that venous thrombi differ from arterial thrombi with respect to both origin and structure. The venous thrombus is the "red thrombus," which closely resembles macroscopically its in vitro counterparts formed in test tubes. Such red thrombi are composed of a fibrin network in which are entrapped the formed elements of the blood. The arterial thrombus is the "white thrombus," in which platelets are the primary component. The red thrombus is the entity with which we must deal in all forms of venous thrombosis and embolism. The white thrombus is the culprit in thrombosis of coronary, cerebral, and renal arteries. These two types of thrombus appear to differ with respect to both the factors which initiate their formation and the factors which promote their propagation.

Stasis of blood flow and coagulation alterations appear to play the primary roles in genesis of the red or venous thrombus. While vascular injury certainly can initiate venous thrombosis, there is now ample evidence that red thrombi can form without such antecedent injury [3]. The extensive studies of Wessler and others have demonstrated that injection of thrombin-free serum can induce thrombosis in a venous segment upon which stasis has been imposed [4,5]. The usual sequence employed experimentally has been serum injection followed by application of atraumatic clamps or ligatures to the vessel of choice. Promptly, a "red" fibrin thrombus develops in the vessel. Thus, thrombosis can take place in vessels not subjected to intimal injury. The thrombi which result from this experimental sequence are faithful morphological counterparts of those encountered in human venous thrombosis [6,7].

Stasis alone does not induce thrombosis. Serum injection (or injection of activated coagulation components) alone will not cause thrombosis. Both factors must coexist. In man, the primary disturbance is likely the activation of appropriate coagulation components in the circulating blood. Once such activation occurs, any static zone is vulnerable to thrombosis. The opportunities for venous stasis are multiple and encompass all of those clinical situations known to be associated with venous thrombosis: the post-operative period, prolonged bed rest for any reason, the post-partum period, long journeys in airplanes or other vehicles during which the subject does not ambulate. Thus, the combination of stasis plus transient release of activated coagulation products fits well with all observations relating to human venous thromboembolism. Thrombus morphology fits. The pathogenetic substrates fit. The in vivo behavior of experimental and clinical "red" thromboemboli appear to be the same. This is not the case with respect to arterial thrombosis. The thrombi in coronary, cerebral, and renal arteries are "white thrombi" composed chiefly of platelets with a modest fibrin component. Even though some red thrombus is often present, careful examination discloses a "white thrombus" nidus upon which the red clot has been engrafted. Thus, morphology alone suggests that major differences exist. Furthermore, in normal arteries supplying vital organs, opportunities for stasis are limited. Neither the high pressure, rapid-flow dynamics of these vessels nor their more rigid architecture would appear to make them as susceptible to stasis as their venous counterparts. Finally, the clinical contexts in which arterial thromboembolism usually occurs do not match those in which venous thrombosis develops. Cerebral thrombosis, for example, strikes "out of the blue" without respect to any activity or inactivity. The same is true of coronary thrombosis.

Thus, the mechanism which explains venous thrombosis so well does not appear applicable to arterial thrombosis. Rather, the primary factor in arterial thrombosis appears to be the third member of the thrombotic triad: vascular injury. Recent investigations have suggested that arterial thrombi are initiated by an intimal injury which exposes circulating platelets to subendothelial collagen [8-13]. The platelets adhere to this exposed "foreign surface." There follows a biochemical-structural sequence involving the platelets which leads to further platelet accretion at the site of injury. Beyond this point, several different fates may befall the platelet nidus. The rapid blood flow may sweep away portions of the incipient thrombus so that only a small mural platelet mass remains and repair of the injury ensues. Or the platelet nidus may grow to completely occlude the vessel, following which red thrombus may propagate in the occluded vessel. Or partial occlusion of the vessel may lead to stasis and local activation of the coagulation system so that red thrombus is then laid down on the initial white thrombus. There is further platelet accretion and red thrombus formation and so forth until total occlusion occurs. Thus, the arterial thrombus begins as a platelet nidus but may finally present either as a pure white thrombus or, more commonly, as a "mixed" thrombus [14,15].

These thrombogenic sequences have major impact upon any attempt to develop thrombolytic agents. A drug capable of inducing the dissolution of fibrin should be effective in dealing with "red" thrombi because their structural integrity depends upon a fibrin matrix. Such fibrinolytic attack, however, will have less effect upon the platelet masses which compose "white" thrombi, since fibrin plays a nominal role in these. Conversely, agents which alter the process of platelet aggregation would not be expected to be therapeutically effective in dealing with red thrombi; but they might be of value in preventing or ameliorating arterial thrombotic disease.

Things are, of course, not quite this "red and white." As indicated above, white thrombi often develop a significant amount of red thrombus either at the site of origin or by propagation. To the extent that red thrombus contributes to the occlusion, a fibrinolytic agent may be of clinical benefit. For example, coronary occlusion may result entirely from "white" thrombosis. But extension proximally and distally is likely to be due to red thrombosis. Dissolution of this red component may limit the extent of myocardial injury. Likewise, a portion of "red thrombus" growth involves surface accretion of platelets. Any agent which would limit such accretion might limit thrombus growth.

C. Other Variations in Thrombus Composition

While the distinction between "red" and "white" thrombi is a critical one, other factors may condition the response of a given thrombus to a specific pharmacologic agent. One such factor is the age of the thrombus. Thrombi are not static entities. Neither the white nor the red thrombus retains its initial architecture indefinitely. Within a few days, each is subject to endothelialization and organization. Endothelial covering of a thrombus serves to exclude the thrombus from the circulating blood. Thus, any circulating therapeutic substance is blocked from its target. Organization of the thrombus converts it from a fibrin or platelet mass into a mass of granulation tissue which will be totally unresponsive to any fibrinolytic agent, regardless of its potency.

The effect of other factors upon thrombolytic efforts is less clear. Red thrombi will have a composition which varies with that of the circulating blood at the time the thrombus forms. Depending on the existing fibrinogen concentration, such thrombi may vary in fibrin content. There is experimental evidence that fibrin-rich thrombi are more resistant to attack than thrombi of normal or low fibrin content [16]. Thrombi also may vary in lipid concentration, and lipid-rich thrombi may be less susceptible to fibrinolytic dissolution [17]. These "details" regarding the composition of thrombi, and their influence upon pharmacological interventions, remain poorly understood. There is limited information, for example, about changes in structure and composition of thrombi during the considerable interval between formation and full organization and whether such changes alter the response of the thrombus to a particular drug [18].

The variable nature of thrombus structure requires consideration as any therapeutic trial is attempted in thromboembolic disease. Marked variation in therapeutic response may reflect variation in the nature of the thrombus, not in the dose, distribution, or action of the drug. The literature dealing with anticoagulant drugs bears witness to this fact. It has long been clear that both heparin and the prothrombinopenic agents were highly effective in treating venous thromboembolic disease, but significantly less valuable in coronary and cerebral thrombosis. The reasons for this now seem clear. The coagulation system plays a major role in the genesis of the "red" venous thrombus so that blockade of this system should have prophylactic value and limit propagation of such thrombi. But vascular occlusion due to platelet accretion — the white, arterial thrombotic sequence — does not initially require coagulation components and can (and does) occur despite the presence of effective anticoagulant therapy. This lesson should not be lost on those developing thrombolytic therapy.

III. THE NATURAL HISTORY OF THROMBOEMBOLIC DISEASE

There are three critical phases in the natural history of thromboembolic disease: initiation, growth, and resolution. The first phase, initiation, has been discussed above. At the end of this phase, a red, white, or "mixed" thrombus has begun within the vessel, but its potential for producing disease remains uncertain. The occurrence and severity of functional impairment depends upon what happens next.

A. The Growth Phase

The mere presence of an intraluminal thrombus does not compromise function. It is the obstruction of blood flow which leads to disease. Thrombosis which does not compromise blood flow does not reach clinical expression. The distinction between the anatomic fact of thrombosis and the potential consequence of obstruction to blood flow may seem an obvious one, but failure to make this distinction is common and can lead to substantial clinical and therapeutic confusion.

The extent to which blood flow through a vessel is compromised by thrombosis depends upon the extent to which the luminal cross-sectional area of the vessel is reduced. There is not, however, a linear relationship between the two. A minor impingement upon luminal area does not cause a slight impairment of blood flow; indeed, a small mural thrombus has virtually no effect on flow through a vessel. The complexities of a system in which there is pulsatile flow through vessels of widely varying structure make broad generalizations imperfect, but some broad guidelines are available to indicate the nonlinearity of the obstruction-flow relationship. In the pulmonary artery, for example, it has been determined that luminal compromise of 60-70 percent is required before blood flow beyond the zone of narrowing is substantially compromised under basal conditions [19]. A similar relationship should obtain in other vessels, including coronary and cerebral arteries. Clinical, angiographic, and post-mortem observations have disclosed that the bulk of red and white thrombi do not completely occlude the vascular

VII. ANTITHROMBOTIC AND THROMBOLYTIC DRUGS 323

lumen. This fact not only means that a thrombolytic agent can be of value even though it removes but a modest percentage of the thrombus, but also means that delivery of the agent to the clot surface via the blood stream is a reasonable maneuver.

These observations have major therapeutic implications. The physician is primarily concerned with preservation or restoration of normal <u>function</u>. In the case of thrombosis, this means preservation or restoration of <u>blood flow</u>. It is apparent that this functional goal can be achieved without requiring total dissolution of a given thrombus. A thrombolytic agent which reduces the extent of luminal obstruction from 80 to 40 percent will have achieved a major functional success even though it has not restored normal luminal patency. Likewise, a regimen which halts a thrombus at a level of 30 percent luminal occlusion will prevent the thrombus from reaching clinical expression. Obsession with <u>total</u> restoration of vascular patency as a criterion for thrombolytic success is not warranted. The objective is return of adequate blood flow, not return to anatomic normality. Failure to achieve the latter cannot be equated with failure to achieve the former.

In terms of disease production, then, the "growth phase" of the thrombus is crucial. Unfortunately, the physician rarely is in a position to alter this phase. Unless clinical manifestations appear, the patient does not seek medical attention and must rely upon his own defenses to halt thrombus growth. Only when his defenses fail and the war is lost does the patient receive his first indication that the battle is being waged. This situation need not be accepted indefinitely, as we shall see. More sensitive detectors of thrombosis are being developed so that therapy can be applied in the early "silent" stages of the battle. And, ultimately, prophylactic measures may be developed to immobilize the forces promoting thrombosis before they can establish a beachhead.

B. The Resolution Phase

Once the thrombus has reached its zenith, the final phase of the thromboembolic story begins. This is usually the point at which the physician enters the picture because the thrombus has caused symptoms by slowing or totally interrupting blood flow. The horse has been stolen, and the physician gallops off in pursuit, after having securely locked the barn door with anticoagulant drugs so that the episode is not repeated.

Three major components can influence the resolution phase: (1) endogenous mechanisms; (2) therapy to halt the progression and recurrence of thrombosis; (3) therapy to remove the existing thrombotic material. Evaluation of success in the latter two categories requires appreciation of the first.

1. The Red Thrombus

We now know that most venous thromboemboli resolve with dispatch in the absence of therapy. The behavior of pulmonary emboli, the most dramatic expression of venous thromboembolism, has been studied in detail. Investigations in man have established, through angiographic and radioisotopic techniques, that most pulmonary emboli completely resolve within a few days to several weeks after lodgement in the pulmonary vasculature [20-22]. Clinical observation of patients with venous thrombosis also indicates that rapid resolution of these thrombi is the rule.

Such observations in man are qualitative rather than quantitative. The investigative tools are crude and many variables cannot be controlled. The age and composition of the embolus in a patient is unknown. Both angiography and scintiphotography have sharp limitations in terms of their ability to quantitate embolic size [23-25]. And, finally, only those patients with symptoms are included in such studies. This latter limitation is a particularly severe one because it is likely that, in many patients, venous thromboembolism does not produce symptoms that lead to medical attention. Indeed, these subclinical episodes of venous thromboembolism probably comprise the great majority. This view seems warranted by studies showing that evidence of previous pulmonary embolism can be detected in more than 60 percent of all patients coming to autopsy [26]. Even this very high figure neglects patients in whom prior emboli may have resolved without trace. Such data strongly suggest that most, if not all, adults have an episode of venous thromboembolism during life, but only a select few reach medical attention as a result.

Investigations in animals have demonstrated the efficient endogenous mechanisms which exist for ridding the pulmonary and venous systems of red thrombi. Wessler demonstrated, in the dog, that fresh pulmonary emboli resolve within hours to days [6]. Aging of thrombi prior to their release as emboli delays their resolution but, within weeks, only a small residual of even these aged emboli can be detected [7]. Recent studies in our laboratory have indicated that fresh venous thromboemboli in the dog are subject to extremely rapid dissolution [27]. Within three hours, the volume of jugular venous thrombi declines by 67 percent. Pulmonary emboli are reduced to 48 percent of their original volume at three hours and 29 percent at the end of 6 hours. This rapid reduction in thrombus volume is due to the action of endogenous fibrinolytic mechanisms. If a residual persists, organization completes the process of resolution. Obviously, the more effective the fibrinolytic attack, the less the residual which remains to undergo organization.

Thus, prompt resolution of red thrombi is the expected outcome. Persistence or extension of thrombosis becomes the exception that must be explained. Some of the factors which delay thrombus resolution — age, thrombus composition — have been identified. Others remain obscure. For instance, it seems clear that patients with congestive heart failure and pulmonary disease resolve pulmonary emboli less well than individuals free of cardiopulmonary disease [28]. Whether this is due to differences in thrombus composition or differences in activation of the endogenous fibrinolytic system is unknown.

VII. ANTITHROMBOTIC AND THROMBOLYTIC DRUGS

2. The White Thrombus

Information regarding the natural history of the white thrombus is much more sparse than that dealing with red thrombi [29, 30]. This is a bit curious since, in terms of morbidity and mortality, the white thrombus far outpaces its "red brother." Unfortunately, inferences regarding the fate of white thrombi cannot be drawn from studies dealing with red thrombi. However, certain parallels do exist. Autopsy observations disclose that thrombosis of coronary, cerebral, renal, and peripheral arterial vessels is an extremely common pathological event which, like its venous counterpart, infrequently produces tissue injury and, even less frequently, brings the patient to medical attention. It also seems likely that many platelet thrombi coat a zone of vascular injury and progress no further.

Investigations of the natural history of the white thrombus are important not only to better understanding of arterial thrombotic disease but also to definition of the potential relationship between arterial thrombosis and atherosclerosis. Does atherosclerosis develop independently, serving only as the source of vascular injury upon which arterial thrombosis is engrafted? Or is the relationship more intimate, as has been suggested [31]? Does atherosclerosis sometimes develop because a thrombus has interfered with intimal nutrition? Is the atherosclerotic lesion in some instances the residual of a previous mural white thrombus? The answers to these questions must remain in the realm of tantalizing speculation at this time.

C. Other Factors Which Determine the Consequences of Thromboembolism

As already stated, the aim of thrombolytic therapy is restoration of function, not removal of the thrombus. Just as partial removal of thrombus may result in therapeutic success with anatomic failure, so may total resolution of thrombus be associated with therapeutic failure. Let us assume at this juncture that a red or white thrombus has grown sufficiently to impair or totally obstruct blood flow. Let us assume further that we possess thrombolytic agents upon which we can rely. Three factors can condition therapeutic success under these circumstances: the specific site of occlusion; the rapidity with which occlusion has developed; and the condition of the patient prior to occlusion.

1. Site of Occlusion

The specific vessel involved heavily conditions the likelihood of therapeutic success because it determines the time-frame during which thrombolysis must occur if function is to be restored. The shortest time-frame is provided when occlusion occurs in an artery supplying a tissue which is highly susceptible to nutrient lack and has poorly developed or nonexisting collateral arterial channels. The longest time-frame is offered by occlusion of a small venous channel in a tissue which is relatively insensitive to reduction in nutrient supply.

A good example of a narrow time-frame is provided by the retinal artery. The retina is extraordinarily sensitive to brief periods of oxygen deprivation. Total oxygen lack for just a few minutes irreparably damages retinal tissue. Furthermore, blockade of this vessel cannot be bypassed through pre-existing collaterals. Therefore, total occlusion means irretrievable loss of retinal function unless thrombolysis is achieved within minutes. This time-frame is so restrictive that, except under the most fortuitous circumstances, thrombolytic therapy cannot be applied in time to exert a beneficial effect. Thrombolytic therapy applied hours later might achieve total dissolution of the offending thrombus; but the patient would remain blind in that eye.

At the other extreme is the red thrombus in a small calf vein. Even total occlusion here would cause only modest functional impairment: that due to edema and slowing of blood egress from a small zone of striated muscle. The patient is at no risk of major injury. Adequate collateral channels exist for drainage and striated muscle is a hardy tissue which can survive mild oxygen deficiency rather nicely. Thus, there is no urgency in achieving thrombolysis. The only danger to the patient is massive extension of the thrombus and detachment of some portion as a pulmonary embolus. Even this danger is a limited one since endogenous mechanisms are likely to resolve the thrombus so that the whole event will pass unnoticed by the victim.

Thus, each specific thrombotic site poses special conditions for therapeutic success. To list these would require a detailed review of the nature of the collateral circulation and nutritive requirements in each instance, an exercise clearly beyond the intent of this chapter. But such a review is essential for any investigator designing a protocol for evaluation of thrombolytic therapy. Unless the investigator is intimately familiar with each disease entity he undertakes to treat, it is likely that his experimental design will be inadequate and his conclusions of doubtful, even negative, value. This requirement for detailed familiarity with the thrombotic entity at issue usually means that interdisciplinary collaboration is needed. The specialist in coronary artery disease is not likely to be familiar with the coagulation phenomena central to thrombolytic therapy. The coagulation expert is equally unlikely to be familiar with the clinical-pathological spectrum of coronary artery disease and thrombosis. Only a pooling of knowledge will produce a rational protocol. Without this, the result must be added confusion — a commodity already in oversupply with respect to the treatment of thrombotic disease.

2. Rapidity of Occlusion

A corollary to the comments made above is that the speed with which thrombus growth occurs will condition thrombolytic success. Sudden, total occlusion of an arterial vessel sets up a tight time-schedule for action. Collaterals do or do not respond immediately. Spontaneous or therapeutic thrombolysis does or does not occur in time. The patient does or does not arrive in the hands of the physician in time. The tissue (and perhaps the patient) does or does not survive. Total arterial occlusion is like the 100

VII. ANTITHROMBOTIC AND THROMBOLYTIC DRUGS 327

yard dash. The issue is settled quickly; there is no margin for error. The same considerations apply to massive pulmonary embolism.

On the other hand, gradual occlusion of a vessel allows the tissue, the patient, and the physician time to maneuver. Partial occlusion of a vessel grants time for potential collaterals to develop, a factor of particular importance in the coronary circulation. Partial occlusion is a pivotal factor in pulmonary embolism, permitting the patient to survive until therapy can be instituted. In deep venous thrombosis, rapidity of occlusion also conditions the clinical course. Slow occlusion of a major vein (even the superior vena cava) may be tolerated with limited symptomatology as collaterals decompress the normal channel [32]. Rapid occlusion of the same vessel may lead to severe edema in the drainage area. If this occurs in the leg, arterial inflow may be compromised with destructive functional consequences [33].

3. The Patient

The state of the patient at the time a given thrombotic event occurs can determine both the urgency and the success of therapeutic intervention. The patient with extensive pre-existing pulmonary disease and an already compromised right ventricle obviously will tolerate pulmonary embolism less well than a patient with a normal cardiopulmonary apparatus. This same principle applies to all other thromboembolic possibilities. The investigator attempting to evaluate thrombolytic therapy cannot preselect the ideal candidates. However, he can — indeed must — take such factors into consideration in establishing criteria for success. For example, superb thrombolytic therapy is not likely to enhance survival in patients with coronary thrombosis admitted in severe, prolonged shock. On the other hand, successful thrombolysis may make a difference in the long-term performance of the left ventricle by limiting the extent of myocardial damage.

Thus, the investigator is obligated to establish reasonable criteria for therapeutic success, based on the patient material studied and the therapeutic benefits which can be expected.

D. Special Considerations

It is already evident that many factors other than the presence of a thrombus will influence the selection of candidates for thrombolytic therapy, the manner in which it is applied, and the anticipated result. Among the factors already enumerated are the nature and site of the thrombus, the extent of occlusion, the rapidity of occlusion, and the patient. Other special concerns merit at least brief mention. For example, thrombolytic therapy in venous thrombosis has a dual purpose: to eliminate the venous obstruction and to remove the threat of potential embolism. The decision to use a thrombolytic agent in venous thrombosis in addition to standard anticoagulant therapy is conditioned more by concern about embolism than by the venous thrombus itself, which poses little risk to the patient. Thus, what a thrombus may do, rather than what it has done, may condition the decision to employ a thrombolytic agent.

In pulmonary embolism, there now seems adequate evidence to indicate that release of serotonin from platelets (on the surface of the "red" thrombus) plays a role in the acute cardiopulmonary symptoms following embolism [34, 35]. Heparin appears to block this effect [36]. In designing a protocol for patients with embolism, it would not be rational (or ethical) to omit prompt application of heparin. To do so would deny a body of convincing data and compromise patient care. Further, since dissolution of the thrombus could not alter effects due to platelet aggregation (until total thrombus dissolution was achieved), omission of heparin certainly would not constitute a "fairer" trial of thrombolytic therapy.

IV. THE DIAGNOSTIC DILEMMA

There is no greater dilemma in attempting to evaluate therapy than that posed by our inability to make a specific diagnosis. This is particularly true in the field of thrombotic disease, in which presumptive diagnoses are fraught with hazard.

Let us begin probing the depths of this dilemma with a deceptively simple example: the design of a protocol for evaluating thrombolytic therapy in patients with acute myocardial infarction. On what diagnostic criteria shall we base selection of candidates? Certainly we cannot use clinical symptoms alone. Many disorders can mimic the symptoms of myocardial infarction, including dissecting aortic aneurysm in which thrombolytic therapy is, to say the least, not indicated. Furthermore, many patients with myocardial infarction present with atypical pain or other "noncharacteristic" symptoms. Obviously, symptoms alone will not do.

How about electrocardiographic changes? Well, this is a somewhat better diagnostic approach, but certainly not ideal. There are patients who have myocardial infarction with equivocal electrocardiographic changes. Shall we omit these? I suppose so, even though it is probable that many patients with borderline EKG changes may have partial occlusion which might be particularly amenable to thrombolytic intervention. What about various enzyme determinations in these borderline cases (CPK, LDH, SGOT)? Again, while these are helpful, they are not specific and they also may be "borderline." Furthermore, while they may become virtually diagnostic if samples are obtained daily for several days, must we wait for such confirmation? Prompt thrombolysis is highly desirable if we are to restore or preserve function. By waiting for enzyme rises, we may miss any therapeutic opportunity. Well, then, why not obtain a coronary arteriogram? Certainly this will establish the presence of an occlusion. Yes, that is true; but even this will not solve our problem. First, because there is reason to question the advisability of coronary angiography in all patients suspected of myocardial infarction. Second, because demonstration of an occlusion is not equivalent to demonstration of thrombosis. Coronary occlusion may be due to atherosclerotic disease alone, with bleeding directly into a plaque often applying the occlusive coup-de-grace. Or occlusion may be due to embolization of

VII. ANTITHROMBOTIC AND THROMBOLYTIC DRUGS

atheromatous material. And how would we know that the occlusion seen is fresh? Might this be an old occlusion not directly related to the patient's current complaints? And what if no occlusion is demonstrated? Does this mean that there was a thrombus which has already fragmented? Or does it mean that the thrombi are in vessels beyond the resolving capability of our radiographic technique? And, regardless of what we decide in this specific case, what are we to do with the literature which debates whether acute thrombosis is a common cause for myocardial infarction [37,38] ? And so on and so on, until the investigator begins to wonder how he became involved in such an impossible problem as the evaluation of thrombolytic therapy.

The diagnosis of other forms of thromboembolic disease is often almost as complex, whether the site is a peripheral vein, a pulmonary artery, or a cerebral artery. What, then, are we to do? Two things, I believe. First, investigative effort must be devoted to the development of improved diagnostic techniques. Second, we should launch therapeutic trials of thrombolytic regimens only in those conditions in which reasonable diagnostic accuracy can be assured. The definition of "reasonable diagnostic accuracy" should incorporate the best clinical and laboratory criteria now available. Institutions which cannot perform critical laboratory investigations should not engage in such studies.

There are "reasonable" techniques now available for establishing the diagnosis of certain thromboembolic diseases. The thromboembolic entity most subject to precise diagnosis at the moment is pulmonary embolism. Pulmonary angiography and ventilation/perfusion scintiphotography, when combined, provide reasonably definitive information regarding the extent and location of embolic material [39,40]. Both procedures have limitations, and of course, cannot provide information regarding embolic age or structure. Nevertheless, the availability of these techniques makes pulmonary embolism a logical first choice for the evaluation of thrombolytic agents. This is true even though thrombolytic therapy may be needed rarely in the management of pulmonary embolism since heparin and endogenous mechanisms are so effective in dealing with it.

The next best candidate for clinical thrombolytic trials is deep thrombosis of peripheral veins. Here venography can be applied with good diagnostic effect if the method is carefully applied and interpreted [41]. Furthermore, the ^{125}Iodine-fibrinogen method may prove a sensitive means of detecting and following venous thrombosis [42,43]. If this method sustains its promise, venous thrombosis will certainly provide a frequent and instructive "testing ground" for thrombolytic agents. Again, unfortunately, effective methods of treatment already exist and the need for thrombolytic therapy in such patients is not likely to be very substantial.

Measurement of fibrin degradation products (F. D. P.) is another highly promising technique for the detection of intravascular coagulation [44-46]. This technique also offers its greatest diagnostic potential in detecting fibrin thrombi, disseminated or focal.

The detection of arterial thrombosis remains a difficult task. New initiatives are needed to solve this problem. Perhaps radioactive techniques for identification of platelet aggregation can be developed. When substantial "red" thrombosis is associated with the platelet thrombus, the ^{125}I-fibrinogen or F. D. P. approaches may prove useful. Miniaturized fiber-optic systems for direct visualization of vascular lesions also are within the realm of possibility. At the moment, however, angiographic techniques, combined with all other clinical and laboratory clues, provide the only diagnostic approach. The multiple pitfalls in these approaches have been enumerated. Until this diagnostic deficit is remedied, thrombolytic evaluation in arterial thrombosis will depend heavily upon observations in animals with experimental arterial thrombosis and in human venous thromboembolism, with the hope that such observations may be in part transferable to human arterial thrombotic disease.

V. THE GOALS OF THROMBOLYTIC THERAPY AND APPROACHES TO ACHIEVING THEM

The primary objectives of thrombolytic therapy are two: prevention of thrombosis and treatment of thrombosis once it has appeared. The basic principles involved in achieving these two objectives are similar since the mechanisms of thrombogenesis determine the points of pharmacological attack in both instances. But the specific techniques will differ because the two objectives differ substantially with respect to the rapidity of effect required, the duration of therapy, and the numbers and types of patients involved. Let us consider first the approach to effective thromboprophylaxis.

A. Prophylaxis

In prophylaxis, the critical time factor often involved in acute thrombolytic therapy is absent. Much more critical is the question, "How shall we identify the population requiring these prophylactic regimens?" The most logical answers can be derived from epidemiological surveys which identify those groups at greatest risk. Further, we would best direct our prophylactic efforts against those thrombotic disorders which extract the highest toll of morbidity and mortality. Most needed are regimens for prevention of arterial thrombosis in the coronary and cerebral circulations. Perhaps next in line would be regimens to prevent pulmonary embolism.

How can we identify these patients? The simplest technique would involve epidemiological surveys using a specific test which identifies a tendency to thrombosis. Attempts to eradicate tuberculosis have been highly successful using the tuberculin skin test in this fashion. Unfortunately, no reliable screening test for thrombotic tendency exists. Multiple approaches are being explored. Platelet adhesiveness ("stickiness") and other tests of the aggregating tendency of platelets may prove to have predictive capability with respect to white thrombus formation [48-51]. The euglobulin lysis time or other measurements of endogenous fibrinolytic activity [52] also may identify patients with a thrombotic tendency, since an impaired fibrinolytic system

VII. ANTITHROMBOTIC AND THROMBOLYTIC DRUGS 331

may permit thrombosis to extend to clinical levels rather than being dissolved promptly [53]. The ability of various agents (e.g., nicotinic acid) to stimulate endogenous fibrinolytic activity may identify individuals at high thrombotic risk [54]. The ^{125}Iodine-fibrinogen and fibrin degradation product (F.D.P.) methods also may provide such information. At this time, however, none of these tests could be accepted as a means for identifying large population groups requiring thrombolytic prophylaxis. The need for such a test (or tests) is great, however, and the search will continue.

If no reliable laboratory means exists for detecting patients needing prophylaxis, we must rely on data derived from other sources. Epidemiological data do exist which would help us to select — by age, sex, degree of obesity, blood pressure, and other identifiers — those individuals most likely to develop myocardial infarction [55,56]. Similar data exist with respect to venous thromboembolism.

Having chosen our population, what pharmacological means might we apply? Since arterial and venous thrombosis differ in their genesis, let us consider them separately.

1. Arterial Thrombosis

If vascular injury plus platelet accretion is the basic sequence here, then our prophylactic options are limited. Until our understanding of intimal injury is further advanced, prevention of arterial thrombosis becomes largely a matter of preventing excessive platelet accretion at sites of injury. We have learned a good deal about the factors underlying platelet adherence, aggregation, and viscous metamorphosis in the recent past [47]. While we have much more to learn, it is already clear that certain drugs alter the tendency of platelets to form white thrombi. Three drugs seem particularly promising in this regard: glyceryl guaiacolate, aspirin, and dipyridamole [57-63]. The first agent, a common ingredient of cough syrups, has an excellent toxicity record to recommend it. Aspirin is acceptable from the toxicity viewpoint and already is widely used on a maintenance basis in several diseases. Dipyridamole is a bit more toxic than the other two, but has been demonstrated to have a promising effect in blocking platelet thrombotic complications following cardiac prosthetic surgery in man [62]. Each of these drugs has the signal advantage of being effective when taken by mouth, though daily use is required. Certainly these agents merit further study. Probably each will serve as a prototype in the search for even more effective pharmacological derivatives.

In addition to such platelet-directed agents, we may consider other pharmacological approaches which are truly thrombolytic. Fibrin is involved in development of the white thrombus, though the magnitude of its contribution remains uncertain [64-66]. Perhaps agents which enhance fibrinolytic activity will prove capable of disrupting the white thrombus matrix or interfering with its growth and stability. More certain is that such enhancement will interfere with development of the red thrombus which contributes to the obstructive potential of most white thrombi. Perhaps preventing this addition of red (fibrin) thrombus will serve the primary goal of thrombolytic therapy — preservation or restoration of blood flow — even though white thrombi continue to form. Drugs which may accomplish this objective must be capable of maintaining enhanced fibrinolytic activity in the patient for prolonged periods. Such drugs will be discussed in the next section.

To summarize, the search for drugs which can prevent arterial thrombosis should include agents directed against both platelet and fibrin thrombus development. Perhaps a regimen directed against both will prove most effective. In the meantime, the prothrombinopenic drugs, despite their known deficiencies, remain the choice for granting some current protection.

2. Venous Thrombosis

Prophylaxis against venous thrombosis is a somewhat less complex problem, chiefly because the mechanisms involved in red thrombus formation and dissolution have been more extensively studied. The primary goal here is to uncover nontoxic drugs capable of maintaining enhanced fibrinolytic activity for prolonged periods in man. Three approaches are worthy of consideration: (1) administration of substances which are directly fibrinolytic; (2) administration of materials which indirectly release endogenous fibrinolytic activity; and (3) delivery of agents which decrease inhibition of endogenous activity.

The first approach has little to recommend it at this time as a prophylactic avenue. The available drugs in this category — plasmin, streptokinase, and urokinase — are not effective unless given intravenously and, therefore, are not suitable for maintenance therapy. The last approach, reduction of inhibitors to components of the fibrinolytic system, is not presently attainable by any known pharmacological maneuver. This leaves the second option as the only feasible prophylactic choice at this time.

A great variety of maneuvers and drugs are known to enhance endogenous fibrinolytic activity. Exercise, for example, accomplishes this; and, no doubt, a reasonable amount of exercise each day is a good antithrombotic prophylactic [67,68]. Nicotinic acid, epinephrine, papaverine, and other vasoactive drugs are known to enhance endogenous activity by releasing plasminogen activator [69-71]. Precisely how they accomplish this is unknown. It is known that the walls of veins contain plasminogen activator [72-75] and it has been demonstrated that such drugs lead to enhanced activator levels in renal venous blood [76], as well as in mixed venous and arterial blood. Whether they lead to release of activator from all veins, or whether only certain venous systems (such as that of the kidney) participate is unsettled. Nor do we know whether such drugs also lead to release of activity from other, nonvascular body stores. But we do know that such drugs cause substantial, although transient, elevations in circulating plasminogen activator activity. Unfortunately, tachyphylaxis develops rather rapidly to each.

Fearnley and his colleagues have demonstrated that a number of other compounds enhance release of endogenous plasminogen activator in man, particularly the sulfonylureas and anabolic steroids [77-79]. Both the sulfonylureas (metformin, phenformin) and anabolic steroids (testosterone, ethyloestrenol) led to elevated circulating fibrinolytic activity, as measured by the euglobulin lysis time and the dilute whole blood clot lysis time [77-79]. Modest declines in plasma fibrinogen concentration occurred concomitantly, suggesting that such fibrinolytic enhancement was exerting a biologic effect. Measurements of F.D.P. were not done.

These promising observations were followed by reports that these drugs lost effectiveness after weeks to months of continuous use [79]. In an effort to overcome such "resistance," these same investigators employed combined sulfonylurea-anabolic steroid regimens. They found that such combined regimens result in sustained fibrinolytic enhancement for periods up to 12 months without evidence of tachyphylaxis [80]. The most effective regimen combined phenformin and ethyloestrenol. Not only did this therapy maintain increased plasminogen activator activity, but it also decreased platelet stickiness [81]. The reduced platelet stickiness was associated with modest elevation of the platelet count, again suggesting that a biologic effect was associated with the laboratory finding. Other interesting aspects of the sulfonylurea-ethyloestrenol therapy included the facts that: (1) the effects required weeks to months for full expression; (2) the effects disappeared rather rapidly when either drug was discontinued; (3) both normal subjects and patients with known arterial occlusive diseases responded to the regimen; and (4) substantial individual variations in responsiveness existed, with a moderate percentage of patients (20 percent) showing no significant response [79].

More recently, synthetic materials of a different structure have been demonstrated to promote fibrinolytic activity in vivo; namely, certain tetrahydroisoquinoline derivatives [82]. Such compounds, administered intravenously, not only enhance activator activity but also promote rapid dissolution of fresh venous thrombi in the dog [54]. These agents may be effective when administered by mouth, and appear to have an acceptable toxicity spectrum in both animals and man. While such preliminary data are promising, the tetrahydroisoquinolines obviously require further study before being considered for broad prophylactic or clinical use.

All of these agents — nicotinic acid, phenformin, tetrahydroisoquinolines, etc. — are totally inactive in vitro and achieve their thrombolytic effect by releasing plasminogen activator in the intact recipient. As already indicated, the exact mechanisms operative remain obscure.

Another promising approach to prevention of thrombosis is provided by materials capable of inducing controlled defibrination. The most widely studied defibrinating agent is a purified venom from the Malayan pit-viper, Arvin [83-85]. The primary effect of this material is to induce defibrination, which may be partial or complete depending on the dose administered. The material is effective by both intravenous and intramuscular routes, although the latter should be avoided because it promotes resistance to the agent, apparently through immunologic mechanisms [86]. The primary defibrination is associated with evidence of enhanced fibrinolytic activity and sharp elevations in circulating fibrin degradation products. Such "secondary" fibrinolysis is now a widely recognized component of intravascular coagulation in animals and in man [87,88]. It also has been shown that Arvin administration in man is followed by resistance to adenosine diphosphate-mediated aggregation of platelets, though platelet adhesiveness is not altered [89]. Indirect evidence relates the inhibition of ADP activity to the presence of fibrin degradation products.

One final approach to chronic enhancement of fibrinolytic activity remains relatively unexplored; namely, blockade of the normal activator clearance mechanisms. It is known that the liver plays a major role in removing activator from the circulating blood, although the exact locus and sequence involved are not understood [90-92]. Blockade of inactivation is an obvious route to enhancement of spontaneous or pharmacologically stimulated levels of fibrinolytic activity. Benemid blockade of renal excretion during penicillin therapy provides a ready parallel. Use of such an approach for maintaining elevated fibrinolytic activity requires greater knowledge of the inactivation-secretion pathways of plasminogen activator. The cirrhotic subject, known to have chronically elevated activator activity and a more prolonged elevation of such activity after pharmacological stimulation, provides an "experiment of nature" indicating that this approach is at least theoretically feasible [90-92].

Some of the pharmacological avenues to prophylaxis of venous thrombosis which have been described here may prove to be "dead-end" streets. Nevertheless, from such a rich list of possibilities, one or more clinically applicable alternatives should arise.

B. Treatment

The search for thrombolytic regimens suitable for acute thrombotic disease is guided by different rules than those applicable to thromboprophylaxis. The most obvious difference is that acute thrombolysis does not afford the luxury of delay, especially in arterial thrombosis. A regimen requiring days or weeks for maximal effect is acceptable for prophylaxis, but not acute therapy. Also, the population under consideration is smaller and more readily identified. The problems of identification (diagnosis) are substantial, as pointed out above; but they are not of the same magnitude as in preventive therapy. Further, the duration of drug therapy is finite, extending to minutes, hours, or days, rather than to months and years as with prophylaxis. Finally, the toxic risks acceptable in acute therapy are higher than those for prophylaxis for we are dealing with patients who have a measurable risk of morbidity or mortality. The points of pharmacological attack, however, are the same as those applicable to prophylaxis. Preformed white or red thrombi must be dismembered and further build-up of platelet or fibrin thrombus prevented. But this must be accomplished within the restricted "time-frames" previously described.

VII. ANTITHROMBOTIC AND THROMBOLYTIC DRUGS

1. Venous Thrombosis

The objective here is prompt attack upon the fibrin matrix. Three approaches are now available: first, administration of agents which directly attack preformed thrombi; second, delivery of agents which are inert *in vitro* but, *in vivo*, can heighten activity of the endogenous plasminogen-plasmin system; and third, agents which compromise the coagulation mechanism in a manner which favors thrombolysis.

a. Proteolytic Enzymes and Direct Activators.

In the first category are plasmin [93] and other proteolytic enzymes, and purified plasminogen activators such as streptokinase [94] and urokinase [95]. These agents have the appeal of therapeutic simplicity. A red thrombus exposed directly to a proteolytic enzyme will be dissolved, regardless of other circumstances operative in the particular patient. The same can be said of urokinase and streptokinase, with the major reservation that these activators will be thrombolytic only if the thrombus or the circulating blood or both contain adequate amounts of plasminogen. With this one reservation, the enzymes and plasminogen activators pose only two problems in application: (1) assurance that the thrombus will be exposed to them in adequate concentration, and (2) proof that such delivery can be achieved with safety.

Plasmin (fibrinolysin) can be prepared in an acceptably pure form and at a cost that is not prohibitive. Plasminogen can be separated from human or animal plasma, then activated to plasmin in several ways [96-98]. The resultant enzyme can be stabilized for prolonged storage prior to use [98]. Thus, technical problems have been solved. Extensive clinical trial of plasmin, however, has been delayed by questions of adequate delivery and toxicity. It is known that there is substantial antiplasmin activity in the blood [99]. The central question has been whether such antiplasmins *irreversibly* bind infused plasmin or whether some serve merely as a convenient carrier for plasmin delivery to the thrombus. If irreversible binding occurs, sufficient plasmin must be infused to totally overcome antiplasmin so that "free plasmin" is available to attack the fibrin thrombus. If some antiplasmin serves a carrier function, however, delivery of plasmin to the clot site can be achieved at much lower doses and without "free" plasmin present. The carrier concept is based on the fact that fibrin has a higher adsorptive affinity for plasmin [100, 101]. Thus, antiplasmin brings plasmin to the fibrin matrix and there yields the plasmin to the material (fibrin) with a higher affinity.

This controversy, unresolved for almost a decade, has delayed clinical trial of plasmin. Retrospectively, the controversy may prove to have had little merit. One concern was economic: irreversible binding would require larger doses of plasmin and higher cost. The major concern, however, was with the effects of "free plasmin." This proteolytic enzyme will digest a number of coagulation components, including fibrinogen [102]. The thesis was that this would induce an uncontrolled, dangerous coagulopathy [103]. This thesis now requires reassessment. Studies in our laboratory with urokinase-activated plasmin have demonstrated that this agent will induce lysis of fresh venous thrombi and pulmonary emboli in the dog [104]. The dose of plasmin required was reduced when heparin was given concomitantly, undoubtedly because heparin blocked thrombus extension while thrombolysis was being achieved [105]. Furthermore, while a coagulopathy was induced when large doses of plasmin, with or without concomitant heparin, were used, no hemorrhagic consequences followed. Plasmin and plasmin-heparin doses which were successful in these animal experiments have been applied to man without induction of a major coagulopathy or hemorrhage [106].

It is clear now that plasmin can induce thrombolysis and that a clinically devastating coagulopathy is not produced. Now that Arvin is being widely studied, the former fears of "hyperplasminemia" appear to have been overdone. Arvin causes a major coagulopathy. Indeed, defibrination and the events that follow are the basis of its therapeutic effect. Arvin therapy not only defibrinates the recipient but leads to a high concentration of F. D. P., one of the "hazards" attributed to "hyperplasminemia." Experience with Arvin has indicated that the profound disturbances which it causes do not lead to serious clinical hemorrhagic phenomena. Thus, the experiences of the last decade may rekindle interest in plasmin itself as a thrombolytic agent.

Of the two "direct" activators — urokinase and streptokinase — urokinase has received the most attention in the United States [95, 107-109]. The ascendancy of urokinase was based on several apparently valid considerations: (1) unlike streptokinase (SK), urokinase (UK) was of human origin, and therefore, not subject to the antigenic problems surrounding the use of SK; (2) UK acts directly to activate plasminogen, whereas SK requires intermediate steps which are still not entirely clear; and (3) UK infusion did not cause fever and SK often did. Thus, UK appeared a better choice, even though SK was substantially less expensive and easier to produce. Again, experience in recent years has raised questions as to the wisdom of concentrating exclusively on UK in this country. European investigators have devised standard SK regimens which appear to achieve adequate thrombolytic activity in patients regardless of their level of preexisting streptokinase-inhibiting antibody [110]. Febrile reactions have been controlled, and the clinical results have been encouraging [111-113]. Meanwhile, UK research has been markedly impeded by the high cost of the material, which has led to tightly controlled investigative distribution. As a result, limited data exist regarding the therapeutic efficacy of the material [95, 108, 109, 114] and difficulties in production becloud its future availability should it prove of value. Understandably, reevaluation of SK is again being discussed seriously [111].

To summarize, then, plasmin, streptokinase, and urokinase all remain worthy of continued investigation in venous thromboembolism, despite the hiatus of interest in the first two in this country in recent years.

b. Indirect Activators. Substantial interest in the development of synthetic pharmacological agents which, though inactive *in vitro*, generate production or release of endogenous activator *in vivo* [82, 115, 116], has been sustained for several reasons: (1) a drug effective by mouth (unlike plasmin,

SK, or UK) would have obvious advantages; (2) a synthetic agent would be simpler to produce in large quantity than the "biologics" discussed above and, therefore, would be much less expensive.

The major synthetic candidates have been discussed in the section dealing with prophylaxis: nicotinic acid, vasocative amines, tetrahydroisoquinoline derivatives, sulfonylureas, and anabolic steroids. However, in dealing with acute venous thrombosis, rather than prophylaxis, our criteria for acceptability change. For example, we need agents capable of <u>rapidly</u> inducing <u>marked</u> elevations of fibrinolytic activity. Therefore, promising prophylactic regimens like phenformin plus ethylestrenol, which require weeks to exert maximal effect, are not suitable. The question which exists with respect to the other synthetics is: Can they induce a level of fibrinolytic activity sufficient to promote acute thrombolysis? Many of the synthetics cause activator release which is detectable by laboratory tests; but what is desired is clot dissolution, not change in a laboratory test. I will have more to say of this below. Suffice it to say here that clinical trial of tetrahydroisoquinoline derivatives seem warranted now in venous thrombosis. Other synthetic materials seem less promising because of toxicity or an inadequate intensity or duration of effect.

c. <u>Arvin.</u> The growing experience with this purified viper venom suggests that it may prove valuable in treating acute venous thrombotic disease [83-85]. Its mechanism of action — defibrination and secondary fibrinolysis — generates understandable trepidation at first encounter. To treat thrombosis by inducing diffuse intravascular coagulation is an idea which requires some psychological adjustment — particularly in the United States where previous agents have been rejected because of the coagulopathy which they might induce. However, investigations to date have disclosed that the agent can be used safely. Therapeutic value remains to be proved. Carefully controlled clinical trials in venous thromboembolism to gather such proof are fully justifiable.

2. <u>Arterial Thrombosis</u>

The pitfalls in launching clinical trials of any acute thrombolytic regimen in arterial thrombosis have been detailed previously. Despite formidable obstacles, however, some reasonable possibilities do exist.

The agents already discussed as candidates for trial in venous thrombosis merit similar trial in arterial thrombosis. In my judgment, however, they should be of proven value in venous thromboembolism before being extended to the more complex areas of coronary and cerebral arterial occlusion. A listing of potentially valuable agents (in no "rank-order") must include plasmin, SK, UK, the tetrahydroisoquinolines, and Arvin. Such thrombolytics would be directed against the red thrombosis component of the arterial thrombus, and, possibly, against the fibrin involved in platelet aggregation. Such agents also may indirectly inhibit platelet aggregation as well. Arvin, for example, appears to inhibit ADP-mediated platelet aggregation [89]. It is not known whether the other fibrinolytics, perhaps by elevating F.D.P. levels, will exert similar effects.

In addition to fibrinolytic thrombolysis, however, arterial thrombosis should be directly attacked by agents known to alter platelet adhesiveness or aggregation. The most promising of these have been enumerated above; aspirin, dipyridamole, and glyceryl guaiacolate. As the true significance of platelet "stickiness" and the sequence of white thrombus development is further understood, other pharmacological agents will undoubtedly present themselves. At the moment, a combined fibrinolytic and "anti-platelet" regimen would appear the most promising one to explore.

VI. LESSONS OF HISTORY AND THE SEARCH FOR THROMBOLYTIC DRUGS

The lessons of history are hard won. Whether the search is for political or scientific solutions, these lessons should be carefully studied before proceeding further. In the case of thrombolytic therapy, we have almost 40 years of history to consider, dating to the discovery of streptokinase in the early 1930's [117]. We have (or should have) learned in this interval how to proceed in the search for thrombolytic agents.

Perhaps the central lesson has been: keep in mind the therapeutic objectives. These objectives have, at times, been obscured. They are: dissolution of preformed intravascular thrombi and, ultimately, thromboprophylaxis. It seems difficult to see how one could lose sight of these obvious objectives. Yet, it has happened frequently in this and other fields. Such deflections have occurred in the history of thrombolytic therapy when concern focused exclusively upon the biochemical alterations induced by a given agent, without attention being directed toward whether or not thrombolysis was being achieved. The use of any _in vitro_ test system to predict what will happen _in vivo_ is fraught with hazard. In my judgment, the most appropriate first step in the investigative sequence of any thrombolytic agent is to determine _whether the agent exerts a thrombolytic effect_. If it does, then the biochemical correlates of successful thrombolysis can be assessed (if, indeed, they exist in _in vitro_ systems).

Elsewhere I have detailed the sequence of investigation which is most likely to yield effective thrombolytic regimens [54]. It consists of four phases: (1) demonstration in animals that the agent in question can lyse thrombi; (2) detailed evaluation of the toxicity of the successful agent in animals; (3) detailed evaluation of the toxicity of the agent in man; and (4) controlled clinical trial of the drug in patients with the particular thrombotic disease in question.

Phase One is, of course, the critical one. If the agent has no thrombolytic activity, it should be discarded early in the game. Detailed study of its effects upon the plasminogen-plasmin system or the coagulation apparatus are meaningless if the agent does not promote thrombolysis. Thus, any promising agent discovered by serendipity in animal or human studies, or by purposeful screening programs, should promptly be submitted to in vivo trial in animals. Naturally, clues to a potential thrombolytic effect may first come by discovering elevated levels of circulating fibrinolytic activity. This is, in fact, what most current pharmacological searches are based upon. But early in the evaluation of such agents, observations regarding thrombolysis should be combined with laboratory tests. This is not difficult in the case of venous thrombosis. Convenient methods exist for inducing venous thrombosis in animals [3]. It is, therefore, a simple matter to carry out studies in which extensive laboratory data and observations regarding thrombolysis are obtained simultaneously. The primary concern at this stage is whether or not thrombolysis occurs, not the behavior of the laboratory tests. There are many pharmacological triumphs in which observation of therapeutic effect long antedated development of laboratory tests which predicted or explained the effects observed. Aspirin, digitalis, and penicillin are notable examples.

Any agent which emerges from animal investigations with established thrombolytic capability and an acceptable toxicity record is then ready for trial in man. In such a sequence, of course, species variability may lead to discard of a potentially valuable substance or study of agents which prove ineffective or toxic in man. In the absence of serendipity, however, such a sequence from animal to man seems the best available. Certainly man cannot be the primary screening animal. However, we can make a concession to species variability by accepting for trial in man agents with a good toxicity record which have modest thrombolytic capability in animals (if the economic questions involved permit such a concession).

The sequence of study in man should, I believe, be the reverse of that in animals; that is, thorough evaluation of toxicity first, followed by clinical thrombolytic trials. The dose regimens chosen for toxicity studies should be those which, in animals, have proven consistently effective in achieving thrombolysis. There can be legitimate debate about the choice of human subjects for toxicity trials. Normal volunteers would seem the logical choice, but the hazards in this approach are quite clear. Patients with the disease who may be aided would be the logical alternative choice, but there are hazards in exercising this option. For example, toxicity testing of a drug using patients with myocardial infarction would be ill-advised. Such seriously ill patients would not tolerate unexpected toxicity well, and their highly variable clinical course may make it difficult to separate toxic responses from naturally occurring events. Obviously, the population studied during this toxicity phase is not easy to choose. Whatever the choice, it cannot be ideal and the investigator must live with that reality.

The final testing phase — controlled clinical trial — should not be hurriedly entered. All available information regarding both the drug regimen and the thrombotic entity should be at hand when the protocol is designed. If this means interdisciplinary collaboration — and it usually will — such collaboration should be sought intensively, not avoided. Furthermore, since each thrombotic disease presents specific problems, each disorder should be studied separately by teams familiar with it.

It should be emphasized, however, that "controlled" studies do not require omission of accepted therapeutic measures. As stressed previously, omission of heparin therapy in thrombolytic studies of pulmonary embolism is a questionable requirement. The ability of heparin to prevent serotonin release from platelets on the red thrombus would make such an omission difficult to justify since thrombolytic agents may not exert a similar effect. In this circumstance, comparison of heparin plus the thrombolytic agent versus heparin alone would seem the logical choice.

VII. CONCLUSIONS

Those who have devoted years to the study of the coagulation-fibrinolytic system need not be reminded of its complexity. Investigations in this field have been plagued by the need to study in vitro delicate substances and reactions which are altered by the very manipulations required to permit laboratory study — ranging from sample withdrawal to contact with foreign surfaces. There was a recent fanciful motion picture in which a team of scientists were placed in a submarine, miniaturized, and injected into a peripheral vein. Their harrowing journey outdid the adventures of Captain Nemo. But what an opportunity to study the problems of coagulation and thrombosis within the proper milieu, the blood stream itself!

Until such a journey is possible, however, we must persist with our attempts to reproduce what occurs in vivo with in vitro or animal models. Such attempts have brought us a substantial distance. We know a good deal about how thrombi form and how we might impede or disrupt such formation. The natural history of thromboembolic diseases beyond their acute phase is better understood. A variety of agents, ranging from such "old standbys" as streptokinase to such new, and unexpected, ones as Malayan pit-viper venom are under active investigation.

The search for thrombolytic agents has been intense and continues. It seems likely that the search is about to uncover multiple agents that will be useful in maintaining the vascular system free of unwanted red, white, and composite obstructing thrombotic masses.

REFERENCES

1. Fibrinolysis, Thrombolysis and Blood Clotting. A Bibliography, compiled by National Heart and Lung Institute, National Institutes of Health in cooperation with the National Library of Medicine, Bethesda, Maryland, 1965-.

2. Webster's Seventh New Collegiate Dictionary, Merriam, Springfield, Massachusetts, 1966.

3. S. Wessler, J. Clin. Invest., 34, 647 (1955).

4. D. Deykin and S. Wessler, J. Clin. Invest., 43, 160 (1964)

5. S. Wessler, S. M. Reimer, and M. C. Sheps, J. Appl. Physiol., 14, 943 (1959).

6. S. Wessler, D. G. Freiman, J. D. Ballon, J. H. Katz, R. Wolff, and E. Wolf, Am. J. Pathol., 38, 89 (1961).

7. D. G. Freiman, S. Wessler, and M. Lertzman, Am. J. Pathol., 39, 95 (1962).

8. J. Hughes, Thromb. Diath. Haemorrhag., 3, 177, (1959).

9. M. D. Zucker and J. Borelli, Proc. Soc. Exptl. Biol. Med., 109, 779 (1962).

10. Y. Bounameaux, Compt. Rend. Soc. Biol., 153, 865 (1959).

11. T. Hovig, Thromb. Diath. Haemorrhag., 9, 248 (1963).

12. T. H. Spaet and M. D. Zucker, Am. J. Physiol., 206, 1267 (1964).

13. J. D. Wilner, H. L. Nassel, and E. C. Le Roy, J. Clin. Invest., 47, 2616 (1968).

14. D. Deykin, Calif. Med., 112, 31 (1970).

15. S. Wessler, B. Alexander, A. C. Beall, Jr., V. De Wolfe, and J. B. Miale, Circulation, 41, A-31 (1970).

16. A. H. Freiman, N. U. Bang, C. E. Grossi, and E. E. Clifton, Am. J. Cardiol., 6, 426 (1960).

17. H. B. W. Greig and I. A. Runde, Lancet, ii, 461 (1957).

18. N. Back, J. L. Ambrus, C. L. Simpson, and S. Shulman, J. Clin. Invest., 37, 864 (1958).

19. K. M. Moser, M. Guisan, P. Harsanyl, and E. Butler, Federation Proc., 27, 578 (1968).

20. H. L. Fred, M. A. Axelrod, J. M. Lewis, and J. K. Alexander, J. Am. Med. Assoc., 196, 1137 (1966).

21. J. E. Dalen, J. S. Banas, H. L. Brooks, G. L. Evans, J. A. Paraskos, and L. Dexter, New Engl. J. Med., 280, 1194 (1969).

22. D. E. Tow and H. N. Wagner, New Engl. J. Med., 276, 1053 (1967).

23. K. M. Moser, P. Harsanyi, G. Rius-Garriga, M. Guisan, G. A. Landis, and A. Miale, Circulation, 39, 663 (1969).

24. J. E. Dalen, V. S. Mathur, H. Evans, F. W. Haynes, A. A. Pur-Shahriari, P. D. Stein, and L. Dexter, Am. Heart J., 72, 509 (1966).

25. H. N. Wagner, D. C. Sabiston, Jr., J. G. McAfee, D. Tow, and S. Stein, New Engl. J. Med., 271, 377 (1964).

26. D. G. Freiman, J. Suyemoto, and S. Wessler, New Engl. J. Med., 272, 1278 (1965).

27. K. M. Moser, M. Guisan, and P. Harsanyi, Clin. Res., 28, 488 (1970).

28. A. Chait, D. Summers, N. Krasnow, and B. M. Wechster, Am. J. Roentgenol. Radium Therapy Nucl. Med., 100, 364 (1967).

29. J. E. French, Ann. Roy. Coll. Surg. Engl., 36, 191 (1965).

30. L. Jorgensen, H. C. Rowsell, T. Hovig, and J. F. Mustard, Am. J. Pathol., 51, 681 (1967).

31. J. B. Duguid, J. Pathol. Bacteriol., 60, 57 (1948).

32. K. P. Klassen, N. C. Andrews, and G. M. Curtis, A.M.A. Arch. Surg., 63, 311 (1951).

33. J. S. Byrne, New Engl. J. Med., 253, 579 (1955).

34. D. P. Thomas, M. Stein, G. Tanabe, V. Rege, and S. Wessler, Am. J. Physiol., 206, 1207 (1964).

35. D. P. Thomas, V. Gurewich, and T. P. Ashford, New Engl. J. Med., 274, 953 (1966).

36. V. Gurewich, M. Cohen, and D. P. Thomas, Am. Heart J., 76, 784 (1968).

37. H. L. Blumgart, M. S. Schlesinger, and D. Davis, Am. Heart J., 19, 1 (1940).

38. W. C. Roberts and L. M. Buja, Ann. Internal Med., 72, 781 (1970).

39. K. M. Moser, M. Guisan, and W. L. Ashburn, Ann. Internal Med., 72, 808 (1970).

40. P. D. Stein, J. F. O'Connor, J. E. Dalen, A. A. Pur-Shahriari, F. G. Hoppin, D. T. Hammond, F. W. Haynes, F. G. Fleishner, and L. Dexter, Am. Heart J., 73, 730 (1967).

41. V. V. Kakkar, C. T. Howe, J. W. Laws, and C. Flanc, Brit. Med. J., 1, 810 (1969).

42. N. Brown and M. Chapman, Brit. J. Surg., 55, 835 (1968).

43. C. Flanc, V. V. Kakkar, and M. B. Clarke, Brit. J. Surg., 55, 742, (1968).

44. C. Merskey, A. J. Johnson, G. J. Kleiner, and H. Wohl, Brit. J. Haematol., 13, 528 (1967).

45. C. Merskey, G. J. Kleiner, and A. Johnson, Blood, 28, 1 (1966).

46. E. Kowalsi, Seminar in Haematol., 5, 45 (1968).

47. A. J. Marcus, New Engl. J. Med., 280, 1213, 1278, 1330 (1969).

48. G. V. R. Born, Nature, 194, 927 (1962).

49. J. R. O'Brien, Ann. Rev. Med., 17, 275 (1966).
50. R. C. Hartman, Seminar in Haematol., 5, 60 (1968).
51. J. R. Hampton, J. Atherosclerosis Res., 7, 729 (1967).
52. P. T. Flute, Brit. Med. Bull., 20, 195 (1964).
53. T. Astrup, Blood, 11, 781 (1956).
54. K. M. Moser, in Chemical Control of Fibrinolysis-Thrombolysis (J. M. Schor, ed.), Wiley (Interscience), New York, 1970, p. 135.
55. T. R. Dauber, F. E. Moore, and G. V. Mann, Am. J. Public Health, 47 (pt. 2), 4 (1957).
56. Coronary Heart Disease in Seven Countries (A. Keys, ed.), Circulation, 41, suppl. 1, 1970.
57. J. L. Silverman and H. A. Wurzel, Am. J. Clin. Pathol., 51, 35 (1968).
58. G. Evans, M. A. Packham, E. E. Nishizawa, J. F. Mustard, and E. A. Murphy, J. Exptl. Med., 128, 877 (1968).
59. J. R. O'Brien, Lancet, i, 779 (1968).
60. P. R. Emmons, M. J. Harrison, A. J. Honour, and J. R. A. Mitchell, Lancet, ii, 603 (1965).
61. J. R. Hampton, M. J. Harrison, A. J. Honour, and J. R. A. Mitchell, Cardiovascular Res., 1, 101 (1967).
62. J. M. Sullivan, D. E. Harken, and R. Gorlin, New Engl. J. Med., 279, 576 (1968).
63. N. L. Browse and J. H. Hall, Lancet, ii, 718 (1969).
64. P. A. Castaldi and J. Caen, J. Clin. Pathol., 18, 579 (1965).
65. M. G. Davey and E. F. Luscher, Biochim. Biophys. Acta, 165, 490 (1968).
66. N. F. Rodman, R. G. Mason, and J. C. Painter, Lab. Invest., 15, 641 (1966).
67. E. Ikkala, G. Myllyla, and H. S. S. Sarajas, Nature, 199, 459 (1963).
68. W. D. Sawyer, A. P. Fletcher, N. Alkjaersig, and S. Sherry, J. Clin. Invest., 39, 426 (1960).
69. M. K. Weiner, K. de Crinis, W. Redisch, and J. M. Steele, Circulation, 19, 845 (1959).
70. R. Holemans, Am. J. Physiol., 208, 511 (1965).
71. S. Sherry, A. P. Fletcher, and N. Alkjaersig, Physiol. Rev., 39, 343 (1959).

72. A. S. Todd, J. Pathol. Bacteriol., 78, 281 (1959).
73. A. S. Todd, Brit. Med. Bull., 20, 200 (1964).
74. T. Astrup and K. Buluk, Circulation Res., 13, 253 (1963).
75. H. C. Kwaan and T. Astrup, Circulation Res., 17, 477 (1965).
76. I. S. Menon, H. A. Dewar, and D. J. Newell, Lancet, i, 785 (1968).
77. G. R. Fearnley, R. Chakrabarti, and C. T. Vincent, Lancet, ii, 622 (1960).
78. G. R. Fearnley and R. Chakrabarti, Lancet, ii, 128 (1962).
79. G. R. Fearnley and R. Chakrabarti, J. Clin. Pathol., 17, 328 (1964).
80. G. R. Fearnley, R. Chakrabarti, E. P. Hocking, and J. F. Evans, Lancet, ii, 1008 (1967).
81. R. Chakrabarti, G. R. Fearnley, and J. F. Evans, Lancet, ii, 1012 (1967).
82. J. M. Schor, in Chemical Control of Fibrinolysis-Thrombolysis (J. M. Schor, ed.), Wiley (Interscience), New York, 1970, p. 113.
83. W. R. Bell, W. R. Pitney, and J. F. Goodwin, Lancet, i, 490 (1968).
84. V. V. Kakkar, C. Flanc, C. T. Howe, M. O'Shea, and P. T. Flute, Brit. Med. J., 1, 806 (1969).
85. H. A. Reid and K. E. Chan, Lancet, i, 485 (1968).
86. W. R. Pitney, P. J. L. Holt, C. Bray, and G. Bolton, Lancet, i, 79 (1969).
87. D. G. McKay, Calif. Med., 111, 186, (1969).
88. D. G. McKay, Therapeutic Implications of Disseminated Intravascular Coagulation — An Intermediary Mechanism of Disease, P. B. Hoeber, New York, 1965.
89. C. R. M. Prentice, A. G. G. Turpie, A. A. Hassanein, G. P. McNichol, and A. S. Douglas, Lancet, i, 644 (1969).
90. A. P. Fletcher, O. Biederman, D. Moore, N. Alkjaersig, and S. Sherry, J. Clin. Invest., 43, 681 (1964).
91. K. M. Moser and G. C. Hajjar, Am. J. Med. Sci., 251, 536 (1966).
92. G. Purcell, Jr., and L. L. Phillips, Surg. Gynecol. Obstet., 117, 139 (1963).
93. C. M. Ambrus, N. Back, and J. L. Ambrus, Circulation Res., 10, 161 (1962).
94. A. P. Fletcher, N. Alkjaersig, and S. Sherry, J. Clin. Invest., 38, 1906 (1959).

95. P. N. Walsh, J. M. Stengle, and S. Sherry, Circulation, 39, 153 (1969).
96. N. Alkjaersig, Biochem. J., 93, 171 (1964).
97. K. H. Slotta and J. D. Gonzalez, Biochemistry, 3, 285 (1964).
98. J. T. Sgouris, J. K. Inman, K. B. McCall, L. A. Hyndman, and H. D. Anderson, Vox Sanguinis, 5, 357 (1960).
99. P. S. Norman, Federation Proc., 25, 63 (1966).
100. C. M. Ambrus and G. Markus, Am. J. Physiol., 199, 491 (1960).
101. L. B. Nanninga and M. M. Guest, Arch. Biochem. Biophys., 108, 542 (1964).
102. V. H. Donaldson, J. Lab. Clin. Med., 56, 644 (1960).
103. A. P. Fletcher, N. Alkaersig, and S. Sherry, J. Clin. Invest., 41, 896 (1962).
104. K. M. Moser, J. Rius-Garriga, P. Harsanyi, and G. C. Hajjar, Circulation, 36, Suppl. II, 193 (1967).
105. K. M. Moser and G. C. Hajjar, Circulation, 34, Suppl. III, 176 (1966).
106. K. M. Moser and G. C. Hajjar, Unpublished observations.
107. J. T. Sgouris, J. K. Inman, and K. B. McCall, Am. J. Cardiol., 6, 406 (1960).
108. D. E. Tow, H. N. Wagner, and R. H. Holmes, New Engl. J. Med., 277, 1161 (1967).
109. A. P. Fletcher, N. Alkjaersig, S. Sherry, E. Genton, J. Hirsch, and F. Bachmann, J. Lab. Clin. Med., 65, 713 (1965).
110. M. Verstraete, J. Vermylen, R. DeVreker, A. Amery, and C. Vermylen, Scand. J. Clin. Lab. Invest., 16, Suppl. 78, 15 (1964).
111. S. Cherry, New Engl. J. Med., 280, 723 (1969).
112. J. Hirsh, G. S. Hale, I. G. McDonald, R. A. McCarthy, and A. Pitt, Brit. Med. J., 4, 729 (1968).
113. H. Poliwoda, K. Alexander, J. Buhl, M. D. Holstein, and H. H. Wagner, New Engl. J. Med., 280, 689 (1969).
114. A. H. Sasahara, J. E. Cannilla, J. S. Belko, R. L. Morse, and H. J. Criss, New Engl. J. Med., 277, 1168 (1968).
115. K. N. von Kaulla, Federation Proc., 25, 57, (1966).
116. K. N. von Kaulla, Chemistry of Thrombolysis: Human Fibrinolytic Enzymes, Thomas, Springfield, Illinois, 1963.
117. W. S. Tillett and R. L. Garner, J. Exptl. Med., 58, 485 (1933).

Chapter VIII

PHARMACOLONGEVITY: CONTROL OF AGING BY DRUGS

Frank S. LaBella

Department of Pharmacology and Therapeutics
University of Manitoba
Faculty of Medicine
Winnipeg, Manitoba, Canada

I.	INTRODUCTION	347
II.	BIOLOGICAL AGING AS A RESULT OF COALESCENCE-ACCRETION-STABILIZATION OF BODY CONSTITUENTS	349
III.	HORMONES	353
IV.	PROCAINE	357
V.	PROCAINAMIDE, DIPHENYLHYDANTOIN, PEMOLINE, AND INOSINE-ALKYLAMINO ALCOHOL COMPLEXES	358
VI.	ANTIOXIDANTS AND FREE RADICAL SCAVENGERS	360
VII.	LATHYROGENS	364
VIII.	CENTROPHENOXINE	367
IX.	IMMUNOSUPPRESSANTS	370
X.	OTHER AGENTS	371
XI.	PROSPECTS FOR PHARMACOLONGEVITY	373
	REFERENCES	377

I. INTRODUCTION

Shortening of the life span of man or animals by the administration of drugs is readily accomplished. Premature or sudden death induced by drugs or other agents is an easily recognized and documented phenomenon. Furthermore, fatal responses can be precisely quantitated and reproducible dose-response curves that relate the incidence of death to the amount of a drug readily constructed. Proven prolongation of life by pharmacological means, on the other hand, is apparently a rare event, if achieved at all. Although legends and anecdotes abound on the topics of elixirs of youth and other means of age retardation or of rejuvenation, it is only in recent years that attempts

Copyright © 1972 by Marcel Dekker, Inc. **NO PART** of this work may be reproduced or utilized in **any form or by any means,** electronic or mechanical, including Xeroxing, photocopying, microfilm, and recording, or by any information storage and retrieval system, without permission in writing from the publisher.

have been made to investigate pharmacological prolongation of life, "pharmacolongevity," by valid scientific approaches.

The assessment of life-prolonging agents involves a commitment to individual experiments which may extend over several years, even in the case of the shortest-lived laboratory mammals. Also, the validity of reported beneficial effects on animal survival or life span depends, on one hand, on the reliability of knowledge of that species' specific, i.e., maximum, life span. This type of data is difficult to come by, because the average or maximum life span of laboratory rodents, for example, reportedly varies from one strain to another, from one laboratory to another, and even at different times in the same laboratory. There are difficulties, however, in relying on the maximum, rather than the average, life span of a given animal population. Average life span can be determined quite accurately, whereas the maximum limit of survival can only be estimated from a few survivors. An extremely wide range of ages at the time of death may be found in very old survivors of a given population.

Inhibition of basic aging processes, whatever these may be, would be expected to increase the maximum life span of a given species. Some recent claims of pharmacolongevity may, in fact, have little to do with aging per se, since average rather than maximum life span has been increased by the so-called "anti-aging" compounds. Average life span may be extended by inhibiting specific morbid processes that ultimately kill the host. Thus, a greater number of protected individuals in the colony at any given time survive to die of "old age."

Many "theories" of aging have been put forth, but only a few have survived even the superficial scrutiny of the scientific method which has been imposed on aging research in relatively recent years. At the present stage of knowledge of the biological aging process, attempts to explain the obvious, deleterious changes that occur with time in all living things must be regarded only as working, premature hypotheses. However, ignorance of the fundamental causes need not preclude therapeutic success in the fight against aging.

In the not too distant past, a scientific reputation could be jeopardized merely by vocal contemplation of the prospects for experimental manipulation of aging. This astounding posture of cynicism by scientists has not yet been completely eradicated. Today, in certain scientific quarters, serious proposals for the studies on fundamental mechanisms of aging and on retardation or reversal of these processes are still regarded as a form of quackery, even when put forth by otherwise competent investigators. Granted, gerontological literature is historically replete with extravagant claims for rejuvenation or aging retardation. However, scientific endeavor has reached the stage where the events of the aging process cannot validly be excluded from the category of biological reactions which may be influenced by drugs or other agents. In recent years, modest beneficial effects of drug administration on the aging animal have been reported, although one's enthusiasm is dampened by the fact that, in practically every case, confirmatory findings from other laboratories have not as yet emerged.

VIII. PHARMACOLONGEVITY: CONTROL OF AGING BY DRUGS

Probably from the time of man's first awareness that the relatively rare individual who did not succumb early in life to diseases or violent death eventually terminated his existence in the state of extreme debility and physical deterioration, humans have attempted to ward off aging. Pharmacotherapy, in the form of extracts or parts of particular plants or animals, was just one of many approaches to the problem. Some of the more imaginative treatments instituted to promote rejuvenation were nonpharmacological but afforded distinct benefits, if not therapeutic success. For example, the heat from the bodies of young virgins was believed to possess special curative and rejuvenating powers. In the First Book of Kings of the Bible, old and stricken King David is treated in this manner, apparently unsuccessfully. However, this significant failure does not seem to have diminished the popularity of this type of therapy. Other therapies recommended that old men suckle at the breasts of healthy young girls. Although these therapeutic regimens may not be amenable to proper scientific control and evaluation, their positive placebo effects should not be underestimated. The anticipation, alone, of impending treatment may well provide the driving force required of the senescent individual to survive from one day to the next.

There have been, of course, innumerable other forms of equally esoteric therapies. Even today, the "royal jelly" obtained from bees, mixtures containing "essential oxidative enzymes and metabolites to replace dwindling body stores," and other irrational and unproved "therapies" are openly promoted in so-called developed nations. Exhibits for these quack medicines may even be seen at national and international medical and gerontological conventions. For the most part, therapy has been directed towards rejuvenation rather than age-retardation. Probably the first example of successful experimental extension of the life span which was adequately documented in recognized scientific literature is the feeding experiments of Osborne et al. [1] and McCay [2-4]. Briefly stated, these experiments, subsequently confirmed by several laboratories ([5,6]; see the review in Ref. [7]) showed that in the albino rat caloric restriction resulted in an extension of mean and maximum life span. It is of significance that the dietary regimen was most successful in the young growing rat and that life extension resulted from "freezing" the animals at this early stage of development. In other words, this was an instance of apparent aging retardation. McCay's results have been generally interpreted to support the premise that underfeeding prolongs life. On the other hand, Le Compte [8] has stated: "From McCay's experiments there is only one conclusion possible, that overfeeding shortens life ...." This latter view is an interesting one and may be the correct interpretation, if one assumes that the usual <u>ad libitum</u> feeding of the confined laboratory rat is an unnatural condition.

II. BIOLOGICAL AGING AS A RESULT OF COALESCENCE-ACCRETION-STABILIZATION OF BODY CONSTITUENTS

The word "aging" still defies attempts at definition in universally acceptable terms. A definition which probably comes closest to general acceptance describes aging as a process in which the individual becomes progressively more susceptible to natural insults and in which the probability of death increases. Although one can find little to argue against in this statement, the definition is notable for its lack of reference to specific biological events. Whereas this rather general description of aging applies to the individual as a whole, a single specific process within that individual should satisfy several criteria before it can be regarded as associated with biological aging. According to Strehler [9], these criteria include (a) universality, (b) progressiveness, (c) intrinsicality, and (d) deleteriousness and apply to changes in the organism which are not due to preventable diseases or other gross accidents.

Hypotheses on the causes of aging are legion, but most have been discarded because they fail to indicate possible experimental means for their validation or because they can be included in more comprehensive proposals. Currently fashionable hypotheses are of more recent vintage and based on modern scientific premises, or are more sophisticated extensions of older ones. Most important, the hypotheses of aging which are popular today appear to have been selected, because each of them delineates specific molecular or cellular events as causes of aging, and each, to some extent, can be tested experimentally or has been supported by experimentation.

Most of the currently attractive hypotheses can apparently be categorized together, for the sake of simplicity, because they appear to encompass similar or identical cellular or molecular processes or both. Thus, for example, hypotheses specifically attributing age-degeneration to crosslinking of structural proteins, to intracellular pigment accumulation, to crosslinking and chemical alteration of nuclear or cytoplasmic nucleic acids, to brain cell degeneration and death, to immunological incompetence or aberration, and to oxidative insult to catalytic molecules, involve three fundamental processes which may be expressed as <u>coalescence,</u> <u>accretion,</u> and <u>stabilization.</u>

Coalescence of lysosomes with other subcellular organelles or fragments thereof probably contributes to pigment accumulation within cells. The residue from normal cellular, digestive processes represents material which is resistant to lysosomal or other intracellular hydrolases. Accretion of various materials on extracellular fibers is indicated by the progressive pigmentation and calcification of collagen and elastin with age. Accretion of organic and inorganic material may contribute to the accumulation of intracellular age pigments. Calcification of cellular membranes may also occur, thereby gradually reducing the proportion of viable membrane surface. Any particulate substance may serve as a nucleus for deposition of soluble molecules and for adsorption of particulate elements, and once initiated, by one mechanism or another, this process of accretion continues indefinitely. Stabilization refers to the process of rendering individual chains of macromolecules physically and chemically less reactive. This may occur by linking adjacent chains of proteins or of nucleic acids through the formation of covalent bonds, or by chemical modification of functional groups on these macromolecules. Thus, structural proteins become less elastic, for example. Enzymes and membrane-transport proteins are inactivated. DNA, including that of immunocompetent cells, is prevented from duplicating itself or is chemically altered so that transcription is faulty. In Table I, the targets for coalescence, accretion, and stabilization and some of the postulated sequelae are categorized.

There is no claim here for a "unified theory" of aging, nor for originality in the hypothesis. It is simply another way of expressing age-related phenomena which may have similar molecular bases and which may be at least partly responsible for aging. The crosslinking hypothesis of aging, which was formulated and developed by Bjorksten [10], embodies many of the features encompassed in coalescence-accretion-stabilization. However, the former hypothesis is somewhat restrictive and excludes phenomena which may be appropriately fitted into the latter. For example, Bjorksten makes a distinction between crosslinking and "clinker" production [10]. Although he correctly points out that crosslinking occurs between theretofore functional molecules, in either case the result is an accumulation of insoluble material as an indirect consequence of the "fires" of cell metabolism. Tappel [11] has stressed the possible role of lipid peroxidation in the age-associated accumulation of intracellular pigment, resulting from coalescence of lysosomes with damaged membranes. Carpenter and Loynd [12] have proposed an "integrated theory of aging" in an attempt to encompass what they feel are the ten "theories" currently in vogue. This "integrated theory" is an elaboration of the crosslinking hypothesis and essentially attempts to attribute all the observable morphological and functional changes occurring with age to this single molecular process. The grouping of these hypotheses into coalescence-accretion-stabilization may be oversimplistic. Obviously, very different agents and specific chemical interactions are involved for each of the afflicted cellular and extracellular components. Furthermore, potential experimental manipulation, i.e., retardation, inhibition, or reversal, of these processes at various cellular sites would no doubt require an equally formidable number of specific pharmacotherapies. However, viewing the panorama of biological aging, specifically mammalian aging, as one of coalescence-accretion-stabilization, emphasizes that with time a greater proportion of the body's irreplaceable and potentially replaceable components become permanently fixed and irreversibly modified. Histological, chemical, and radioisotopic studies do, in fact, support this contention. On one hand, there is interference with structural, catalytic, or informational function by direct attack to macromolecules, and, on the other, a degeneration in the organizational capability of cells due to the effects on specific macromolecules and to the physical presence of accumulated materials in, on, and around the cells. Shock [13] feels that impairment in humans with advancing age is due to (a) dropping out of functional units in key organ systems, (b) some impairments in the functional capacities of cells remaining in the body of the aged, and (c) breakdown of neural and endocrine integrative functions in the individual. These events may be readily interpreted as arising from coalescence-accretion-stabilization phenomena, occurring in both dividing and nondividing cells and in intercellular components.

TABLE I

Coalescence–Accretion–Stabilization Hypothesis of Aging

Targets	Effects
Normally replaceable cellular structures Plasma membrane Cytoplasmic organelles Soluble components	Impairment of intracellular diffusion, membrane transport, and catalytic and metabolic functions of macromolecular constituents. Formation and accumulation of "foreign" proteins.
Genetic apparatus including that of immunocompetent cells	Inactivation or impairment of transcription. Somatic mutation leading to alterations in the number and properties of replaceable molecules, or to formation of abnormal, deleterious molecules. Antibody formation to self.
Extracellular permanent structures Collagen, elastin Some components of the ground substance	Pigmentation, calcification, fragmentation, loss of elasticity and mechanical strength. Impairment of intercellular diffusion. Foci for pathological changes, e.g., atherosclerosis. Formation and accumulation of "foreign" proteins.

Quantitative chemical estimates of age which can be used to assess the possible effects of various regimens on the aging process are rare. One of the more widely used techniques is the measurement of the physicochemical properties of individual tail tendons from the rat. Verzar [14] showed that the rat tail tendon exhibits well-defined increases with age in tensile strength and the temperature required for shrinkage, and progressive decrease in the amount of labile, hydroxyproline-containing peptide released during thermal contraction. The tail tendon is an almost pure preparation of collagen, and physical changes with age in this tissue are consistent with a progressive covalent crosslinking between constituent collagen molecules. LaBella and co-workers [15, 16] showed in the human that over the entire life span there is a linear increase in visible fluorescence in purified aortic elastin and Achilles tendon collagen; these observations have been confirmed by others [17, 18]. The increased fluorescence with age may not necessarily reflect changes in the elastin molecule per se, but there is evidence that it may be a property of material which appears to become covalently bound to elastin with time [89]. This may also be true for tendon collagen in the human. The regular accumulation of "age pigment," lipofuscin, in postmitotic cells [19, 20] is another of the few chemical measures of age. It should be pointed out that, with the exception of the permanent structural proteins, no adequate data are available to show cumulative deterioration of catalytic, informational, and other functional macromolecules. In contrast, it is quite clear that lifelong accretion of insoluble proteins and associated substances and continuous chemical modifications of these materials occur both intra- and extracellularly. Although there is no proof for a causal relationship between coalescence-accretion-stabilization and aging, the correlation alone would seem to afford a sufficiently sound basis for initiating attempts at pharmacolongevity on a molecular or cellular level.

III. HORMONES

It is probably safe to assume that the rate of animal aging, and hence life span, is regulated to some extent by the endocrine glands. Because the life span of a species is apparently genetically "programmed," to use an overworked gerontological cliché, the program no doubt comprises every aspect of organismal function, including endocrine status. Thus, removal and dysfunction of endocrine tissues or administration of their secretory products to intact individuals would be expected to modify the aging processes typical of the species. There is evidence, in the case of the pituitary gland particularly, that endocrine manipulation or dysfunction does apparently retard or accelerate a number of age-related changes (see review in [21]). There are few endocrine data available, however, bearing on the most important criterion of age-retardation, i.e., increase in specific life span.

Removal of the pituitary gland from laboratory animals is reported to retard the aging process in the ovary and connective tissue and prevent the experimental development of certain diseases typical of old age (see review in [21]). However, the role of multiple collaborating hormones and of interlocking metabolic processes in establishing the rate of aging in a species is underlined by the fact that hypophysectomy generally shortens life span [21]. Conversely, administration of pituitary growth hormone [22] or thyroxine [23] to the aging rat, or pituitary extract to the aging mouse [24], had no effect on life span. The biological age of the tail tendons in hypophysectomized 800-day old rats, however, corresponded to that of the 400-day old sham-operated animals [25]. Similarly, decreased tensile strength of tail tendon was reported for adult rats of both sexes castrated early in life [26].

Friedman and his co-workers [27-30] have reported that the chronic administration of neurohypophysial hormones (as posterior pituitary powder or extract) to rats as old as 24 months prolongs average life span. Representative survival data from Friedman's laboratory are shown in Fig. 1. The general condition of the treated animals was reported to be conspicuously improved. Fur condition was better, muscle tone was increased as evidenced during handling, and there were fewer ulcerated lesions on the feet (Fig. 2). Furthermore, hormone therapy improved the old animals' ability to perform work, inhibited the senescence-related increase in the weights of several organs, and restored ionic gradients and water turnover towards values of

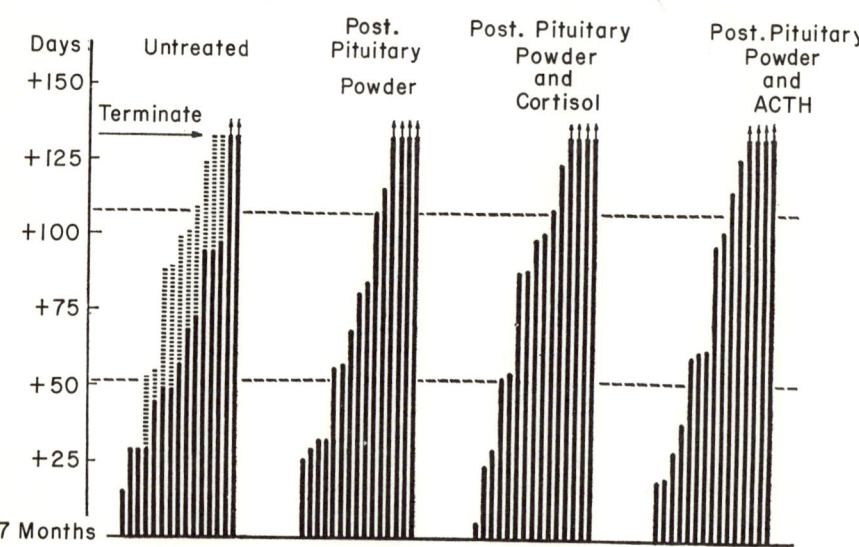

Fig. 1. Effect of posterior pituitary principles on survival of rats. Each animal is indicated by a black bar and survivors at the time of termination of the experiment by arrows. As an aid for comparison, those cortisol-treated animals surviving more than 50 days are superimposed as dotted lines on the untreated group. The experiment began with male albino rats of the Wistar strain, aged 27 months. (From Friedman et al. [27].)

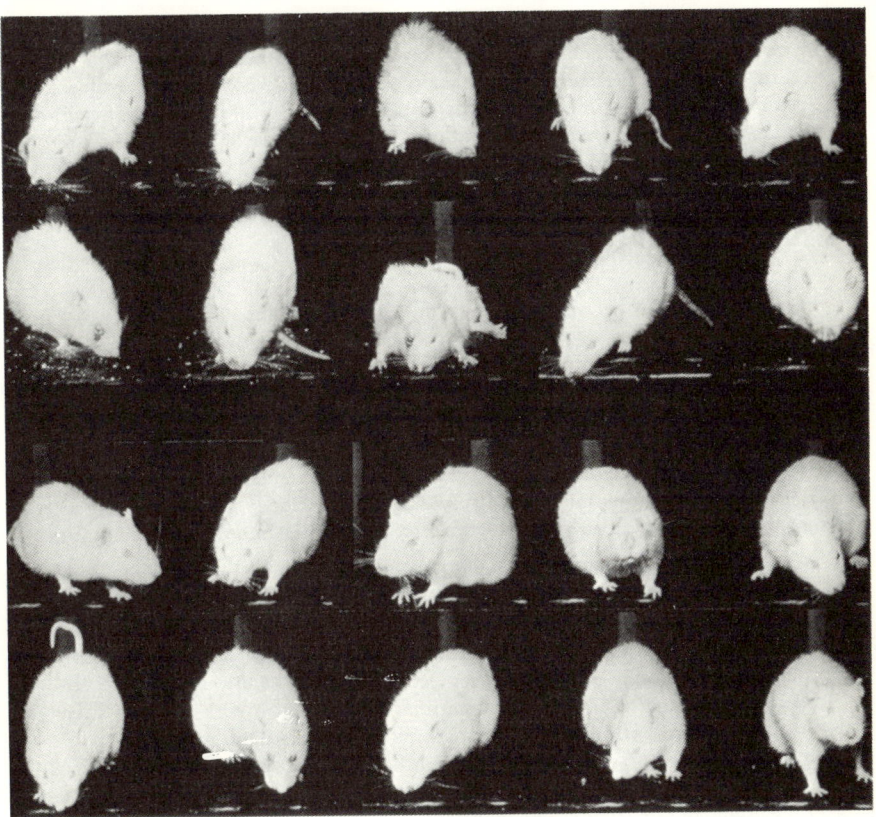

Fig. 2. The appearance of 10 unselected untreated rats (top two rows) compared with that of 10 unselected old rats treated with posterior pituitary powder and cortisol for 41 days (bottom two rows). At this time, there were 11 untreated and 12 treated survivors. At the start of the experiment, male albino rats were 24 months old. (From Friedman et al. [27].)

younger animals. There is physiological and histological evidence for age-related deterioration of neurohypophysial function in the rat (see [27]), and Friedman's findings are compatible with a hormone-replacement function of posterior pituitary extracts. The addition of glucocorticoid to the neurohypophysial therapy appeared to enhance the beneficial effects of the posterior pituitary extract.

There are several problems in the interpretation of these findings. First, although there appears to have been some reproducible effect of the pituitary extract on mean survival [27, 28, 31], relatively few animals are involved and maximum life spans are not reported. Secondly, purified vasopressin itself was without benefit and, in fact, may have decreased survival [27, 31]. Factors other than the known neurohypophysial peptide hormones in gland extracts may be responsible for the observed changes. Also, the improved appearance of the old animals is stated to be obvious after 31 days of therapy, but no differences could be seen between treated and control rats after 79 days. This last observation suggests that the beneficial effects of hormone treatment are transient or reversible with time or that deterioration in all animals progresses very rapidly at some later stage.

Bellamy [32] reported a doubling or more of the life span of a short-lived strain of mice by addition of prednisolone phosphate (2.1 µg/ml) to the drinking water. Beneficial effects of the steroid on survival were obtained with both males and females of a closely inbred strain of mice with a well-defined maximum life-span of about one year (Fig. 3). In this series, many of the experimental animals were still alive at 680 days. Steroid-treated mice showed a reduced rate of growth (body weight), although they eventually achieved the maximum body size. The rate of accumulation of tissue collagen, decline in liver respiratory capacity, decrease in kidney ATPase, and rise of calcium to collagen ratio in bone were reduced in prednisolone treated mice.

The experiment of Bellamy confirms the well-known property of adrenal steroids to inhibit growth of animals. In this connection, there may be a relation between growth inhibition by steroids and by caloric restriction and life extension. Bellamy states that there was no significant difference between untreated and prednisolone treated mice in food and water intake related to body weight. Several explanations may be put forth; Bellamy speculates that the anti-inflammatory properties of prednisolone may inhibit autoimmune processes that contribute to the short life span of this strain of mice. It is equally plausible that this particular animal is or becomes unusually deficient in adrenocortical function.

The cell density of radiation-arrested primary human amnion cultures was found to be consistently higher than control cultures when grown in the presence of hydrocortisone, suggesting that the steroid prolonged the average post mitotic life span of the cells [33]. In addition, culture degeneration occurred several months later in the presence of steroid than in its absence [34]. Steroids with an 11-OH, but not those with 11-keto, delayed cell degeneration [35]. Prolongation of the life span of human embryo fibroblasts in cultures by cortisone has also been reported [36]. Yuan et al. [37] suggest that adrenal steroids prevent cell death in cultures by an action on the cell membrane. Leith [38] has proposed alternatively that the beneficial effects of steroids on aged cells may be due to their depressing activity on RNA synthesis. He cites reports of (a) a firmer DNA-histone binding and diminished RNA synthesis in old cells, (b) the stimulatory effect of steroids on RNA synthesis in many types of cells, and (c) the binding of steroids to histones and DNA, to support his hypothesis.

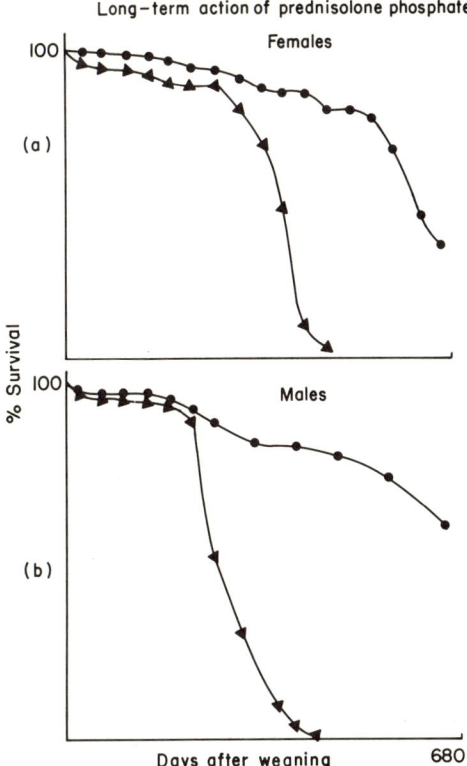

Fig. 3. Effect of corticosteroid on the mortality rate of mice. Prednisolone phosphate was incorporated into the drinking (tap) water (2.1 μg/ml) of 3-week-old animals throughout the remainder of the life span. Animals were kept in groups of 10 (400 mice of each sex) in metal cages at $25°C$ with a 12-hour photoperiod (from Bellamy [32]). ▲-normal; ●-prednisolone treated.

IV. PROCAINE

In 1956 Aslan and colleagues [39-41] in Romania first reported that repeated intramuscular injections of procaine hydrochloride produced remarkable changes in aged and debilitated humans. Although these reports deal with several thousands of subjects, the clinical design and therapeutic evaluation leave much to be desired. The Romanian workers make unrestrained claims for rejuvenation of senescent individuals. They report that procaine therapy provides ameliorative and even curative effects in arthritis, psychoses, Parkinsonism, hypertension, arteriosclerosis, and many other states of physical and mental deterioration. With regard to the rejuvenating properties of the drug, Aslan went so far as to say that "Procaine reduces the biological age of the individual below his chronological age." Procaine injections are still widely prescribed in Europe, and there the drug (Gerovital H_3) has widespread popular appeal to the layman. Many well-known statesmen, artists, and other prominent people are reported to have journeyed to Romania for procaine therapy. Substantiating reports of beneficial effects of procaine therapy have been published almost exclusively in European journals, but all of these studies suffer from lack of scientific control and evaluation (see review in [42]). In contrast, well-controlled studies, including those incorporating a placebo group, showed no beneficial effect of the drug [43-47]. Workers reporting improvement in senescent individuals by administration of procaine (or, for that matter, strychnine, pentylenetetrazol, Vitamin B_{12}, etc.) have apparently been generally ignorant of the powerful benefits of placebo alone. Any drastic environmental change in the usually uneventful life of an institutionalized or otherwise restricted, aged individual is bound to improve his mental and, perhaps to a lesser extent, physical status.

In an abstract, Aslan and colleagues [48] reported beneficial effects of Gerovital H_3 on rat survival. In a series of 1416 rats of the Wistar strain, oral or parenteral administration of the preparation increased mean life span of males of about 20% and of females by about 7%. In contrast, Verzar [49] injected large doses of procaine or its hydrolysis products, para-aminobenzoic acid and diethylethanolamine, to year-old rats for 14 to 30 months. There was no difference between control and treated animals in survival, body weight, or general appearance. In addition, no differences were found in a reliable age test, the thermic contraction of isolated tail tendon fibres.

Gordon and co-workers [50] reported that, in a double-blind study on aged humans, "procaine with additives" (Gerovital H_3; Chimimport, Bucharest) but not procaine alone (Abbott Laboratories), "significantly improved behavioral functioning" after 6 months of chronic injection. Although there were some slight changes induced by the drugs, they were not of enough significance, according to the investigators, to justify the use of either procaine preparation as a eutrophic treatment in the aged.

V. PROCAINAMIDE, DIPHENYLHYDANTOIN, PEMOLINE, AND INOSINE-ALKYLAMINO ALCOHOL COMPLEXES

Citing the suggestions of others that deterioration of function in the aged brain may be partly due to development of domains of hyperexcitability, Gordon [51] proposed that diphenylhydantoin (DPH) and procainamide (PA) might be useful in the aged. DPH and PA presumably exert therapeutic effects in convulsive and cardiac disorders by decreasing hyperexcitability in brain cells and heart cells, respectively. PA was reported to be very effective in ameliorating age-related deficits in avoidance behavior in experimental animals [51]. More recently [52], these workers reported in

VIII. PHARMACOLONGEVITY: CONTROL OF AGING BY DRUGS

controlled "blind" studies that DPH and PA improved behavior and learning deficits in aging rats, and in aged human subjects certain subtle aspects of mentation were apparently improved by drug administration.

The progressive inability of individual cells during aging to maintain homeostasis, thereby reducing the organism's resistance to environmental stress, no doubt reflects the gradual deterioration of genetic and metabolic machinery of the cell. A concept arising from these considerations is that aging is associated with defective internal information flow. Gordon [52a, 52b] reports that with age "organizational entropy of brain polyribosomes markedly increases" in rats. Entropy increase (disorder) in polyribosomes is reflected presumably in alterations in the distribution of RNA forms between double helix, base stacked, and random coil and related categories. An obvious consequence of conformational disturbances in polyribosomes would be errors in amino acid incorporation into proteins, resulting, as one example, in disturbances of learning and memory. Gordon [52a] reviews the findings which support the hypothesis that changes in the protein synthetic machinery take place with age; these changes include those of rate and accuracy.

Gordon [52a, 53, 54] reports that DPH prevents polyribosomal disaggregation and renders RNA more resistant to hydrolysis by RNAse. Thus, DPH fosters organization of polyribosomes in the aged towards the state of aggregation found in young animals. In recent brief reports and in a review, Gordon and co-workers [52a, 55-57] described pharmacological and biochemical effects of other compounds which were shown to alter the structure of polyribosomes; these "inosine-alkyl-amino alcohol complexes" (IAC) are apparently unrelated chemically to either DPH or PA. IAC was reported to produce several changes in polyribosomes of liver and brain of aged rats, including an increased content and hypochromicity of RNA, decreased susceptibility of RNA to RNAse, and marked changes in RNA and amino acid turnover and incorporation. IAC enhanced acquisition and retention of avoidance paradigms in 12- and 24-month-old rats and enhanced learning in 2 to 3-month-old rats. These workers hypothesized that learning was enhanced in rats through an action of IAC on neuronal polyribosomal structure. The ribosomal site of action of IAC was supported by an antiviral action of the drug observed in mice and in tissue culture; there were indications that IAC altered the structure of the host ribosomes so as to preserve their synthetic functions. It is claimed that IAC is more effective than DPH in restoring age-related alterations in polyribosomal structure and function to the younger patterns, and, thus, more effectively "reverses biochemical aging in animals" [52a, 54].

A structural relative of diphenylhydantoin, pemoline (2-imino-5-phenyl-4-oxazoledinone), with central nervous stimulant rather than depressant actions, has been reported to enhance memory and learning of both animals and man. It is said to increase levels of brain RNA in animals. This compound has been marketed for use in man under the trade name Cylert (pemoline plus magnesium hydroxide; Abbott Laboratories). Magnesium pemoline enhanced performance over placebo of subjects carrying out a fatiguing, repetitive cognitive task, but was no better than caffeine, methylphenidate, or amphetamine [58, 59]. The drug also reportedly improved performance on I.Q. tests, only after several weeks of administration, of subjects suffering from age-related memory defects [60]. This study was apparently without adequate controls, however. In a double-blind study, no effect of the drug was found on learning, memory, and performance of normal adult males [61]. The relationship of the purported benefits of pemoline administration to a specific role in brain RNA metabolism is rendered doubtful by observations that facilitation of learning can also be promoted by amphetamine, nicotine, caffeine, strychnine, physostigmine, pentylenetetrazol, and many other drugs [62].

Several reports have suggested that acquired information can be transferred to naive animals by administration of purified material (presumably containing RNA) from the brains of trained animals. These reports of positive findings have been disputed by others in which transfer of information in extracts could not be demonstrated. In humans, Cameron [63] claimed that intravenous administration of RNA ameliorates memory disturbances in the elderly. There is abundant evidence to indicate a role for RNA in molecular processes concerned with memory and learning [64, 65]. It is not known whether nucleotide sequences store processed information, much as they determine transfer and utilization of genetic information, or whether they reflect the primary role of newly synthesized proteins concerned with information storage.

VI. ANTIOXIDANTS AND FREE RADICAL SCAVENGERS

Harman [66, 67] has suggested that aging may be the result, at least in part, of destructive side reactions arising from free radicals, which are continually produced by tissue metabolism. A free radical is a transient form of an atom or functional group of a molecule which contains an unpaired electron. Free radicals are highly reactive species and are ubiquitous and numerous in biological systems [68.69]. A typical free radical reaction that can be expected to be of significance in biology [70] is shown in Fig. 4. Harman [70] suggests that there may occur among the free radical-induced deleterious changes occurring with age, (a) accumulative oxidative alterations in the long-lived molecules of collagen, elastin, and chromosomal material, (b) breakdown of mucopolysaccharides through oxidative degradation, (c) accumulation of metabolically inert material such as ceroid and age pigment through oxidative-polymerization reactions involving lipids, particularly polyunsaturated lipids, and proteins, (d) changes in membrane characteristics of mitochondria, lysosomes, and other organelles, due to lipid peroxidation, and (e) arteriolocapillary fibrosis due to peroxidation products of serum and vessel wall components, probably largely lipids, acting as vessel wall irritants. He points out, also, the deleterious effects of whole-body ionizing radiation, Vitamin E deficiency, and oxygen toxicity, conditions in which the level of random free radical reactions is increased. Furthermore, in support of the free radical theory of aging a correlation has been pointed out between the degree of radiation resistance and life span of strains in mice [71].

VIII. PHARMACOLONGEVITY: CONTROL OF AGING BY DRUGS

Initiation $RH + O_2 \xrightarrow{Cu} R\cdot + HO_2\cdot$

Propagation $R\cdot + O_2 \rightarrow RO_2\cdot$

      $RO_2\cdot + RH \rightarrow R\cdot + ROOH$

Termination $R\cdot + R\cdot \rightarrow R{:}R$

Fig. 4. Reaction of molecular oxygen with organic compounds (RH) and catalyzed by copper (Cu).

These observations are consistent with the hypothesis that resistance to the actions of free radicals protects against both the ravages of time and of radiation.

Harman [70, 72, 73] has tested several antioxidants for antiaging activity (estimated from survival data). This class of compounds is capable of reacting with free radicals and thereby sparing endogenous molecules from attack. Butylated hydroxytoluene (BHT) was found to be among the most effective agents in increasing survival in animal colonies. BHT is believed to react with free radicals as depicted in Fig. 5.

Representative results for the action of BHT and 2-mercapto-ethylamine (2-MEA) on survival of young LAF_1 mice are shown in Fig. 6. Both agents increased the mean life span but had no significant effect on maximum life span. In this same series cysteine, propyl gallate, 2,6-di-tertbutylhydroquinone, and hydroxylamine were without effect [72]. Harman suggests that the antioxidants which are ineffective in increasing survival may be less capable of inhibiting in vivo free radical reactions or may have achieved inadequate tissue distribution and concentration or both.

Harman's studies [72] also pointed out the marked effects of diet on animal survival. The mortality rate of LAF_1 male mice was much greater in animals on a synthetic diet than in those on a commercial diet. He attributes the adverse effects of a synthetic diet to its propensity to enhance the production of amyloidosis in those animals: Histologically, an incidence of 60% of the pathology was noted in mice on the synthetic diet compared with 20% in those on the commercial diet. Female C3H mice and male Sprague

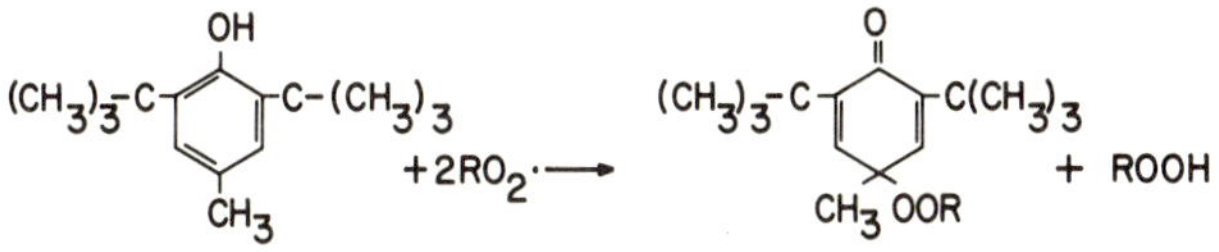

Fig. 5. Postulated reaction of BHT with free radical (RO_2).

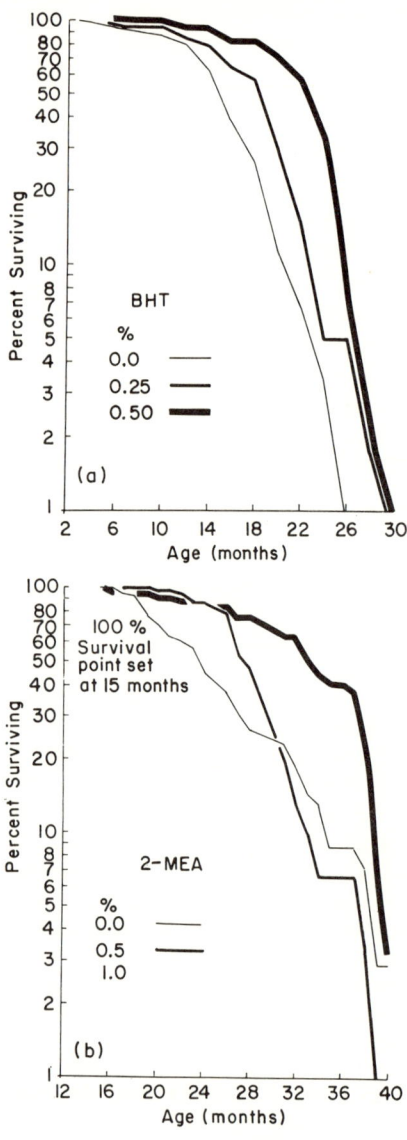

Fig. 6. Effect of BHT and 2-MEA on survival of 2-month-old male LAF_1 mice. The drugs were added to the diet which was available ad libitum. (a) Effect of BHT added to a commercial, powdered mouse diet. (b) Effect of 2-MEA added to a semisynthetic diet. The 100 percent survival point was set at 15 months. (From Harman [72].)

Dawley rats, on the other hand, showed similar survival on either diet. Thus, the adverse effect of the synthetic diet reflected an unusual susceptibility of the LAF_1 strain. Harman's studies [70] suggested, also, that survival of mice and rats was enhanced at lower dietary levels of unsaturated fat. This observation is pertinent, since unsaturated lipids are more liable than the saturated variety to participate in free radical reactions.

The inability of BHT and 2-MEA to alter the specific (maximum) life span suggests that these agents have little effect on the fundamental aging process in mice. The increase in mean life span may reflect a fortuitous beneficial effect of the drugs on some unknown disease process.

Tappel [11] stressed the role of unsaturated lipids as a source of free radicals, and, like Harman, suggests that regulation of the intake of unsaturated lipids and administration of antioxidants might slow the aging process. Unsaturated lipids readily undergo peroxidation, a reaction which involves direct participation of oxygen plus lipid to form free radical intermediates and semistable peroxides. Peroxidation can presumably occur in free and membrane-bound lipids and could lead to rupture of lysosomes and other organelles, to crosslinking of catalytic and structural proteins, and to accumulation of insoluble protein-lipid complexes. Furthermore, release of lysosomal enzymes may exert deleterious hydrolytic actions on a variety of essential tissue substrates. Blood platelets have been reported to accumulate lipid peroxides during platelet aging [74]. Enhancement of lipid peroxidation by heavy metals was greater in aged platelets, suggesting loss of defense against peroxidation with time. Tappel [11] emphasized the importance of Vitamins E and C and selenium in animal and human nutrition. Vitamin E serves as a general biological antioxidant in body metabolism, and its lack results in a wide variety of biochemical lesions. A synergistic antioxidant action occurs between Vitamins E and C. Tappel [11] suggested possible anti-aging therapy by the administration of one or more antioxidants including Vitamins E and C, selenium, sulfur amino acids, glutathione, and a variety of synthetic compounds.

It is of interest in this regard that augmenting the diet with essential fatty acids and other lipids reduced the life-shortening effects of ionizing radiation in mice [75]. There is considerable controversy as to the relevance of radiation sequelae to spontaneous aging; although they have many features in common, certain important differences cast doubt on claims that radiation produces a state of accelerated aging [76]. An impressive study in this regard is that by Lindop and Rotblat [77] who concluded, on the basis of extensive postmortem examinations, that the early death of irradiated mice apparently occurred from the same causes that lead to the death of normal senescent animals. The protective effect of added dietary lipid [75] is compatible with the hypothesis that endogenous essential lipids are being spared from the oxidizing action of radiation.

VII. LATHYROGENS

Kohn [78, 79] and LaBella [80, 81] proposed that agents which interfere with crosslinking of peptide chains in the fibrous connective tissue macromolecules might retard biological aging, and they have initiated experimental work along these lines. The basis of this proposal resides in the assumption that aging of the permanent structural proteins, mainly collagen and elastin, significantly determines aging of the animal, including man, as a whole.

There is almost universal agreement that the physical properties of connective-tissue-rich tissues, such as tendons and skin, change with aging in a manner that is consistent with the progressive accumulation of covalent crosslinks between polypeptide chains of the component structural proteins. Thus, with aging, solubility, extensibility, and swelling of the tissues decreases, and tensile strength and the temperature for shrinkage increase. Furthermore, artificial crosslinking of proteins in various tissues, by aldehydes, quinones, or other reagents, mimics the effects of spontaneous in vivo aging, with respect to the physical properties of the tissue (see review in [82]). About 30 to 40% of total body protein is made up of collagen and elastin, and a large proportion of these fibrous, structural proteins is permanently consolidated in the tissues early in life. Histological, and even gross, observations indicate that deleterious change is continually taking place in arteries, skin, and joints, for example. Sobel [83] has postulated a more general role of connective tissues in the aging process, in stressing that an increased fiber to gel ratio and other changes in the ground substance lead to diminished nutrient exchange between blood and parenchyma.

Because of the apparent importance of time related alterations in connective tissue as a causative factor in aging of the organism as a whole, interference with crosslinking of the fibrous proteins might retard aging in the animal to some extent. Lathyrogens were the first pharmacological agents found to interfere with the formation of crosslinks and, thus, fiber maturation in collagen and elastin. The first lathyrogen, so-called because of its presence in Lathyrus odoratus, a variety of sweet pea, to be isolated was β-aminopropionitrile (BAPN) (Fig. 7). Subsequently, a large number of compounds with certain structural similarities were also shown to be capable of inducing a state of lathyrism in young growing animals: semicarbazide and penicillamine are two other examples. Lathyrism in animals is characterized by the occurrence of skeletal deformities, dissecting aortic aneurysms, and other abnormalities. The syndrome is most prominent in young animals, in which active fibrous connective tissue protein synthesis is occurring.

The basic defect in lathyrism was gradually elucidated and shown to be a failure in the processes which govern formation of crosslinks derived from lysine in both collagen and elastin ([84-86]; see review in [82]). BAPN inhibits an amine oxidase which oxidatively deaminates the ε-amino group of lysine residues in collagen and elastin, converting the side chain to an aldehyde. Other lathyrogens prevent the formation of this type of crosslink by inhibiting the enzyme or by combining with the resulting aldehyde group or

VIII. PHARMACOLONGEVITY: CONTROL OF AGING BY DRUGS

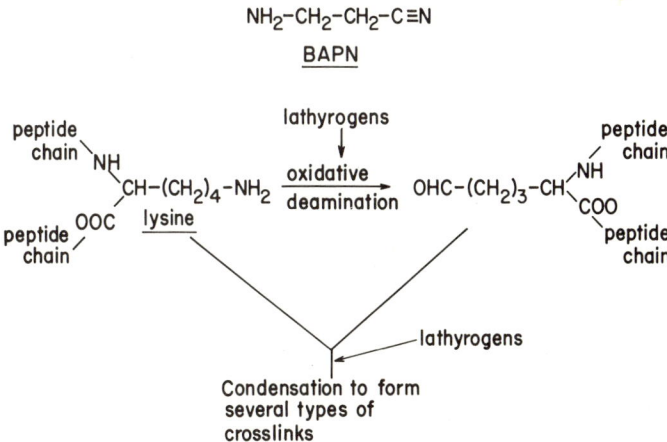

Fig. 7. Diagrammatic summary of lysine-derived crosslinks in collagen and elastin, and the site of action of lathyrogens. See Ref. [82].

both (Fig. 7). Conversion of lysine side chains to aldehydes is the first step in the condensation of lysine residues on different peptide chains to form characteristic crosslinks (Fig. 7). Both LaBella and Kohn initiated their studies on chronic lathyrogen administration before the exact nature of the crosslinks had been elucidated. There was some evidence that in collagen intramolecular crosslinking (within the triple strands of a single molecule) and intermolecular crosslinking (between collagen molecules) were competitive and continuous processes [87, 88]. Maturation and aging of collagen probably is governed largely by the latter process. Thus, the rationale for instituting lathyrogen treatment as a possible inhibitor of aging was based on the hypothesis that, given to the young adult animal, the drug would prevent or delay further deleterious crosslinking. Lysine-derived crosslinks, at least in elastin, do not appear to be involved in aging, since their density is constant from childhood to old age [89]. In unpublished work, LaBella detected no significant decrease with age in the lysine content of insoluble collagen from human tendon. Thus, other types of chemical bonds must be operative in the presumed crosslinking of collagen and elastin with age. However, profound changes in solubility and other properties of polymers may occur by the institution of an extremely small number of crosslinks which elude detection. For example, a single crosslink between two chains of a synthetic polymer, each composed of 30,000 monomer units, was reported to result in insolubility of the polymer [90].

Kohn's study [79], performed with weanling, pathogen-free rats, was marred by the death of most of his animals, presumably due to air-conditioning failure in the animal house. No increase in longevity by chronic administration of BAPN was found in the few surviving rats. However, he did report that high doses of the drug caused irreversible stunting of growth of the animals, and for a shorter period had a delayed effect on growth, manifested by weight loss late in life. The animals showed signs of lathyrism while on the drug, and they survived for 104 to 154 weeks.

In LaBella's study [81] several hundred male albino rats (Holtzman Company) of various ages were fed BAPN, semicarbazide, or penicillamine at varying levels (Fig. 8). These findings must be regarded as preliminary; no systematic study was made of food intake, body weight, or incidence of pathological conditions. The study was designed only to obtain estimates of satisfactory levels of drug, using survival as the basic criterion. The only

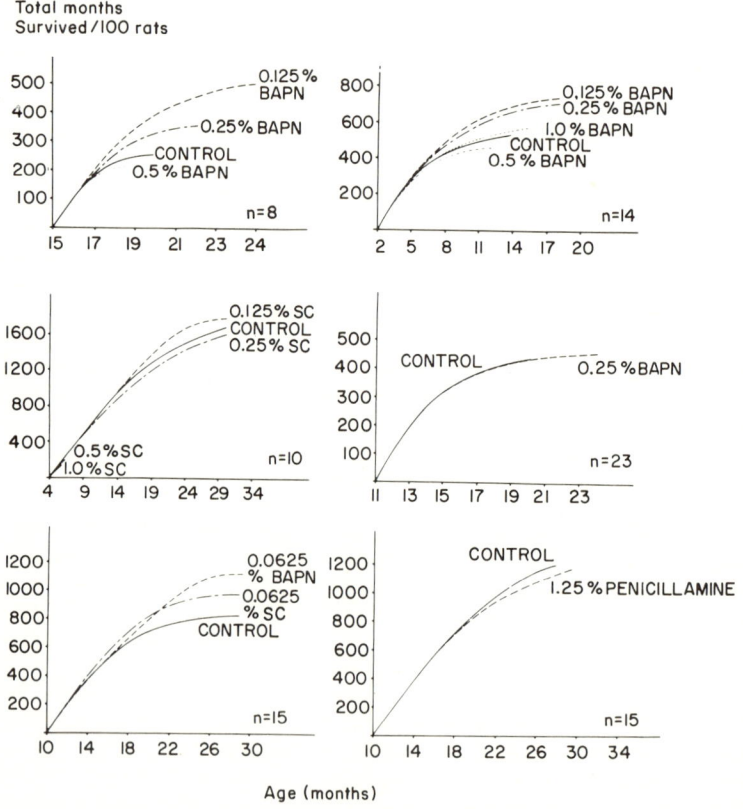

Fig. 8. The effect of β-aminopropionitrile (BAPN), semicarbazide (SC), and penicillamine on survival of male rats. The drugs were administered in the diet at the levels indicated throughout the entire period and the experiment continued until all the animals were dead. N = number of animals in each group.

instances in which maximum life span was increased by lathyrogen treatment occurred in those experiments where control animals died at an unusually early age (Fig. 8). The lathyrogens, in these cases, may have inhibited some morbid disease process which caused premature death of the animals. However, in other experiments (Fig. 8) there was evidence of increased average life span but not of maximum life span. The beneficial effects of lathyrogens added to the diet were evident in animals aged 2 to 15 months at the start of the drug administration.

Nitriles and other lathyrogens are highly reactive chemical species. Their action in enhancing survival may be related to the similar action of antioxidants in Harman's studies. LaBella [91] showed that lathyrogens form covalent bonds with aromatic amino acid residues in elastin during ultraviolet irradiation of the purified protein in vitro, presumably due to the formation of free radical intermediates. Thus, the salutary effect of lathyrogens may be related to free radical trapping, rather than to a specific connective tissue protein target. Clearly, more work is required to elucidate the mechanism whereby the lathyrogens induced the modest enhancement of survival in these series.

Because of their pronounced action on the physical state of collagen and elastin, lathyrogens have been administered empirically to humans suffering from various collagen diseases. The drugs were administered despite the knowledge that significant effects on the fibrous proteins could only be produced in very young animals and prior to the elucidation of molecular mechanisms of lathyrism. Penicillamine was reported to improve several serological parameters in rheumatoid arthritics [92]. Alterations were reported in the solubility of collagen from patients with Wilson's disease or scleroderma treated with penicillamine [93].

VIII. CENTROPHENOXINE

It appears that centrophenoxine (Fig. 9) was instituted as a geriatric therapeutic agent because it is structurally related to natural plant auxins which have been shown to retard senescence in leaves. These botanical observations would hardly appear to be sufficient grounds for extrapolation to the senescent human. Uncontrolled evaluation of centrophenoxine in geriatric patients with various types of mental deterioration led French workers [94, 95] to conclude that the drug was extremely beneficial in these clinical conditions. Improvement was reported after several weeks treatment (400-800 mg drug per day) in the majority of patients suffering from confusional states, Parkinsonism, and a variety of other states. These unimpressive, subjective reports apparently provided a sufficient basis for initiating studies concerned with possible salutary effects of the drug on the neurocytological deterioration in brain which is characteristic of senescent animals [96].

Accumulation of intracellular deposits, "age pigment," is a characteristic feature of nonreplaceable postmitotic cells, e.g., striated muscle and brain neurons. Bondareff [97] has stated that, of the numerous

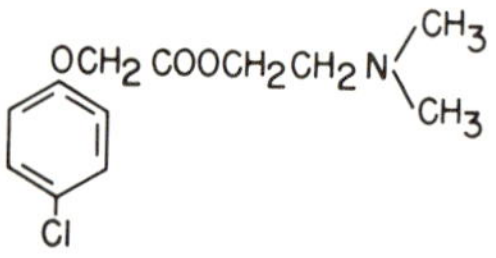

$$\text{OCH}_2\text{COOCH}_2\text{CH}_2\text{N} \begin{matrix} \text{CH}_3 \\ \text{CH}_3 \end{matrix}$$

(benzene ring with Cl substituent)

Fig. 9. Structure of centrophenoxine.

neurocytological events correlated with aging, accumulation of this pigment, lipofuscin, is one of the most consistent. The pigment is present as granules which can be seen in unstained tissue sections by virtue of their fluorescence (see Fig. 10). Fluorescence is probably due to the presence of oxidized lipid in the pigment. It is not known whether the pigment affects the functional integrity of nerve cells in the living animal. However, Bondareff cited some positive evidence in studies on cultured ganglion cells [98]: cells containing the pigment failed to migrate, as did other cells, and nuclei in the pigmented cells lost their characteristic staining properties. Strehler et al. [19] estimated that in the human myocardium the pigment increased at a rate of about 0.6% of the total intracellular volume per decade. The rate of pigment accumulation in the dog myocardium was estimated to be five times greater than in the human [20]. It is of significance that the average age of the human subjects was about 52 years [19] and about 10 years for the dogs [20].

The origin of lipofuscin is uncertain. Strehler [99] favors its derivation from the endoplasmic reticulum, although others have implicated various cell organelles. It appears that this pigment, which chemically and histochemically has been found to contain lipid, protein, nucleic acid, carbohydrate, and enzymes, is probably a conglomerate of residues of several organelles. It has been demonstrated in cells in general that fusion of lysosomes with other cellular organelles and digestion of these organelles is a normal process. Insoluble lipid-protein residues commonly result from this process (see [100]). It appears likely that lipofuscin represents, at least in part, accumulated, insoluble residues of intracellular digestion. Furthermore, this residue might act as a catch basin for the accretion of both soluble and particulate cellular elements. Thus, the histochemical observations [99] and analysis of isolated lipofuscin particles [101, 102] are compatible with the presence of a mass of oxidized lipid, proteins, and a wide variety of other cell constituents, covalently linked to form an insoluble sludge.

A number of experimental procedures have been reported to increase pigment accumulation, such as the administration of several antipyretic analgesics [103], hypoxia [104], and Vitamin E deficiency [105]. Nandy's report [96] is apparently the first to claim a drug-induced reduction in age pigment. He claimed that the administration of centrophenoxine daily for at least 10 weeks caused a reduction in pigment of brain neurons, as determined histologically, in guinea pigs aged 6 months to 6 years. There was an apparent reduction, also, in the activity of a number of oxidative enzymes, as determined histochemically. Nandy suggested that the drug promoted

VIII. PHARMACOLONGEVITY: CONTROL OF AGING BY DRUGS 369

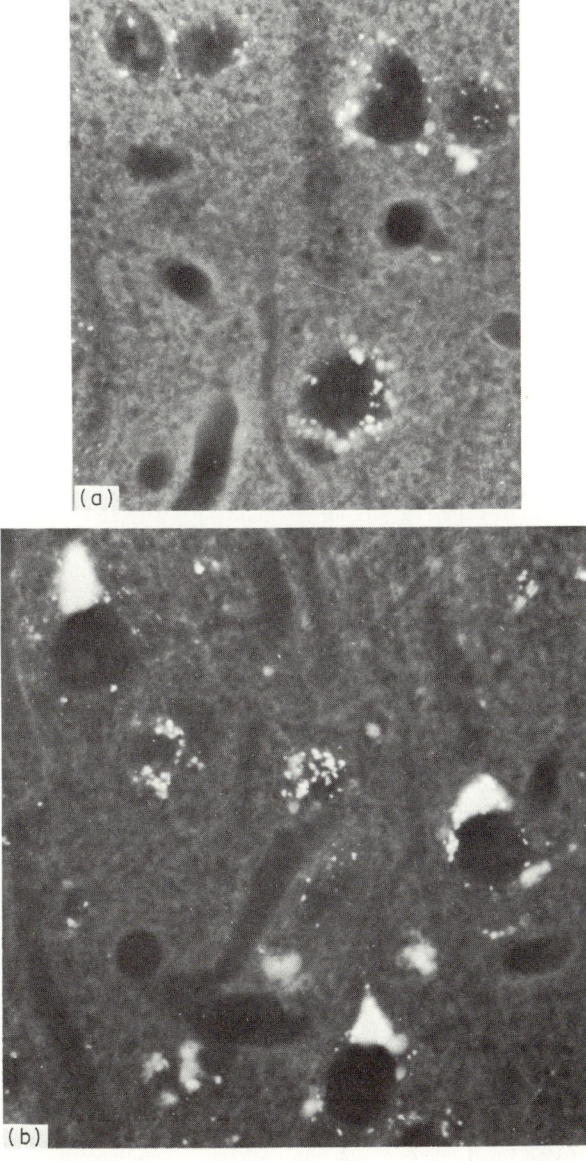

Fig. 10. Photomicrographs of unstained sections under blue light fluorescence, illustrating lipofuscin pigment in neuron stomata in lamina V of rat cerebral cortex. (a) Young adult rat (about 100 days old). (b) Aged rat (about 700 days old). Magnif. x720 (from Brizee et al. [105].)

diversion of glucose metabolism to the pentose cycle, resulting, in some way, in the elimination of accumulated pigments.

Although Nandy's report is of possible great significance, the study's major failing is the lack of statistical or controlled procedures for quantitative estimates of histochemical parameters. An adequate study would utilize a double-blind procedure in both the performance of the histochemical tests and the histological evaluation of sections from treated and untreated animals. Randomization of selection of tissue sections and of areas within a section for evaluation would be essential, also. Furthermore, some objective criteria are absolutely necessary for estimates of enzyme activity and pigment density.

In a recent abstract, Harman [105a] reported that incorporation of centrophenoxine into the diet of Swiss male mice was deleterious. Mean life span (months $\pm$ S.D.) for mice fed 0, 0.25, or 0.5% of the drug (percent weight of the diet) was 16.5 ± 5.5, 16.0 ± 6.3, and 10.6 ± 4.6, respectively.

IX. IMMUNOSUPPRESSANTS

Walford [106, 107] has developed a "theory" which proposes that "aging is due to long-term-minor-grade histo-incompatibility reactions among the body's populations of cells." Others, also, have considered the possibility that aging may be an autoimmune disease [108, 109]. Walford stresses "minor-grade reactions," because the postulated immune reactions responsible for aging would have to exist over a significant portion of the animal's life before becoming manifest. A further postulate is that lymphocytes undergo immunogenetic diversification with age (probably due to somatic mutation) and these diversified cells "recognize the body as foreign across weak loci and react against it." In this context, Walford regards aging as a minor-grade transplantation reaction. He attempts to reconcile with his immunologic hypothesis several environmental factors that drastically alter the normal average life span of a given species [107]. For example, the diet-restricted animals show a particularly marked loss of weight of lymphoid organs; thus, life prolongation by this regimen could be a result of diminished autoimmune reactions. The well-known shortening of life by radiation may reflect the equally well recognized sensitivity of lymphoid cells to the destructive properties of this agent.

A preliminary study was carried out by Walford [110] to examine the effect of an immunosuppressant on the survival of mice. Sixty-nine 1-year old mice (C3H X C57Bl F_1 hybrid) were divided into 3 groups and for the remainder of the life span fed a control diet or one containing 100 or 200 mg azathioprine (Imuran)/kg diet. The higher level of the drug proved toxic and resulted in an accelerated mortality rate, associated with liver necrosis. The mice on 100 mg/kg showed a mean survival time 10 weeks longer than the controls; all animals in both groups expired by 135 to 140 weeks of age. This marginal increase in survival afforded by Imuran may not be significant, considering the relatively few animals involved. Furthermore, the maximum life span was not affected; in fact, the last survivors of the control group were the longest-lived mice in the experiment. Reference was made to unpublished data that administration of 100 mg Imuran/kg to 2-year old mice caused an accelerated mortality rate, as occurred with 200 mg/kg in year-old animals.

Albright et al. [110a] reported that spleen cells of aged (C57BL/6 x C3HF$_1$), mice, when transferred into middle-aged mice of the same strain, severely reduced the survival of the recipients. This life-shortening effect became progressively greater with increasing age of the donor mice. In contrast, splenectomy of mice of interjacent ages nearly doubled the remaining life expectancy. Although there are valid theoretical reasons why rejuvenating the immune system of aging animals by transference of competent progenitor cells might prolong life, spleen cells from juvenile mice failed to have a beneficial effect, presumably due to the presence of deleterious spleen factors in the old recipients. The authors suggest that deleterious factors from spleens of older animals might, in fact, be leukemic cells. These workers suggest that transfer of "young" immunocompetent cells might prolong life in aged animals whose spleens have been removed.

X. OTHER AGENTS

The profound effect of dietary restriction on the life span of experimental animals has already been alluded to. Caloric restriction in the rat apparently retarded one of the few physicochemical parameters quantitatively correlated with age. The tail tendons of the restricted rats behaved like those from normally fed animals [111]; the rate of crosslinking of collagen in this tissue was apparently reduced, as determined indirectly by thermal shrinkage and tensile strength. Conversely, an atheroma-inducing diet apparently enhanced collagen crosslinking [112]. Harman [70] reported that increasing the dietary level of unsaturated fat, a regimen which is expected to yield more free radical reactions, had a detrimental effect on rat survival.

The administration of nucleic acid preparations from yeast or various animal tissues has been reported to have a number of salutary effects on laboratory animals. Thus, the addition of thymic nuclei to the diet was reported to increase the life span of mice, more so in females than in males [113]; injected preparations of purified nucleic acid reacted similarly [114]. It is difficult to see how these observations could be due to a specific action of exogenous nucleic acids, considering the heterogeneous nature of the preparations and their probable degradation in the alimentary tract. Beneficial effects on survival may have been due to the general nutritive supplement of these preparations. Gardner [114], however, believes that the basic diet of animals in Robertson's studies [113, 115], in which oral RNA prolonged life, was nutritionally adequate. Yeast RNA has been ingested by man, including Gardner who ate 5 gm/day for several weeks, with no adverse effects (nor with any obvious benefits) [114-116]. More recently, injections of purified yeast RNA have been reported to improve learning and memory in young and old rats [117-119]. Assuming the validity of these observations on mentation and life span, the observed benefits may derive from some nonspecific factors in the administered preparations. Nucleic acids of heterologous sources and heterogeneous composition may conceivably provide substrates for endogenous synthesis of RNA and DNA, since they obviously cannot serve as a source of specific information for learning and memory in the recipient animal.

Oeiru [120] has attributed a major role to disulfide accumulation in the generation of senescence. He catalogues data bearing on the reduction in sulfhydryl groups and increase in disulfide groups with age in the tissues of man, animals, and plants. Disulfide accumulation, Oeiru presumes, is associated with increased stability of proteins in general and, thereby, with the inactivation of certain enzymes. Theoretically, exogenous sulfhydryl compounds should protect the organism against oxidative reactions which ordinarily attack functional groups on endogenous proteins and other molecules. Indeed, sulfhydryl compounds are known to protect against oxidative reactions which attack functional groups. Sulfhydryl compounds are known to protect against radiation, and, if spontaneous free radical formation contributes to aging, these compounds should retard the aging process. Harman [70, 72, 121], in fact, reported that chronic administration of cysteine or 2-mercaptoethylamine increased mean life span by about 20%. Oeiru [120] provides data which indicate that the administration of sulfhydryl compounds to old rats restores the amino acid profiles in various tissues towards those of younger animals. He also claims restoration of enzyme levels and protein turnover rates, and that the action of exogenous sulfhydryl compounds is enhanced by coadministration of Vitamins B6, B12, or folic acid. Unfortunately, no detailed observations were reported on the physical state of treated animals nor on their life span. In an abstract, Oeiru [122] reported increased survival by treating rats and guinea pigs with cysteine. Intramuscular injections of cysteine or cysteine plus folic acid daily for several weeks had no effect on the thermic contraction of tail tendons from either young or old rats [123]. In another study, the administration of cysteine plus folic acid enhanced the incorporation of ^{35}S into connective tissue and decreased the level of serum mucoprotein in 12- and 16-month-old rats [124]. Thus, certain changes occurring with age were apparently reversed by the drug therapy.

Aging in higher plants is partly under hormonal control. Plant hormones, auxins, have been reported to retard aging in leaves. For example, a synthetic auxin, 2,4-dichlorophenoxyacetic acid, applied to green leaves early in autumn, prevents the color change and subsequent falling-off of the leaves [125]. Centrophenoxine represents one attempt to test the antiaging effects of plant auxins on animals and man. Indole-3-acetic acid, another plant growth hormone, has been tested in animals with contradictory effects on growth [126]. This compound is a normal metabolite in animals and probably represents an end-product of the metabolism of endogenous indole compounds. Because of the reported effects on animal growth, Everitt [126] injected or fed indole-3-acetic acid to aging male rats (about 400 days old) and detected no effect on body weight and life span.

XI. PROSPECTS FOR PHARMACOLONGEVITY

There is presently sufficient basis for optimism that the life span of man can be extended by one means or another. Extension of life span, however, is more often than not regarded with abject horror. The major objection resides in a general assumption that prolonging life necessitates an extension only of the period of senescence. It is likely that, if the rate of aging is reduced, the entire mortal continuum will be expanded. It appears on the basis of present evidence that retardation of biological processes at an early life stage is essential for life prolongation. The debilitated and vulnerable state that leads to mortality in contemporary man at about the seventh or eighth decade would do so at whatever age this state is attained. Therefore, age-retardation, by definition, involves expansion of the nonsenescent period. Life-extension programs which are initiated in the senescent individual imply attempts at rejuvenation, since the statistical probability of death is already near the maximum.

The feeding experiments of McCay established the foundations for the hope that the maximum life span of animals and man was not unalterably determinate and not unlikely to be significantly extended in any foreseeable period of time. Life-extension by manipulation of the diet, unlike that reported for other regimens, has been amply confirmed and documented in the scientific literature. The feeding experiments indicate that inhibition of growth and development, achieved by minimizing the intake of calories but not of essential nutrients, is accompanied by retardation of aging as well. This is not surprising if one regards growth, maturation, and aging as a continuum, and that deleterious events occurring late in life result from the progression of processes initiated very much earlier. For example, crosslinking or "tanning" of connective tissue proteins may represent an evolved mechanism for creating optimal structural tissue components, but apparently leads to deleterious changes if it proceeds indefinitely. The increased survival of cultured cells or mice treated with adrenal corticoids supports the concept that delayed growth and development and inhibition of the aging process are concomitants. However, although life prolongation appears to necessitate expansion of the entire continuum of life, it is equally apparent that inhibition of growth often occurs without retardation of the aging process.

Although the most dramatic experimental extension of life span has been achieved by dietary means, extrapolation of this technique to the human is not particularly desirable, even if it can be shown to be effective in man. There is an apparent general retardation of growth and metabolism as a whole in diet-restricted animals. Maximum life prolongation may not be attainable short of total metabolic deceleration. On the other hand, selective inhibition at certain critical loci might result in significant age-retardation without the necessity for severe dietary restriction and its associated problems. The latter goal is probably most readily achieved by the use of specific drugs. McCay [127, 128], himself, ventured into the area of pharmacolongevity by testing life-long administration of coffee on survival of rats. His unimpressive finding that the life span of rats was not influenced by this regimen may at least offer some small degree of reassurance to the inveterate and overindulgent caffeine devotee.

The problems in reversing profound and cumulative tissue deterioration of long standing, i.e., in rejuvenation, seem infinitely more formidable than in preventing the development of this deterioration. Moreover, certain phenomena, such as the extensive cell death which the old individual has experienced, cannot be rectified. Bjorksten [129] has repeatedly urged the search for enzymes that are capable of degrading the crosslinks in the structural proteins of the aged individual. He postulates the presence of certain microorganisms in soil which contain the necessary enzymes; otherwise, he points out, the earth would be covered by a blanket of insoluble crosslinked protein. Collagen and elastin undergo many degradative processes, including calcification and fragmentation; this deterioration may or may not be a consequence of excessive crosslinking. Nevertheless, selective cleavage of crosslinks, even if this could be achieved, could hardly reverse the other age-related alterations of the proteins. The claims of Nandy [96], Gordon et al. [53,54], and Friedman et al. [27-30], if substantiated, would indicate that reversal of at least some age-related phenomena is feasible; in these instances, pharmacological removal of intracellular pigment, reorganization of polyribosomal structures to the youthful pattern, and restitution of the age-related shift in ionic concentrations, respectively. It is also a recognized clinical fact that replacement therapy in hormone-deficiency states can reverse profound physiological and biochemical disturbances.

Attempts at pharmacolongevity in the human would appear to be feasible now, if only restricted to hormonal therapy. It has already been demonstrated in the human female that estrogen administration postmenopausally can reverse or retard several of the conditions apparently arising from ovarian insufficiency. Amelioration of some cardiovascular, skin, and epithelial disturbances in these women has been amply documented. Perhaps, other more fundamental disturbances are salutarily influenced by estrogen replacement therapy. Certainly, replacement of other hormones that can be shown to be in low titer in a given individual would appear to be a rational approach. It appears that initiation of hormonal therapy should begin long before gross signs of deficiency are evident, which is usually in the elderly person. For example, excretion of 11-deoxy-17-ketosteroids diminishes linearly with age in both men and women, and this reduction is evident as early as the third decade of life [130].

Pharmacolongevity directed at aging chromosomes is of potentially great significance. The modification of long-lived macromolecules which is to be expected in the aging organism would include crosslinking and oxidation of DNA, thereby restricting its transcriptional and self-replicating activities. An increased thermal stability of DNA in aged animals has been reported, and it was suggested that with age an increase in the irreversible binding of protein to DNA occurs, thereby impairing the availability of genetic information [131]. Interference with the genetic program by deletion of segments of the codon could arise from rupture or crosslinking of the DNA molecule and by chemical modification of its functional groups. Thus, one may hypothesize that aging may be a result of somatic mutations induced in dividing cells, or a consequence of cumulative damage to the genome in fixed, nondividing cells, or both (see Table I). Both types of genetic aberration probably contribute to the aging process; in either case, therapeutic prophylaxis and reversal of DNA deterioration may strike at a basic determinant of biological aging.

Drugs which are capable of significantly retarding the aging process, and thereby extending the most viable period in the lifetime of the individual, may be as prevalent as the manifold chemical processes which as a group contribute to biological aging. The frequency with which instances of positive pharmacolongevity are being reported suggests that a variety of unidentified sensitive sites are being successfully attacked. It is hard to accept that in each case the postulated target was, in fact, the locus of salutary drug effect. This somewhat skeptical attitude derives from acceptance of two basic principles: first, that aging represents a composite of countless simultaneous and interlocking processes, and second, that any drug interacts to varying degrees with each of the fundamental components of protoplasm in general. Acknowledgment of both of these assumptions need not promote undue pessimism regarding the prospects for human pharmacolongevity. There is at hand evidence for successful life extension in experimental animals. Extrapolation of certain of these effective therapies to man may be difficult but not insurmountable. It seems likely that random screening of chemical agents in general could uncover agents capable of extending life span of experimental animals; conceivably, a larger number of drugs would be found that shorten life span. Although a screening program of this type may seem to be inefficient, there does not appear to be at present any better approach, in view of the fact that no single cause of biological aging has been unmasked with any degree of certainty. Furthermore, random screening programs for cancer chemotherapeutic agents have provided several compounds with varying degrees of effectiveness. As our understanding of aging mechanisms develops, specific drug design will follow.

The severely restricted animals of McCay were stunted, scrawny, and of unattractive general appearance. However, less drastic restriction of food intake also increased survival and resulted in animals that were more youthful in appearance and healthier than those on an <u>ad libitum</u> diet [132, 133]. Restricted animals also showed decreased incidence of tumors, cardiovascular lesions, and other pathological conditions (see review in [134]). Regulation of the diet of man would appear to afford definite benefits on longevity. An optimum regimen will probably also include regular exercise. Ordy et al. [135] showed an increased survival of mice forced to exercise. Palmore [136] in a longitudinal study of aging men concluded that the factors which were predictive of longevity were as follows: (a) maintenance of a useful and satisfying role in society, (b) maintenance of a positive view of life, (c) maintenance of good physical function, and (d) avoidance of smoking. Most of us, no doubt, intuitively acknowledge this regimen as one capable of maximizing the probability of surviving to the limit of the specific life span

TABLE II

Draft Test Battery for Physiological Age in Man[a]

Hair-graying score	Protein-bound iodine	W.A.I.S. tests (automated set)
Skin elasticity	Serum-copper	Similarities
Systolic blood pressure	Serum-elastase	Digit span
Diastolic blood pressure	Serum-RNAase	Vocabulary
Heart size	Nail calcium content	Digit symbol
Thorax size	Stature	Block design
Total vital capacity	Seated stature	Digit copying
Tidal volume	Trunk height	Tapping test
One-second expiratory volume	Biacromial diameter	Reaction-time, ruler test
Hand-grip strength	Metacarpal osteoporotic index	Reaction-time, light
Light extinction test	Lymphocyte RNA : DNA ratio	Flicker-fusion frequency
Vibrometer	Explant latency	Taste sensitivity
Visual acuity	Serum growth-promotion (tissue culture)	Total 5-year mortality
Audiometry (200 c.p.s.)	Biopsy healing: contraction	Organ weights
Audiometry (4000 c.p.s.)	Clonal further viability	Disease-specific mortalities
Serum-cholesterol	Leucocyte aneuploidy	Tumor incidence, living
Total serum-albumin	Autoantibody titres	Tumor incidence, necropsy
Albumin-globulin ratio	Skin melanocyte count	Amyloidosis, stainable
Plasma water		Lipofuscin accumulation
Mean venous pressure		Aortic calcium
		Collagen contractility
		Collagen fluorescence

[a] From Comfort [137].

of our species. Not included in the above list is the genetic factor, which is probably of greater predictive significance in determining life span, i.e., the longevity of the parents.

The potential versatility of pharmacolongevity among various regimens, promises the greatest degree of life prolongation in man. The biological age of the individual is the result of many concomitant processes. Each of these aging processes progresses at its own characteristic rate, but all are probably interdependent. It seems unlikely that a single agent would retard all aging processes to the same extent (severe caloric restriction is a possible exception). Thus, sulfhydryl compounds are reported to increase the life span of rats [70, 72, 121], but do not affect the currently most fashionable index of age in this species, i.e., physical properties of the tail tendon [123]. Sulfhydryl compounds do, however, apparently reverse some other age-related changes [124]. Effective pharmacolongevity will probably entail a multiplicity of agents, each constructed to act at a specific site, and perhaps even for a specific life phase. Retardation of any one process should contribute to life prolongation. Predictive evaluation of pharmacolongevity requires access to several objective parameters known to be age-related. Without some objective measure of biological age, at least one generation must elapse for the assessment of a potential, life-prolonging agent in man. Comfort [137] believes that it is now possible to make short-term measurement of the rate of aging in the human. He states that the technique "could transfer much nonhazardous fundamental research on the slowing of age changes from animals to man: It would provide important experience with, and knowledge of, aging variables other than mortality, and it would offer a method of attacking the real possibility that drugs and environmental agents already current may affect that rate — a side effect inherently undetectable with present resources." Comfort proposes a battery of tests (Table II) based on that proposed by others to measure the rate of aging in Hiroshima survivors, but he acknowledges that a final battery will evolve from the efforts of both gerontologists and clinicians.

REFERENCES

1. T. B. Osborne, L. B. Mendel, and E. L. Ferry, Science, 45, 294 (1917).
2. C. M. McCay, L. A. Maynard, G. Sperling, and L. C. Barnes, J. Nutr., 18, 1 (1939).
3. C. M. McCay, in Cowdry's Problems of Aging (A. I. Lansing, ed.), Williams and Wilkins, New York, 1952, p. 139.
4. C. M. McCay, G. Sperling, and L. L. Barnes, Arch. Biochem., 2, 469 (1943).
5. B. N. Berg and H. S. Simms, J. Nutr., 71, 255 (1960).
6. A. J. Carlson and F. Hoelzel, J. Nutr., 31, 363 (1946).

7. M. Silberberg and R. Silberberg, Physiol. Rev., 35, 347 (1955).
8. H. LeCompte, J. Am. Geriat. Soc., 14, 334 (1966).
9. B. L. Strehler, Time, Cells, and Aging, Academic Press, New York, 1962, p. 12.
10. J. Bjorksten, J. Am. Geriat. Soc., 16, 408 (1968).
11. A. L. Tappel, Geriatrics, 23, 97 (1968).
12. D. G. Carpenter and J. A. Loynd, J. Am. Geriat. Soc., 16, 1307 (1968).
13. N. W. Shock, in Aging, Some Social and Biological Aspects (N. W. Shock, ed.), Amer. Assoc. Adv. Sci., Washington, D.C., 1960, p. 241.
14. F. Verzar, Intern. Rev. Connective Tissue Res., 2, 244 (1964).
15. F. S. LaBella and G. Paul, J. Gerontol., 20, 54 (1965).
16. F. S. LaBella and W. G. Lindsay, J. Gerontol., 18, 111 (1963).
17. J. Blomfield and J. F. Farrar, Cardiovascular Res., 3, 161 (1969).
18. I. Banga, in International Symposium on Biochemistry of the Vascular Wall, Fribourg, 1969, p. 202.
19. B. L. Strehler, D. D. Mark, A. S. Mildvan, and M. V. Gee, J. Gerontol., 14, 430 (1959).
20. J. F. Munnell and R. Getty, J. Gerontol., 23, 154 (1968).
21. A. V. Everitt, Gerontol. Geriatrics, 7, No. 6 (1964).
22. A. V. Everitt, J. Gerontol., 14, 415 (1959).
23. A. V. Everitt, Gerontologia, 3, 37 (1959).
24. T. B. Robertson and L. A. Ray, J. Biol. Chem., 37, 427 (1919).
25. Z. Deyl, A. V. Everitt, and J. Rosmus, Exptl. Gerontol., 2, 249 (1967).
26. Z. Hruza, M. Chvapil, and V. Kobrle, Physiol. Bohemoslov., 10, 290 (1961).
27. S. M. Friedman, M. Nakashima, and C. L. Friedman, Gerontologia, 11, 129 (1965).
28. S. M. Friedman and C. L. Friedman, Exptl. Gerontol., 1, 37 (1964).
29. S. M. Friedman, C. L. Friedman, and M. Nakashima, Am. J. Physiol., 199, 35 (1960).
30. S. M. Friedman, F. A. Sreter, and C. L. Friedman, Gerontologia, 7, 65 (1963).
31. S. M. Friedman and C. L. Friedman, Nature, 200, 237 (1963).

32. D. Bellamy, Exptl. Gerontol., 3, 327 (1968).
33. G. C. Yuan, J. B. Little, and R. S. Chang, J. Gerontol., 20, 522 (1965).
34. R. S. Chang, J. Nat. Cancer Inst., 40, 491 (1968).
35. G. C. Yuan and R. S. Chang, J. Gerontol., 24, 82 (1969).
36. A. Maciera-Coelho, Experientia, 22, 390 (1966).
37. G. C. Yuan, R. S. Chang, J. B. Little, and G. Cornil, J. Gerontol., 22, 174 (1967).
38. J. D. Leith, Gerontologist, 7, 244 (1967).
39. A. Aslan and N. David, Therapiewoche, 8, 1 (1957).
40. A. Aslan and N. David, Fourth International Congress on Gerontology, Firenze, 1959, p. 81.
41. A. Aslan, Therapiewoche, 7, 14 (1956).
42. J. Brozek and E. Simonson, Geriatrics, 17, 464 (1962).
43. L. Gitman, Fifth International Congress on Gerontology, San Francisco, 1960, p. 54.
44. R. H. May, M. B. Ruland, N. D. Bylenga, and H. H. Peppel, Geriatrics, 17, 161 (1962).
45. S. R. Fee and A. N. G. Clark, Brit. Med. J., No. 5268, 1680 (1961).
46. J. A. W. Berryman, H. A. W. Forbes, and R. Simpson-White, Brit. Med. J., No. 5268, 1683 (1961).
47. J. Hirsh, Brit. Med. J., No. 5268, 1684 (1961).
48. A. Aslan, A. Vrabiescu, and C. Domilescu, Gerontologist, 4(3) (II), 33 (1964).
49. F. Verzar, Gerontologia, 3, 351 (1959).
50. P. Gordon, J. J. Fudema, G. L. Snider, A. Abrams, S. S. Tobin, and J. D. Kraus, J. Gerontol., 20, 144 (1965).
51. P. Gordon, Recent Advan. Biol. Psychiat., 10, 121 (1968).
52. P. Gordon, S. S. Tobin, B. Doty, and M. Nash, J. Gerontol., 23, 434 (1968).
52a. P. Gordon, Advan. Gerontol. Res., 3, in press.
52b. P. Gordon, Gerontologist, in press.
53. P. Gordon, Eighth International Congress on Gerontology, Vol. 1, 1969.
54. P. Gordon, Postgrad. Med., in press.

55. B. Doty and P. Gordon, Federation Proc., 29, 684 (1970).
56. P. Gordon and B. Ronsen, Federation Proc., 29, 684 (1970).
57. E. R. Brown and P. Gordon, Federation Proc., 29, 684 (1970).
58. M. H. Orjack, C. L. Taylor, and C. Kornetsky, Psychopharmacologia, 13, 413 (1968).
59. S. Gelfand, L. D. Clark, E. W. Herbert, D. N. Gelfand, and E. D. Holmes, Clin. Pharmacol. Therap., 9, 56 (1968).
60. D. E. Cameron, Science, 157, 958 (1967).
61. R. G. Smith, Science, 155, 603 (1967).
62. J. L. McGaugh, Science, 153, 1351 (1966).
63. D. E. Cameron, Brit. J. Psychiat., 109, 325 (1963).
64. B. W. Agranoff, Perspectives Biol. Med., 9, 13 (1965).
65. G. R. Van Sickle and R. H. McCluer, Perspectives Biol. Med., 9, 425 (1966).
66. D. Harman, J. Gerontol., 11, 298 (1956).
67. D. Harman, Radiation Res., 16, 753 (1962).
68. I. Isenberg, Physiol. Rev., 44, 487 (1964).
69. R. B. Mesrobian and A. V. Tobolsky, in Autoxidation and Antioxidants (W. O. Lundberg, ed.), Vol. 1, Interscience, New York, 1961, pp. 55-106.
70. D. Harman, Agents and Actions, 1, 3 (1969).
71. D. Grahn, Proceedings of the Second United Nations International Conference on Peaceful Uses of Atomic Energy, Geneva, 1958, 394.
72. D. Harman, J. Gerontol., 23, 476 (1968).
73. D. Harman, J. Gerontol., 16, 247 (1961).
74. M. Okuma, M. Steiner, and M. Baldini, Blood, 34, 712 (1969).
75. P. Alexander, D. I. Connell, A. Brohult, and S. Brohult, Gerontologia, 3, 147 (1959).
76. G. W. Casarett, Advan. Gerontol. Res., 1, 109 (1964).
77. P. J. Lindop and J. Rotblat, Proc. Roy. Soc., Ser. B, 154, 332 (1961).
78. R. R. Kohn, in Reproduction: Molecular, Subcellular and Cellular, (M. Locke, ed.), Academic Press, New York, 1965, p. 291.
79. R. R. Kohn and A. M. Leash, Exptl. Mol. Pathol., 7, 354 (1967).
80. F. S. LaBella, Gerontologist, 6, 46 (1966).

81. F. S. LaBella, Gerontologist, 8, 13 (1968).
82. F. S. LaBella, in Treatise on Skin (H. Elden, ed.), Vol. I, Wiley, New York, in press.
83. H. Sobel, Advan. Gerontol. Res., 2, 205 (1967).
84. E. J. Miller, G. R. Martin, C. E. Mecca, and K. A. Piez, J. Biol. Chem., 240, 3623 (1965).
85. B. L. O'Dell, D. F. Elsden, J. Thomas, and S. M. Partridge, Nature, 209, 401 (1966).
86. M. E. Nimni, J. Biol. Chem., 243, 1457 (1968).
87. A. Veis and J. Anesey, J. Biol. Chem., 240, 3899 (1965).
88. P. Bornstein, G. R. Martin, and K. A. Piez, Science, 144, 1220 (1964).
89. F. S. LaBella, S. Vivian, and D. P. Thornhill, J. Gerontol., 21, 550 (1966).
90. H. Staudinger, Zur Entwicklung der Chemie der Hochpolymeren, Verlag Chimie, Berlin, 1937, p. 152.
91. F. S. LaBella, Seventh International Congress on Gerontology, Vol. 1, Vienna, 1966, p. 153.
92. I. A. Jaffe, Arthritis Rheumat., 8, 1064 (1965).
93. E. D. Harris, Jr., and A. Sjoerdsma, Lancet, ii, 707 (1966).
94. H. Destrem, Presse Med., 69, 1999 (1961).
95. L. F. Fichez, G. Boureq, and G. Nedelec, Gaz. Hop. (Paris), 133, 1137 (1961).
96. K. Nandy, J. Gerontol., 23, 82 (1968).
97. W. Bondareff, Advan. Gerontol. Res., 1, 1 (1964).
98. M. R. Murray and A. P. Stout, Am. J. Anat., 80, 225 (1947).
99. B. L. Strehler, Advan. Gerontol. Res., 1, 343 (1964).
100. D. Brandes, in Topics in the Biology of Aging (P. Krohn, ed.), Interscience, New York, 1966, p. 149.
101. S. Bjorkerud, Advan. Gerontol. Res., 1, 257 (1964).
102. D. D. Hendley, A. S. Mildvan, M. C. Reporter, and B. L. Strehler, J. Gerontol., 18, 250 (1963).
103. C. Haudenschild, Pathol. Microbiol., 33, 193 (1969).
104. N. M. Sulkin and P. Srivanij, J. Gerontol., 15, 2 (1960).
105. K. R. Brizzee, P. A. Cancilla, N. Sherwood, and P. S. Timiras, J. Gerontol., 24, 127 (1969).

105a. D. Harman, Gerontologist, in press.

106. R. L. Walford, J. Gerontol., 17, 281 (1962).

107. R. L. Walford, Exptl. Gerontol., 1, 67 (1964).

108. M. Burnet, Brit. Med. J., 2, 720 (1959).

109. A. Comfort, Am. Heart J., 62, 293 (1961).

110. R. L. Walford, in Topics in the Biology of Aging (P. Krohn, ed.), Interscience, New York, 1966, p. 163.

110a. J. F. Albright, T. Makinodan, and J. W. Deitchman, Exptl. Gerontol., 4, 267 (1969).

111. M. Chvapil and Z. Hruza, Gerontologia, 3, 241 (1959).

112. Z. Hruza and M. Chvapil, Physiol. Bohemoslov., 11, 423 (1962).

113. T. B. Robertson, Australian J. Exptl. Biol. Med., 47 (1928).

114. T. S. Gardner, J. Gerontol., 1, 445 (1946).

115. T. B. Robertson, C. S. Hicks, and H. R. Marston, Australian J. Exptl. Biol. Med. Sci., 4, 125 (1927).

116. C. S. Hicks, Australian J. Exptl. Biol. Med. Sci., 4, 151 (1927).

117. D. F. Cameron, V. A. Kral, L. Solyum, S. Sved, B. Wainrib, C. Beaulieu, and H. Enesco, in Macromolecules and Behaviour (J. Gaito, ed.), Appleton-Century-Crofts, New York, 1966, p. 129.

118. L. Cook, A. B. Davidson, D. J. Davis, H. Green, and E. J. Fellows, Science, 141, 268 (1963).

119. J. Corson and H. Enesco, Psychonom. Sci., 5, 217 (1966).

120. S. Oeriu, Advan. Gerontol. Res., 1, 23 (1964).

121. D. Harman, J. Gerontol., 11, 298 (1956).

122. S. Oeiru, Sixth International Congress on Gerontology, Copenhagen 1963.

123. S. Oeriu and F. Verzar, Gerontologia, 8, 242 (1963).

124. Z. Hruza, V. Hlavackova, and A. Babicky, Exptl. Gerontol., 2, 9 (1966).

125. H. M. Hallaway, New Scientist, 10, 1243 (1960).

126. A. V. Everitt, Gerontologia, 3, 65 (1959).

127. C. M. McCay, G. Sperling, F. E. Lovelace, L. L. Barnes, C. H. Liu, C. A. M. Smith, and J. A. Saxton, Jr., J. Gerontol., 7, 161 (1952).

128. G. A. Sperling, J. K. Loosli, L. L. Barnes, and C. M. McCay, J. Gerontol., 1, 426 (1946).

129. J. Bjorksten, J. Am. Geriat. Soc., 10, 125 (1962).
130. C. N. Gherondache, L. P. Romanoff, and G. Pincus, in Endocrines and Aging (L. Gitman, ed.), Thomas, Springfield, Illinois, 1967, p. 76.
131. H. P. von Hahn and F. Verzar, Gerontologia, 7, 105 (1963).
132. B. N. Berg, J. Nutr., 71, 242 (1960).
133. B. N. Berg and H. S. Simms, J. Nutr., 71, 255 (1960).
134. M. H. Ross, Federation Proc., 18, 1190 (1959).
135. J. M. Ordy, T. Samorajski, and C. Rolsten, Seventh International Congress on Gerontology, 1966, p. 197.
136. E. Palmore, Gerontologist, 9, 247 (1969).
137. A. Comfort, Lancet, ii, 1411 (1969).

Chapter IX

DRUGS AFFECTING FACILITATION OF
LEARNING AND MEMORY

Walter B. Essman

Queens College
The City University of New York
Flushing, New York

I.	INTRODUCTION	385
II.	RNA	389
III.	URIC ACID	392
IV.	MALONONITRILE DERIVATIVES	392
V.	MAGNESIUM PEMOLINE	394
VI.	CENTRAL NERVOUS SYSTEM STIMULANTS AND ANALEPTICS	397
VII.	CHOLINERGIC AGENTS	399
VIII.	ELECTROLYTES	400
IX.	STATUS OF BEHAVIORAL FACILITATION AND SEARCH FOR NEW DRUGS	401
	REFERENCES	402

I. INTRODUCTION

The ambitious title given to this overview should not mislead the reader into the often implied view that there is a direct relationship between certain psychotropic drugs and learned behavior or more stable memory patterns. Several reviews of the literature in this area have appeared exploring some of the problems of drug evaluation and behavioral methodology [1-4]. There are indeed several problems that confront the researcher as well as the academician, both of whom hope to sort out the significance (empirically as well as conceptually) of presumed relationships between drug action and behavioral facilitation. Some of these problems focus upon the central action of drugs, raising questions regarding the central mechanisms involved in the induction of, or the increased probabilities for, behavioral facilitation.

Other problems pertain to the evaluation of research literature in the general area of drug effects and behavior. To what extent do acute versus chronic drug treatments bear upon applicability or generality of the emerging findings?. For example, if single administration of a drug leads to behavioral responses that by definition are in some way "superior" to those made by appropriate "control" subjects, then this may constitute facilitation. If, however, multiple dose administration of the same drug fails to produce facilitation, then how are these findings to be resolved? Problems such as this may, and frequently do, arise out of variables in the pharmacological parameters, the biochemical complexities, or the behavioral conditions. The latter appears to contribute appreciably to inter- and intra-experimental variability, particularly in instances where screening or evaluation or both of new drugs are involved.

The issue of applicability, especially where compounds possessing specific learning and memory facilitatory potential are involved, appears to reside in clinical areas, basic mechanisms research, or philosophical curiosity. I would like to put the first and last of these aside to the extent that this becomes permissible, and focus upon applicability in terms of basic mechanisms. This referent suggests that learning and memory, as processes mediated by complex cellular events in the central nervous system, can potentially be altered through the direct or indirect action of a drug. By one or another criterion the compounds which have been reported to induce or mediate facilitation of learning and/or memory are generally mood-altering agents or central nervous system stimulants. The generality of the classes to which such compounds are assigned is perhaps another clue as to the multivaried effects that they may initiate, and as such probably limits the similarities in both central and behavioral action that they possess.

The purpose of this overview is to present, as fairly and critically as the work itself allows, the present status of facilitation of learning and memory by drug action. It is often difficult to assess a scientist's goal in initiating and reporting a piece of research. One may ask whether reported "facilitation" adds to our knowledge of the basic mechanisms involved in drug action, learning and memory, or the corresponding central processes common to one or both. What advantage lies in the approach whereby acceptance of an existing theory or hypothesis regarding central corollaries of learning and/or memory influences the search for "facilitated behaviors" that coincide exclusively with the predictions of the theory? Such textbook pharmacologizing, as contrasted with laboratory pharmacology, has in part accounted for a literature that has become sizable enough to warrant reviewing. Finally, there have been studies that are so empirically based that they force the reader to make his own theoretical inferences or to independently test hypotheses that emerge as a consequence of rather than a basis for the study.

On the behavioral side of the issue of "facilitation" are the questions of what is facilitated, what is defined as facilitation, and what are the limitations or generalities for such behavior. What is facilitated raises some serious methodological problems for the precise definition of learning and/or memory — allowing for, but limiting by design or definition, the cross-contaminating effects of performance, motivational factors, social conditions, nutritional contributions, cyclical and seasonal variation, endogenous conditions, and any number of independent physiological changes which individually or interactively can contribute to any of the above. The operational nature of many behavioral studies concerned with "facilitation" is itself a limiting factor. If an animal treated with a drug requires fewer trials than a placebo-treated animal to acquire a response in a maze (to a criterion of a given number of successively correct responses), does such operationally defined facilitation imply "better learning," or are there other alternatives (e.g., reduced fatigue, enhanced motivation, sharpened sensory input, altered stimulus thresholds, etc.). Admittedly, any combination of such alternatives can certainly constitute a foundation upon which the building blocks of facilitation can be fitted into place and matched with the appropriate pharmacological, biochemical, and physiological mortar. More commonly the foundation represents a questionable hypothesis upon which building blocks of irrelevant data are applied.

Generally, theoretical positions on the processes of learning and/or memory have been concerned with either structural or cellular events in the brain. These depend for proper integration of information (i.e., its acquisition, registration, storage, and retrieval capacity) upon morphological, electrical, or metabolic events that have in turn been ascribed variously to membrane changes, cell body alteration, variations in axoplasmic transport, changes in dendritic orientation or function, nerve ending conditions, etc. Consideration has also been accorded the synthesis, storage, release, and functional character of a number of molecules either directly concerned with synaptic transmission or having direct biological effects which can regulate such transmission. It is therefore not surprising to note that the basis for investigation of a particular drug regarding "facilitation" effects can be related to one or more of these possible mechanisms. Occasionally, however, such theoretical parallelism can be adapted to a very convenient homeostatic-like position within which drug-induced facilitation can be interpreted as maximization of interacting systems (enzyme-substrate, effector-receptor). The adequacy of such a conceptualization for learning and memory would appear to be dependent upon a careful dose-response evaluation and systematic manipulation of such relevant behavioral variables as drive level, stimulus complexity, temporal aspects of trials and reinforcement.

A further, and perhaps final, distinction should be made between drugs of known structure, the character, dose, potency, absorption, and metabolism of which can be reasonably determined, specified, and replicated and those compounds of unknown or speculated makeup. This distinction arises out of the controversial area of intra-animal information transfer through ingestion or injection of tissue extracts from trained animals. Numerous reports have appeared in the literature of the past five years and the progress of this approach has been summarized in two recent volumes [5,6]. It is not the purpose of this chapter to review or comment extensively upon presumed "learning" or "memory-transfer" by brain extracts, since adequate replicability, methodological consistency, and neurobiological logic and adequacy still constitute major problems in this approach. The positive behavioral effects that occur after treatment with an extract of brain tissue cannot be interpreted as facilitation of learning and/or memory until the following experimental conditions are clarified: titrations of dose, variations of injection or ingestion times, evaluation of differences in route of administration, differences in duration of treatment regimen, and analysis of possible immunological components in long term studies.

As mentioned earlier, central nervous system stimulants appear to affect the induction or mediation of processes leading to (a) enhanced learning ability, as inferred from more rapid learning or from fewer response errors recorded during acquisition, and (b) memory for acquired behavior, as exemplified by more efficient retrieval, a greater reservoir for its storage, or greater stability within the behavioral repertoire (temporal as well as competitive survival of the presumed memory trace). Inadequate knowledge of the nature of just what is stimulated centrally by such compounds (structurally, physiologically, or metabolically) remains as a methodological as well as a conceptual barrier to effective guiding principles in the search for new drugs.

To a considerable extent the rationale underlying a hypothesis of "facilitation" in behavioral investigation has derived partially from presumed processes. The inherent danger in speculating about such processes is obvious; nonmeasurable corollaries of biological events or elegant labels constitute weak bases for processes that one attempts to facilitate with drugs. There are instances, however, when the behavioral effect of a drug (the theoretical basis for the choice of which may be weak or poorly substantiated) is dramatic.

Most of those pharmacological agents presumably facilitating some aspect of learning or memory have emerged because of their anticipated central actions. Their effects may range from the modification of macromolecular constituents in some area(s) of the central nervous system to alterations of the electrical excitability of the cerebral cortex. Although these general examples may involve agents of diverse chemical structure and dissimilar pharmacological effects, the systems affected may be common under both circumstances.

Electroconvulsive shock (ECS) can lead to regionally specific changes in macromolecular content [7,8], biogenic amine levels [9,10], acetylcholine levels [11], and electrical activity alterations over several regions of the central nervous system [12, 13]. One methodological approach toward the identification of pharmacological agents whose central effects may presumably account for facilitation of memory is to titrate such compounds against the amnesic effect of post-training electroshock. Under such conditions "facilitation" may represent either acceleration of some central process with which the disruptive effect of ECS is no longer temporally compatible, or prevention by drug effect of a central change by ECS that accounts for part of the amnesic phenomenon. Either alternative can certainly implicate multiple effects in several systems that may be related in a number of ways to the processes of learning and memory.

II. RNA

Hypotheses suggesting that macromolecular structure, function, or interaction in brain cells may constitute a basis for information input, storage, and retrieval have given further impetus to pharmacological studies in which the macromolecules themselves or agents which alter their synthesis, content, or degradation have been considered. One such macromolecule, ribonucleic acid (RNA), has received considerable attention in the past decade. Hyden [14] suggested that the stability of nitrogenous bases on the RNA molecule was affected by changes in cytoplasmic ionic equilibrium attending frequency-modulated inputs to the central nervous system. Alterations in RNA structure due to stimulation or conditions of "learning" could result in the synthesis of substances that modify interneuronal communication. Effects on the release of neurotransmitters or on the responsiveness of synaptic effector sites are possibilities for pharmacological investigation and may represent a significant approach in the search for new centrally active drugs.

Another early theoretical model for learning and memory proposed that experience-specific nucleoproteins constitute a lattice representing a memory trace [15].

The administration of RNA as a means of inducing facilitation of learning or memory is open to many questions, one of which involves the capability of the intact RNA molecule to survive as such when introduced outside of the central nervous system [16, 17]. It seems apparent that any effects upon learning or memory initiated by systemic RNA treatment must be accounted for by (1) entry into the brain of only a very few such molecules, (2) entry of portions of the molecule, or (3) effects mediated through the peripheral effects of either the molecule itself, its nitrogenous bases, or intermediates in the metabolism of these bases, or combinations of the enumerated possibilities.

One of the first studies in which the facilitative properties of RNA were reported was conducted in a geriatric population with yeast-RNA administered both orally and intravenously [18]. When given over a three month period, this substance led to improved retention and enhanced interest and alertness. In another study [19], smaller amounts of yeast-RNA given orally to senile and senescent patients did not result in improvement of these functions. The implied premise of such studies is based on the view that RNA represents a "memory molecule," and that exogenous RNA can either directly or indirectly stimulate those molecular substrates within which information is presumably encoded. It may not be appropriate to compare the first study with the second; the former, a double-blind investigation, allowed for a summated dosage of 700 g over three months. Significant improvement in memory function was observed at an approximate ED 50 of 540 g. In the latter study, senescent patients free of neurological or psychiatric signs were compared with senile patients (senile dementia, arteriosclerotic brain disease, or amnestic syndrome) on pre- and post-treatment tests of memory. Thirty-nine patients received a total of 42 g of RNA over 7 days and 12 patients were given placebos. Comparative memory scores, although generally improved after RNA treatment, were not significantly different between groups. These studies do suggest that RNA treatment tends to improve the performance of persons with diffuse retention disorders although such improvement may result from central nervous system stimulation, a local metabolic effect, or an antifatigue action of yeast-RNA. Furthermore, it does not clearly indicate whether registration, storage, or retrieval of information is modified through RNA treatment.

In rats, the chronic administration of yeast-derived RNA (160 mg/kg/day for 53 successive days) led to enhancement of the rate of acquisition and prolongation of retention for a conditioned avoidance pole-climbing response [20]. Solyom et al. [21] demonstrated that old and young rats, maintained on a schedule of reinforcement, had an increased rate of responding after RNA treatment. In another study [22], rats trained to lever press for food pellet reinforcement reached twice the level of lever pressing of that shown by controls when injected daily with 160 mg/kg of RNA over a 30 day period. This finding offers some support for the hypothesis that presumed learning and/or memory facilitation by exogenous RNA may be related to the stimulatory effects of the drug -- either directly, or indirectly -- perhaps through metabolic intermediaries or possibly as a stimulus to enzyme induction in the liver.

In a more recent series of studies, Cook [23, 24] has essentially replicated and extended his initial findings regarding the effect of yeast-RNA on learning and memory in rats. After 53 days of consecutive yeast-RNA injection (160 mg/kg/day, i.p.), rats reached 100% criterion of conditioned pole jumping by 10 trials, as compared with 36 trials for controls. Even with shorter periods of pretraining RNA injections (28 to 30 days), a more rapid rate of acquisition occurred and extinction was more prolonged than that of controls. The prolonged rate of extinction suggests that this phenomenon, often viewed as a type of learning or mode of adaptive behavior, might be expected to progress more rapidly if learning were consistently "facilitated." Independent of the possible contribution of differences in acquisition rate, Cook [17] reported that rats trained to criterion and then given RNA for two weeks had slower rates of extinction than controls. These findings may be explained by differences in conditioned stimulus (CS) or unconditioned stimulus (US) responsivity, or both, or reaction time to CS onset, or threshold differences in US.

Cook and Davidson [24] considered a number of dose and behavioral parameters relating to the apparent facilitatory effect of yeast-RNA. Previously reported enhancement of pole-climbing responses and prolongation of extinction by RNA treatment were confirmed as was enhancement of acquisition and retention of simultaneous or delayed conditioned responses. Prolonged retention among RNA-treated rats was also shown to be independent of the effects related to acquisition. When rats given a lever-pressing task were maintained on a schedule of continuous shock avoidance, no facilitation of lever-pressing was achieved with yeast-RNA; and yet rats responding for positive reinforcement (food) showed enhanced rates of acquisition of discrimination behavior. Treatment of rats with yeast-DNA (500 mg/kg/day for 3 weeks) or with guanylic acid (300 mg/kg/day for 3 weeks) enhanced conditioned avoidance pole-climbing and prolonged the rate of extinction of this response; the prolongation of extinction has been taken as an indication of prolonged retention. If drug-induced enhancement of acquisition implies a greater number of nonreinforced acquisition responses, these animals (compared with controls) should have different rates of extinction based upon reinforced acquisition trials. Since these are not comparable it would appear that there are differences in the extinction behavior that are both drug-dependent as well as possibly reinforcement-dependent. Another consideration in these studies is that the percent criterion measure used to evaluate differences in acquisition and extinction is based upon the number of rats that show the response. It would be of considerable interest to know whether those rats that do not show conditioned avoidance under control conditions have a more rapid avoidance onset after RNA treatment than untreated controls. Individual differences between animals (i.e., fast versus slow learners) may be as significant a factor in accounting for the facilitative effects of RNA (or other drugs) as are other interindividual differences in animals and man (e.g., bright-dull, deficient-enriched, senile-normal, retarded-normal, etc.).

Somewhat contrasting results have been obtained by other investigators. Wagner et al. [25] found that yeast-RNA had no effect upon acquisition of a discrimination response in a maze when rats were trained on food reinforcement; however enhancement of acquisition and prolonged extinction rates were observed in yeast-RNA treated rats trained on the pole-climbing task. This finding suggests that positively versus negatively reinforced acquisition tasks or the nature of the discriminative stimulus utilized may determine whether RNA treatment exerts a positive change in task acquisition or retention. Corson and Enesco [26] replicated the facilitation of pole-climbing acquisition by yeast-RNA treatment in rats, but in spatial and temporal discrimination tasks reinforced by shock, no effect was observed. Boissier et al. [27] found RNA ineffective in modifying acquisition and retention of a discrimination maze. In Y-maze acquisition by mice, yeast-RNA had no apparent effect [28]. Voronin et al. [29] showed that direct administration of RNA into the central nervous system of rabbits through implanted cannulae produced reversible conditioned response inhibition when applied to the hippocampus (80%), motor cortex (17.7%), and visual cortex (20%). The selectivity of these effects suggests that the direct central effect of this macromolecule is probably quite different from secondary or tertiary effects mediated by peripheral administration.

Yeast-RNA has also been investigated in the context that facilitation of memory may be reflected in the rate at which the neural memory trace is fixated [30]. The drug was given to mice (50 mg/kg or 100 mg/kg) in a single i.p. dose 60 min prior to training for one-trial passive avoidance response; training was followed, within 10 sec, by administration of electroconvulsive shock (ECS), which under control conditions produced a retrograde amnesia (failure to show passive-avoidance behavior in 90% of the animals). In the case of the RNA-treated mice, 80-90% showed amnesia, suggesting that under these experimental conditions, there was no decrease in the incidence of ECS-amnesia either by acceleration of memory fixation or through antagonism of the amnesic effect of ECS.

III. URIC ACID

Uric acid has been proposed as a mediator of the facilitatory or stimulatory effects of systemically administered RNA. It is formed by the deamination and oxidation of purines and has established central nervous system stimulant properties. Uric acid may be involved in cognitive and intellectual functioning [31], intelligence test performance [32], and achievement [33]. The facilitative effect of RNA (extracted from mouse brain tissue) on the maze acquisition rate and error incidence of mice was partially attributed to elevated serum uric acid levels [34]. In human senile and senescent patients given yeast-RNA orally for 7 days (6 g/day), substantial increases in serum uric acid occurred with some slight, but not statistically significant improvement in memory test scores [19]. In a series of studies [30] concerned with the relationship between RNA, uric acid, and the processes of learning and memory in mice, it was shown that mouse brain RNA produced a significant elevation (274%) in plasma uric acid beyond the smaller significant elevation (5%) produced by the same dose of yeast-RNA. Treatment of mice with intraperitoneal injections of uric acid (75 mg/kg) prior to training in a water-escape maze caused reduced escape latencies and fewer errors during acquisition and reversal of the escape response. Pretreatment with uricase sufficient to reduce endogenous serum uric acid levels resulted in longer escape latencies and more errors during acquisition and reversal trials as compared to controls.

While these studies do not necessarily point to a causal relationship between changes in endogenous uric acid and brain RNA, they do suggest that biologically active molecules such as uric acid may be important for those conditions under which behavioral facilitation by drugs can occur. These considerations and the possibility that learning and memory can be enhanced when the RNA molecule is in some way increased, changed, or synthesized more efficiently have led to a number of studies in which compounds affecting the RNA molecule in brain have been investigated.

IV. MALONONITRILE DERIVATIVES

Some degree of controversy exists concerning the relationship between drug-induced changes in brain RNA levels and learning and memory. Derivatives of malononitrile have apparently altered the RNA content of the brain without affecting the activity of DNA-dependent RNA polymerase.

Early studies indicated that malononitrile stimulated large central nervous system neurons increasing their production of nucleic acid and protein. Later studies seemed to show improvement of psychiatric patients treated chronically with malononitrile [35,36]. The active constituent of this compound is the dimer 1,1,3-tricyano-2-amino-1-propene, or tricyanoaminopropene (TCAP), which was shown to increase the RNA and nucleoprotein content of single neurons in the rabbit brain [37]. TCAP was studied in maze learning and avoidance conditioning wherein the retention of the latter was apparently enhanced without any contribution toward the effects of emotionality or arousal; maze learning was not affected [38].

The suggestion that neuronal RNA production is increased by TCAP and decreased by an amnesic event (ECS) led to studies concerned with the temporal character of this interaction and its relationship to the memory consolidation process [8,39]. It was shown that elevation of brain RNA with TCAP (20 mg/kg/day, i.p. for 3 days) in mice led to antagonism of the brain RNA decrease produced by ECS; furthermore, the amnesic effect of the ECS was significantly reduced. ECS also produced a retrograde amnesia for a passive avoidance response in 72% of saline-treated control mice, but only in 27% of the TCAP-treated mice. The two areas of the brain showing the greatest ECS-induced RNA decrements were the corpus callosum and the limbic system (7% and 3%, respectively), both of which were unmodified when TCAP treatment preceded ECS.

Talland et al. [40] compared the effects of TCAP and placebo on learning capacity and memory function in a cross-over study on 23 senile patients. They found no significant differences between drug and placebo. The state of deterioration of the subject population chosen and the possible confounding of results by the presence of a practice effect make this study difficult to interpret. The absence of any motor task or motor component involved in either the acquisition or memory tasks introduces the problem of baseline evaluation for purely cognitive tasks in an already cognitive-deficient population.

Whereas some studies have indicated that TCAP administration leads to enhanced acquisition of discrimination learning in rats [41,42] and to faster rates of water maze acquisition with fewer errors in mice [10], other studies have demonstrated a lack of TCAP effect on active avoidance and water maze learning [43], on acquisition and extinction of a conditioned emotional response [44], on maze learning [45], and on passive-avoidance learning [46]. The difficulty in comparing these apparently conflicting results is due to differences in dosage and to the duration of drug administration. There is little evidence, for example, of a direct relationship between TCAP treatment, brain RNA effects, and changes in learning and/or memory. It has been shown that chronic TCAP treatment in adult mice (10 to 60 mg/kg) led to increases in whole brain RNA level as a function of dose, but did not produce any consistent change in locomotor activity or affect the rate of water maze acquisition or error incidence [47]. In that study it was suggested that water maze acquisition, involving motor learning, could affect the extent to which the drug interacts with cognitive cues in maze learning. Mice were therefore given motor training in the maze, without any opportunity for a choice discrimination or escape response. Chronic TCAP treatment (10-60 mg/kg/day, i.p., for 3 days) led to dose-related facilitation of maze learning on subsequent trials. These findings argue against a strictly motor-stimulation or antifatigue role for TCAP, since by minimizing motor learning involved in maze acquisition through prior motor training, the effects of TCAP would be expected to be chiefly nonmotor.

Utilizing a trimer of malononitrile, 2-cyanomethyl-1,1,3,3-tetracyanopropene (T4CAP), the rate of maze acquisition and habit reversal in a water maze was considerably accelerated in mice given daily intraperitoneal injections of 10 to 30 mg/kg; higher doses of this compound were shown to be toxic [43]. In a more extensive series of studies with T4CAP, mice given 20 mg/kg/day, i.p., for either 1, 2, or 3 days prior to being trained to a passive avoidance response plus ECS exposure had 35, 60, and 76% retention of that response, respectively, whereas saline controls had only 10% retention. A statistically significant increase in cortical RNA content was also noted in the T4CAP-treated mice [49]. These findings have been interpreted as reflecting a drug-induced enhancement of memory consolidation through an action upon the molecular complex (RNA-5-hydroxytryptamine?) modified by the amnesic properties of ECS. Such enhancement is viewed as either acceleration of the rate at which the memory fixation process occurs or attenuation of the central changes associated with memory disruption.

Whereas it has been previously indicated that compounds such as the malononitrile derivatives affect brain RNA without altering the activity of DNA-dependent RNA polymerase, there is some question as to the role this relationship may play in learning and memory. Agents that decrease DNA dependent RNA polymerase in brain, i.e., actinomycin D, presumably have no obvious effect upon memory [50] whereas other agents, notably magnesium pemoline which increases brain RNA polymerase, have generated a rather controversial literature in regard to their merits as facilitators of learning and memory.

V. MAGNESIUM PEMOLINE

The equimolar combination of pemoline (2-imino-5-phenyl-4-oxazolidinone), a mild stimulant, and magnesium hydroxide has generated a series of studies concerned with the potential effects of this compound, magnesium pemoline (MP), on learning and memory. In initial reports, MP was reputed to selectively stimulate rat brain RNA polymerase under in vivo and in vitro conditions [51]. Coincident with this report was another in which MP was reported to enhance the acquisition and retention of a conditioned response in rats [52]. The conditioning situation consisted of a 15 sec buzzer with a 5 sec overlapping foot shock with avoidance achieved by jumping from a box to a platform in order to escape the shock. The increased rate of learning observed following drug treatment was not changed when trials were given on the following day in the absence of the drug. The simultaneity of these reports suggested that MP, by its apparent RNA polymerase effect, also served to facilitate learning and memory. The theoretical or logical basis for this inference, which apparently served as a basis for generating a considerable number of subsequent studies, is extremely vague and probably unfounded. Subsequent attempts to replicate the biochemical observations have not yielded positive results [53, 54] and the entire issue is currently under question.

In subsequent behavioral studies, Plotnikoff [55, 56] observed that rats, classified as "fast-learners" on an avoidance task, showed a more rapid relearning of avoidance responding after ECS when pretreated with MP. The return to the pre-ECS level of avoidance responding was not achieved by the control group (unidentified as to treatment conditions), whereas there was a dose-dependent return to pre-ECS levels in the MP-treated rats.

In early reports of the efficacy of MP in human subjects, a geriatric population with signs of intellectual deterioration was considered improved after treatment [57]. In patients with clearly established memory defects of organic origin, 25 to 125 mg/day of MP was given over a two month period with a battery of memory tests given before, during, and after treatment. By the end of one month of treatment, there were statistically significant differences between drug and placebo-treated groups on the Wechsler Memory Quotient, the former showing a point gain of approximately 10% above initial scores.

Other investigators have reported essentially negative results for MP in learning and memory facilitation. Smith [58] in a double-blind study with normal adult men given 25 and 37.5 mg orally 3 hours before verbal and motor learning tasks, found that MP treatment did not facilitate learning, memory, or performance. When tested among a group of college students in a double-blind study, a single oral dose (6.25, 12.5, or 25 mg) of MP 2.5 hours before a learning task had no facilitatory effect upon acquisition [59]; the response, a discrimination of light cues shown by key-pressing, was actually acquired at a faster rate by placebo-treated subjects. It is perhaps unfair on several grounds to compare the success reported by Cameron and the negative findings of the latter studies; the comparison involves elderly senescent subjects, in whom improvement on specific retention tasks was only clearly apparent after one week at daily doses of 25 mg or more as opposed to healthy, young adult subjects given an acute dose of MP shortly before perceptual-motor tasks.

Errorless field tracking performance and task recall were only minimally affected when MP (25 mg, p.o.) was given to young adults 90 min before testing [60]. In a series of experiments with patients in the chronic stage of the Korsakoff syndrome, MP was given in both single and daily doses (over three weeks) of 25 and 50 mg. Performance over a range of memory tasks was, except for a few isolated instances, not benefited by the drug.

It has been suggested that MP has a dual effect in behavioral situations maintained by shock avoidance [61]. Mice given stimulant or nonstimulant oral doses of MP (as determined by the locomotor activity effect) showed facilitation of acquisition of an active avoidance response but not a passive avoidance response. This can be interpreted as drug-induced stimulation of locomotor excitation as well as possibly increased reactivity to shock. Although the latter possibility may represent an alternative to avoidance learning as a function of facilitation, it has not yet been tested experimentally. In another study, MP-injected rats responded more frequently and had shorter latencies in response to a buzzer followed by shock [62]. Buzzer-avoidance prevailed over shock-avoidance, however, and increased responsivity to auditory stimuli could explain the apparently enhancing effect of MP under these circumstances; i.e., the conditioned stimulus actually acquires aversive properties. This explanation was not supported by experiments in which rats pretreated with oral MP showed a greater number of avoidance responses and faster running times whether subjected to buzzer or light CS [63]. The possibility still exists, however, that MP induces a threshold change to foot shock.

When MP was tested in two different strains of rats conditioned to a pole-climbing response, it was found that Long-Evans rats had impaired acquisition whereas Sprague-Dawley rats showed prolonged extinction [64]. Perhaps such strain differences reflect variations between "emotionality" and its interaction with the drug in acquisition tasks dependent upon avoidance behavior. When a rate discrimination was imposed upon trained rats (schedule of differential reinforcement of low rates of response), MP significantly impaired such behavior [65].

In studies utilizing positive reinforcement, MP has sometimes been indicated as mediating enhanced performance or learning. MP was administered (5, 10, 15, or 20 mg/kg, i.p.) to rats 30 min prior to trials in a T-maze (light cues) using goal box food reinforcement. Those rats given 10 mg/kg reached criterion (9 out of 10 correct responses) significantly faster than controls [66]. The possibility of drug-appetitive behavior interaction was not studied or considered. The interaction of a wide range of central nervous system stimulants and appetitive behavior is well known. Furthermore, the specificity of a 10 mg/kg dose, without observed effects at lower or higher doses, suggests that the 30 min drug-training interval was perhaps too short to adequately test differences in dosage. The effect of MP (20 mg/kg, i.p.) upon repeated acquisition and extinction of a bar-press response in rats on schedules of water reinforcement indicated that resistance to extinction, as measured by response rate, was somewhat better maintained [67]. Repeated exposure to the acquisition-extinction sequence reduced the possibly facilitative effects of MP. In rats treated with MP (20 mg/kg) and trained to acquire a Y-maze brightness discrimination task reinforced with sucrose, significantly better performance was obtained [68]. Significant differences from controls were obtained for running speed, response latency, trials to criterion, reinforcements to criterion, and the percent of correct choices.

The administration of MP prior to training of rats on a passive-avoidance task was effective in attenuating the amnesic effect usually attending ECS [69]. This finding bears several similarities with previous studies cited

[55,56] in that it may be partially explained by the anticonvulsant action of MP. It also raises the question of whether an anticonvulsive effect alone is sufficient to reduce the amnesic effect of ECS. In partial answer to this question, anticonvulsive effects do not reduce amnesic effects [70] and reduction of the RNA-depleting effect in brain through anticonvulsant action does not necessarily reduce the amnesic effect [71]. In human patients, learning and memory after electroconvulsive therapy were somewhat facilitated by MP treatment [72]. This apparent facilitative effect is difficult to reconcile with the suggestions that MP acts as a nonspecific central nervous system stimulant or as an antifatigue agent. The nature of the motivation underlying the learning task and the contribution of the task to performance variability constitute basic steps toward the evaluation of the cognitive processes affected by MP. Another consideration is the extent to which this compound proves to be more efficient as a possible "learning and memory drug" than other stimulants; for example, it has been shown that subjects required to perform a nonmotivated continuous attention task showed an increase in errors under placebo conditions whereas there was no such increase with MP (50 mg), caffeine (200 mg), or methylphenidate (15 mg) [73].

Data from behavioral and biochemical studies with MP lend weak support to the hypothesis that this compound exerts a facilitative effect upon learning and memory through its brain RNA effect. There remains a need for replicability of (1) both behavioral methods as well as results, (2) pharmacological dose, (3) frequency of dosage, (4) time course, (5) biochemical effect, (6) central uptake, (7) time course of central action, and (8) central locus of any presumed chemical change.

An increase in nucleic acid, nucleotide, or nucleoprotein level in brain can be brought about in several ways — sometimes by endogenous means and perhaps more indirectly by drug action. It is perhaps relevant to consider what RNA's, which proteins, and at what regional, cellular, subcellular, and organelle sites such changes become relevant to the processes of learning or memory. As of this date, the appropriate pharmacological and behavioral studies relevant to facilitation of learning and/or memory have not been carried out.

VI. CENTRAL NERVOUS SYSTEM STIMULANTS AND ANALEPTICS

Several stimulant and analeptic drugs have been reported as exerting "facilitative" effects upon measures of learning, largely in animal studies. Results are usually based on a single, acute treatment under rather idealized experimental circumstances. Notable among the central nervous system stimulants in this realm are the amphetamines. A number of studies have been concerned with the possibility of their facilitative effects and these have been reported for (1) discriminated avoidance responding in the rat [74], (2) improved temporal discrimination involved in the shift of interresponse time to avoid shock [75], (3) increase in the response rate and decrease in the number of punishing shocks in acquisition of a temporal schedule of operant responding [76], (4) facilitation of acquisition of avoidance behavior in rats [77] without any effect upon escape latency [78], and (5) discriminated learning in hamsters [79, 80]. When administered immediately after training to rats, amphetamine facilitated the acquisition of one-way conditioned avoidance responding in a shuttle box, discriminated avoidance responding, and reversal of discriminated avoidance behavior. The extent of the facilitative effect was reduced with increased training-drug treatment intervals and older animals showed a greater drug effect [81].

In man, the enhancement of performance by the amphetamines has been critically reviewed [82] and more recent studies of possible facilitative effects have been few. Intellectual capacity, as defined by performance on tests of abstract reasoning, free association, sentence completion, addition, writing speed, etc., was enhanced by dextroamphetamine sulfate given for ten days [83]. Disjunctive reaction time was decreased when d-amphetamine was given two hours prior to an experimental session [84], and in subjects that were moderately fatigued from sleep deprivation, there was a drug-related increase in the number of problems solved under high motivation and a decrease in the number of errors [85].

Amphetamine is believed to exert its effects indirectly through release of norepinephrine from adrenergic neurons. Brain norepinephrine levels are decreased by 6 to 8 hours after amphetamine treatment in rodents and remain low for 24 hours, or more. There has been little in the way of behavioral investigation to which the catecholamine effect of the amphetamines has been related. It should be pointed out that perhaps the time course of the central adrenergic effect of the amphetamines is relevant to drug-behavior time intervals. In consideration of catecholamine depletion by other pharmacological means, it has been shown that avoidance learning is markedly impaired and the degree of such disrupted acquisition relates directly to the extent to which brain catecholamines are depleted [86, 87]. The possible relationship between mechanism of action and mediation of facilitative processes (i.e., by norepinephrine release) and subsequent depletion of the amine (and behavioral impairment) suggests the need for further study of the time course over which the presumed facilitatory effects of amphetamines are observed behaviorally; this obvious variable has not been systematically applied in behavioral studies with amphetamines.

Probably the most repeatedly investigated of the analeptic drugs in learning and memory studies has been strychnine, an agent initially reported to facilitate the maze acquisition behavior of rats [88]. This effect, and the dichotomous effects of low doses (facilitatory?) and high doses (disruptive?) for some, but not all, rats has been tangentially related to the possible depression of postsynaptic inhibitory synapses and the in vitro inhibition of cholinesterase [89]. Some studies [90] have apparently demonstrated strychnine-induced behavioral facilitation, but the cholinergic concept is no longer popular as a working hypothesis underlying continued facilitative effects (see reviews [1, 91, 92]. Most of these results have been interpreted as drug-induced facilitation of a temporally labile phase of memory trace consolidation; as such this could involve cholinergic as well as macromolecular effects. It has been shown, in this latter regard, that whole brain RNA level was elevated by 27% after six daily intraperitoneal injections of strychnine. This, however, does not completely explain the behavioral results [93].

A variety of other analeptic agents such as pentylenetetrazol and picrotoxin have also been reported as presumably facilitating behaviors similar to those studied with strychnine. Nicotine and caffeine have also enhanced the "learning" capacity of rodents possibly via brain 5-hydroxytryptamine metabolism [94]. Moreover, the release of brain acetylcholine by nicotine has been suggested as an adjunct of its central action [94, 95].

Facilitation of those behavioral responses taken as criteria of learning and/or memory by central nervous system stimulants remains questionable. The central events basic to the processes of learning and memory are not known. It is clear that central nervous system stimulants are not, as a class, consistently facilitatory. Their behavioral effects vary within and among species especially when administered chronically. Clarification of some of these issues is essential before guidelines can be generated for the selection of other stimulants as potential "facilitators."

VII. CHOLINERGIC AGENTS

Pharmacological agents that effect the transmission of impulses across cholinergic synapses, presumably through modification of the ratio of acetylcholine to its hydrolyzing enzyme, acetylcholinesterase, have been suggested as providing facilitation of learning. It has never been perfectly clear what brain pool of acetylcholine need be affected or what degree of effect is required to evoke behavioral facilitation. One approach toward optimizing central cholinergic transmission is the use of precursors of acetylcholine that penetrate the blood-brain barrier more effectively than choline; a compound suggested in this regard has been deanol (2-dimethylaminoethanol). There is no evidence for any change in brain acetylcholine levels after administration of this compound [96]. Moreover, its stimulant-like effects upon the reticular system in bringing about electroencephalographic and behavioral arousal [97] resemble closely the effects seen with compounds that stimulate the adrenergic system. In rats trained to respond to light on an elevated T-maze, deanol given two hours prior to training had no effect [98]. When deanol was administered during the tasks, a significant increase in performance occurred during the initial states of each task, with correspondingly longer response latencies.

The concept that cholinergic mediation of learning and/or memory may be responsive to pharmacological agents that inhibit cholinesterase and thereby reduce the rate of acetylcholine destruction has been tested experimentally. One such agent, physostigmine (eserine), reversibly competes with acetylcholine for cholinesterase and predictably prolongs the effects of acetylcholine liberated at cholinergic nerve endings. The acquisition of simple discriminative avoidance learning was reported to be facilitated with administration of eserine [99]. In two strains of rats ("maze-bright" and "maze-dull"), daily trials in a Lashley III maze followed by posttrial physostigmine caused facilitation of maze acquisition at lower doses (0.50 to 0.75 mg/kg) and disruption of performance at higher doses (0.75 to 1.00 mg/kg); a higher dose within each dose range was required to produce facilitation or disruption, respectively, in the "maze-dull" rats [100]. In rats trained to learn a simple discriminative avoidance response, posttrial physostigmine treatment led to facilitation of response acquisition as a function of age and difficulty of the task [101]. Enhancement of discrimination learning [102] and maze learning in mice [103] has also been reported. The irreversible combination with cholinesterase by di-isopropylfluorophosphonate (DFP) has been indicated, in at least two studies, as providing for enhancement of learning; this phenomenon, however, appears to be highly specific to the nature of the initial learning and the time course over which the direct central effect of DFP occurs. On one hand, it was shown that direct injection of DFP into the hippocampus can produce amnesia for a learned habit, whereas when the same habit is forgotten, DFP injection can lead to enhancement of memory [104]. The apparent rationale of this approach is that drug-induced prevention of acetylcholine destruction promotes the depolarization of postsynaptic membranes especially in those conditions wherein low levels of synaptic conductance prevail. If, as has been assumed, synaptic conductance is increased after training, increased with learning, and decreased with forgetting, then the enhancement of memory for a forgotten habit by DFP may be due to increased acetylcholine levels superimposed upon hypothetically low synaptic conductance. In a subsequent study [105], the injection of DFP resulted in enhancement of the recall of a partially learned habit, also lending support to the premise that synaptic transmission has been altered to account for facilitation.

Some attention has already been given to nicotine regarding its capacity to effect the release of acetylcholine. Analysis of this factor and others related to a possible facilitatory role of nicotine, its metabolites, and analogs have been reviewed [95].

VIII. ELECTROLYTES

The effect of specific electrolytes upon the processes of learning and memory has been sparingly investigated. Because of the profound cognitive deficits associated with clinically observed electrolyte imbalance, there has been little impetus for the study of this issue. Possible facilitation of avoidance acquisition was observed when potassium chloride was injected intraventricularly in cats [106]. There was a decrease in both the response variability during training when the electrolyte was administered 10 min after training trials, and also a decrease in the number of trials to acquisition.

Lithium salts have recently appeared on the psychoactive drug scene as offering potential chemotherapeutic value in the treatment of affective disorders. A series of combined biochemical and behavioral studies in mice indicated that intraperitoneal injections of lithium carbonate showed a partial (30.5%) reinstatement of retention for a conditioned avoidance response, after amnesia for this response had been produced by ECS [94]. Brain tissue lithium uptake was fairly rapid (within 15 min), and this treatment resulted in statistically significant increases in brain magnesium levels. In several respects, the behavioral effects of lithium salts resemble those of antidepressant compounds, and because of their currently accepted clinical use, further exploration of learning and memory facilitation by lithium salts appears warranted.

IX. STATUS OF BEHAVIORAL FACILITATION AND SEARCH FOR NEW DRUGS

The one obvious conclusion emerging after consideration of all of the potential candidates as "facilitators" of learning and memory is that no single compound presents unique credentials that qualify it over any others. The foundation for the selection of a potential drug appears to rest upon theoretical assumptions regarding the central processes mediating learning and memory; perhaps this has been a critical limiting factor in drug selection. Disregard for either central mechanisms or central action has occasionally produced compounds of questionable central action, which, nevertheless, exert, either by operational or inferential definition, a "facilitative" effect upon learning and/or memory. The actions of such compounds could establish the requirements for reliable, reproducible, and valid behavioral tasks. These tasks, in turn, may provide the basis for the learning of one or more responses (distinguishable from one another, either temporally, spatially, or by stimulus specificity) and for the conditions under which the retention of such a response(s) is carried out. Answers are needed to such questions as whether drug-induced "more rapid learning" (facilitation?) is consistent with "more stable learned performance" of a response (also facilitation?), or whether memory as defined by the number of animals showing criterion performance of a learned response is compatible with reduced error performance after a criterion of learning has been reached.

The necessary prerequisites for new drug selection in the areas of learning and memory include the ability (1) to specify the limits of those techniques by which such behaviors are assessed, (2) to undertake comparative pharmacological investigation within the scope of the same behavioral procedure, and (3) to specify, a priori, the requisites for facilitation of those processes potentially mediated by drug action. The search for new drugs that lead to facilitation of learning and/or memory appears, therefore, to depend upon a search for more sound hypotheses concerning the central interaction of drugs with the processes of learning and memory and for better techniques by which learning and memory and drug-induced facilitation may be defined.

REFERENCES

1. J. L. McGaugh and L. Petrinovich, Intern. Rev. Neurobiol., 8, 139 (1965).
2. A. Weissman, Intern. Rev. Neurobiol., 10, 167 (1967).
3. G. C. Quarton, in The Neurosciences (G. C. Quarton, T. T. Melnechuk, and F. O. Schmitt, eds.), Rockefeller Univ. Press, New York, 1967, pp. 744-755.
4. B. Weiss and V. G. Laties, Ann. Rev. Pharmacol., 9, 297 (1969).
5. W. L. Byrne, Molecular Approaches to Learning and Memory, Academic Press, New York, 1970.
6. G. Adám, Biology of Memory, Akademiai Kiado, Budapest, 1970.
7. L. Mihailović, B. D. Jankovic, M. Petrovic, and K. Isakovic, Experientia, 14, 144 (1958).
8. W. B. Essman, Proc. XXIII Intern. Congr. Physiol. Sci., Tokyo, 1965, p. 470.
9. S. Garattini and L. Valzelli, Serotonin, Elsevier, Amsterdam, 1967.
10. W. B. Essman, Proc. Vth Intern. Congr. of the Collegium Intern. Neuropsychopharmacologicum, Washington, 1966, in Excerpt. Med, 185-190 (1967).
11. D. Richter and J. Crossland, Am. J. Physiol., 159, 257 (1949).
12. M. Fink and M. A. Green, Diseases Nervous System, 19, 227 (1958).
13. R. B. Aird, A. M. A. Arch. Neurol. Psychiat., 75, 371 (1956).
14. H. Hydén, in Proc. 4th Intern. Congr. Biochem., Vienna, 1958, Pergamon Press, London, 1959, Vol. 3.
15. J. J. Katz and W. C. Halstead, Comp. Psychol. Monogr., 20, 1 (1960).
16. P. M. Roll, G. B. Brown, F. J. DiCarlo, and A. S. Schultz, J. Biol. Chem., 180, 333 (1949).
17. S. Sved, Can. J. Biochem., 43, 949 (1965).
18. D. E. Cameron and L. Solyom, Geriatrics, 16, 74 (1961).
19. V. A. Kral, L. Solyom, and H. E. Enesco, J. Am. Geriat. Soc., 15, 364 (1967).
20. L. Cook, A. B. Davidson, D. J. Davis, H. Green, and E. T. Fellows, Science, 141, 268 (1963).
21. L. Solyom, H. E. Enesco, and C. Beaulieu, J. Gerontol., 22, 1 (1967).
22. H. Brown, Psychol. Rec. 16, 173 (1966).

23. L. Cook, in Animal Behaviour and Drug Action (H. Steinberg, ed.), Little, Brown, Boston, 1964, pp. 23-43.
24. L. Cook and A. B. Davidson, in Psychopharmacology, A Review of Progress, 1957-1967 (D. H. Efron, ed.), U. S. Govt. Printing Office, Washington, D. C., 1968.
25. A. R. Wagner, J. B. Carder, and W. W. Beatty, Psychon. Sci., 4, 33 (1966).
26. J. A. Corson and H. E. Enesco, Psychon. Sci., 5, 217 (1966).
27. J. R. Boissier, P. Simon, and J. M. Lwoff, J. Pharm. Pharmacol., 18, 687 (1966).
28. S. H. Barondes and H. D. Cohen, Science, 151, 594 (1966).
29. L. G. Voronin, N. A. Tushmalova, I. I. Kazennova, Z. Vysshei Nerv. Deyat., 18, 3 (1968).
30. W. B. Essman, in Molecular Approaches to Learning and Memory (W. L. Byrne, ed.), Academic Press, New York, 1970, pp. 307-323.
31. E. Orowan, Nature, 175, 683 (1955).
32. D. Stetton and S. Z. Heron, Science, 129, 1737 (1959).
33. G. W. Brooks and E. Mueller, J. Am. Med. Assoc., 195, 415 (1966).
34. W. B. Essman and G. M. Lehrer, Federation Proc., 26, 263 (1967).
35. H. Hydén and H. Hartelius, Acta Psychiat., Suppl. 48, 1 (1948).
36. H. Hartelius, Am. J. Psychiat., 107, 95 (1950).
37. E. Egyhazi and H. Hydén, J. Biophys. Biochem. Cytol., 10, 403 (1961).
38. T. J. Chamberlain, G. H. Rothschild, and R. W. Gerard, Proc. Nat. Acad. Sci., 52, 918 (1964).
39. W. B. Essman, Psychopharmacologia, 9, 426 (1966).
40. G. A. Talland and G. C. Quarton, Psychopharmacologia, 1, 379 (1965).
41. D. Daniels, Psychon. Sci., 1, 5 (1967).
42. M. J. Schmidt and J. W. Davenport, Psychon. Sci., 1, 185 (1967).
43. F. R. Brush, J. W. Davenport, and V. J. Polidora, Psychon. Sci., 4, 183 (1966).
44. L. Solyom and H. M. Gallay, Intern. J. Neuropsychiat., 2, 577 (1966).
45. L. McNutt, Proc. 75th Ann. Conv. Am. Psychol. Assoc., 2, 77 (1967).

46. E. M. Gurowitz, J. F. Lubar, B. R. Ain, and D. A. Gross, Psychon. Sci., 8, 19 (1967).
47. S. Lewis, Paper presented at meeting of Eastern Psychological Assoc., Boston, April 1967.
48. S. Lewis and W. B. Essman, Unpublished material, 1967.
49. W. B. Essman and S. G. Essman, Pharmakopsychiat.-Neuropsychopharmkol., 12, 28 (1969).
50. S. H. Barondes, J. Neurochem., 11, 187 (1964).
51. A. J. Glasky and L. N. Simon, Science, 151, 502 (1966).
52. N. Plotnikoff, Science, 151, 703 (1966).
53. N. R. Morris, G. K. Aghajanian, and F. E. Bloom, Science, 155, 1255 (1967).
54. H. H. Stein and T. O. Yellin, Science, 157, 96 (1967).
55. N. Plotnikoff, Federation Proc., 25, 262 (1966).
56. N. Plotnikoff, Life Sci., 5, 1495 (1966).
57. D. E. Cameron, Presidential address, Society of Biological Psychiatry Meeting, Washington, D. C., 1966.
58. R. G. Smith, Science, 155, 603 (1967).
59. J. T. Burns, R. F. House, F. C. Fensch, and J. G. Miller, Science, 155, 849 (1967).
60. G. A. Talland and M. T. McGuire, Psychopharmacologia, 10, 445 (1967).
61. C. Wimer, S. Donner, and D. Martin, Psychon. Sci., 12, 23 (1968).
62. G. Beach and D. P. Kimble, Science, 155, 698 (1967).
63. R. F. Ritzmann, L. Miller, and R. W. Bell, Psychon. Sci., 14, 103 (1969).
64. J. A. Corson, Psychon. Sci., 5, 217 (1966).
65. R. W. Thompson and M. E. Meyers, Psychol. Rept., 24, 425 (1969).
66. B. R. Cooper, W. Potts, D. L. Morse, and W. C. Blank, Psychon. Sci., 14, 225 (1964).
67. P. M. Adams, F. T. Crawford, and W. G. Lee, Psychon. Sci., 14, 101 (1964).
68. J. G. Bridge and G. I. Hatton, Psychon. Sci., 15, 52 (1966).
69. D. G. Stein and J. J. Brink, Psychopharmacologia, 14, 240 (1969).
70. W. B. Essman, Psychol. Rept., 22, 929 (1968).

71. W. B. Essman, Physiol. Behavior, 3, 549 (1968).
72. I. F. Small, P. Sharpley, and J. G. Small, Am. J. Psychiat., 125, 837 (1968).
73. M. H. Orzack, C. L. Taylor, and C. Kornetsky, Psychopharmacologia, 13, 413 (1968).
74. E. Hearst and R. E. Whalen, J. Comp. Physiol. Psychol., 56, 124 (1963).
75. T. A. Verhave, Federation Proc., 20, 395 (1961).
76. N. A. Sidley and W. N. Schoenfeld, J. Exptl. Anal. Behavior, 6, 293 (1963).
77. K. Keleman and D. Bovet, Acta Physiol. Acad. Sci. Hung., 19, 143 (1961).
78. G. L. Gatti and D. Bovet, in Psychopharmacological Methods (Z. Votava, M. Horvath, and O. Vinar, eds.), Pergamon Press, London, 1963, pp. 50-57.
79. R. Rensch and H. Rahmann, Pfluegers Arch. Ges. Physiol., 271, 693 (1960).
80. H. Rahmann, Pfluegers Arch. Ges. Physiol., 272, 263 (1961).
81. B. A. Doty and L. A. Doty, Psychopharmacologia, 9, 234 (1966).
82. B. Weiss and V. G. Laties, Pharmacol. Rev., 14, 1 (1962).
83. H. Nash, J. Nervous Mental Disease, 134, 203 (1962).
84. W. O. Evans and A. Jewett, Psychopharmacologia, 3, 124 (1962).
85. A. R. Holliday, Federation Proc., 24, 328 (1965).
86. R. H. Rech, H. K. Borys, and K. E. Moore, J. Pharmacol. Exptl. Therap., 153, 412 (1966).
87. W. B. Essman, Trans. N. Y. Acad. Sci., 32, 948 (1970).
88. K. S. Lashley, Psychobiology, 1, 141 (1917).
89. D. Nachmansohn, Seanc. Soc. Biol., 129, 941 (1938).
90. J. L. McGaugh, Psychol. Rev., 8, 99 (1961).
91. J. L. McGaugh, Science, 153, 1351 (1966).
92. J. L. McGaugh, in Psychopharmacology, A Review of Progress, 1957-1967 (D. H. Efron, ed.), U. S. Govt. Printing Office, Washington, D. C., 1968, pp. 891-904.
93. G. R. S. Carlini and E. A. Carlini, Med. Pharmacol. Exptl., 12, 21 (1965).

94. W. B. Essman, in Drugs, Development and Cerebral Function (W. L. Smith, ed.), Charles Thomas, Springfield, Ill., 1971, in press.
95. A. K. Armitage and G. H. Hall, Nature, 214, 977 (1967).
96. G. Pepeu, D. X. Freedman, and N. J. Giarman, J. Pharmacol. Exptl. Therap., 129, 291 (1960).
97. L. Goldstein, J. Pharmacol. Exptl. Therap., 128, 392 (1960).
98. A. J. Karoly and L. J. Hunt, Federation Proc., 24, 196 (1965).
99. B. Cardo, J. Physiol. (Paris), 53, 1 (1961).
100. L. O. Stratton and L. Petrinovich, Psychopharmacologia, 5, 47 (1963).
101. B. A. Doty and M. M. Johnston, Psychon. Sci., 6, 101 (1966).
102. J. M. Whitehouse, Psychopharmacologia, 9, 183 (1966).
103. L. O. Stratton and L. F. Petrinovich, Psychopharmacologia, 10, 204 (1967).
104. J. A. Deutsch and S. F. Leibowitz, Science, 153, 1017 (1966).
105. J. A. Deutsch and H. Lutzky, Nature, 213, 742 (1967).
106. E. Sachs, Federation Proc., 20, 339 (1961).

AUTHOR INDEX

Numbers in parentheses are reference numbers and indicate that an author's work is referred to although his name is not cited in the text. Underlined numbers show the page on which the complete reference is listed.

A

Aagaard, P., 124(56), 178
Ablondi, F.B., 173(513), 199
Abrams, A., 358(50), 379
Achor, R.W.P., 265(39), 281
Ackerman, G.L., 32(75), 107
Adam, G., 387(6), 402
Adams, P.M., 396(67), 404
Adams, S.S., 4(6), 27(59), 103, 106
Adamson, R.H., 301(62), 302(62, 63, 64), 303(69), 304(71), 305(71), 313, 314
Adelardi, C.F., 171(498), 198
Adesola, A.O., 136(199), 137(199), 170(199), 184
Adkins, R.B., 157(387), 158(387), 193
Adler, R., 156(376), 193
Adlersberg, D., 272(138), 286
Aghajanian, G.K., 395(53), 404
Agranoff, B.W., 360(64), 380
Ahlquist, R.P., 233(4), 235(4, 6, 7), 236(12), 237(12), 257, 258
Ahmed, Q., 154(339), 191
Ain, B.R., 393(46), 404
Aird, I., 128(84), 134(163), 179, 182
Aird, R.B., 388(13), 402
Airth, G.R., 133(139), 181
Alaupovic, P., 275(179), 287
Albright, F., 141(262), 187
Albright, J.F., 371(110a), 382

Albrink, M.J., 265(30), 281
Alderman, S.J., 138(244), 186
Alexander, B., 320(15), 341
Alexander, H.L., 4(29), 30(29), 105
Alexander, J.K., 324(20), 341
Alexander, K., 336(173), 345
Alexander, P., 363(75), 380
Alexander, W.R.M., 4(23), 104
Alfin-Slater, R.B., 263(17), 280
Al-Hussaini, M.K., 305(74), 314
Ali, S.Y., 94(227), 113
Alivirta, P., 278(206), 289
Alkjaersig, N., 332(68, 71), 334(90), 335(94, 96, 103, 109), 343, 344, 345
Allen, A., 131(97), 180
Allison, A.G., 295(16), 311
Almy, T.P., 170(493), 175(493), 198
Alonso, D., 120(14), 131(14), 176
Alphin, R.S., 157(382), 171(501), 175(501), 193, 198
Altschul, R., 272(124, 139), 285, 286
Alvarez-Amezquita, J., 306(90), 315
Alvarez, T.R., 65(127), 109
Ambrose, C.T., 98(237), 114
Ambrus, C.M., 335(93, 100), 344, 345
Ambrus, J.L., 321(18), 335(93), 341, 344
Amery, A., 336(110), 345
Amselem, A., 275(178), 287
Amure, B.O., 160(405), 194

Anastasi, A., 118(435), 164(432, 435), 195
Anderson, H.D., 335(98), 345
Anderson, W., 134(158), 152(316), 182, 190
Andersson, S., 121(16), 122(16, 21), 176
Andre, C., 133(151), 134(151), 156(368), 170(151), 182, 192
Andreassen, M., 124(56), 178
Andrews, N.C., 327(32), 342
Andriole, V.T., 20(39), 105
Andrus, S.B., 263(19), 280
Anesey, J., 365(87), 381
Angeletti, P.U., 172(505), 198
Angulo, M., 171(499), 198
Anitschkow, N., 262(12), 278(194), 280, 288
Anthony, W.L., 172(507), 199
Aono, S., 268(70), 282
April, S.A., 241(29), 258
Aramazi, Y., 267(62), 282
Aranow, L., 253(45), 259
Armitage, A.K., 399(95), 400(95), 406
Arnold, A., 255(51), 258
Art, C.P., 156(364), 157(364), 192
Arunlakshana, O., 249(43), 259
Aschoff, L., 263(15), 280
Ash, A.S.F., 160(408), 194
Ashburn, W.L., 329(39), 342
Ashford, T.P., 328(35), 342
Ashworth, C.T., 6(32), 105
Aslan, A., 357(39, 40, 41), 358(48), 379
Asofsky, R., 304(71), 305(71), 314
Astrup, T., 331(53), 332(74, 75), 343, 344
Atherden, L.M., 149(278), 188
Atkinson, M., 140(260), 143(260), 187
Atsumi, T., 273(156, 157), 283
Atwater, J.S., 143(264), 187
Auerbach, M., 274(159), 286
Augier, D., 169(485), 198
Augur, N.A., 123(37), 143(37), 177
Aurbach, G.D., 136(205), 184

Aures, D., 162(413), 163(422), 174(423a, 423b), 194, 195
Avery, F., 133(136), 181
Avery Jones, F., 129(89), 179
Avigan, J., 265(36), 281
Avoy, D.R., 270(111), 284
Axelrod, M.A., 324(20), 341
Azarnoff, D.L., 270(107, 112), 284

B

Babicky, A., 372(124), 377(124), 382
Babouris, N., 138(248), 186
Bachmann, F., 336(109), 345
Bachrach, W.H., 140(256), 155(346), 186, 191
Back, K.D., 156(357), 158(358), 192
Back, N., 321(18), 335(93), 341, 344
Baddeveley, R.M., 149(288), 188
Baker, B.L., 135(197), 136(215), 184, 185
Baker, B.R., 68(134, 135, 136), 99(242), 110, 114
Baker, J.W., 154(331), 190
Baldini, M., 363(74), 380
Balenzina, T., 306(102), 315
Balestrieri, C., 135(182), 183
Balis, M.E., 156(370), 192
Ball, P.A.J., 133(42), 181
Ballard, H.S., 137(224), 185
Ballon, J.D., 319(6), 324(6), 341
Banas, J.S., 324(21), 341
Banaski, D., 85(171), 111
Bancroft, F.C., 98(236), 114
Bang, N.U., 321(16), 341
Banga, I., 353(18), 378
Bank, S., 151(298), 189
Barboriak, J.J., 273(150), 286
Barborka, C.J., 127(68), 178
Barenfus, M., 155(342), 191
Barile, M.F., 77(151), 110
Barnardo, D.E., 133(140), 181
Barnes, C.G., 27(63), 106
Barnes, J.M., 306(90), 315
Barnes, L.C., 349(2, 4), 377
Barnes, L.L., 373(127, 128), 382
Barnes, V.R., 132(125), 181

AUTHOR INDEX

Barnhart, M.I., 68(138), 110
Baron, J.H., 132(117), 149(282, 285), 151(282), 153(285), 180, 188
Baron, S., 292(2, 4, 5, 6, 7), 293(4, 5, 6, 9, 10), 294(2, 4, 5, 7, 10), 295(12, 14, 16, 22, 23), 296(7), 298(7), 301(14, 22), 303(70), 309(107, 108), 311, 312, 314, 316
Barondes, S.H., 391(28), 394(50), 403, 404
Barr, D.P., 269(81, 82), 283
Barr, G.A., 270(112), 284
Barrett, W.E., 156(355), 192
Bass, P., 168(468, 469, 470, 475, 476), 197
Bauer, W., 26(53), 106
Baum, J., 27(62), 106
Baume, P.E., 140(258), 187
Beach, G., 396(62), 404
Beall, A.C., Jr., 320(15), 341
Beathard, G.A., 35(89), 108
Beatty, W.W., 391(25), 403
Beaulieu, C., 371(117), 390(21), 382, 402
Bechtol, L.D., 269(90), 283
Beck, C., 74(145), 110
Beck, P., 133(130), 181
Bedi, B.S., 167(458), 168(461), 196
Beer, B., 218(25), 232
Beeston, D., 154(333), 191
Bektemirov, T.A., 306(89), 315
Belko, J.S., 336(114), 345
Bell, R.W., 396(63), 404
Bell, W.R., 333(83), 337(83), 344
Bellamy, D., 356(32), 357(32), 379
Bellanti, J., 307(105), 316
Bencosme, S.A., 137(228), 170(228), 185
Bencze, W.L., 266(53), 271(115), 274(53), 282
Bennett, A., 165(439, 449), 195, 196
Bennett, J.C., 27(61), 106
Benson, J.A., Jr., 136(217), 185
Bentall, H.H., 128(84), 134(163), 179, 182
Bentley, P.H., 118(515), 199

Berenbaum, M.C., 82(166), 111
Berg, B.N., 345(5), 375(132, 133), 377, 383
Berg, G., 136(208), 184
Berg, M., 155(347), 158(347), 191
Bergen, S.S., 268(75), 283
Berger, F.M., 274(159, 160, 161, 164), 286, 287
Bergmann, W., 266(54), 282
Bergström, S., 92(212), 113, 165(436), 195
Berk, J.E., 148(274), 187
Bernard, C., 133(145), 182
Bernardi, L., 118(435), 164(435), 195
Bernheim, B.C., 306(94), 315
Bernick, S., 263(17), 280
Bernsten, C.A., 27(57), 33(57), 106
Berryman, J.A.W., 358(46), 379
Berson, S.A., 164(424), 195
Bertaccini, G., 118(435), 164(433, 435), 195
Berthet, L., 136(202), 184
Bertino, J.R., 82(167), 111
Best, M.M., 270(97), 284
Bevans, M., 278(200), 288
Bhayan, B.K., 303(68), 314
Bianchi, R.G., 156(353), 167(457), 192, 196
Bianchine, J.L., 271(118), 285
Bieber, S., 34(82), 107
Biederman, O., 334(90), 344
Biggs, M.W., 265(44), 265(45), 281
Billiau, A., 295(22, 23), 301(22), 303(70), 312, 314
Billingham, M.E.J., 93(218, 219), 113
Bindra, D., 209(11), 231
Bjorkerud, S., 368(101), 381
Bjorksten, J., 351(10), 374(129), 378, 383
Black, B.M., 137(223), 185
Black, J.W., 236(10, 11), 258
Black, P.H., 298(37), 312
Blackwell, R.Q., 92(213), 113
Blair, D.W., 139(250), 160(250), 186
Blair, M., 135(194), 184
Blanchette, E.J., 267(63), 282

Bland, J.H., 26(54), 106
Blank, W.C., 396(66), 404
Blatrix, C., 93(223), 113
Blomfield, J., 353(17), 378
Bloom, F.E., 395(53), 404
Bluestone, R., 21(40), 105
Bluhn, G.B., 68(138), 110
Blumenthal, I.S., 123(44), 124(44, 46), 177
Blumgart, H.L., 329(37), 342
Bocci, V., 300(50, 52), 313
Bockus, H.L., 145(272), 187
Bodey, G.P., 4(20), 19(20), 21(20), 22(20), 73(20), 104
Bogdanski, D.F., 135(185), 183
Bogomolova, N., 295(22), 301(22), 312
Boissier, J.R., 391(27), 403
Bokisch, V.A., 66(131), 109
Boldt, H.A., Jr., 137(219), 185
Boler, K., 154(327), 190
Bollet, A.J., 94(232), 114
Bollman, J.L., 272(41), 286
Bolton, G., 333(86), 344
Bonanni, R., 309(107), 316
Bondareff, W., 367(97), 381
Bonfils, S., 156(359, 362, 375), 157(359, 362), 192, 193
Booner, K.O., 253(47), 256(47), 257(47), 258
Borelli, J., 320(9), 341
Borisov, Yu.V., 306(102), 315
Born, G.V.R., 330(48), 342
Born, Max, 3(1a), 4(1a), 103
Bornstein, P., 365(88), 381
Borys, H.K., 398(86), 405
Bosisio, G., 118(435), 164(435), 195
Bostrom, H., 131(101), 180
Boucek, R.J., 65(127), 109
Bough, R.G., 27(59), 106
Bounameaux, Y., 320(10), 341
Boureq, G., 367(95), 381
Bournique, C., 275(176), 287
Bovet, D., 398(77, 78), 405
Bower, E.M., 203(6), 231
Bower, R.J., 154(334), 191

Boyd, G.S., 269(83), 283
Boyd, W.C., 135(190), 184
Boyle, D.E., 135(190), 184
Boyle, E.J., 272(137), 285
Boylston, A.W., 90(200), 112
Bradley, D.F., 160(406), 194
Bradley, P.B., 209(13), 231
Bradley, W.H., 90(195), 112
Bragdon, J.H., 278(196), 288
Bralow, S.P., 124(45), 128(45), 136(216), 156(45), 163(45), 177, 185
Branceni, D., 94(224), 113
Brandes, D., 368(100), 381
Brattsand, R., 272(143), 286
Braun, W., 305(72), 314
Braunwald, E., 234(13), 237(13, 16, 17), 258
Bray, C., 333(86), 344
Breen, J.J., 156(366), 192
Brekhman, I.I., 170(494), 198
Bridge, J.G., 396(68), 404
Bridgman, R.M., 136(215), 185
Brink, J.J., 396(69), 404
Bristow, M., 253(46), 255(46), 256(46), 257(46), 259
Brizee, K.R., 368(105), 369(105), 381
Broderick, F.L., 154(333), 191
Brodie, B.B., 23(44, 45), 63(121), 105, 109
Brodie, D.A., 25(47), 105, 126(61), 131(102), 133(144), 135(61), 155(61, 345), 156(61, 345, 349, 358, 360, 376), 157(61, 358, 381, 190), 158(61, 392), 178, 180, 181, 191, 192, 193
Brody, M., 140(256), 186
Brohult, A., 363(75), 380
Brohult, S., 363(75), 380
Brooks, A.M., 170(492), 175(492), 198
Brooks, F.P., 158(399, 401), 159(401), 160(404), 169(483), 193, 194, 197
Brooks, G.W., 392(33), 403
Brooks, H.L., 324(21), 341

Brown, D.F., 265(32, 33), <u>281</u>
Brown, D.M., 156(354), <u>192</u>
Brown, E., 270(95), <u>284</u>
Brown, E.R., 359(57), <u>380</u>
Brown, G.B., 389(16), <u>402</u>
Brown, H., 90(196), <u>112</u>, 390(22), <u>402</u>
Brown, I.N., 82(166), <u>111</u>
Brown, J.H., 58(118), <u>109</u>
Brown, N., 329(42), <u>342</u>
Brown, R.A., 265(40), 266(46), <u>281</u>
Brown, T.G., Jr., 255(51), <u>258</u>
Brown, W.V., 270(102), <u>284</u>
Browse, N.L., 331(63), <u>343</u>
Brozek, J., 358(42), <u>379</u>
Brun, C., 34(85), <u>107</u>
Brunori, F., 272(144), <u>286</u>
Brush, F.R., 393(43), 394(43), <u>403</u>
Buch, J., 131(109), <u>180</u>
Buchanan, K.D., 137(227), <u>185</u>
Buchanan, P.J., 172(507), <u>199</u>
Buchanan, W.W., 27(60), <u>106</u>
Buchko, M., 277(182), <u>287</u>
Buchschacher, P., 85(172), <u>111</u>
Buchwald, H., 266(47), <u>281</u>
Buckler, C.E., 292(7), 294(7), 295(12, 22, 23), 296(7), 298(7), 301(22), 303(70), <u>311</u>, <u>312</u>, <u>314</u>
Buckwalter, J.A., 135(179), <u>183</u>
Buhl, J., 336(173), <u>345</u>
Buja, L.M., 329(38), <u>342</u>
Bullock, B.C., 263(20), <u>280</u>
Bullough, W.S., 91(207), 92(211), <u>113</u>, 135(195), 171(195), 172(195), <u>184</u>
Buluk, K., 332(74), <u>344</u>
Burberi, S., 90(197), <u>112</u>
Burke, D., 297(28), <u>312</u>
Burnett, C.H., 141(262), <u>187</u>
Burnett, M., 370(108), <u>382</u>
Burns, J.J., 23(44, 45), 63(121), <u>105</u>, <u>109</u>, 240(22, 23, 24), 241(28), <u>258</u>
Burns, J.T., 395(59), <u>404</u>
Burton, A.F., 98(238), <u>114</u>
Butcher, R.W., 136(201, 206), <u>184</u>

Butler, D.E., 168(468, 469), <u>197</u>
Butler, E., 322(19), <u>341</u>
Byers, S.O., 278(197), <u>288</u>
Bylenga, N.D., 358(44), <u>379</u>
Byrne, E.B., 306(98), <u>315</u>
Byrne, J.S., 327(33), <u>342</u>
Byrne, W.L., 387(5), <u>402</u>
Bywaters, E.G.L., 4(30a), <u>105</u>

C

Caen, J., 331(64), <u>343</u>
Cain, W.A., 47(110), <u>109</u>
Calabresi, P., 38(95, 97), 82(167), <u>108</u>, <u>111</u>
Callahan, M., 25(51), <u>106</u>
Callahan, S., 34(82), <u>107</u>
Cameron, D.E., 360(60, 63), <u>380</u>, 389(18), 395(57), <u>402</u>, <u>404</u>
Cameron, D.F., 371(117), <u>382</u>
Camiener, G.W., 87(181), <u>111</u>
Cammarata, P.S., 152(317), <u>190</u>
Canales, C.C., 35(89), <u>108</u>
Cancilla, P.A., 368(105), 369(105), <u>381</u>
Canelos, G., 309(108), <u>316</u>
Cannilla, J.E., 336(114), <u>345</u>
Cantagalli, P., 300(52), <u>313</u>
Cantell, K., 300(58), 305(75), <u>313</u>, <u>314</u>
Cantor, H., 304(71), 305(71), <u>314</u>
Cantwell, N.H.R., 25(47), <u>105</u>
Capelik, J., 245(44), 246(44), 247(44), 253(44), <u>259</u>
Capper, W.M., 133(139), <u>181</u>
Carbone, P., 309(108), <u>316</u>
Card, W.I., 124(52), <u>178</u>
Carder, J.B., 391(25), <u>403</u>
Cardo, B., 400(99), <u>406</u>
Caren, J.F., 162(413), <u>194</u>
Carey, T.F., 265(39), <u>281</u>
Carlini, E.A., 399(93), <u>405</u>
Carlini, G.R.S., 399(93), <u>405</u>
Carlson, A.J., 349(6), <u>377</u>
Carlson, L.A., 165(436), <u>195</u>, 265(31), 266(48), 272(48, 127), 273(127), <u>281</u>, <u>285</u>
Carne, S., 154(332), <u>190</u>

AUTHOR INDEX

Caroli, J., 6(31), 105
Caroline, N.L., 303(66), 306(100), 314, 315
Carpenter, D.G., 351(12), 378
Carr, A.J., 139(250), 160(250), 186
Carter, W.A., 298(31, 34), 312
Casarett, G.W., 363(76), 380
Case, R.M., 120(12), 176
Cassel, W.A., 306(101), 315
Castaigne, A., 275(178), 287
Castaldi, P.A., 331(64), 343
Castor, C.W., 74(144), 110
Casula, P.L., 168(466, 467), 197
Catalano, L., 307(105), 316
Catanese, B., 90(197), 112
Caulin, C., 156(359), 157(359), 192
Cayer, D., 143(264), 152(310), 187, 190
Chaikoff, I.L., 267(58), 268(72, 73), 282, 283
Chait, A., 324(28), 342
Chakrabarti, R., 333(77-81), 344
Chakravarti, R.N., 278(198), 288
Chalatow, S., 262(12), 280
Chamberlain, T.J., 393(38), 403
Chan, K.E., 333(85), 337(85), 344
Chandler, J.G., 138(244), 186
Chang, R.S., 356(33, 34, 35, 37), 379
Chany, C., 300(53), 305(53, 76), 313, 314
Chapman, B.L., 131(105), 180
Chapman, M., 329(42), 342
Chase, B.J., 131(102), 133(144), 157(390), 180, 181, 193
Chase, L.R., 136(205), 184
Chassary, A., 306(94), 315
Chen, J.K., 156(350), 191
Cheney, F.D., 143(264), 187
Chenkin, T., 23(44), 105
Chevillard, I., 275(176), 287
Chrisman, O.D., 94(228), 114
Chvapil, M., 354(26), 371(111, 112), 378, 382
Cirri, G., 300(50, 52), 313
Clark, A.N.G., 358(45), 379
Clark, D.H., 131(108), 137(108), 180

Clark, L.D., 360(59), 380
Clark, R.H., 135(197), 184
Clark, W.G., 163(422), 174(423a, 423b), 194, 195
Clarke, C.A., 124(51), 134(51, 164, 169), 135(51), 178, 182, 183
Clarke, M.B., 329(43), 342
Clarke, S.D., 136(199), 137(199, 231), 170(199), 184, 185
Clarkson, E.M., 140(254), 186
Clarkson, S., 263(14), 280
Clarkson, T.B., 263(20), 265(42), 280, 281
Clayman, C.B., 153(324), 168(324), 190
Cleave, T.L., 128(86), 179
Clemmer, D.J., 306(95), 315
Cliff, J.M., 151(303), 189
Cliffe, E.E., 27(59), 106
Clifton, E.E., 321(16), 341
Clifton, J.A., 169(481), 197
Clody, D.E., 218(25), 232
Cobb, R., 4(6), 47(6), 103
Coceani, F., 165(440, 441), 195
Cochrane, C.G., 66(131), 75(147), 109, 110
Cocking, J.B., 151(290), 188
Code, C.F., 133(150), 134(150, 157), 163(419), 182, 194
Coghill, N.F., 135(191), 184
Cohan, E.L., 151(296), 189
Cohen, H.D., 391(28), 403
Cohen, N., 154(338), 191
Cohen, R.M., 269(89), 283
Colcher, H., 154(336), 191
Colin-Jones, D.G., 151(304), 189
Collier, H.O.J., 27(66c), 106, 168(475), 197
Colman, D., 265(45), 281
Colville, K.I., 240(22, 23, 24), 258
Comfort, A., 370(109), 376(137), 377(137), 382, 383
Commons, R.R., 141(262), 187
Congdon, R.H., 135(190), 184
Conn, J.W., 151(296), 189
Connell, A.M., 151(291), 168(459), 188, 196
Connell, D.I., 363(75), 380

AUTHOR INDEX   413

Connor, W.E., 267(63), 282
Conolly, M.E., 237(15), 258
Constantinides, P., 278(199), 288
Cook, D.L., 152(314, 317),
    156(353), 167(457),
    168(462), 190, 192, 196
Cook, L., 371(118), 382, 390(20,
    23, 24), 402, 403
Cooke, A.R., 136(209, 210),
    169(480), 184, 197
Cooper, B.R., 396(66), 404
Cooperband, S.R., 90(201, 204),
    112
Copeman, W.S.C., 4(24), 26(24),
    104
Copp, D.H., 92(213), 113
Coppey, J., 295(13), 300(47, 57),
    303(13), 311, 313
Corley, C.C., 34(84), 107
Cornfield, J., 274(168), 287
Cornill, G., 356(37), 379
Correll, J.W., 275(175), 287
Corson, J., 371(119), 382
Corson, J.A., 391(26), 396(64),
    403, 404
Cory, M., 68(134, 137), 110
Cottet, J., 265(43), 281
Courvoisier, S., 209(16), 231
Couzens, E.A., 270(113), 284
Cowan, W.K., 134(164), 182
Cox, A.J., Jr., 132(45, 116), 180,
    181
Cox, G., 152(320), 190
Cox, G.E., 263(22), 278(203),
    280, 289
Cox, H.T., 127(62), 135(62), 178
Cox, S.V., 25(47), 105
Craig, J.M., 278(202), 288
Crawford, F.T., 396(67), 404
Creamer, B., 137(234), 153(234),
    185
Crean, G.P., 132(124), 133(124,
    127, 149), 181, 182
Crim, J.A., 87(180), 111
Criss, H.J., 336(114), 345
Cristofalo, V.J., 270(109), 284

Croft, D.N., 131(96), 135(191),
    180, 184
Crossland, J., 388(11), 402
Crowther, A.F., 236(11), 258
Cullum, V.A., 255(52), 257(52),
    258
Cummings, B.L., 168(475), 197
Curling, T.B., 157(380), 193
Currey, H.L., 27(63), 86(173),
    106, 111
Curt, J.R., 134(162), 182
Curtis, G.H., 37(94), 108
Curtis, G.M., 327(32), 342

D

Dale, H.H., 233(3), 257
Dalen, J.E., 324(21, 24), 329(40),
    341, 342
Dalton, C., 272(135), 273(135), 285
Damin, G.J., 33(80), 107
Daniels, D., 393(41), 403
Dardymov, I.V., 170(494), 198
Da Re, G., 168(466, 467), 197
Datko, L.J., 58(116), 86(176), 109,
    111
Dauber, T.R., 331(55), 343
Daughaday, W.H., 94(229), 114
Davenport, H.W., 120(10), 122(10),
    123(10), 131(93, 95), 132(10),
    133(95, 143), 139(10), 154(10),
    157(95), 176, 179, 180, 181
Davenport, J.W., 393(42, 43),
    394(43), 403
Davey, M.G., 331(65), 343
David, N., 357(39, 40), 379
Davidson, A.B., 371(118), 382,
    390(20, 24), 402, 403
Davidson, J.D., 278(200), 288
Davies, D.T.P., 75(148), 110
Davies, G.E., 88(186), 112
Davis, D., 124(47), 159(47), 178,
    329(37), 342
Davis, D.J., 371(118), 382,
    390(20), 402
Davis, G.E., 25(48), 106

Davis, J.M., 204(8), <u>231</u>
Davis, J.S., 170(497), <u>198</u>
Davis, R.C., 90(201, 204), <u>112</u>
Dawber, T.R., 265(28, 29, 34), 274(28, 29), <u>280</u>, <u>281</u>
Dayton, P.G., 63(121), <u>109</u>
Dayton, S., 278(204), <u>289</u>
Dazziano, L., 100(247), <u>114</u>
De, V.N., 278(198), <u>288</u>
Dean, A.C.B., 151(291a), <u>188</u>
Dean, P.D.G., 149(281), 151(281), <u>188</u>
Debas, H.T., 168(461), <u>196</u>
DeBeer, E.J., 216(21), <u>231</u>
deBono, Edward, 3(1b), 4(1b), <u>103</u>
de Castiglione, R., 118(435), 164(435), <u>195</u>
Decker, J.L., 4(25), <u>104</u>
DeConti, R.C., 82(167), <u>111</u>
deCrinis, K., 332(69), <u>343</u>
Defelice, S., 273(152), <u>286</u>
DeFina, E., 273(146), <u>286</u>
DeGraef, J., 133(148, 152), 134(148, 152), 170(148, 152), 175(148, 152), <u>182</u>
Deitchman, J.W., 371(110a), <u>382</u>
de la Rosa, C., 158(394), <u>193</u>
Dell'Omodarme, G., 272(144), <u>286</u>
Demand, H.A., 136(208), <u>184</u>
Dempsey, M.E., 267(61), <u>282</u>
Denborough, M.A., 135(181), <u>183</u>
Deodhar, S.D., 35(88), <u>107</u>
DeRenzo, E.C., 173(513), <u>199</u>
Desai, H.G., 154(340), <u>191</u>
Descos, L., 133(151), 134(151), 170(151), <u>182</u>
de Stevens, G., 266(53), 274(53), <u>282</u>
Destrem, H., 367(94), <u>381</u>
Deutsch, J.A., 400(104, 105), <u>406</u>
DeVita, V., 309(108), <u>316</u>
De Vrecker, R., 336(110), <u>345</u>
Dewar, H.A., 332(76), <u>344</u>
de Wardener, H.E., 140(254), <u>186</u>
De Wolfe, V., 320(15), <u>341</u>
Dexter, L., 329(40), <u>342</u>
Deykin, D., 319(4), 320(14), <u>341</u>
Dianzani, F., 295(23), 309(107), <u>312</u>, <u>316</u>

DiBona, B.R., 74(146), <u>110</u>
DiCarlo, F.J., 389(16), <u>402</u>
Dick, A., 133(131), <u>181</u>
Dick, G.W.A., 306(93), <u>315</u>
Dingle, J.H., 306(87), <u>315</u>
DiPasquale, G., 39(99), 93(216), <u>108</u>, <u>113</u>
Dixon, F.J., 75(147), <u>110</u>
Dixon, W.J., 278(204), <u>289</u>
Djahanguiri, B., 157(386), <u>193</u>
Dlin, B., 137(238), <u>186</u>
Dodson, W.H., 27(61), <u>106</u>
Doebel, K.J., 4(10, 11), <u>104</u>
Dogra, J.R., 128(83), <u>179</u>
Doll, R., 124(50), 129(50, 89), 130(90), 131(50, 109, 110), 134(165, 170, 173), 138(90), 149(286, 287), 151(286, 287), 153(90, 286, 322), 171(286, 287), <u>178</u>, <u>179</u>, <u>180</u>, <u>182</u>, <u>183</u>, <u>188</u>, <u>190</u>
Dollery, C.T., 237(15), <u>258</u>
Domenjoz, R., 4(5), 28(5), 94(233), <u>103</u>, <u>114</u>, 172(511), <u>199</u>
Domilescu, C., 358(48), <u>379</u>
Donaldson, V.H., 335(102), <u>345</u>
Donegan, W.L., 137(221), <u>185</u>
Doniach, D., 133(141), <u>181</u>
Donner, S., 395(61), <u>404</u>
Donnorso, R.P., 135(182), <u>183</u>
Donohoe, W.T.A., 133(149), 134(175), <u>182</u>, <u>183</u>
Dornhorst, A.C., 236(11), <u>258</u>
Dorstewitz, E.L., 74(144), <u>110</u>
Doshi, J.C., 154(340), <u>191</u>
Doskotch, R.W., 88(184), <u>112</u>, 173(514), <u>199</u>
Dotevall, G., 136(207), <u>184</u>
Doty, B., 358(52), 359(55), <u>379</u>, <u>380</u>
Doty, B.A., 398(81), 400(101), <u>405</u>, <u>406</u>
Doty, L.A., 398(81), <u>405</u>
Douglas, A.S., 334(89), 338(89), <u>344</u>
Douglas, F.C., 6(32), <u>105</u>
Douglas, J.F., 274(160, 161, 164), <u>287</u>
Douthard, R.J., 295(24), 298(24), <u>312</u>

AUTHOR INDEX

Downie, W.W., 27(60), 106
Doyle, J.T., 265(33), 281
Dragstedt, L.R., 121(17, 18),
    132(114), 158(394), 176, 180,
    193
Drane, H., 134(170), 183
Dreilling, D.A., 137(229),
    154(338), 185, 191
Drill, V.A., 152(314), 190
Drury, R.A.B., 133(136), 181
Dubarry, J.J., 132(111), 180
Dubrasquet, M., 156(375), 193
Dubois, E.L., 30(71), 33(71), 107
Dubuc, J., 265(37), 281
duBuy, H., 303(70), 314
Duchkova, M., 38(96), 108
Duersch, F., 274(159), 286
Duff, G.L., 263(16), 280
Duggan, J.M., 131(105), 180
Duguid, J.B., 325(31), 342
Duhamer, J., 132(111), 180
Dujovne, C.A., 271(118), 285
Dull, H.B., 306(79), 314
Dumonde, D.C., 69(140), 110
Duncan, C.H., 270(97), 284
Duncan, G.G., 270(100), 284
Duncan, T.G., 270(100), 284
Dunlop, D., 244(37), 259
Dunn, W.L., 98(238), 114
Dunne, J.F., 27(63), 106
Dunphy, J.E., 171(503), 198
duPlessis, D.J., 133(137), 181
Durbin, R.P., 165(447), 196
Duthie, H.L., 122(28, 29), 177
Duthie, J.J.R., 4(23), 104
Dvornik, D., 265(37), 281

E

Eagleton, G.B., 152(318, 319),
    157(385), 190, 193
East, J., 45(101), 108
Ebringer, A., 38(98), 108
Edwards, J.W., 134(164, 169),
    182, 183
Eggen, D.A., 263(21), 280
Egyhazi, E., 393(37), 403
Eich, S., 152(317), 190

Eiseman, B., 125(59), 155(59),
    157(59), 178
Elion, G.B., 21(41), 34(82, 83),
    77(157), 105, 107, 110
Elis, J., 38(96), 108
Elkes, J., 209(14), 231
Elliott, F.A., 270(100), 284
Elliott, G.A., 279(211), 289
Elliott, H., 263(23), 264(24), 280
Ellis, L.F., 295(20), 312
Ellison, E.H., 132(118), 137(226),
    180, 185
Elsden, D.F., 364(85), 381
Elwin, C.-E., 120(8), 176
Emås, S., 131(103), 157(389),
    180, 193
Emmons, P.R., 331(60), 343
Endean, R., 164(432, 433), 195
Endo, M., 268(69, 70), 282
Enesco, H.E., 371(117, 119), 382,
    389(19), 390(21), 391(26),
    392(19), 402, 403
Engel, F.L., 136(213), 184
Engelberg, H., 271(123), 285
Englert, E., Jr., 90(196), 112
Englert, M.E., 265(40), 281
Ennis, R.S., 30(70), 107
Epps, L., 162(412), 194
Epstein, S.E., 237(16, 17), 258
Erasian, S., 133(126), 136(126), 181
Erickson, E.H., 68(136), 110
Eriksson, S., 270(94), 283
Ermolieva, Z.V., 306(102), 315
Erspamer, V., 118(435), 432, 433,
    435), 195
Ertel, N.H., 19(37), 105
Essman, S.G., 394(49), 404
Essman, W.B., 388(8, 10), 391(30),
    392(30, 34), 393(8, 10, 39),
    394(49), 397(70, 71), 398(87),
    399(94), 401(94), 402-406
Estes, J.W., 170(488), 175(488),
    198
Etévé, J., 6(31), 105
Etherington, D.J., 122(34), 177
Evans, D.A.P., 133(149), 134(174,
    175), 135(180), 182, 183
Evans, G., 331(58), 343

Evans, G.L., 324(21), <u>341</u>
Evans, H., 324(24), <u>341</u>
Evans, J., 149(288), <u>188</u>
Evans, J.F., 333(80, 81), <u>344</u>
Evans, L., 94(227), <u>113</u>
Evans, W.O., 398(84), <u>405</u>
Evanson, J.M., 74(146), <u>110</u>
Everitt, A.V., 353(21), 354(21, 22, 23, 25), 372(126), <u>378</u>, <u>382</u>
Evrard, E., 268(80), <u>283</u>
Eylar, E.H., 86(174), <u>111</u>
Eyssen, H., 268(70), <u>283</u>

F

Fabro, S., 301(62), 302(62, 63), <u>313</u>, <u>314</u>
Failey, R.B., Jr., 270(95), <u>284</u>
Fain, J.N., 240(25), <u>258</u>, 272(133), <u>285</u>
Falcoff, E., 295(13), 300(47, 53, 57), 303(13), 305(53, 76), <u>311</u>, <u>313</u>, <u>314</u>
Falcoff, R., 295(13), 300(47, 53), 303(13), 305(53), <u>311</u>, <u>313</u>
Fantes, K.H., 298(33), <u>312</u>
Farmer, J.B., 255(52), 257(52), <u>258</u>
Farquhar, J.W., 267(61), <u>282</u>
Farrar, J.F., 353(17), <u>378</u>
Fearnley, G.R., 333(77-81), <u>344</u>
Fee, S.R., 358(45), <u>379</u>
Feldman, D., 33(80), <u>107</u>
Fellows, E.J., 371(118), <u>382</u>
Fellows, E.T., 390(20), <u>402</u>
Fels, S.S., 155(348), <u>191</u>
Fensch, F.C., 395(59), <u>404</u>
Fenton, B., 152(312), <u>190</u>
Fenton, B.H., 134(160), 154(333), <u>182</u>, <u>191</u>
Ferguson, R.H., 22(42), <u>105</u>
Fernandez, L.A., 90(191), <u>112</u>
Ferrier, J.-P., 156(359), 157(359), <u>192</u>
Ferris, A.J., 27(66b), <u>106</u>
Ferry, E.L., 349(1), <u>377</u>
Fiasse, R., 134(157), <u>182</u>
Fichez, L.F., 367(95), <u>381</u>

Field, A.K., 295(17, 18, 19, 21), 299(17), 301(17, 18, 21), <u>311</u>, <u>312</u>
Field, E.J., 45(103), <u>108</u>
Field, H., Jr., 267(59), 277(191), 282, <u>288</u>
Fink, B.A., 299(44), 302(44), <u>313</u>
Fink, M., 388(12), <u>402</u>
Finstad, J., 47(110), <u>109</u>
Finter, N.B., 292(8), 296(8), 300(51), <u>311</u>
Fischer, J., 80(163), <u>111</u>
Fischer, J.E., 163(415), <u>194</u>
Fish, A., 47(110), <u>109</u>
Fish, J.C., 35(89), <u>108</u>
Fisher, J.M., 136(211), <u>184</u>
Firkin, B.G., 69(139), <u>110</u>
Fitts, C.T., 156(364), 157(364), <u>192</u>
Fitzgerald, J.D., 237(18), <u>258</u>
Flanc, C., 329(41, 43), 333(84), 337(84), <u>342</u>, <u>344</u>
Fleishner, F.G., 329(40), <u>342</u>
Fletcher, A.P., 332(68, 71), 334(90), 335(94, 103), 336(109), <u>343</u>, <u>344</u>
Fletcher, D.G., 157(379), <u>193</u>
Fletscher, J., 138(248), <u>186</u>
Flint, S.F., 82(168), <u>111</u>
Flute, P.T., 330(52), 333(84), 337(84), <u>343</u>, <u>344</u>
Fodor, O., 134(171), 135(171), <u>183</u>
Fontaine, D., 295(13), 300(47, 57), 303(13), <u>311</u>, 313
Fontaine, D., 300(47, 57), <u>313</u>
Forbes, H.A.W., 358(46), <u>379</u>
Forbes, J.C., 93(221), <u>113</u>
Ford, D.K., 6(33), <u>105</u>
Ford, S.H., 165(450), <u>196</u>
Forestier, J., 29(68), <u>107</u>
Forscher, B.K., 4(16), <u>104</u>
Forster, G., 271(117), <u>285</u>
Fosdick, L.S., 92(213), <u>113</u>
Fosdick, W.M., 27(64), 83(169), <u>106</u>, <u>111</u>
Fournier, F., 300(53), 305(53, 76), <u>313</u>, <u>314</u>

Fowler-Bergfeld, W., 37(94), 108
Fox, J.P., 306(95), 315
Frame, B., 137(220, 224), 185
Frankland, M., 140(261), 187
Franklin, T.J., 88(185), 112
Franko, B.V., 157(382), 193
Fraumeni, J.F., Jr., 23(46), 105
Fred, H.L., 324(20), 341
Fredrickson, D.S., 265(42), 270(102), 275(169, 170, 171, 173), 276(170), 281, 284, 287
Freedman, D.X., 399(96), 406
Freibrun, J.L., 269(88), 283
Freiman, A.H., 321(16), 341
Freiman, D.G., 319(6, 7), 324(6, 7, 26), 341, 342
French, J.E., 325(29), 342
French, J.M., 137(225), 185
Freyberg, R.H., 27(57), 33(57), 106
Freyhan, F.A., 204(9), 231
Frezzotti, R., 309(107), 316
Fried, J., 165(450), 196
Friedlander, P.H., 143(265), 187
Friedman, C.L., 354(27, 28, 29, 30), 255(27, 28), 356(27, 31), 274(27, 29, 30), 378
Friedman, G.A., 133(135), 135(135), 136(135), 181
Friedman, G.D., 265(34), 281
Friedman, M., 278(197), 288
Friedman, M.H.F., 122(23), 177
Friedman, R.M., 293(9), 295(12), 297(29), 311, 312
Friedman, S.M., 354(27, 28, 29, 30), 355(27, 28), 356(27, 31), 374(27, 29, 30), 378
Friedmann, C.A., 165(439), 195
Friend, D.G., 143(269), 187
Frisk, Å., 133(134), 134(134), 181
Frost, D.V., 265(24), 280
Frost, P., 37(93), 108
Fudema, J.J., 358(50), 379
Fujinami, T., 171(504), 198
Fujita, T., 273(153, 156), 286
Fukushima, H., 268(67, 69, 70), 282
Fukushima, M., 35(89), 108

Furchgott, R.F., 253(49), 254(49), 255(49), 258
Furman, R.H., 275(177, 179), 287

G

Gabrielson, A.E., 77(154), 110
Gaffey, H.W., 267(57), 282
Gagnon, J., 100(247), 114
Galbraith, J.E.K., 305(74), 314
Gallay, H.M., 393(44), 403
Gallo, B., 135(182), 183
Galloway, R., 149(275, 280), 151(294), 187, 188, 189
Galton, D.J., 272(133), 285
Garapin, A., 304(71), 305(71), 314
Garattini, S., 388(9), 402
Gardner, F., 90(194), 112
Gardner, T.S., 271(114), 382
Garner, R.L., 338(117), 345
Garrett, R.E., 306(101), 315
Garrido-Klinge, G., 128(82), 179
Garrod, A.B., 19(38), 105
Gatti, G.L., 398(78), 405
Gatti, R.A., 47(110), 109
Gaudry, R., 265(37), 281
Gaut, Z.N., 273(148), 286
Gee, M.V., 353(19), 368(19), 378
Geisel, A., 160(403), 194
Gelfand, D.N., 360(59), 380
Gelfand, H.M., 306(95), 315
Gelfand, S., 360(59), 380
Geller, I., 218(24), 232
Genton, E., 336(109), 345
Gerard, R.W., 393(38), 403
Gerring, E.L., 171(501a), 198
Gershey, E.L., 89(187), 112
Getty, R., 353(20), 368(20), 378
Gherondache, C.N., 374(130), 383
Ghosh, P.B., 88(183), 112
Giarman, N.J., 399(96), 406
Gibbons, A.J., 87(179), 111
Gilgore, S., 273(152), 286
Gillespie, G., 167(458), 168(461), 196
Gillespie, I.E., 122(26), 167(458), 168(461), 177, 196

Gilman, A., 19(36), 21(36), 23(36), 25(36), 27(36), 31(36), 34(36), 37(36), 105
Gilsdorf, R.B., 138(239), 186
Ginsburg, M., 160(405), 194
Girerd, R.S., 93(216), 113
Gitman, L., 358(43), 379
Gius, J.A., 135(190), 184
Givner, M., 265(37), 281
Gladner, J.A., 98(235), 114
Glasgow, L.A., 295(15), 311
Glasky, A.J., 394(51), 404
Glass, G.B.J., 123(40), 133(148, 152), 134(148, 152, 157), 135(179), 170(148, 152), 175(148, 152), 177, 182, 183
Glassman, J.M., 154(329), 190
Glassock, R.J., 33(80), 107
Glazer, A.N., 98(240), 114
Glazko, A.J., 27(58), 106
Glenn, E.M., 58(115), 87(178), 89(188), 94(225), 109, 111, 112, 113
Glennon, W.E., 265(34), 281
Glovsky, M., 68(137), 110
Glynn, L.E., 4(28), 105, 134(176), 183
Gobbel, W.G., Jr., 157(387), 158(387), 193
Goffredo, O., 118(435), 164(435), 195
Gofman, J.W., 263(24), 264(24), 265(45), 280, 281
Goia, A., 134(171), 135(171), 183
Goldberg, A., 127(63), 178
Goldman, A., 23(44), 105
Goldman, H., 156(363, 373), 192
Goldman, I.M., 253(47), 256(47), 257(47), 258
Goldsmith, G.A., 268(79), 272(132), 283, 285
Goldstein, A., 253(45), 259
Goldstein, L., 399(97), 406
Gonin, J., 94(224), 113
Gonzalez, J.D., 335(97), 345
Good, R.A., 47(110), 77(154), 109, 110

Goodier, T.E.W., 151(294, 295), 189
Goodman, L.S., 19(36), 21(36), 23(36), 25(36), 27(36), 31(36), 34(26), 37(36), 105
Goodman, M.L., 171(504), 198
Goodwin, J.F., 333(83), 337(83), 344
Goodwin, S., 23(45), 105
Gorbatow, O., 170(495), 175(495), 198
Gordon, F.B., 298(40), 312
Gordon, P., 358(50-54), 359(55, 56, 57), 374(54), 379, 380
Gore, I., 171(504), 198
Gorham, J.R., 45(102), 108
Gorinsky, P.D., 168(463), 196
Gorlin, R., 331(62), 343
Gould, R.G., 270(111), 277(192), 284, 288
Gowans, J.L., 36(90a), 108
Grady, H., 270(107), 284
Graeme, M.L., 4(11), 104
Grahn, D., 360(71), 380
Gralnick, H., 309(108), 316
Granda, J.L., 30(70), 107
Grant, L., 4(15), 104
Gray, G.D., 87(180), 111
Gray, J., 94(225), 113
Gray, S.J., 127(71), 136(217), 171(498), 179, 185, 198
Grayzel, A.I., 74(145), 110
Green, A.G., 136(218), 185
Green, H., 371(118), 382, 390(20), 402
Green, K.G., 270(99), 284
Green, L., 90(192), 112
Green, M.A., 388(12), 402
Green, R.D., 253(46), 255(46), 256(46), 257(46), 258
Greenwood, B.M., 91(206), 113
Gregory, F.J., 82(168), 111
Gregory, H., 118(516, 517, 518, 519), 199
Gregory, R.A., 120(9), 122(9), 137(225), 167(9, 464), 176, 185, 197
Greig, H.B.W., 321(17), 341
Greig, M.E., 87(179), 111

Gresser, I., 295(13), 300(47, 57), 303(13), 306(79, 82), 311, 313, 314
Griffin, D., 67(132), 109
Griffin, D.M., 170(496), 198
Griffins, J.A., 149(288), 188
Griffith, E.M., 134(160), 182
Grigas, E.O., 165(450), 196
Grigg, D.I., 156(366), 192
Gristina, A., 100(245), 114
Grizzle, J.E., 153(325), 190
Gross, A., 151(298), 189
Gross, D.A., 393(46), 404
Grossi, C.E., 321(16), 341
Grossman, M.I., 117(2), 120(3, 4, 6, 7), 122(22, 24, 26), 123(43), 128(77), 131(2), 135(183), 136(209), 139(2, 252), 140(259), 143(270), 155(346), 157(389), 159(402), 163(2), 164(434), 166(453, 454), 167(24, 453, 456), 169(479, 482, 483, 484), 170(482, 492), 175(492), 176, 177, 179, 183, 184, 186, 187, 191, 193-198
Grosz, C.R., 157(378), 193
Gruenfeld, N., 4(11), 104
Gruenstein, M., 133(133), 155(348), 181, 191
Grummer, J.W.P., 124(53), 128(53), 131(53), 132(53), 173(53), 178
Gryboski, W., 134(161), 182
Guerken, N., 149(282), 151(282), 188
Guerra, R., 309(107), 316
Guest, M.J., 265(35), 281
Guest, M.M., 335(101), 345
Guggenheim, M.A., 308(106), 316
Guisan, M., 322(19), 324(23, 27), 329(39), 341, 342
Guiss, L.W., 132(120), 180
Gulbenkian, A., 131(106), 136(106), 180
Gurewich, V., 328(35, 36), 342
Gurian, H., 272(138), 286
Gurowitz, E.M., 393(46), 404

Guth, P.H., 135(187), 183
Gutman, A.B., 63(121), 109
Gutmann-Auersperg, N., 278(199), 288
Gutova, M., 38(96), 108
Györkey, F., 31(73), 76(73), 107
Györkey, P., 31(73), 76(73), 107

H

Haddock, D.R.W., 134(169), 183
Hagen, P., 162(410), 194
Hahn, P.F., 271(121), 285
Hajjar, G.C., 334(91), 336(104, 105, 106), 344, 345
Håkanson, R., 162(411), 194
Häkkinen, I.P.T., 131(99), 134(168), 180, 183
Hale, E.H., 140(259), 187
Hale, G.S., 336(112), 345
Hall, G.H., 399(95), 400(95), 406
Hall, J.H., 331(63), 343
Hall, K., 94(230), 114
Hall, P., 135(187), 183
Hall, W.H., 138(240), 186
Hallaway, H.M., 372(125), 382
Hallenbeck, G.A., 122(27), 137(230), 177, 185
Hallum, J.V., 297(27), 312
Halsall, T.G., 149(281), 151(281), 188
Halstead, W.C., 389(15), 402
Hamerman, D., 74(143), 110
Hamilton, J.G., 268(79), 272(132), 283, 285
Hammer, C., 94(229), 114
Hammerl, H., 272(145), 286
Hammond, D.T., 329(40), 342
Hamor, G.H., 174(423a), 195
Hampton, J.R., 330(51), 331(61), 343
Handler, J.S., 136(200, 204), 184
Hansch, C., 44(100), 108
Hansky, J.H., 133(316), 181
Hanson, H.M., 156(376), 157(381), 158(392), 193
Hanson, M.A., 58(117), 109

Haot, J., 157(386), <u>193</u>
Hardy, J.D., 133(126), 136(126), <u>181</u>
Hardy, P.M., 118(516), <u>199</u>
Harken, D.E., 331(62), <u>343</u>
Harkins, H.N., 154(335), <u>191</u>
Harman, D., 360(66, 67, 70),
　361(70, 72, 73), 362(72),
　370(105a), 371(70), 372(70, 72,
　121), 377(70, 72, 121), <u>380</u>, <u>382</u>
Harman, R.E., 25(48), <u>106</u>
Harris, E.D., Jr., 74(146), <u>110</u>,
　367(93), <u>381</u>
Harris, J.B., 120(14), 131(14), <u>176</u>
Harrison, M.J., 331(60, 61), <u>343</u>
Harrison, R.C., 121(19), <u>176</u>
Harsanyi, P., 322(19), 324(23, 27),
　336(104), <u>341</u>, <u>342</u>, <u>345</u>
Hartelius, H., 393(35, 36),
　<u>403</u>
Hartiala, K., 169(479), <u>197</u>
Hartman, R.C., 330(50), <u>343</u>
Hartmann, G., 271(117), <u>285</u>
Hartsock, R.J., 137(224), <u>185</u>
Hartzell, R.W., Jr., 277(180, 193),
　<u>287</u>, <u>288</u>
Hashim, G.A., 86(174), <u>111</u>
Hashim, S.A., 268(76), <u>283</u>
Hashimoto, S., 278(204), <u>289</u>
Hassanein, A.A., 334(89), 338(89),
　<u>344</u>
Hatton, G.I., 396(68), <u>404</u>
Haubrich, W.S., 137(220), <u>185</u>
Haudenschild, C., 368(103), <u>381</u>
Hausmann, W., 149(283), 151(283),
　<u>188</u>
Hauss, W.H., 94(234), <u>114</u>
Haverback, B.J., 135(185), <u>183</u>
Hay, L., 132(122), <u>181</u>
Hayes, C., 92(210), <u>113</u>
Haynes, F.W., 324(24), 329(40),
　<u>341</u>, <u>342</u>
Haynes, R.C., Jr., 136(202), <u>184</u>
Hazard, J.B., 35(88), <u>107</u>
Hazleman, B.L., 27(63), <u>106</u>
Healey, L.A., 25(49), <u>106</u>
Hearst, E., 397(74), <u>405</u>
Heatley, N.G., 133(153), <u>182</u>

Heinken, T.S., 152(309), <u>190</u>
Heins, J.N., 94(229), <u>114</u>
Helyer, B.J., 155(343), 158(343),
　<u>191</u>
Hempel, K.H., 90(191), <u>112</u>
Hench, P.S., 90(193), <u>112</u>
Henderson, E.D., 100(244), <u>114</u>
Hendley, D.D., 368(102), <u>381</u>
Henson, J.B., 45(102), <u>108</u>
Henzel, J.H., 172(508), <u>199</u>
Herbert, E.W., 360(59), <u>380</u>
Hernandez, H.H., 267(58), <u>282</u>
Heron, S.Z., 392(32), <u>403</u>
Herrick, E.M., 91(206), <u>113</u>
Herring, V., 263(23), 264(23), <u>280</u>
Herriott, R.M., 77(153), <u>110</u>,
　122(32), <u>177</u>
Herrmann, R.G., 277(185), <u>288</u>
Hersh, E.M., 4(20), 19(20), 21(20),
　22(20), 73(20), <u>104</u>
Hess, H.-J., 165(442), 166(442),
　168(442), <u>196</u>
Hess, R., 266(52, 53), 270(106,
　108), 271(115), 274(53), <u>282</u>,
　<u>284</u>, <u>285</u>
Hewitt, J., 263(23), 264(24), <u>280</u>
Heyman, R.L., 125(59), 155(29),
　157(29), <u>178</u>
Hicks, C.S., 371(115, 116), <u>382</u>
Higginson, B., 88(185), <u>112</u>
Hightower, N.C., 153(325), <u>190</u>
Hill, A.G.S., 4(26), <u>104</u>
Hill, D.F., 27(64), 83(116), <u>106</u>, <u>111</u>
Hill, R.A., 168(459), <u>196</u>
Hilleman, M.R., 295(17, 18, 19, 21),
　299(17), 300(55), 301(17, 18, 21,
　61), <u>311</u>, <u>312</u>
Himizu, J., 165(450), <u>196</u>
Hinobara, M., 306(81), <u>314</u>
Hirsch, E.Z., 270(113), <u>284</u>
Hirschmann, R., 85(172), <u>111</u>
Hirschowitz, B.I., 122(31, 35),
　123(31, 38), 133(38), 137(219),
　139(35), <u>177</u>, <u>185</u>
Hirsh, J., 336(109, 112), 358(47),
　<u>345</u>, <u>379</u>
Hislop, I.G., 133(138), <u>181</u>

AUTHOR INDEX

Hitchings, G.H., 21(41), 34(82, 83), 77(157), 105, 107, 110
Hlavackova, V., 372(124), 377(124), 382
Ho, M., 300(49), 313
Ho, R.S., 271(119, 120), 285
Hochstein, F.A., 273(152), 286
Hocking, E.P., 333(80), 344
Hodes, M.E., 270(95), 284
Hoezel, F., 349(6), 377
Hoffer, A., 272(124), 285
Hofmann, A.F., 133(140), 181
Hogg, D.F., 132(124), 133(124), 181
Holborow, E.J., 134(176), 183
Holemans, R., 332(70), 343
Holland, G.F., 273(152), 286
Holland, J.F., 307(104), 316
Hollander, F., 133(146), 139(251), 154(336), 182, 186, 191
Hollander, J.L., 4(22), 12(22), 26(22), 29(22), 30(22), 31(22), 36(22), 104
Holliday, A.R., 398(85), 405
Holmes, E.D., 360(59), 380
Holmes, J.H., 33(79), 107
Holmes, R.H., 336(108), 345
Holmgren, A., 94(230), 114
Holmström, B., 133(134), 134(134), 181
Holstein, M.D., 336(173), 345
Holt, P.J.L., 333(86), 344
Homan, E.R., 301(62), 302(62), 313
Honour, A.J., 331(60, 61), 343
Hooper, C.S., 135(194), 184
Hopkins, C.E., 269(84), 283
Hoppin, F.G., 329(40), 342
Horgan, E.S., 306(93), 315
Horlick, L., 272(129), 285
Horning, E.C., 23(45), 105
Horton, E.W., 165(448), 196
Horwich, L., 134(174, 175), 135(180), 149(280), 151(294), 183, 188, 189
Hoshino, M., 306(81), 314
Hoskins, L.C., 134(159), 182
Hostetler, D.D., Jr., 306(94), 315
Hotchin, J., 45(105a), 108

Houck, J.C., 4(16, 18), 98(235), 104, 114
House, R.F., 395(59), 404
Hovig, T., 320(11), 325(30), 341, 342
Howard, J.E., 141(262), 187
Howard, R.P., 275(177), 287
Howe, C.T., 329(41), 333(84), 337(84), 342, 344
Howel-Evans, A.W., 134(164, 169), 182, 183
Howie, J.B., 155(343), 158(343), 191
Howson, W.T., 69(140), 110
Hruza, Z., 354(26), 371(111, 112), 372(124), 377(124), 378, 382
Hsu, J.M., 172(507), 199
Huang, C.Y., 45(104), 108
Huang, K.Y., 298(40), 312
Hucker, H.B., 25(47), 105
Hudyma, G.M., 154(329), 190
Huebner, P.J., 303(70), 314
Hueck, W., 262(13), 280
Hughes, J., 320(8), 341
Hume, D.M., 33(81), 107
Hundley, J.M., 156(351), 191
Hunt, J.H., 140(258), 187
Hunt, J.N., 143(270), 187
Hunt, L.J., 399(98), 406
Hunt, T., 151(299), 189
Hunt, T.C., 151(302), 189
Hunter, J., 133(132), 181
Hunter, J.D., 272(140), 286
Hurlbut, J.A., 68(135), 110
Hurst, A.F., 128(72), 179
Hyde, G., 265(45), 281
Hyde, H.A., 121(19), 176
Hydén, H., 389(14), 393(35, 37), 402, 403
Hyndman, L.A., 335(98), 345
Hynie, S., 245(44), 246(44), 247(44), 253(44), 259

I

Iencica, R., 134(171), 135(171), 183
Iggo, A., 121(20), 176

Ignarro, L.J. , 4(11), <u>104</u>
Ignatowski, A. , 262(9), <u>280</u>
Ikkala, E. , 332(67), <u>343</u>
Ilea, V. , 134(171), 135(171), <u>183</u>
Imagawa, R. , 275(177), <u>287</u>
Imai, Y. , 267(62, 64), 268(70), <u>282</u>
Imondi, A.R. , 156(370), <u>192</u>
Impiccatore, M. , 118(435), 164(433, 435), <u>195</u>
Ingenito, E.F. , 278(202), <u>288</u>
Inman, J.K. , 335(98), 336(107), <u>345</u>
Innes, I.R. , 145(271), <u>187</u>
Iorio, I.C. , 253(47), 256(47), 257(47), <u>258</u>
Ireson, H. , 133(129), <u>181</u>
Irwin, S. , 202(1, 2, 3), 205(10), 209(15, 17), 213(19, 20), 215(3), 216(1), 217(10, 22), <u>231</u>, <u>232</u>
Isaacs, A. , 292(1, 2, 3), 293(3), 294(2, 3), 295(3, 16), 296(3), 297(28), <u>311</u>, <u>312</u>
Isakovic, K. , 388(7), <u>402</u>
Isenberg, I. , 360(68), <u>380</u>
Isenberg, J. , 170(492), 175(492), <u>198</u>
Ishii, Y. , 152(308), <u>189</u>
Ishimori, A. , 135(179), <u>183</u>
Ishioka, I. , 273(156), <u>283</u>
Ishioka, T. , 273(157), <u>286</u>
Isokane, N. , 273(157), <u>286</u>
Ito, M. , 267(63), <u>282</u>
Ito, Y. , 128(76), <u>179</u>
Iversen, O.H. , 92(208), <u>113</u>
Iveson, P. , 149(289), <u>188</u>
Ivy, A.C. , 155(346), 169(479), <u>191</u>, <u>197</u>

J

Jack, D. , 255(52), 257(52), <u>258</u>
Jackson, A.M. , 149(282), 151(282), <u>188</u>
Jackson, G.G. , 306(77), <u>314</u>
Jackson, R.A. , 143(264), <u>187</u>
Jacobs, A. , 133(129), <u>181</u>
Jacobsen, T.N. , 156(357), 158(357), <u>192</u>

Jaffe, B.M. , 164(430, 431), <u>195</u>
Jaffe, I.A. , 367(92), <u>381</u>
Jahiel, R.I. , 298(38), <u>312</u>
Jao, R. , 306(77), <u>314</u>
Jankovic, B.D. , 388(7), <u>402</u>
Janowitz, H.D. , 137(229), 154(336, 338), <u>185</u>, <u>191</u>
Janssen, P.A.J. , 219(26, 27), <u>232</u>
Jaraskova, L. , 305(72), <u>314</u>
Jasani, M.K. , 27(60), <u>106</u>
Jasinski, B. , 94(231), <u>114</u>
Jasmin, G. , 45(107), <u>108</u>
Jaworski, A.A. , 306(98), <u>315</u>
Jaworski, R.A. , 306(98), <u>315</u>
Jefferson, N.C. , 160(403), <u>194</u>
Jerzy Class, G.B. , 174(522), <u>199</u>
Jewett, A. , 398(84), <u>405</u>
Jiminez, L. , 305(72), <u>314</u>
Johansson, R. , 131(99), <u>180</u>
Johnson, A. , 329(45), <u>342</u>
Johnson, A.J. , 329(44), <u>342</u>
Johnson, F.R. , 151(293), <u>189</u>
Johnson, G.D. , 134(176), <u>183</u>
Johnson, H.D. , 124(55), 134(166, 167), <u>178</u>, <u>183</u>
Johnson, L.R. , 162(413), 164(434), 166(454), 167(456), <u>194</u>, <u>195</u>, <u>196</u>
Johnson, M.L. , 303(70), <u>314</u>
Johnston, D. , 122(28, 29), <u>177</u>
Johnston, I.D.A. , 153(321, 326), <u>190</u>
Johnston, M.M. , 400(101), <u>406</u>
Joklik, W.K. , 298(35), <u>312</u>
Jones, B.R. , 305(74), <u>314</u>
Jones, D.S. , 118(516), <u>199</u>
Jones, F.A. , 124(50, 53), 128(53, 81), 129(50), 131(50, 53), 132(53), 173(53), <u>178</u>, <u>179</u>
Jones, H.B. , 265(45), <u>281</u>
Jones, J.H. , 151(304), <u>189</u>
Jones, R.J. , 277(192), <u>288</u>
Jorgensen, L. , 325(30), <u>342</u>
Jori, G.P. , 135(182), <u>183</u>
Jorpes, J.E. , 118(451, 452, 520), 119(452), 166(451, 452), <u>196</u>, <u>199</u>

AUTHOR INDEX

Joynes, C., Jr., 267(60), <u>282</u>
Juergens, J.L., 272(141), <u>286</u>
Julien, C., 6(31), <u>105</u>
Junge-Hülsing, G., 94(234), <u>114</u>

K

Kabakjian, J.R., 270(109), <u>284</u>
Kadatz, R., 156(357), 158(357), <u>192</u>
Kagan, A., 265(28, 29), 274(28, 29), <u>280</u>
Kagan, H., 275(176), <u>287</u>
Kahlson, G., 65(126), 76(126), 99(126), <u>109</u>, 163(416), 168(460), <u>194</u>, <u>196</u>
Kahn, D.C., 157(384), 158(384), <u>193</u>
Kahn, J.R., 132(112), 138(112), <u>180</u>
Kajander, A., 100(248), <u>114</u>
Kakkar, V.V., 329(41, 43), 333(84), 337(84), <u>342</u>, <u>344</u>
Kalbhen, D.A., 94(233), <u>114</u>, 172(511), <u>199</u>
Kalman, S.M., 253(45), <u>259</u>
Kanazawa, K., 267(62), <u>282</u>
Kannel, W.B., 265(28, 29, 34), 274(28, 29), <u>280</u>, <u>281</u>
Kantor, T.G., 100(245), <u>114</u>
Kappas, A., 89(189), <u>112</u>
Kapusta, M.A., 91(203), <u>112</u>
Karkins, H.N., 157(379), <u>193</u>
Karoly, A.J., 399(98), <u>406</u>
Karstad, L., 45(104), <u>108</u>
Karvonen, M.J., 278(206), <u>289</u>
Karzel, K., 94(233), <u>114</u>, 172(511), <u>199</u>
Kassarich, J., 58(116), 86(176), <u>109</u>, <u>111</u>
Katz, J.H., 319(6), 324(6), <u>341</u>
Katz, J.J., 389(5), <u>402</u>
Katz, L.N., 269(85, 86), 278(201), <u>283</u>, <u>288</u>
Kause, P., 170(495), 175(495), <u>198</u>
Kay, A.W., 132(115), <u>180</u>
Kaye, M.D., 133(128, 129, 130), <u>181</u>
Kazennova, I.I., 391(29), <u>403</u>
Keaty, E.C., 275(177), <u>287</u>
Keiter, J.E., 138(244), <u>186</u>

Keleman, K., 398(77), <u>405</u>
Kellgren, J.H., 36(91), <u>108</u>
Kellner, A., 275(175), <u>287</u>
Kellock, T.D., 131(110), 137(236), <u>180</u>, <u>185</u>
Kelly, L.A., 271(119, 120), <u>285</u>
Kelly, P., 137(233), <u>185</u>
Kendall, F.E., 278(200), <u>288</u>
Kenner, G.W., 118(515, 516), <u>199</u>
Kensler, C.J., 25(50, 51), <u>106</u>
Kent, P.W., 131(97), <u>180</u>
Kerley, T.L., 156(357), 158(357), <u>192</u>
Kerr, R., 135(193), <u>184</u>
Khan, M.H., 149(277), 151(277), <u>187</u>
Kier, L.B., 65(128, 129), <u>109</u>, 160(407), 174(407), <u>194</u>
Kijima, M., 128(76), <u>179</u>
Kikuchi, S., 267(62, 64), <u>282</u>
Kilby, J.O., 133(139), <u>181</u>
Kim, Y.S., 135(193), 158(396), <u>184</u>, <u>193</u>
Kimble, D.P., 396(62), <u>404</u>
Kinch, S.H., 265(33), <u>281</u>
King, J.S., Jr., 265(41), <u>281</u>
Kippen, I., 21(40), <u>105</u>
Kirchgessner, T., 236(9), <u>257</u>
Kirk, J.E., 277(190), <u>288</u>
Kirsner, J.B., 133(147), 138(245), 152(313), 153(323, 324, 325), 157(383), 168(324), <u>182</u>, <u>186</u>, <u>190</u>, <u>193</u>
Klassen, K.P., 327(32), <u>342</u>
Klein, D.F., 204(7, 8), <u>231</u>
Kleiner, G.J., 329(44, 45), <u>342</u>
Kleinschmidt, W.J., 295(20, 24), 298(24), 299(43), <u>312</u>, <u>313</u>
Kleinsmith, L.J., 89(187), <u>112</u>
Klinenberg, J.R., 21(40), <u>105</u>
Kobayashi, T., 267(62), <u>282</u>
Kobrle, V., 354(26), <u>378</u>
Koch, M.A., 306(90), <u>315</u>
Kohn, R.R., 364(78, 79), 365(79), <u>380</u>
Kohonen, J., 134(168), <u>183</u>
Komarov, S.A., 133(133), 136(216), 155(348), <u>181</u>, <u>185</u>, <u>191</u>

Kono, R., 306(81), <u>314</u>
Konttinen, A., 270(101), <u>284</u>
Konturek, S., 122(24), 167(24), <u>177</u>
Konturek, S.J., 169(487), <u>198</u>
Korabelnikova, N.I., 306(102), <u>315</u>
Korn, E.D., 271(122), <u>285</u>
Kornetsky, C., 211(18), <u>231</u>, 360(58), <u>380</u>, 397(73), <u>405</u>
Kothari, M.L., 154(340), <u>191</u>
Kottke, B.A., 272(41), <u>286</u>
Kovacev, V.P., 272(133), <u>285</u>
Kowalczyk, T., 155(341), <u>191</u>
Kowalsi, E., 329(46), <u>342</u>
Kowalski, C., 272(136), 273(136), <u>285</u>
Kral, V.A., 371(117), <u>382</u>, 389(19), 392(19), <u>402</u>
Kramel, M., 265(37), <u>281</u>
Kramer, P., 154(337), <u>191</u>
Krane, S.M., 74(146), <u>110</u>
Kränzl, C., 272(145), <u>286</u>
Krasner, L., 203(5), <u>231</u>
Krasnow, N., 324(28), <u>342</u>
Kraus, J.D., 358(50), <u>379</u>
Krawitt, E.L., 169(481), <u>197</u>
Kritchevsky, D., 262(2), 265(26, 40, 44, 45, 46), 266(2, 49, 50), 268-275(49, 50, 66, 87, 91, 93, 109, 110, 116, 130, 158, 162, 163, 165, 179, 181, 182), 277(183, 186, 187, 193), <u>279-288</u>
Krueger, R.F., 299(45), 302(45), <u>313</u>
Kubikova, M., 38(96), <u>108</u>
Kudchodkar, B., 272(129), <u>285</u>
Kuehl, F.A., Jr., 25(48), <u>106</u>
Kühn, R., 271(123), <u>285</u>
Kuklinca, A.G., 35(88), <u>107</u>
Kumagai, F., 128(76), <u>179</u>
Kunitz, M., 122(32), <u>177</u>
Kuo, P.T., 267(60), <u>282</u>
Kupiecki, F., 273(151), <u>286</u>
Kuron, G.W., 268(74), <u>283</u>
Kurz, L., 124(56), <u>178</u>
Kuzell, W., 4(3), <u>103</u>
Kuzma, O.T., 269(84), <u>283</u>
Kwaan, H.C., 332(75), <u>344</u>

Kyle, J., 136(199, 214), 137(199), 170(199), <u>184</u>, <u>185</u>

L

LaBella, F.S., 353(16, 17, 89), 364(80, 81, 82), 365(82, 89), 366(81), 367(91), <u>378</u>, <u>380</u>, <u>381</u>
Labusquiere, R., 306(94), <u>315</u>
Lack, C.H., 47(113), 94(227), <u>109</u>, <u>113</u>
Ladd, A.T., 275(175), <u>287</u>
Laden, C., 92(213), <u>113</u>
Lakey, W.H., 121(19), <u>176</u>
Lallouette, P., 93(217), <u>113</u>
Lambert, G.F., 265(24), <u>280</u>
Lambert, R., 133(151, 154), 134(151), 170(154), 170(151, 154), <u>182</u>, <u>192</u>
Lamblin, P., 306(94), <u>315</u>
Lambling, A., 156(362, 375), 157(362), <u>192</u>, <u>193</u>
Lambooy, J.P., 158(396), <u>193</u>
Lampson, G.P., 295(17, 18, 19, 21), 299(17), 300(55), 301(17, 18, 21), <u>311</u>, <u>313</u>
Lande, K., 29(67), <u>107</u>
Landis, G.A., 324(23), <u>341</u>
Landor, J., 121(17), <u>176</u>
Landor, J.H., 138(243), <u>186</u>
Lands, A.M., 255(51), <u>258</u>
Landy, M., 72(141), <u>110</u>
Langan, J., 269(91), <u>283</u>
Langley, J.N., 233(1, 2), <u>257</u>
Langman, M.J.S., 133(136), 134(173), 149(286, 287), 151(286, 287, 295a, 304), 153(286, 322), 171(286, 287), <u>181</u>, <u>183</u>, <u>188</u>, <u>189</u>, <u>190</u>
Larke, R.P.B., 303(65), 306(83, 100), <u>314</u>, <u>315</u>
Larsen, W.E., 34(84), <u>107</u>
Larson, S.J., 174(521), <u>199</u>
Lasagna, L., 271(118), <u>285</u>
Lashley, K.S., 398(88), <u>405</u>
Laster, L., 164(428), <u>195</u>
Laties, V.G., 385(4), 398(82), <u>402</u>, <u>405</u>

Laughlin, R.C., 265(39), 281
Laulajainen, M., 170(495), 175(495), 198
Laurence, E.B., 135(195), 171(195), 172(195), 184
Laurin, C.A., 100(247), 114
Law, L.W., 303(67), 314
Lawrence, H.S., 72(141), 110
Lawrence, E.B., 92(211), 113
Lawrence, I.H., 151(301, 305), 189
Laws, J.W., 329(41), 342
Lazar, H.P., 127(68), 178
Lazarus, S.S., 137(228), 170(228), 185
Leary, T., 278(195), 288
Leash, A.M., 364(79), 365(79), 380
LeBlanc, D.R., 306(95), 315
LeCompte, H., 349(8), 378
Lee, D., 93(220), 113
Lee, W.G., 396(67), 404
Lee, Y.H., 158(400), 194
Lees, R.S., 275(169, 170), 276(170), 287
Lefkowitz, E., 38(95), 108
Legerton, C.W., Jr., 143(264), 187
Lehner, N.D.M., 263(20), 280
Lehtosuo, E.J., 278(206), 289
Leibowitz, S.F., 400(104), 406
Leith, J.D., 356(38), 379
Lembeck, F., 168(463), 196
Lemberger, L., 241(28), 258
Lemoine, G., 274(166), 287
Lengsfeld, H., 272(131), 285
Lennander, K.G., 127(67), 178
Lennard-Jones, J.E., 151(304), 189
Lenon, H.L., 68(138), 110
Leonard, A.S., 138(239), 156(365), 157(365), 186, 192
Leonard-Jones, J.E., 124(53), 128(53), 131(53), 132(53), 138(248), 143(263), 173(53), 178, 186, 187
Lepori, L., 168(466), 197
Leren, P., 278(207), 289
Le Roy, E.C., 320(13), 341
Lertzman, M., 319(7), 324(7), 341
Lessel, B., 27(59), 106
Lessner, H.E., 34(84), 107

Levey, S., 152(315), 190
Levi-Montalcini, R., 172(505), 198
Levin, W.C., 35(89), 108
Levine, L., 98(236), 114
Levine, R.J., 156(367), 163(417, 418, 420), 192, 194
Levy, B., 235(5, 6, 7), 236(12), 237(12), 238(40), 239(5), 241(27, 30, 31, 33, 35), 243(30), 245(39), 247(40), 249(27, 41), 251(27), 252(33), 253(48), 254(48), 255(39), 257, 258, 259
Levy, G.P., 255(52), 257(52), 259
Levy, H.B., 292(5, 7), 293(5), 294(5, 7), 295(22), 296(7), 298(7, 31, 34), 300(56), 301(22), 303(67), 304(71), 305(71), 308(106), 309(108), 311-314, 316
Levy, L., 47(112), 87(177), 109, 111
Levy, R.I., 270(102), 275(170, 171, 172, 173), 276(170), 284, 287
Lewis, D.O., 151(200), 189
Lewis, J.M., 324(20), 341
Lewis, R.M., 45(106), 108
Lewis, S., 393(47), 404
Liepa, E., 137(228), 170(228), 185
Limbosch, J.M., 168(477), 197
Lin, C.H., 165(450), 196
Lin, T.M., 170(490), 198
Lincova, J., 245(44), 246(44), 247(44), 253(44), 259
Lindahl, U., 94(230), 114
Lindenmann, J., 292(1), 297(28), 311, 312
Lindgren, F., 263(23), 264(23), 280
Lindgren, F.T., 265(45), 281
Lindner, A.E., 154(338), 191
Lindsay, A.C., 137(227), 185
Lindsay, L.A., 240(23, 24), 258
Lindsay, W.G., 353(16), 378
Lipkin, M., 135(193), 151(292), 156(369, 370), 184, 188, 192
Lipman, M.O., 26(56), 106
Lippmann, W., 165(446), 168(473), 196, 197

Lipsett, M.B., 32(76), 107
Little, J.B., 356(33, 37), 379
Liu, C.H., 373(127), 382
Loane, R.A., 151(291), 188
Lockart, R.Z., 297(30), 312
Loehry, C.A., 137(234), 153(234), 185
Lofland, H.B., 263(20), 280
Logan, J.B., 265(40), 266(46), 281
Logan, J.S., 136(214), 185
Lojda, Z., 277(188), 288
Loosli, J.K., 373(128), 382
Lorenzen, I., 34(85), 107
Love, A.H.G., 134(166), 183
Lovelace, F.E., 373(127), 382
Lowe, R.D., 241(26), 258
Loynd, J.A., 351(12), 378
Lu, G.G., 274(161), 287
Lubar, J.F., 393(46), 404
Lubbe, R.J., 270(97), 284
Luduena, F.P., 255(51), 258
Ludwig, B.J., 274(159, 160, 161, 164), 283, 287
Ludwig, W., 151(292), 188
Ludwig, W.M., 156(369), 192
Lundholm, L., 272(143), 286
Lunsford, C.D., 157(382), 193
Luscher, E.F., 331(65), 343
Lutzky, H., 400(105), 406
Lwoff, J.M., 391(27), 403
Lyon, E.S., 121(17), 176
Lyon, T.P., 263(23), 264(23), 265(45), 280, 281

M

Määttä, K., 89(190), 112
MacCaig, J.N., 151(290), 188
MacCallum, F.O., 90(194, 195), 112
Maciera-Coelho, A., 356(36), 379
Macleod, I.B., 168(459), 196
MacDonald, R.A., 135(186), 183
MacDougall, J.D.B., 139(250), 160(250), 186
MacGregor, R.R., 32(76), 107
MacKaness, G.B., 46(109), 109
MacKay, I.R., 38(98), 108, 133(138), 181

Mackey, H.K., 58(118), 109
MacMahon, B., 124(49), 129(49), 178
Madden, J., 156(351), 191
Maezawa, H., 273(156), 286
Magee, D.F., 123(41), 166(455), 169(486), 171(41), 175(486), 177, 196, 198
Mailhe, H., 277(180, 193), 287, 288
Main, I.H.M., 165(448), 196
Makin, M., 100(246), 114
Makinodan, T., 371(110a), 382
Malawista, S.E., 20(39), 105
Malhotra, S.L., 128(87, 88), 171(500), 179, 198
Malinov, M.R., 273(154), 286
Mallon, J., 272(135), 273(135), 285
Malmo, R.B., 209(12), 231
Malmros, H., 263(18), 265(25), 280
Manderson, W.G., 137(227), 185
Mangold, R., 124(54), 178
Mann, F.C., 155(344), 156(344), 158(393), 168(478), 191, 193, 197
Mann, F.D., 168(478), 197
Mannick, J.A., 90(201, 204), 112
Manolo-Estrella, P., 263(22), 280
Mansi, M., 135(182), 183
Manton, D.J., 151(301, 305), 189
Mantz, W., 263(23), 264(23), 280
Manzano, C., 158(394), 193
Maragoudakis, M.E., 270(114), 284
Marchand, F., 262(7), 280
Marchiero, T.L., 33(79), 107
Marcus, A.J., 331(47), 342
Marcus, P.I., 298(36), 312
Marcus, R., 152(318, 319), 157(385), 190, 193
Margetts, G., 270(99), 284
Margolin, S., 274(160, 164), 287
Margolis, S., 271(118), 285
Mark, D.D., 353(19), 368(19), 378
Markarian, B., 154(337), 191
Marks, I.N., 124(52), 132(52, 121), 133(121), 151(298), 178, 180, 189
Markus, G., 335(100), 345
Marmor, L., 36(92), 108
Marmorston, J., 269(84), 283

AUTHOR INDEX

Marray, H.L., 58(118), <u>109</u>
Martin, D., 395(61), <u>404</u>
Martin, E.M., 298(33), <u>312</u>
Martin, F., 133(151, 154),
    134(151), 156(368), 170(151, 154), <u>182</u>, <u>192</u>
Martin, G.R., 364(84), 365(88), <u>381</u>
Martinelli, M., 278(202), <u>288</u>
Marschhaus, C., 272(135), 273(135), <u>285</u>
Marshall, M.W., 133(127), <u>181</u>
Marshall, N.B., 273(151), <u>286</u>
Marston, H.R., 371(115), <u>382</u>
Mason, M., 27(63), <u>106</u>
Mason, R.G., 331(66), <u>343</u>
Masserman, J.H., 203(4), <u>231</u>
Masters, Y.F., 134(161), <u>182</u>
Mathivat, A., 265(43), <u>281</u>
Mathur, V.S., 324(24), <u>341</u>
Matsuo, T., 267(64), <u>282</u>
Matsukawa, T., 267(62), <u>282</u>
Matthew, M., 69(140), <u>110</u>
May, P.R.A., 230(28), <u>232</u>
May, R.H., 358(41), <u>379</u>
Mayer, G.D., 299(44), 302(44), <u>313</u>
Mayer, S., 240(25), <u>258</u>
Maynard, L.A., 349(2), <u>377</u>
Mazzacca, G., 135(182), <u>183</u>
McAfee, J.G., 324(25), <u>341</u>
McAuliff, J.P., 255(51), <u>258</u>
McCall, K.B., 335(98), 336(107), <u>345</u>
McCandless, R.F.J., 265(40), <u>281</u>
McCarthy, R.A., 336(112), <u>345</u>
McCarty, D.J., 4(21), <u>104</u>
McCaugh, J.L., 398(90, 91, 92), <u>405</u>
McCaw, P.A., 273(149), <u>286</u>
McCay, C.M., 349(2, 3, 4),
    373(127, 128), <u>377</u>, <u>382</u>
McClosky, R.V., 295(12), <u>311</u>
McCluer, R.H., 360(65), <u>380</u>
McCluskey, R.T., 4(.5), <u>104</u>
McConnell, 124(51), 133(149),
    134(51, 164, 169, 172, 174, 175), 135(51), <u>178</u>, <u>182</u>, <u>183</u>
McCusker, V.I., 168(461), <u>196</u>
McDonald, I.G., 336(112), <u>345</u>

McDonald, S.J., 140(254), <u>186</u>
McDougall, E., 39(99), <u>108</u>
McGaugh, J.L., 360(62), 385(1), 398(1), <u>380</u>, <u>402</u>
McGregor, D.D., 36(90a), <u>108</u>
McGuigan, J.E., 164(425, 429, 430, 431), <u>195</u>
McGuire, M.T., 395(60), <u>404</u>
McHardy, G., 143(330), 153(325), 154(330), 160(330), <u>190</u>
McHardy, R.J., 143(330), 154(330), 160(330), <u>190</u>
McHugh, P.R., 156(372), <u>192</u>
McKay, D.G., 334(87, 88), <u>344</u>
McKiddie, M.T., 137(227), <u>185</u>
McLaughlin, P., 273(155), <u>286</u>
McIlrath, D.C., 122(27), <u>177</u>
McNamara, P.M., 265(34), <u>281</u>
McNew, J.J., 158(400), <u>194</u>
McNichol, G.P., 334(89), 338(89), <u>344</u>
McNutt, L., 393(45), <u>403</u>
McNutt, S.H., 155(341), <u>191</u>
McShane, W.K., 253(47), 256(47), 257(47), <u>258</u>
Meade, R.C., 273(150), <u>286</u>
Mecca, C.E., 364(84), <u>381</u>
Mecs, E., 298(33), <u>312</u>
Medawar, P.B., 78(159), <u>111</u>
Mehigan, J.A., 134(163), <u>182</u>
Mehta, J.M., 154(340), <u>191</u>
Meisinger, M.A.P., 25(48), <u>106</u>
Mellors, R.C., 45(104), <u>108</u>
Melrose, A.G., 133(131), 143(266), <u>181</u>, <u>187</u>
Mendel, L.B., 349(1), <u>377</u>
Mendelson, J., 91(203), <u>112</u>
Mendl, K., 151(301, 305), <u>189</u>
Menguy, R., 123(39, 42), 131(42), 133(42), 134(161), 136(42), 156(374), 171(42), <u>177</u>, <u>182</u>, <u>192</u>
Menon, I.S., 332(76), <u>344</u>
Menon, M.K., 174(423b), <u>195</u>
Meranze, D., 155(348), <u>191</u>
Merigan, T.C., 297(27), 298(35, 39), 299(42), 300(56), 301(59), 306(85, 92, 88), 307(42), <u>312</u>, <u>313</u>, <u>315</u>

Merkel, J., 204(9), 231
Merrill, C.R., 160(406), 194
Merrill, J.P., 33(80), 107
Merskey, C., 329(44, 45), 342
Mertz, D.P., 120(13), 176
Mesrobian, R.B., 360(69), 380
Meyer, H.M., Jr., 306(94), 315
Meyer, K., 123(36), 177
Meyer, R.F., 168(475), 197
Meyers, M.E., 396(65), 404
Meyers, W.C., 132(119), 180
Meynell, M.J., 270(103), 284
Miale, A., 324(23), 341
Miale, J.B., 320(15), 341
Michaels, R.H., 306(90), 315
Michal, F., 69(139), 110
Mickelson, M.M., 87(180), 111
Miescher, P.A., 4(30), 105
Miettinen, M., 278(206), 289
Miettinen, T.A., 270(96), 272(128), 284, 285
Mihailović, L., 388(7), 402
Miho, O., 128(76), 179
Mildvan, A.S., 353(19), 368(102), 368(19), 378, 381
Miller, E.J., 364(84), 381
Miller, G., 152(320), 190
Miller, J.G., 395(59), 404
Miller, J.P., 265(24), 280
Miller, L., 396(63), 404
Miller, O.N., 268(79), 272(132), 283, 285
Mills, R.F.N., 27(59), 106
Milton, J.D., 90(200), 112
Mims, C.A., 300(48), 313
Min, K-W., 31(73), 76(73), 107
Miner, N., 298(32), 312
Mirsky, A.F., 211(18), 231
Misher, A., 168(472), 197
Misiewicz, J.J., 151(304), 189
Mitchell, J.R.A., 331(60, 61), 343
Mitchell, M.S., 82(167), 111
Mitchell, R.D., 143(270), 187
Mody, G.D., 128(88), 179
Moll, W., 12(34), 105
Monson, R.R., 124(49), 129(49), 178
Montgomery, R.D., 151(297, 301, 305), 189

Moore, A.E., 306(99), 315
Moore, D., 334(90), 344
Moore, F.J., 269(84), 283
Moore, K.E., 398(86), 405
Moore, P.F., 253(47), 256(47), 257(47), 258
Moore, R.D., 303(66), 314
Moore, T.C., 33(81), 107
Moorhead, J.F., 92(210), 113
Moran, N.C., 237(14, 19), 240(25), 241(34), 258
Morin, R.J., 263(17), 280
Morley, J., 69(140), 110
Morley, J.S., 118(519), 164(426, 427), 174(427), 195, 199
Morris, N.R., 395(53), 404
Morse, D.L., 396(66), 404
Morse, R.L., 336(114), 345
Morton, L.T., 4(30a), 105
Moser, K.M., 322(19), 324(23, 27), 329(39), 331(54), 333(54), 334(91), 336(104, 105, 106), 338(54), 341-344
Moses, C., 262(3), 266(3), 279
Mosettig, E., 265(36), 281
Moskowitz, R.W., 26(55), 106
Motomiya, T., 273(157), 286
Mowbray, J.F., 90(200), 112
Moyer, A.W., 265(40), 266(46), 281
Moynihan, B.G.A., 127(65), 178
Moynihan, J.L., 269(91), 283
Mrhova, O., 277(188), 288
Mueller, E., 392(33), 403
Mueller, J.H., 268(71), 282
Mueller, M.N., 89(189), 112
Muggenburg, B.A., 155(341), 191
Mukerji, B., 278(198), 288
Müller-Eberhard, H.J., 66(130, 131), 109
Müller, H.J., 4(30), 105
Munnell, J.F., 353(20), 368(20), 378
Murphy, B.R., 295(15), 311
Murphy, E.A., 331(58), 343
Murphy, E.B., 295(20, 24), 298(24), 312
Murray, J.G., 165(449), 196
Murray, M.R., 368(98), 381

AUTHOR INDEX

Mustard, J.F., 325(30), 331(58), 342, 343
Mutt, V., 118(451, 520), 166(451), 196, 199
Myant, N.B., 270(92), 283
Myerson, R.M., 154(334), 191
Myhill, J., 139(253), 140(253), 186
Myllyla, G., 332(67), 343

N

Nabarro, J.D.N., 149(282, 285), 151(282), 153(285), 188
Nachmansohn, D., 398(89), 405
Naficy, K., 306(82), 314
Nakamura, M., 169(486), 175(486), 198
Nakamura, Y., 268(70), 282
Nakano, M., 305(72), 314
Nakashima, M., 354(27, 30), 355(27), 356(27), 374(27, 30), 378
Nakatani, H., 265(65), 268(67, 69), 282
Nakijima, S., 166(455), 169(486), 175(486), 196, 198
Nandy, K., 367(96), 368(96), 374(96), 381
Nanninga, L.B., 335(101), 345
Nash, H., 398(83), 405
Nash, M., 358(52), 379
Nasio, J., 137(232), 185
Nassel, H.L., 320(13), 341
Nathan, F.F., 100(244), 114
Navarret, E.E., 138(241), 186
Necheles, H., 135(188), 183
Nedelec, G., 367(95), 381
Neill, D.W., 136(214), 137(231), 185
Neklyudova, L.J., 306(89), 315
Nelson, B., 67(132), 109
Nelson, D.S., 73(142), 110
Nemes, M.M., 295(17, 19), 299(17), 300(55), 301(17), 311, 313
Nestel, P.J., 270(113), 284
Newburgh, L.H., 263(14), 280
Newbould, B.B., 86(175), 111
Newell, A.C., 134(165, 170), 182, 183

Newell, D.J., 332(76), 344
Newman, W.P., 263(21), 280
Newton, W.T., 164(430, 431), 195
Nezamis, J.E., 133(156), 165(443, 444), 182, 196
Nichols, C.W., Jr., 266(56), 268(73), 282, 283
Nickerson, M., 145(271), 187
Nicoloff, D.M., 156(365), 157(365), 192
Niemegeers, C.J.E., 219(26, 27), 232
Nigon, K., 120(14), 131(14), 176
Nimi, M.E., 364(86), 381
Nimni, M., 67(133), 110
Nishikawa, K., 267(64), 282
Nishizawa, E.E., 331(58), 343
Nokoneczna, I., 93(221), 113
Nolan, C.M., 32(75), 107
Norman, A., 137(237), 185
Norman, P.S., 335(99), 345
Northover, B.J., 99(243), 114
Northrop, J.H., 122(32), 177
Norton, S., 216(21), 231
Norton, W.L., 31(72), 76(72, 150), 107, 110
Nowinski, W.W., 120(11), 176
Numano, F., 273(153, 155), 286
Nussenzweig, R., 298(38), 312
Nutter, P.B., 132(113), 138(113), 180
Nyberg, L.O., 170(495), 175(495), 198
Nye, E.R., 273(149), 286
Nyhus, L.M., 154(335), 168(477), 191, 197

O

Oberhelman, H.A., Jr., 121(18), 176
O'Brien, J.R., 330(49), 331(59), 343
O'Brien, W.M., 25(52), 106
O'Connor, J.F., 329(40), 342
O'Dell, B.L., 364(85), 381
Oeriu, S., 372(120, 122, 123), 377(121), 382

O'Gara, R.W., 301(62), 302(62), 313
Ogden, D.A., 33(79), 107
Oi, M., 128(76), 179
Ojha, K.N., 154(339), 191
Okabe, S., 157(377), 193
Okuma, M., 363(74), 380
Oliver, M.F., 269(83), 278(210), 283, 289
Olsen, R.T., 265(24), 280
Olson, R.E., 265(27), 280
Ono, S., 162(410), 194
Ordy, J.M., 375(135), 383
Oren, B.G., 143(264), 187
Orjack, M.H., 360(58), 380
Orloff, J., 136(200, 204), 184
Orloff, M.J., 138(244), 186
Oro, L., 266(48), 272(48), 281
Orowan, E., 392(31), 403
Orzack, M.H., 397(73), 405
Osborne, T.B., 349(1), 377
O'Shea, M., 333(84), 337(84), 344
Ott, W.H., 268(74), 283
Overholt, B.F., 133(144), 181
Owensby, J., 273(150), 286
Owen Williams, G.E., 270(103), 284
Owman, C., 162(411), 194
Oxman, M.N., 298(37), 312

P

Pace, N., 100(245), 114
Pace-Asciak, C., 165(440, 441), 195
Packham, M.A., 331(58), 343
Padgett, G.A., 45(102), 108
Painter, J.C., 331(66), 343
Palmer, E.D., 135(189), 183
Palmer, P.E., 151(298), 189
Palmer, W.L., 127(69, 70), 132(113), 138(113), 154(69, 70), 153(324), 168(324), 178, 180, 190
Palmore, E., 375(136), 383
Paloheimo, J., 270(101), 284
Panayi, G.S., 69(140), 110
Paoletti, R., 275(174), 287

Paraskos, J.A., 324(21), 341
Paraskova-Tschernozenska, E., 92(210), 113
Parbhoo, S.P., 153(321), 190
Park, J., 303(70), 314
Park, J.H., 295(14), 301(14), 311
Parke, D.V., 149(279, 289), 188
Parmenter, K., 236(9), 257
Parsons, J.L., 27(64), 83(169), 106, 111
Parsons, W.B., Jr., 272(125, 126, 136), 285
Partridge, S.M., 364(85), 381
Pascal, J.P., 169(485), 198
Patel, Y.M., 98(235), 114
Paterson, J.W., 237(15), 258
Paterson, P.Y., 58(117), 109
Path, M.C., 133(129), 181
Patterson, M.A., 168(468, 469, 470, 476), 197
Paucker, K., 299(46), 313
Paul, G., 353(15), 378
Pavlov, I.P., 121(15), 176
Pearce, E., 26(56), 106
Pearce, M.L., 278(204), 289
Pearl, J.M., 138(239), 186
Pearson, C.M., 35(90), 36(92), 72(90), 91(202), 108, 112
Peek, N.F., 267(57), 282
Pelon, W., 306(90), 315
Pendleton, R.G., 168(472), 197
Peña, L., 128(82), 179
Pepeu, G., 399(96), 406
Peppel, H.H., 358(44), 379
Pereira, J.N., 273(152), 286
Perey, D.Y., 47(110), 109
Perkins, M.E., 237(19), 258
Perley, A., 273(154), 286
Perris, A.D., 76(149), 98(239), 110, 114
Perry, H.O., 265(38), 281
Persellin, R.H., 30(69), 90(191), 107, 112
Peter, E.T., 138(239), 156(365), 157(365), 186, 192
Peter, J.B., 36(92), 108
Peters, C.M., 158(395), 193

AUTHOR INDEX

Peterson, D.W., 266(55, 56), 267(57), 282
Petillo, J.J., 131(106), 136(106), 180
Petralli, J.K., 306(88, 92), 315
Petrinovich, L., 385(1), 398(1), 400(100, 103), 402, 406
Petrovic, M., 388(7), 402
Pevsner, L., 120(4), 176
Pfeiffer, C.J., 158(395), 193
Phillips, J.P., 133(156), 165(443, 444), 182, 196
Phillips, L.L., 334(92), 344
Phillips, M.J., 157(384), 158(384), 193
Phillips, S.F., 133(140), 181
Pichler, O., 272(145), 286
Pick, R., 269(85), 278(201), 283, 288
Pickering, G.W., 127(66), 178
Piez, K.A., 364(84), 365(88), 381
Pilatskata, E.P., 306(102), 315
Piliero, S.J., 4(2, 11), 103, 104
Pilkington, T.R.E., 241(26), 258
Pincus, G., 374(130), 383
Pincus, I.J., 122(23), 177
Pinkerton, I.W., 143(266), 187
Pinson, R., 273(152), 286
Piper, D.W., 124(333), 134(160), 139(253), 140(253), 152(312), 182, 186, 190, 191
Pirrie, A.J., 92(210), 113
Pisot, C., 132(111), 180
Pitney, W.R., 333(83, 86), 337(83), 344
Pitt, A., 336(112), 345
Plotnikoff, N., 394(52), 395(55, 56), 397(55, 56), 404
Plummer, A.J., 156(355), 192
Polacek, M.A., 137(226), 185
Polidora, V.J., 393(43), 394(43), 403
Poliwoda, H., 336(173), 345
Pollard, H.M., 123(37), 137(219), 143(37), 177, 185
Poller, L., 127(62), 135(62), 178
Polley, H.F., 22(42), 105
Pollock, D.J., 135(191), 184

Popescu, S., 134(171), 135(171), 183
Pories, W.J., 172(508), 199
Porter, K.A., 33(79), 107
Porterfield, J.F., 138(243), 186
Portet, R., 275(176), 287
Portman, O.W., 263(19), 280
Posey, E.L., Jr., 154(327), 190
Posey, L., III., 154(327), 190
Posner, A.S., 30(70), 107
Possanza, G.J., 58(119), 109
Postic, B., 300(49), 313
Potash, L., 306(95), 315
Potts, W., 396(66), 404
Powell, C.E., 235(8), 237(8), 257
Pradham, S.N., 168(471), 197
Prentice, C.R.M., 334(89), 338(89), 344
Preshaw, R.M., 136(209), 184
Prévot, A.R., 6(31), 105
Price, Evans, D.A., 124(51), 134(51), 135(51), 178
Prichard, R.W., 263(20), 280
Pringle, R., 134(162), 182
Probst, G.W., 299(43), 313
Prudden, J.F., 172(510), 199
Puletti, E.J., 127(68), 178
Pulvertaft, C.N., 128(85), 136(218), 179, 185
Pur, L., 244(38), 259
Purcell, G., Jr., 334(92), 344
Purdon, R.A., 168(468, 469, 476), 197
Pur-Shahriari, A.A., 324(24), 329(40), 341, 342
Pygott, F., 129(89), 179

Q

Quarfordt, S.H., 270(102), 284
Quarton, G.C., 385(3), 393(40), 402, 403
Quincke, H., 128(73), 179
Quintana, C., 68(138), 110

R

Rabson, A.S., 303(67), 314
Radious, N., 92(209), 113

Ragan, C., 26(56), 106
Rahmann, H., 398(79, 80), 405
Rainsford, K.D., 131(98), 180
Rall, T.W., 136(203), 184
Ramos-Alvarez, M., 306(90), 315
Ramsburg, H.H., 156(351), 191
Ramsey, C., 136(217), 185
Ramwell, P.W., 165(437, 438), 195
Rand, M.J., 244(38), 259
Randall, L.O., 139(249), 186
Räsänen, T., 135(196), 184
Raskova, H., 38(96), 108
Rassaert, C.L., 39(99), 108
Ratcliffe, H.L., 279(211, 212), 289
Ratnoff, O.D., 172(512), 199
Ratti, G., 273(146), 286
Raunio, V., 134(168), 183
Ray, L.A., 354(24), 378
Ray, W.J., Jr., 298(32), 312
Reber, K., 266(51), 281
Rech, R.H., 398(86), 405
Redisch, W., 332(69), 343
Rege, V., 328(34), 342
Regelson, W., 299(41, 42), 301(61), 302(41), 307(41, 42, 104), 313, 316
Rehfuss, M.E., 122(23), 177
Reichenthal, J., 23(45), 105
Reid, H.A., 333(85), 337(85), 344
Reinfenstein, R.W., 136(217), 185
Reigel, D.H., 174(521), 199
Reilly, M.A., 65(123, 124), 109, 164(423), 194
Reimer, S.M., 319(5), 341
Reinhardt, W.O., 268(72), 282
Remington, J.S., 298(39), 312
Remington, L., 25(51), 106
Remmers, A.R., 35(89), 108
Rensch, R., 398(79), 405
Reporter, M.C., 368(102), 381
Resnick, R.H., 127(71), 171(498), 179, 198
Revotskie, N., 265(28, 29), 274(28, 29), 280
Reynell, P.C., 124(57), 131(57), 178
Reynolds, E.S., 33(80), 107
Reynolds, R.C., 6(32), 105
Reynolds, W.E., 26(53), 106

Rheault, M.J., 154(335), 191
Rhim, J.S., 306(90), 315
Rhodes, J., 133(130, 140), 181
Ribet, A., 169(485), 198
Rich, S.T., 155(342), 191
Richelle, M., 157(386), 193
Richmond, C., 266(46), 281
Richou, H., 93(217), 113
Richou, R., 93(217), 113
Richter, D., 388(11), 402
Riddle, J.M., 68(138), 110
Riess, W., 270(106, 108), 284
Riley, F., 304(71), 305(71), 314
Rimmer, D.G., 140(261), 187
Rindani, T.H., 92(215), 113
Rinzler, S.H., 278(205), 289
Rita, G., 300(52), 309(107), 313, 316
Ritchie, W.B., 138(239), 186
Richie, W.P., Jr., 156(366), 192
Ritzmann, R.F., 396(63), 404
Ritzmann, S.E., 35(89), 108
Rius-Garriga, G., 324(23), 341
Rius-Garriga, J., 336(104), 345
Rob, C.G., 172(508), 199
Robert, A., 133(156), 137(233), 165(443, 444, 445), 182, 185, 196
Roberts, J.A.F., 134(163), 182
Roberts, W.C., 329(38), 342
Robertson, A.L., 35(88), 107
Robertson, T.B., 354(24), 371(113, 115), 378, 382
Robin, G., 100(246), 114
Robinson, B.F., 241(26), 258
Robinson, B.V., 93(218, 219), 113
Robinson, G.A., 136(201), 184
Robinson, L.B., 76(150), 110
Robson, J.M., 93(218, 219), 113
Rodbard, S., 278(201), 288
Rodman, N.F., 331(66), 343
Roen, P., 269(88), 283
Roenigk, H.H., Jr., 37(94), 108
Rogers, L., 25(50), 106
Rogers, K.S., 93(221), 113
Rogers, N.C., 134(166), 183, 306(94), 315

Roine, P., 278(206), <u>289</u>
Roitt, I.M., 133(141), <u>181</u>
Rokitansky, C., 262(6), <u>279</u>
Roll, P.M., 389(16), <u>402</u>
Rolsten, C., 375(135), <u>383</u>
Romanoff, L.P., 374(130), <u>383</u>
Ronsen, B., 359(56), <u>380</u>
Rose, H.M., 26(56), <u>106</u>
Rose, R.K., 23(44, 45), <u>105</u>
Rosen, H., 138(244), <u>186</u>
Rosenberg, A., 156(361), <u>192</u>
Rosenberg, L.T., 67(132), <u>109</u>
Rosengren, E., 65(126), 76(126), 99(126), <u>109</u>, 163(416), 168(460), <u>194</u>, <u>196</u>
Rosenstein, B.J., 306(98), <u>315</u>
Rosenthal, S.R., 274(167), <u>287</u>
Rosenthale, M.E., 58(116), 86(176), <u>109</u>, <u>111</u>
Rosmus, J., 354(25), <u>378</u>
Rosoff, C.B., 156(363, 373), <u>192</u>
Ross, M.H., 375(134), <u>383</u>
Roth, J.L.A., 145(272), <u>187</u>
Rothblat, G.H., 277(180, 181, 182, 186, 193), <u>287</u>, <u>288</u>
Rothschild, G.H., 393(38), <u>403</u>
Rotstein, J., 4(27), <u>104</u>
Rovati, A.L., 168(465, 466, 467), <u>197</u>
Rovelstad, R.A., 127(64), 133(140), <u>178</u>, <u>181</u>
Rovner, D.R., 151(296), 189
Rowe, W.P., 298(37), <u>312</u>
Rowlands, E.N., 140(260), 143(260), <u>187</u>
Rowsell, H.C., 325(30), <u>342</u>
Rubin, B., 165(450), <u>196</u>
Ruelius, H.W., 82(168), <u>111</u>
Ruffin, J.M., 143(264), <u>187</u>
Rufin, J.M., 152(310), 153(325), <u>190</u>
Ruland, M.B., 358(41), <u>379</u>
Rumball, J.M., 143(264), <u>187</u>
Rumsey, R.D.E., 132(124), 133(124, 127), <u>181</u>
Runcie, J., 152(307), <u>189</u>
Runde, I.A., 321(17), <u>341</u>

Rundles, R.W., 21(41), 34(82), <u>105</u>, <u>107</u>
Rune, S.J., 122(30a), <u>177</u>
Ruotsi, A., 100(248), <u>114</u>
Russell, P.S., 35(87), <u>107</u>
Russell, R.I., 127(63), 133(131), <u>178</u>, <u>181</u>
Russi-Sorce, M., 300(50, 52), <u>313</u>
Rutledge, R., 156(355), <u>192</u>
Rutstein, D.D., 278(202), <u>288</u>
Ryan, T.J., 151(300), <u>189</u>
Ryan, W.L., 87(182), <u>111</u>
Ryder, R.J.W., 90(198), <u>112</u>

S

Sabin, A.B., 306(90, 91, 97), <u>315</u>
Sabiston, D.C., Jr., 324(25), <u>341</u>
Sachs, E., 400(106), <u>406</u>
Sachs, M.L., 269(91), <u>283</u>
Saigal, O.N., 128(88), <u>179</u>
St. Clair, R., 263(20), <u>280</u>
Sakuma, A., 273(157), <u>286</u>
Salaman, M.H., 91(205), <u>112</u>
Salaman, M.N., 78(161), <u>111</u>
Salb, J.M., 298(36), <u>312</u>
Sallata, P., 270(109, 110), 274(163), <u>284</u>, <u>287</u>
Salter, R.H., 131(94), <u>180</u>
Saltykow, S., 262(10), <u>280</u>
Salvador, R.A., 240(23, 24), 241(29), <u>258</u>
Samorajski, T., 375(135), <u>383</u>
Samter, M., 4(29), 30(29), <u>105</u>
Samuel, O.W., 171(502), 173(502), <u>198</u>
Samuel, P., 268(77, 78), <u>283</u>
Samuels, B.M., 27(60), <u>106</u>
Sances, A., Jr., 174(521), <u>199</u>
Sanders, H.J., 4(14), <u>104</u>
Santhanakrishnan, T.S., 165(450), <u>196</u>
Sarajas, H.S.S., 332(67), <u>343</u>
Sarles, H.E., 35(89), <u>108</u>
Sarma, P., 303(70), <u>314</u>
Sasahara, A.H., 336(114), <u>345</u>
Sato, T.L., 163(418), <u>194</u>

Sawyer, W.D., 332(68), 343
Saxton, J.A., Jr., 373(127), 382
Schapiro, H., 154(328), 170(488, 489), 175(488, 489), 190, 198
Schatonoff, J., 270(100), 284
Schayer, R.W., 64(122), 65(123, 124, 125), 109, 162(409), 164(423), 194
Scheagren, J.M., 32(76), 107
Schellekens, K.H.L., 219(26), 232
Scherrer, R.A., 4(13), 104
Schild, H.O., 160(408), 194, 249(42, 43), 259
Schlesinger, M.S., 329(37), 342
Schlesinger, R.B., 148(273), 187
Schleissner, L.A., 269(88), 283
Schmidt, M.J., 393(42), 403
Schneider, F., 58(116), 86(176), 109, 111
Schoch, H.K., 278(209), 289
Schoenfeld, W.N., 397(76), 398(76), 405
Schofield, B., 120(5), 176
Schools, P.E., Jr., 277(191), 288
Schor, J.M., 333(82), 336(82), 344
Schroeder, E.T., 140(255), 142(255), 186
Schulert, A., 23(44), 105
Schultz, A.S., 389(16), 402
Schultz, W.W., 298(40), 312
Schwartz, A., 93(217), 113
Schwartz, J., 156(371), 192
Schwartz, N.L., 58(118), 109
Schwartz, R.S., 62(120), 77(155), 90(198), 109, 110, 112
Schwarz, K., 128(74), 179
Scobie, B.A., 127(64), 178
Scratcherd, T., 120(12), 176
Scriabine, A., 253(47), 256(47), 257(47), 268
Seay, P.H., 156(356), 192
Sébald, M., 6(31), 105
Sebrell, W.H., 268(75), 283
Segal, H.L., 157(388), 193
Seifter, J., 154(329), 190, 218(24), 232
Seirafi, R., 158(398), 193

Semb, L.S., 154(335), 191
Senay, E.C., 156(367), 192
Sercek, V., 38(96), 108
Seronde, J., 158(397), 193
Sewing, K.-F., 168(463), 196
Seyle, Hans, 3(1), 4(1), 103
Sgouris, J.T., 335(98), 336(107), 345
Shanks, R.G., 235(20), 236(11), 239(20, 21), 244(37), 258, 259
Sharma, V.K., 98(235), 114
Sharpley, P., 397(72), 405
Shaw, J.E., 165(437, 438), 195
Shawdon, H.H., 149(286, 287), 151(286, 287), 152(286), 153(286, 322), 171(286, 287), 188, 190
Shay, H., 128(75), 132(75, 121), 133(133, 201), 136(216), 137(75, 238), 155(348), 179, 180, 181, 185, 186, 191
Shea, S.M., 156(352), 192
Sheinfeld, S., 152(315), 190
Shen, T.Y., 4(9, 12), 164
Sheppard, P.M., 124(51), 134(51, 164, 169), 135(51), 178, 182, 183
Sheppard, R.C., 118(515), 199
Sheps, M.C., 319(5), 341
Sherlock, S., 138(242), 186
Sherman, J.L., 135(189), 183
Sherman, R., 170(488), 175(489), 198
Sherrod, T.R., 253(46), 255(46), 256(46), 257(46), 258
Sherry, S., 332(68, 71), 334(90), 335(94, 95, 103), 336(95, 109, 111), 343, 344, 345
Sherwood, N., 368(105), 369(105), 381
Sheth, U.K., 154(340), 191
Shetlar, M.R., 275(177), 287
Shils, M.E., 168(474), 197
Shimamoto, T., 273(153, 155, 156, 157), 286
Shneour, E.A., 266(56), 267(57), 282
Shock, N.W., 351(13), 378

AUTHOR INDEX

Short, C.L., 26(53), 106
Shull, H., 153(325), 190
Shulman, S., 321(18), 341
Shupe, J.L., 45(108), 108
Sidley, N.A., 397(76), 398(76), 405
Sidman, M., 218(23), 232
Siegel, H., 268(74), 283
Siegenthaler, P., 272(142), 286
Silber, R., 85(172), 111
Silberberg, M., 349(7), 378
Silberberg, R., 349(7), 378
Silverman, J.L., 331(57), 343
Silvestrini, B., 90(197), 112
Simkin, P.A., 25(49), 106
Simler, M., 156(371), 192
Simms, H.S., 349(5), 377
Simon, E.H., 298(32), 312
Simon, L.N., 394(51), 404
Simon, P., 391(27), 403
Simons, E.L., 90(196), 112
Simonson, E., 358(42), 379
Simpson, C.L., 321(18), 341
Simpson, L.O., 155(343), 158(343), 191
Simpson-White, R., 358(46), 379
Sines, J.O., 156(376), 193
Singleton, J.W., 170(491), 198
Siperstein, M.D., 265(35), 268(72, 73), 281, 282, 283
Siplet, H., 133(133), 181
Sircus, W., 122(25), 132(123), 133(149), 137(225), 167(25), 168(459), 177, 181, 182, 185, 196
Siurala, M., 170(495), 175(495), 198
Sjöerdsma, A., 163(418), 194, 367(93), 381
Sjovall, J., 277(184), 288
Skeith, M.D., 25(49), 106
Skidmore, I.F., 4(8), 99(241), 104, 114
Skoryna, S.C., 128(78), 157(78), 179
Slater, I.H., 235(8), 237(8), 257
Slater, J.D.H., 149(285), 153(285), 188
Slavick, M., 38(96), 108
Sloan, H.R., 270(102), 284

Slotta, K.H., 335(97), 345
Smadel, J.E., 306(94), 315
Small, I.F., 397(72), 405
Small, J.G., 397(72), 405
Smallwood, R.A., 137(222), 185
Smith, C., 74(143), 110
Smith, C.A.M., 373(127), 382
Smith, G.P., 138(240), 156(372), 186, 192
Smith, L.A., 124(48), 178
Smith, M.J.H., 27(66a), 106, 131(98), 180
Smith, P.K., 27(66a), 106
Smith, R.E., 267(61), 282
Smith, R.G., 360(61), 380, 395(58), 404
Snider, G.L., 358(50), 379
Snyder, R.L., 279(212), 289
Snyder, S.H., 160(406), 162(412, 415), 194
Sobel, H., 364(83), 381
Sodeman, W.A., Jr., 123(37), 143(37), 177
Sodhi, H.S., 272(129), 285
Sokoloff, L., 36(92a), 108
Soloviev, V.D., 300(54), 305(54), 306(89), 313, 315
Solyom, L., 389(18, 19), 390(21), 392(19), 393(44), 402, 403
Solyum, L., 371(117), 382
Somani, P., 244(36), 259
Sonnabend, J.A., 297(29), 298(33), 312
Sorkin, E., 77(156), 110
Sorkin, S.Z., 136(212), 184
Sornsen, H.C., 87(182), 111
Southam, C.M., 306(99), 315
Spaet, T.H., 320(12), 341
Spigland, I., 306(90), 315
Spiro, H.M., 137(221), 185
Spector, W.G., 3(1C), 4(1C, 17), 47(114), 73(17), 103, 104, 109
Sperling, G., 349(2, 4), 373(127, 128), 377, 282
Sperry, W.M., 266(54), 282
Spray, G.F., 170(490), 198
Sreter, F.A., 354(30), 374(30), 378

Srivanij, P., 368(104), <u>381</u>
Srivastava, L., 94(229), <u>114</u>
Stainthorpe, E., 94(227), <u>113</u>
Stamler, J., 269(85, 86), 278(201), <u>283</u>, <u>288</u>
Stanton, H.C., 236(9), <u>257</u>
Staple, E., 272(130), <u>285</u>
Staples, R., 168(472), <u>197</u>
Starr, P., 269(88), <u>283</u>
Starzl, T.E., 33(79), 35(86), <u>107</u>
Stastny, P., 47(111), <u>109</u>
Staübli, W., 270(106, 108), <u>284</u>
Staudinzer, H., 365(90), <u>381</u>
Steele, J.M., 332(69), <u>343</u>
Steelman, S.L., 85(172), <u>111</u>
Steigmann, F., 148(273), <u>187</u>
Stein, D.G., 396(69), <u>404</u>
Stein, H.H., 395(54), <u>404</u>
Stein, M., 328(34), <u>342</u>
Stein, P.D., 329(40), <u>342</u>
Stein, S., 324(25), <u>341</u>
Steinberg, D., 265(36, 42), 272(134), <u>281</u>, <u>285</u>
Steinbuch, M., 93(223), <u>113</u>
Steiner, A., 268(77), <u>283</u>
Steiner, M., 363(74), <u>380</u>
Steinman, M., 271(123), <u>285</u>
Stengle, J.M., 335(95), 336(95), <u>345</u>
Stening, G.F., 164(434), 166(454), 169(483, 484), <u>195</u>, <u>196</u>, <u>197</u>, <u>198</u>
Stephen, J.D., 272(124), <u>285</u>
Stephenson, J.S., 236(10), <u>258</u>
Sternby, N.H., 263(18), <u>280</u>
Stetton, D., 392(32), <u>403</u>
Stewart, A., 90(194), <u>112</u>
Stewart, F.W., 132(120), <u>180</u>
Stewart, P.B., 58(119), <u>109</u>
Stiglitz, R.A., 273(150), <u>286</u>
Stinebring, W.R., 297(26), <u>312</u>
Stjernsward, J., 78(160), <u>111</u>
Stock, J.A., 79(165), <u>111</u>
Stokes, J., 265(29), 274(29), <u>280</u>
Storr, J.M., 98(238), <u>114</u>
Stout, A.P., 368(98), <u>381</u>
Storz, J., 45(108), <u>108</u>
Strachan, R.G., 85(172), <u>111</u>
Strander, H., 305(75), <u>314</u>

Strain, W.H., 172(508), <u>199</u>
Straton, L.O., 400(100, 103), <u>406</u>
Straughn, J., 133(155), <u>182</u>
Streeten, D.H.P., 137(219), <u>185</u>
Strehler, B.L., 350(9), 353(19), 368(19, 99, 102), <u>378</u>, <u>381</u>
Strickland, I.D., 27(63), <u>106</u>
Strickland, R.G., 136(211), <u>184</u>
Strisower, B., 263(23), 264(23), <u>280</u>
Strisower, E.H., 270(104, 105), <u>284</u>
Strong, J.P., 263(21), <u>280</u>
Stuckey, N.W., 262(11), <u>280</u>
Studer, A., 266(51), <u>281</u>
Studlar, M., 272(145), <u>286</u>
Subrahmanyan, T.P., 300(48), <u>313</u>
Sulica, L., 134(171), 135(171), <u>183</u>
Sulkin, N.M., 368(104), <u>381</u>
Sullivan, F.M., 149(277), 151(277), <u>187</u>
Sullivan, J.M., 331(62), <u>343</u>
Summers, D., 324(28), <u>342</u>
Sun, D.C.H., 128(79), 131(104), 136(79), 143(79, 267, 268), 152(311), 156(350), <u>179</u>, <u>180</u>, <u>187</u>, <u>190</u>, <u>191</u>
Sun, D.H., 137(238), <u>186</u>
Sunaga, T., 273(156), <u>283</u>
Suolanen, R., 89(190), <u>112</u>
Susser, M., 128(80), <u>179</u>
Sutherland, E.W., 136(201, 203, 206), <u>184</u>
Suyemoto, J., 324(26), <u>342</u>
Suzuoki, Z., 267(64), <u>282</u>
Svahn, D., 163(416), <u>194</u>
Sved, S., 371(117), 389(17), 390(17), <u>382</u>, <u>402</u>
Svensson, S.E., 168(460), <u>196</u>
Svoboda, D., 270(107), <u>284</u>
Sweetnam, P.M., 133(130), <u>181</u>
Swell, L., 267(59), 277(191), <u>282</u>, <u>288</u>
Swynnerton, B.F., 134(165), <u>182</u>
Swyryd, E.A., 270(111), <u>284</u>
Szego, C.M., 170(496, 497), <u>198</u>
Szulman, A.E., 134(177), <u>183</u>

T

Tabachnick, I.I.A., 131(106), 136(106), 180
Tachibana, D.K., 67(132), 109
Tainter, M.L., 27(66b), 106
Takagi, K., 152(308), 189
Takogi, K., 157(377), 193
Talbott, J.H., 19(35), 21(35), 105
Talland, G.A., 393(40), 395(60), 403, 404
Tanabe, G., 328(34), 342
Tanaka, N., 174(522), 199
Tanaka, Y., 45(102), 108, 128(76), 171(504), 179, 198
Tappel, A.L., 351(11), 363(11), 378
Tárnoky, A.L., 149(283), 151(283), 188
Tashjian, A.H., Jr., 98(236), 114
Taylor, C.B., 263(22), 278(203), 280, 289
Taylor, C.L., 360(58), 380, 397(73), 405
Taylor, J., 293(11), 297(11), 311
Taylor, K.B., 136(211), 184
Taylor, W.H., 122(34), 177
Taylor, W.J.R., 273(148), 286
Tazelaar, A.P., Jr., 156(356), 192
Teir, H., 135(198), 184
Telford, J.M., 162(414), 194
Tennent, D.M., 268(74, 75), 283
Tepper, S.A., 265(26), 268(66), 269(91), 270(109, 110), 271(116), 273(158), 274(162, 163), 275(179), 277(186), 280, 282-288
Terasaki, P.I., 33(79), 107
Tesar, W.C., 265(40), 266(46), 281
Tesler, M.A., 152(320), 190
Tewari, S.N., 156(306), 189
Texter, E.C., Jr., 127(68), 143(264), 178, 187
Thein, P., 120(5), 176
Thomas, D.P., 328(34, 35, 36), 342
Thomas, J., 368(85), 381
Thomas, J.E., 122(23), 177
Thomas, P.J., 6(32), 105
Thompson, A.E., 123(39), 177
Thompson, C.J., 165(448), 196
Thompson, J.C., 116(1), 118(1), 164(1), 176
Thompson, J.H., 130(91, 92), 140(257), 158(400), 171(499), 179, 186, 194, 198
Thompson, M.J., 265(36), 281
Thompson, R.W., 396(65), 404
Thomson, J.M., 127(62), 135(62), 178
Thomson, T.J., 152(307), 189
Thornbill, D.P., 353(89), 365(89), 381
Thorp, J.M., 270(98), 284
Thrasher, J.D., 135(192), 155(342), 184, 191
Thunberg, R., 163(416), 194
Tillets, W.S., 338(117), 345
Timiras, P.S., 368(105), 369(105), 381
Timms, A.R., 271(119), 285
Titterington, E., 241(26), 258
Tobin, S.S., 358(50, 52), 379
Tobolsky, A.V., 360(69), 380
Todd, A.S., 332(72, 73), 344
Toivanen, P., 89(190), 112
Toki, K., 265(65), 268(67, 68), 282
Tomeczek, K., 274(159), 286
Tomiyama, Y., 160(403), 194
Tomiyasu, U., 278(204), 289
Tommila, V., 300(58), 313
Tow, D.E., 324(22, 25), 336(108), 341, 345
Townsend, S.F., 126(60), 178
Tozzi, S., 241(27), 249(27), 250(27), 251(27), 258
Trach, B., 132(122), 181
Tracy, H.J., 118(519), 137(225), 185, 199
Trapold, J.H., 271(119), 285
Trautschold, I., 94(226), 113
Treadwell, C.R., 267(59, 63), 277(191), 282, 288
Trembalowicz, F.C., 152(306), 189
Trevett, D., 133(129), 181
Trethewie, E.R., 163(421), 104
Triopathy, S.P., 46(109), 109

Trnavsky, K., 4(8), 104
Trout, E.C., Jr., 267(59), 282
Trudeau, W.L., 164(425), 195
Trueheart, R.E., 278(203), 289
Truelove, S.C., 124(57), 131(57), 137(235), 153(235), 178, 185
Tucker, D.R., 270(112), 284
Tuffley, R., 149(285), 153(285), 188
Turpeinen, O., 278(206), 289
Turpie, A.G.G., 152(307), 189, 334(89), 338(89), 344
Turk, J.L., 80(162), 111
Turner, D.H., 156(354), 192
Turner, M.D., 122(33), 177
Turner, R., 38(95, 97), 108
Tushmalova, N.A., 391(29), 403
Tykkläinen, R., 89(190), 112
Tyrrell, D.A.J., 296(25), 312
Tyson, K.R.T., 35(89), 108
Tytell, A.A., 295(17, 18, 19, 21), 299(17), 300(55), 301(17, 18, 21), 311, 312, 313

U

Uhlendorf, C., 295(23), 312
Ullman, L.P., 203(5), 231
Underdahl, L.O., 137(223), 185
Underwood, E.J., 172(506), 198
Urbach, G.I., 90(192), 112
Urcan, S., 134(171), 135(171), 183
Uvnäs, B., 120(8), 122(21), 176

V

Vagne, M., 169(483), 197
Vahouny, G.V., 267(63), 282
Vaidya, A.B., 154(340), 191
Valitski, L.S., 156(360), 192
Valzelli, L., 388(9), 402
Vanderberg, J., 298(38), 312
Vander Brook, M.J., 156(356), 192
Vanderhaeghe, H., 268(80), 283
VanDeripe, D.R., 241(34), 258
Vane, J.R., 165(439), 195
Van Eldik, E., 151(298), 189
Van Frank, R.M., 295(20), 312

Van Itallie, T.B., 268(75, 76), 283
Van Loghem, J.J., 77(152), 110
Van Rossum, J.M., 254(50), 258
Van Sickle, G.R., 360(65), 380
Vantrappen, G.R., 127(68), 178
Varco, R.L., 132(122), 181
Varis, K., 170(495), 175(495), 198
Vaughan, J., 27(62), 106
Vaysse, N., 169(485), 198
Veis, A., 365(87), 381
Velayos, E.E., 76(150), 110
Veldkamp, W., 156(356), 192
Ventzke, L.E., 135(183), 183
Verbruggen, F.J., 219(27), 232
Verhave, T.A., 397(75), 405
Vermylen, C., 336(110), 345
Verymylen, J., 336(110), 345
Verstraete, M., 336(110), 345
Verzar, F., 348(49), 353(14), 372(123), 374(131), 377(123), 378, 379, 382, 383
Vestea, S., 134(171), 135(171), 183
Videbaek, A., 34(85), 107
Vidt, D.G., 35(88), 107
Vilcek, J., 298(38), 312
Vincent, C.T., 333(77), 344
Virchow, R., 135(184), 183, 262(5), 279
Virtanen, S., 134(168), 183
Viskum, K., 122(30a), 177
Visscher, F.E., 156(356), 192
Vivian, S., 353(89), 365(89), 381
Vocac, J.A., 171(501), 175(501), 198
Vogel, J., 264(4), 279
Vogel, J.R., 218(25), 232
Vogel, R., 94(226), 113
Voller, A., 91(206), 113
Volta, F., 165(440), 195
Von Hahn, H.P., 374(131), 383
Von Heimburg, R.L., 137(230), 185
Von Kaulla, K.N., 336(115, 116), 345
Von Rechenberg, H.K., 23(43), 105
Voronin, L.G., 391(29), 403
Voroshilova, M.K., 306(80), 314
Vouillon, G., 133(151), 134(151), 170(151), 182
Vrabiescu, A., 358(48), 379
Vroman, H.E., 265(36), 281

AUTHOR INDEX 439

W

Wacker, L., 262(13), 280
Wade, M.E., 82(167), 111
Wagner, A.R., 391(25), 403
Wagner, H., 94(234), 114
Wagner, H.H., 336(173), 345
Wagner, H.N., 324(22, 25), 336(108), 341, 345
Wagner-Jauregg, T., 80(163), 111
Wainrib, B., 371(117), 382
Wakimura, A., 268(69), 282
Wallace, S.L., 19(37), 105
Wallach, S., 90(196), 112
Wale, J., 244(38), 259
Walford, R.L., 370(106, 107, 110), 382
Wallensten, S., 133(134), 134(134), 181
Walpole, S., 132(122), 181
Walsh, J.H., 164(428), 195
Walsh, P.N., 335(95), 336(95), 345
Walton, K.W., 4(19), 45(19), 104
Wangensteen, O.H., 132(122), 156(365, 366), 157(365), 181, 192
Ward, J.W., 157(382), 193
Ward, J.T., 136(199), 137(199), 170(199), 184
Wares, E., 127(63), 178
Waring, W.S., 270(98), 284
Warner, W.L., 269(90), 283
Warnock, N.H., 265(41), 281
Warren, G.H., 82(168), 111
Wasley, J.W.F., 4(11), 104
Wasserman, M., 249(41), 259
Watkins, J., 131(98), 180
Watkins, W.M., 134(178), 173(178), 183
Watkinson, G., 124(58), 131(107), 133(58), 149(276), 178, 180, 187
Watson, G.I., 306(97), 315
Watt, J., 152(316, 318, 319), 157(385), 190, 193
Way, L., 165(447), 196
Weaver, L.C., 156(357), 158(357), 192

Wechsler, R.L., 145(272), 187
Wechster, B.M., 324(28), 342
Weeks, J.R., 165(436), 195
Weichmann, K., 136(208), 184
Weigel, W., 94(231), 114
Weiner, J., 269(84), 283
Weiner, M., 4(2), 103
Weiner, M.K., 332(69), 343
Weinstein, G.D., 37(93), 108
Weiss, B., 385(4), 398(82), 402, 405
Weiss, E., 137(238), 186
Weiss, P., 271(118), 285
Weissman, A., 385(2), 402
Weissman, G., 75(148), 110
Weksler, M., 90(200), 112
Welbourn, R.B., 136(199, 214), 137(199, 231), 170(199), 184, 185
Welch, G.E., 143(330), 154(330), 160(330), 190
Wenke, M., 245(44), 246(44), 247(44), 253(44), 259
Werle, E., 94(226), 113
Wessler, S., 319(3, 4, 5, 6, 7), 320(15), 324(6, 7, 26), 328(34), 339(3), 340, 341, 342
West, G.B., 162(144), 194
West, H.F., 138(246), 186
Westling, H., 136(207), 184
Whalen, R.E., 397(74), 405
Wheelock, E.F., 303(65, 66), 306(77, 78, 86, 87, 100), 314, 315
White, T.T., 123(41), 171(41), 177
Whitehouse, D.J., 35(90), 72(90), 108
Whitehouse, J.M., 400(102), 406
Whitehouse, M.W., 4(7), 35(90), 65(129), 68(137), 72(90), 80(164), 88(164, 183, 184), 93(222), 99(241), 103, 108-114, 131(100, 101), 149(281), 151(281), 173(514), 180, 188, 199, 272(130), 285
Whitfield, J.F., 76(149), 98(239), 110, 114
Wigand, G., 265(25), 280

Wigzell, H., 90(199), 112
Wilbur, J.R., 306(88, 92), 315
Wilder, W.T., 137(220), 185
Wilkenfeld, B.E., 241(35), 245(39), 253(48), 254(48), 255(39), 259
Williams, A.W., 155(343), 158(343, 391), 191, 193
Williams, R.C., 31(74), 107
Williams, R.T., 149(289), 188
Williamson, C.S., 158(393), 193
Williamson, J.M., 127(63), 178
Willoughby, D.A., 3(1C), 4(1C), 47(114), 103, 109
Wilner, J.D., 320(13), 341
Wimer, C., 395(61), 404
Wingate, H.W., 168(471), 197
Winkelmann, R.K., 265(38), 281
Winter, C.A., 4(4), 47(4), 103
Wirth, W., 94(234), 114
Wissler, R.W., 277(192), 288
Wittenborn, J.R., 230(28), 232
Wohl, H., 329(44), 342
Wolf, E., 319(6), 324(6), 341
Wolf, F.J., 268(74), 281
Wolf, H.H., 140(260), 143(260), 187
Wolf, P.L., 92(209), 113
Wolfe, L.S., 165(440, 441), 195
Wolff, R., 319(6), 324(6), 341
Wolff, R.A., 152(313), 190
Wolff, S.M., 32(76), 107
Wolff, W.S., 138(243), 186
Wolstencroft, R.A., 69(140), 110
Wong, L.C., 272(140), 286
Wood, F.D., 91(202), 112
Wood, P.H.N., 131(96), 180
Woodrow, J.C., 134(164), 182
Woodward, E.R., 121(17, 18), 154(328), 158(394), 176, 190, 193
Woolner, L.B., 137(223), 185
Wormsley, K.G., 120(3), 122(22, 30), 176, 177
Wright, P.M., 165(448), 196
Wruble, L.D., 170(488, 489), 175(488, 489), 198
Wu, K.-T., 157(378), 193
Wurzel, H.A., 331(57), 343

Wyatt, A.P., 134(166), 183
Wyllie, J.H., 165(449), 168(477), 196, 197
Wyngaarden, J.B., 21(41), 105
Wynn, V., 149(284), 188

Y

Yajima, Y., 305(72), 314
Yalow, R.S., 164(424), 195
Yamashita, S., 273(157), 286
Yamazaki, H., 273(156), 286
Yeh, S.D.J., 168(474), 197
Yellin, T.O., 395(54), 404
Yerasimides, T.G., 279(211), 289
Yesair, D.W., 25(50, 51), 106
Yonkman, F.F., 156(355), 192
Yoshida, K., 128(76), 179
Yoshikawa, K., 128(76), 179
Yoshimura, S., 299(45), 313
Youdale, T., 98(239), 114
Youngner, J.S., 297(26, 27), 312
Yu, T.F., 63(121), 109
Yuan, G.C., 356(33, 35, 37), 379

Z

Zacchei, A.G., 25(47), 105
Zajdela, A., 295(13), 303(13), 303(13), 311
Zalmanzon, E.S., 306(112), 315
Zamcheck, N., 134(159), 182
Zanetti, M.E., 268(74), 283
Zeitlenok, N.A., 306(103), 315
Zeleznick, L.D., 303(68), 314
Zeller, W., 273(147), 286
Zemplenyi, T., 277(188, 189), 288
Zendzian, R., 301(62), 302(62), 313
Ziff, M., 30(69), 47(111), 107, 109
Zimmerman, G.R., 169(481), 197
Zimmon, D.S., 152(320), 190
Zollinger, R.M., 132(118), 180
Zubiran, J.M., 121(18), 176
Zucker, M.D., 320(9, 12), 341
Zweifach, B.W., 4(15), 104
Zydeck, F.A., 92(209), 113

SUBJECT INDEX

A

Acetylcholine, 388, 399-400
Acetylcholinesterase, 399-400
Acetylsalicylic acid, see Aspirin
ACTH, see Adrenocorticotropic hormone
Actinomycin D, 394
Addisons disease, 136
Adiphenine, 145
Adjuvant arthritis (rat), 58, 86, 95; see also Lymphocytes
  estrogens in, 89
  prevention of induction, 81
  suppression by conventional anti-inflammatory drugs, 81
  suppression by poly I: poly C copolymers, 89
  thiazolidinone in, 86
Adrenocorticosteroids, 7, 31, 58, 90, 97, 133, 158, 355, 373
  as anti-inflammatory agents, 32
  effect on immune processes, 32
  side effects, 31
  tissue anabolism by, 98
  tissue repair, 11
Adrenocorticotropic hormone, 32, 131, 133, 136
Age pigment, 360, 367-368
Aging, 349-375
  clinker theory of, 351
  coalescence-accretion-stabilization, 349-352
  crosslinking theory of, 350-351
  diet and, 349, 361, 371, 373, 375
  integrated theory of, 351
  theories, 349-374
  theory of autoimmunity and, 356
  theory of brain and, 350-351, 358-360, 368, 372
  theory of endocrine and, 353-357
  theory of growth and, 349, 356, 373
  theory of intracellular pigment and, 350-351, 353
  theory of nucleic acids and, 350, 356, 359-360, 374
  theory of radiation and, 360, 363, 367, 370
ALG, see Antilymphocyte globulin
Alkyl sulfates, 152
Allergic encephalomyelitis, 58, 86; see also Lymphocytes
Allergic thyroiditis, 58, 86; see also Lymphocytes
Allopurinol, 21
  inhibition of purine oxidation by, 22
Alpha adrenergic receptors, 233-235, 239
  activators, 239
  antagonists, 235, 239
  classification, 235
Alpha methyl INPEA, 244
Aluminum hydroxide, 141
Amethopterin, see Methotrexate
Aminocaproic acid, 173
Amitriptyline, 221-228
Amnesia, 392
Amphetamine, 209, 211, 398
Amprotropine, 145
Amyloidosis, 361
Amylopectin sulfate, 152
Analgesics, 220
Anaphylotoxins, 62, 66
Antacids, 139-142, 169
  action, 139
  adverse effects (see individual drugs)
  classification, 140
  clinical use, 140
  milk-alkali syndrome and, 141

principles of use, 139
Anti-(acute) inflammatory agents, 63
Antibody production, 62
Anticoagulants, 322, 328
   heparin, 322, 328
   prothrombinopenic agents, 322
Antidepressants, 209, 220-228
Antigen recognition, chemical
   nature of, 73
Antihistamines, 139, 160
Anti-inflammatory agents,
   naturally occurring, 96
Anti-inflammatory drug design, 75
   assay methods for, 77, 96, 102
   "chromosomal pharmacology", 98
   chronic inflammatory states, 40,
      54, 56, 57
   for clinical use, 102
   efficacy in chronic human disease,
      102
   eradicative agents, 76
   induced repression of RNA
      synthesis, 98
   induction of drug metabolism, 97
   latent drugs, activation in situ,
      100
   mediators of tissue injury, 64
   mediators of tissue repair, 75
   metabolism in small animals, 97
   moderation of tissue injury
      response, 11, 47
   narrow spectrum agents, 96
   potency in, 40, 96
   to prevent initial tissue injury,
      10, 46
   replacement therapy, 95
   restorative agents, 11, 76
   retrospective survey, 96
   role of endogenous anti-
      inflammatory factors, 93
   role of large molecules, 89
   role of non-functional chemical
      compounds, 89
   therapeutic effect and toxicity, 97
   therapeutic goals, 8, 52, 55
   therapeutic index, 97
Anti-inflammatory drug screening,
   40-50, 73, 87, 97

anti-etiologic agents, 44
disease models, 44, 48, 49, 50
in vitro, 41-44, 73, 87
infection versus host's natural
   defenses, 46
random tests of chemicals, 88
Anti-inflammatory drugs, 4, 7; see
   also individual agents
counterirritant action, 92
definition, 6
effect on polymorphonuclear
   leukocytes, 20
evaluation of anti-etiologic agents,
   47, 51
evaluation of classical anti-
   inflammatory agents, 51
evaluation of drugs for prevention
   of tissue injury, 51
evaluation in man, 47
as lymphokine antagonists, 72
potency, 7
role of adrenals, 62
role of thymus, 62
as sensitization inhibitors, 7, 10,
   40, 52
therapeutic effect and toxicity of,
   7, 10, 40, 52
therapeutic goals, 5
Anti-injury factors, 93, 95
   antinuclease activity, 93
   antiprotease activity, 93-94
   globulin increase, 93-94
Antilymphocyte globulin, 35, 73
Antimetabolites, 99; see also
   Azaribine, Cycloleucine,
   Methotrexate
   as immunosupressors, 80, 82
   potential antiviral activity of, 83
Antimitotic agents (natural), see
   Chalones
Antimuscarinic drugs,
   139, 142-145, 164, 175
   action, 143
   adverse effects, 145
   classification, 143
   principles of use, 143
Antinuclear antibodies, 22
Antioxidants, 360-363

SUBJECT INDEX

Antipepsins, 152, 170, 175
  amylopectin sulfate, 152
Antiplasmin, 335
Antiproliferative drugs, 79; see
  also Cytostatic agents
Antithrombotic therapy, 331-332
  in arterial thrombosis, 331
  aspirin, 331, 338
  dipyridamole, 331, 338
  glyceryl guaiacolate, 331, 338
  in venous thrombosis, 332
Antitumor and immunosuppressive
  drugs, 79
Antiurease compounds, 168
Antiviral drugs, 173
Antral chalone, 121
Arthritis, 36, 45, 58, 93; see also
  Gout, Rheumatoid Arthritis,
  Psoriasis, Osteoarthritis,
  Systemic Lupus Erythematosus
  in animals, see Adjuvant
    arthritis (rat)
  articular cartilage, 36, 94
  folk remedies, 93
  loss of function, 58
  mycoplasmal infections in, 45
Arvin, 333, 337
Aryloxy aliphatic acids, 270-271
  ethyl α-(p-chlorophenoxy)
    isobutyrate, 270; see also
    CPIB, Clofibrate, Atromid-S
  1-methyl-4-piperidyl bis
    (p-chlorophenoxy) acetate,
    271
  2-methyl (p-1, 2, 3, 4-
    tetrahydro-1-naphthylphenoxy)
    propionic acid, 271
Aspirin, 27-29, 96, 131, 133, 157,
  331, 338
  anti-inflammatory effects of, 28
  epithelial cell exfoliation and,
    131, 135
  mucous secretion and, 131
Atherosclerosis, 262
  definition of, 262
  in rabbits, 262
Atromid-S, 270; see also CPIB,
  Clofibrate

Atropine, 143, 164
Aurothioglucose, 98
Aurothiomalate, see Gold sodium
  thiomalate
Aurothiosulfate, 30
Auto-allergic inflammatory diseases
  (experimental), 72; see also
  Lymphocytes
Autoantigens, 84
  immunogenic amino acid sequences,
    86
Autoimmunity, 26, 356
Autoimmunoregulation, 90
Azaribine, 38
Azathioprine, 27, 34-35, 100

B

Bacterial lipopolysaccharides, 168
Behavioral analyses, 202-212
  arousal, 208-209
  desired subjective state, 209
  individual control, 205-208
  normal and abnormal, 202-203
  operant response, 210-212
  response to stimuli, 209
  target-diagnosis, 204
  target-function, 205-212
  target-symptom, 205
Behavioral research philosophy 212,
  214-215
  principles of exclusion and
    inclusion, 212
  strategy and tactics, 214-215
  system analysis, 212
Beta adrenergic receptors, 233-256
  activators, 245-246, 248-249, 255
  antagonists, 235-237, 240-242,
    245-250, 253, 256
  classification, 235, 246-247,
    254-255
  selective activators, 255-256
  selective antagonists, 241-244,
    246, 250
Beta-aminopropionitrile, 364
Biogastrone, 149
bis-DEAE-fluorenone, 300, 302
Brocresine, 163
Brunner's glands, 169
Butoxamine, 241, 244, 247-248, 250,
  253, 255-256

Butazolidin, see Phenylbutazone
Butylated hydroxytoluene, 361

C

Caerulein, 164
Caffeine, 374, 397
Calcification, 350, 374
Calcium carbonate, 141
Caloric restriction, 349, 356, 371, 373, 375, 377
Carbofluorene, 145
Carbonic anhydrase inhibitors, 139, 154, 160
Cartilage erosion, 94; see also Osteoarthritis
Cartilage regeneration factors, 94
Cell lysins, 62
Centrophenoxine, 367-370, 372
Chalones, 47, 91-92, 95
　specificity of, 91-92
Chemical synovectomy, 100
Chemotaxins, 62, 66
Chlorpromazine, 209
Cholecystokinin-pancreozynin, 122, 162, 166
Cholestane-3β, 5α, 6β-triol, 267
Cholesterol absorption and inhibition, 266-268
　cholestane-3β, 5α, 6β-triol, 267
　cholestyramine, 268
　ergosterol, 267
　ferric chloride, 268
　linoleic acid amides, 267
　neomycin, 268
　sitosterol, 266
　soybean sterols, 266
　stigmasterol, 267
Cholestyramine, 268
Chondrocytes, biosynthesis of cartilage matrix by, 94
Chronic inflammatory states, 5, 27, 77, 103
　autoantibodies in, 6
　control mechanisms, 6
　etiology, 5, 6, 8, 10, 77
　methods of current drug research, 103
　pharmacological approach, 8, 77
　role of normal defense mechanisms, 77
　spontaneous remissions, 27
　suppressive therapy in, 27
CI-588, 168
Cinchophen, 131, 157
Clofibrate, 270, 278; see also CPIB, Atromid-S
Coalescence-accretion-stabilization, see Aging
Colchicine, 19-20
Collagen, 350, 353, 356, 360, 364-365, 367, 371, 374
Collagenase synthesis, 98
Complement, 65-68
　activation of, 67
　inhibition of, 68
　regulation of, 66
　role in body defenses, 65
Conditioned avoidance, 390-391, 393, 396-399
　active avoidance, 393, 396
　buzzer, 396
　discriminated avoidance, 397, 398, 399
　extinction, 390-391, 396
　passive avoidance, 392-393, 396
　pole-jumping, 390
　retention, 390
　shuttle box, 398
Cortex, 391
Corticosteroids, see Adrenocorticosteroids
CPIB, 270; see also Clofibrate, Atromid-S
Cortisone, see Adrenocorticosteroids
Crosslinking, 350-351, 363-364, 371, 373-375
Crypto-antigen, screening for, 84
Cushings disease, 136
Cyclic AMP, 136, 165, 170
Cycloheximide, 168
Cycloleucine, 82
Cyclosphosphamide, 27, 100
　use in rheumatoid arthritis, 81
Cysteine, 361, 372
Cytarabine, 87

SUBJECT INDEX

Cytolysin, 66, 68
Cytosar, see Cytarabine
Cytostatic agents, 27, 29, 80
   development of drug-resistance to, 81
   development of locally active, 85
   effect on the immune response, 31, 80
   inhibition of nucleic acid synthesis, 83
   Methotrexate, 37
   oncogenic effect of, 80
   toxicity, 27, 37-38, 80
Cytotoxins, 69
Cytoxan, see Cyclophosphamide

D

Deanol, 399
Degenerative joint disease, see Osteoarthritis
Depression, 220
Diagnosis of thrombotic disease, 328-331
   arterial, 330
   fibrin degradation products, 329, 331
   ^{125}Iodine-fibrinogen, 329, 331
   myocardial infarction, 328
   pulmonary embolism, 329
   venography, 329
Dibenamine, 235
Dibozane, 239
Dichloroisoproterenol (DCI), 235-237, 240-241, 247, 255
Dicyclomine, 145
Diisopropylfluorophosphate (DFP), 400
Dimethyl isopropylmethoxamine (DIMA), 241
Diphenylhydantoin, 358
Dipyridamole, 331, 338
Disulfides, 372
Diuretic drugs, 154
DNA, 37, 78, 88, 391
   blockade of nuclear transcription, 88
   blockade of synthesis, 78, 88
   precursors, 37
   synthesis, 78, 88
Drug-induced ulceration, 157
Duogastrone, 149

E

Elastin, 350, 353, 360, 364, 367, 374
Electroconvulsive shock (ECS), 388, 392-393, 395, 396
Electrolytes, 400-401
   lithium salts, 400-401
   magnesium, 401
   potassium chloride, 400
Endogenous fibrinolytic activity, 332, 336-337
   drugs which enhance, 332, 336-337
Endothelial cells, 74; see also Inflammation
   histamine, 75
   kinin, 75
   permeability, 75
   serotonin, 75
   specialization by function, 75
Enterogastrone, 122, 166, 167
Epinephrine, 135, 136, 157
Epithelial cell renewal, 131, 135, 171, 175
   corticosteroids and, 131
   5-fluorouracil and, 131
Ergosterol, 267
Estrogens, 89, 153, 170, 269, 374
Ethyl α-(p-chlorophenoxy) isobutyrate, 270; see also CPIB, Atromid-S, Clofibrate
Evaluation of behavioral drugs, 206-230
   drug-drug interaction, 219
   instrumental assessment, 212, 218
   observational assessment, 212, 215-217, 221-223
   physiological state, 206
   predictability, 202, 212-213, 218
   psychosocial state, 207
   side effect assessment, 227-228
   therapeutic objectives, 202, 229-230
   subjective state, 225-226
Experimental design, 326

F

Ferret, use as ulcer model, 158
Fibrin degradation products, see Diagnosis of thrombotic disease
Fibrinolysin, 172
Fibrinogen synthesis, 62
Fluorescence, 353, 368
Flufenamic acid, 131
Folic acid, 37; see also Methotrexate
Free radicals, 360-363, 367, 371-372
Freund's adjuvant, 91; see also Adjuvant arthritis (rat)
Furosemide, 154

G

Gastric freezing, 153
Gastric irradiation, 153
Gastric mucin, 123, 145
Gastric secretion, 116-123, 134, 160-169, 174
    gastric mucous, 123
    hydrochloric acid, 117
    inhibition of, 121, 134, 160-169, 174
    interprandial, 120
    pepsin, 122-123
    pepsinogen, 122
    postprandial, 120
Gastrin, 121-122, 162, 164, 174
    antibodies to, 164
    inhibitors of, 164
    SC-15396, 167
Gastrone, 134
Gerovital H_3, 358
Glucagon, 136, 137, 170, 175
Glutathione, 363
Glyceryl guaiacolate, 331, 338
Glycoproteins, 92; see also Chalones
Gold preparations, 29, 85
    biosynthesis in vivo of mucopolysaccharides, 98
    possible mode of action, 40
    therapy, 27, 29
    toxicity, 29, 30
Gold sodium thiomalate, 30
Gout, 19, 21
    pathogenesis of, 19
    therapy of hyperuricemia, 21
    therapy of inflammation, 22
Ground substance, 364
Growth hormone, 133, 354
Guanylic acid, 391

H

H 29/50, 245-246
H 35/25, 241, 245-246
Heparin, 135, 271
Hippocampus, 391
Histamine, 65, 93, 135, 160
Histidine decarboxylase, 64, 131, 149, 161, 174
    activation in lymph nodes, 65
    inhibitors of, 161, 174
Hormones and aging, 353-357, 374
Hydrocortisone, 356
5-Hydroxytryptamine 93, 135, 157, 171, 328, 399
    antagonists of, 131, 171
5-Hydroxytryptophan, 135, 157, 171
Hyperlipemia, 274-275
    electrophoretic classification of, 274
Hypnotics, 212
Hypophysectomy, 354

I

I^{131}, 169
Immune response, 55, 73, 91
    control by inhibition of end-product, 91
    control with synthetic drugs, 73
    endogenous inhibitors, 90
    exogenous inhibitors, 90
    inhibition by L-asparaginase, 87
    leukocytes in, 69
    natural regulators, 89, 94
    normal, 55
    polynuclear benzenoid hydrocarbons, 88
Immunological tolerance, 82, 84, 90
Immunosuppressive drugs, 35, 78, 81, 370
    adaptation for clinical use, 83
    antilymphocyte globulin, 35, 78
    anti-Rh antiserum, 78

assays, 87; see also Allergic
encephalomyelitis, Allergic
thyroiditis, Adjuvant
arthritis (rat)
  biodistribution of, 85
  chemical species for investigation, 86
  contraindication for clinical use, 39
  development of new agents, 78
  efficacy, 82
  fundamental action of, 81
  intra-articular injection of, 84
  local activation in tissue, 85
  nucleic acid complexes, 90
  potency, 82
  properties of, 81
  therapy, 27
  toxicity of, 37, 38, 82, 83
Imuran, see Azathioprine
Indocin, see Indomethacin
Indole acetic acid, 372
Indomethacin, 25-26, 131, 133, 157
Inflammation, 7; see also Synovial cells
  animal models of, 47
  causes of, 5, 12, 55
  complement system, 65
  definition, 4
  endothelial cells, 75
  inflammagenic factors, 72, 93, 99
  inflammalytic agents, 59, 68
  leukocytes in, 69
  microvascular histamine synthesis, 64
  natural inhibitors of, 47
  natural regulators of, 55, 62, 89
  pathophysiology of, 60-61
  proteolysis, role of, 68
  purpose of, 75
  in rheumatoid arthritis, 26
  suppression of acute response, 89
Inflammatory disease, 4; see also individual diseases
  available therapy, 12
  clinical conditions, 11
  diet in, 93
  drug design for, 40
  epidemiology, 95
  natural regulators of, 89
  skin, 37
  therapy, 9, 33, 39, 101, 102
Inflammatory exudates, 93; see also Rindani agents
Inflammatory response, 44, 55, 92
  hormonal regulators of, 92
  in vitro, 44
  normal (protective), 55, 59
Inosine-alkylamino complexes, 358
INPEA, 244
Intelligence, 392
Interferon, 59, 72, 294-310
  antitumor activity, 303-305
  antiviral activity, 297-299
  biological properties, 296-297
  clinical trials, 305-306
  ideal inducer of, 311
  induction of, 295, 296, 299-305, 306-310
  mechanism of action, 297-299
  molecular weight, 296
Intrinsic factor, 123
Ion exchange resins, 142
Iritis, 22, 26
Isopropylmethoxamine, 240-241
Isoproterenol, 245-246, 248-249, 255

J

Jaundice, 90
Joint cartilage, 12

K

Kinins, 62, 66, 93, 98
Korsakoff syndrome, 395

L

Lathyrogens, 364-367
Learning, 392-393
  discrimination, 393
  field-tracking performance, 395
Leukocyte pharmacology, 69-73
Licorice derivatives, 139, 148-152, 171, 173
  carbenoxolone sodium, 139, 148-151, 171, 173
  deglycyrrhizinated licorice, 148, 151
Lignosulfonates, 171

Linoleic acid amides, 267-268
  cyclohexylamine, 267
  α-methylbenzylamine, 268
  α-phenyl-β-(p-tolyl) ethylamine, 268
Lipids, 360, 363, 368
Lipofuscin, 353, 368
Lipolysis, inhibition of, 272-273
  3,5-dimethylpyrazole, 273
  5-methylpyrazole-3-carboxylic acid, 273
  5-(3-pyridyl)tetrazole, 273
  nicotinic acid, 272
Lipoproteins, 263-265, 274
  chemical composition of, 263
  electrophoresis of, 274
  metabolism, 265
Local anesthetics, 154
Lymphocytes, 33, 69, 72, 85
  delayed hypersensitivity, 35
  depletion of, 35
  rejection of homografts, 33
  role in adjuvant arthritis (rat), 72
  role in allergic thyroiditis, 72
  role in allergic encephalomyelitis, 72
  in tissue injury, 72
Lymphokines, 69, 73
Lysosomes, 20, 62, 350, 360, 363

M

Macrophages, 73
Magnesium antacids, 141
Magnesium pemoline, 358, 394-397
Major tranquilizers, 209, 211, 220
Malononitriles, 392-394
  2-cyanomethyl-1, 1, 3, 3-tetracyanopropene, 394
  tetracyanopropene (T4CAP), 394
  tricyanoaminopropene (TCAP), 393-394
Mann-Williamson ulcer, 158, 169
Maximum life span, 356, 361, 367, 370, 373

Maze, 391, 393-394, 396
  T-maze, 396
  water, 394
  Y-maze, 396
Meckels, diverticulum, 124
Memory, 389-393, 395, 399
  consolidation, 393, 399
  Wechsler Memory Quotient, 395
Mercaptoethylamine, 361, 372
6-Mercaptopurine, 34
Methotrexate, 37-38
Methoxamine, 239-241, 246
Methylphenidate, 397
1-Methyl-4-piperidyl bis(p-chlorophenoxy)acetate, 271
2-Methyl(p-1, 2, 3, 4-tetrahydro-1-naphthylphenoxy)propionic acid, 271
Microvascular histamine synthesis, 64
  regulation by drugs, 65
Minor tranquilizers, 212, 220
Mitogens, 72
Monarticular juvenile rheumatoid arthritis, 26
Mucopolysaccharide synthesis, 94, 98; see also Cartilage regeneration factors, Gold preparations
Mucous, 133, 170
  carbenoxolone sodium and, 151
  5-hydroxytryptamine and, 171
  secretion of, 170
Musculotropic antispasmodic drugs, 145
Myochrysin[R], see Gold sodium thiomalate

N

Natural history, thromboembolic disease, 322-324
  growth phase, 322
  luminal compromise, 322
  resolution phase, 323-324
  therapeutic implications, 323
  therapeutic implications with congestive heart failure, 324

SUBJECT INDEX

therapeutic implications with
pulmonary disease, 324
Neomycin, 268
Nerve growth factor, 172
Neurohypophysial hormones, 354
Nicotine, 400
Nicotinic acid, 272-273, 278
 antilipolytic activity of, 272
 derivatives of, 273
 esters of, 272
 homologs of, 273
 mechanisms of action of, 272
Nicotinyl alcohol, 273
Non-steroid anti-inflammatory
 drugs, 7, 24
Norepinephrine, 398
Nucleic acids, 87, 90, 94, 371

O

Observational procedures, 212-218,
 221-228
 animal models, 213-214, 217-218
 disadvantages of, 216
 humans, 221-228
Operant behavior, 203, 209-212, 218
 approach, 210
 avoidance, 210, 212
 catatonic schizophrenic, 211
 escape, 210
 manic-depressive, 210
 methods, 218
 mode of response, 210-212
 paranoid schizophrenic, 212
 reward and punishment, 210
Osteoarthritis, 36, 37
 role of inflammation in, 36
Oxethazine, 154
Oxyphenbutazone, 23

P

pA_2, 249
Pannus, 94
Penicillamine, 364, 367
Pentylenetetrazol, 399
Peptic ulcer, 123-174
 ACTH and, 131, 133, 135

adrenal medulla and, 136
age and, 131
alcohol and, 129, 131
amylopectin sulfate in treatment
 of, 152
antacids in treatment of, 139-142
antihistamines in treatment of,
 139
antimuscarinic drugs in treatment
 of, 139
antipepsin drugs in treatment of,
 139, 152
antrectomy in treatment of, 138
aspirin and, 131, 133
association with other diseases,
 138
autoimmunity and, 133
barbiturates and, 153
blood group substances and, 133,
 134
carbenoxolone sodium in treatment
 of, 149-151
carbonic anhydrase inhibitors in
 treatment of, 139
cinchophen and, 131
constitutional factors and, 131
corticosteroids and, 131, 133, 136
definition of, 124
diet in treatment of, 128, 138
diuretic drugs in treatment of, 154
endocrine glands and, 136
environmental factors in, 128
epinephrine and, 135, 136
epithelial cell renewal and, 131,
 135
estrogens in treatment of, 153
etiology of, 128
fibrinolysis, 135
5-fluoruracil and, 131
flufenamic acid and, 131
formation in animals, 155
fungal injection and, 133
gastric freezing in treatment of,
 153
gastric irradiation in treatment of,
 153
gastric mucin in treatment of, 145
gastritis and, 133

gastrone and, 133
hemorrhage and, 126
heparin and, 135
heredity in, 131
histamine and, 135
histidine decarboxylase and, 131
hydrochloric acid secretion in, 132
5-hydroxytryptamine and, 131, 135
5-hydroxtryptamine antagonists and, 131
5-hydroxytryptophan and, 135
indomethacin and, 131, 133
local anesthetics in treatment of, 154
menopause and, 131
mucosal blood flow and, 135
mucosal resistance and, 133
nucous and, 133
musculotropic antispasmodic drugs in treatment of, 145
nutritional deficiencies and, 133
occupation and, 129
ovary and, 137
oxethazine in treatment of, 154
pancreas and, 137
pantothenate deficiency and, 158
parathyroid gland and, 137
parietal cells and, 132
pathology of, 125
penetration of, 127
perforation of, 127
phenylbutazone and, 131, 133
pituitary gland and, 136
pregnancy and, 131
pyloric stenosis and, 127
race and, 131
riboflavin deficiency and, 158
sedatives in treatment of, 138
sex incidence of, 131
stress and, 137
symptoms of, 127
thyroid gland and, 137
tobacco and, 129
treatment of, 138-154
vagotomy in treatment of, 138
vascular diathesis in, 135
xanthine alkaloids and, 131, 136

Peroxidation, 351, 360, 363
Phenoxybenzamine, 235
Phentolamine, 235
Phenylbutazone, 23, 97, 131, 157
Phenylephrine, 239
N-α-Phenylpropyl-N-benzyloxy acetamide, 274
Physostigmine, 399
Picrotoxin, 399
Pitressin, 136
Pituitary gland, 136, 353
Plant sterols, 267
Plasmin, 332, 335
  in venous thrombosis, 335
Platelets, 69, 319-321, 330-332, 337
  aggregation of, 330-331, 337
Podophyllotoxin derivative, 85
Poly I: Poly C, 89, 299, 304-305, 307-310
Polymeric antacids, 142
Polymorphonuclear leuokocytes, 20, 26
  chemotactic response, 20
  kinin generation, 20
  phagocytosis, 20
  role in rheumatoid arthritis, 26
Polyribosomes, 359, 374
Portocaval shunt, 158
Practolol, 244, 246, 248, 250, 253, 255-256
Prednisolone, 356
Prednisone, 35
Probenecid, 21
Procainamide, 358
Procaine, 357-358
Pronethalol, 236-237, 241, 247, 253, 255
Propranolol, 236-237, 241, 247-248, 250, 253, 255
Proresid, see Podophyllotoxin derivative
Prostaglandins, 92, 165, 171, 174
Psoriasis, 37
  azaribine, 38
  clinical aspects, 37
  methotrexate, 37
Pulmonary embolism, 324, 328-329

angiography in, 324
diagnosis of radioisotopic technics in, 324
resolution of, 324
Pylorus-ligated rat, 155
Pyran co-polymer, 299, 307
Pyridinol carbamate, 273

Q

Quinterenol, 256-257

R

Radiation, 360, 363, 367, 370
Radiation therapy, 168
Rapidity of vascular occlusion, 326-327
  arterial, 326
  significance of, 326
  vein, 327
Red thrombus, see Thrombogenesis
Rejuvenation, 347-349, 357, 371, 373-374
Reserpine, 131, 157
Renal transplantation, 33
  anti-inflammatory therapy, 33-34
  azathioprine, 34
  immunosuppressive therapy, 33-34
  lymphocyte depletion, 35
Rheumatoid arthritis, 26; see also Synovial cells
  remission during jaundice, 90
  remission during pregnancy, 89
  role of estrogens, 95
  systemic manifestations, 26
  therapy, 27
Rheumatoid factor, 22, 26-27
Rheumatoid variants, 22, 24
  indomethacin, 25
  phenylbutazone, 24
Rindani agents, 47, 92, 93, 94
Royal jelly, 349
RNA, 37, 389-392, 397
  brain-RNA, 392, 397
  precursors, 37
  yeast - RNA, 389-392
Rumalon, 94, 96

S

Salbutamol, 255-257
Salicylates, 27-29
SC-15396, 167
Scopolamine, 143
Scurvy, 127
Secretin, 122, 169
Sedatives, 138, 160
Selenium, 363
Semicarbazide, 364
Serotonin, see 5-Hydroxytryptamine
Shay rat, 155
Sialic acid, 123, 133
Site of occlusion, 325-326
  calf vein, 326
  eye, 326
  significance of, 325
Sitosterol, 266
Skin diseases, 38, 39
  adrenocorticosteroid therapy, 38, 39
  antimalarial drug therapy, 38, 39
  circulating antibodies in, 38
  immunosuppressive therapy in, 38
  inflammatory reactions in, 38
Sodium bicarbonate, 141
Solganol, see Aurothioglucose
Somatotrophin, 94
Sotalol, 236-237, 241, 247, 253
Soybean sterols, 266
Specific life span, 348, 353, 363, 375
Stigmasterol, 267
Stimulants, 209, 211, 220
Stomach, 116
  anatomy, 116
  secretion, 116-123
Streptokinase, 332, 335-336
  in venous thrombosis, 335
Stress-induced gastric ulcer, 156
Strychnine, 398, 399
Sulfated polysaccharides, 152
"Sulfation factor", 94, 96
Sulfinpyrazone, 21
Sulfhydryl compounds, 372, 377
Synovial cells, 74, 76
  in vitro cultures, 74
  respnse to hydrocortisone, 74

resistance to viral infection, 74
Synovial fluid enzymes, 69
Synovial membrane, 12
Systemic lupus erythematosus, 30-33
   adrenocorticosteroids, 31-33
   etiology, 31
   immunological abnormalities, 30
   therapy, 31

T

Tail tendon, 353-354, 358, 371-372, 377
Tandearil, see Oxyphenbutazone
Theories of aging, see Aging
Thiazolidinone, 86
Thrombogenesis, 319-321, 323, 325
   coagulation alterations and, 319
   fibrin matrix in, 321
   platelets in, 320
   red thrombus, 319, 323
   serum injection, 320
   stasis, 319
   three major factors, 319
   vascular injury, 320
   white thrombus, 319, 325
Thrombolytic therapy, 327-330, 337-340
   in arterial thrombosis, 337-338
   objectives of, 330, 338
   in pulmonary embolism, 328
   selection for, 327
   sequence of investigation, 338-340
   in venous thrombosis, 327, 335-337
Thrombosis, 318-322, 325, 330, 334-338
   and atherosclerosis, 325
   prophylaxis of, 330
   semantic considerations, 318
   treatment of, 334-338
Thrombus, 321-322
   composition, 321
   endothelialization, 321
   fibrin content, 321
   growth, 321
   organization, 321
Thyrocalcitonins, 92
Thyroid hormone, 269-270, 278, 354
   D-thyroxine, 269, 278
   L-thyroxine, 269, 354
   D-triiodothyronine, 269
   L-triiodothyronine, 269
   mechanism of action, 270
Tilorone, see bis-DEAE-fluorenone
Tissue cultures, 277-278
   cholesterol deposition in, 278
   cholesterol uptake by, 277
Tissue factors, 91
Triacetyl-6-azauridine, see Azaribine

U

Urate lowering drugs, 21-22; see also Gout
   inhibitors of urate synthesis, 21
   uricosurics, 21
Uric acid, 392
Urogastrone, 171
Urokinase, 332, 335-336
   in venous thrombosis, 335

V

Vagotomy, 133
Vasculitis, 27, 38, 74; see also Endothelial cells, Skin diseases
Vasopressin, 356
Viral disease, 292-294
   course of, 292-293
   recovery from, 293-294
Vitamin C, 363
Vitamin E, 360, 363, 368

W

White thrombus, see Thrombogenesis

X

Xanthine alkaloids, 131
Xylamide, 168

Z

Zinc, 172
Zollinger-Ellison syndrome, 132, 137, 163, 164, 169

DATE DUE			
OCT 29 1980			

DEMCO 38-297